Clinical Anesthesia Procedures of the Massachusetts General Hospital

Sixth Edition

Clinical Anesthesia Procedures of the Massachusetts General Hospital

Sixth Edition

Department of Anesthesia and Critical Care
Massachusetts General Hospital
Harvard Medical School

Senior Editor
William E. Hurford, M.D.

Associate Editors
Michael T. Bailin, M.D.
J. Kenneth Davison, M.D.
Kenneth L. Haspel, M.D.
Carl Rosow, M.D.
Susan A. Vassallo, M.D.

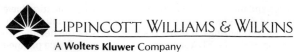

LIPPINCOTT WILLIAMS & WILKINS
A **Wolters Kluwer** Company
Philadelphia · Baltimore · New York · London
Buenos Aires · Hong Kong · Sydney · Tokyo

Acquisitions Editor: R. Craig Percy
Developmental Editor: Erin McMullan
Production Editor: Emily Lerman
Manufacturing Manager: Colin J. Warnock
Cover Designer: Christine Jenny
Compositor: Maryland Composition
Printer: Vicks Lithograph

Library of Congress Cataloging-in-Publication Data
ISBN: 0-7817-3718-4

Care has been taken to confirm the accuracy of the information
presented and to describe generally accepted practices. However,
the authors, editors, and publisher are not responsible for errors or
omissions or for any consequences from application of the information in this book and make no warranty, expressed or implied, with
respect to the currency, completeness, or accuracy of the contents
of the publication. Application of this information in a particular
situation remains the professional responsibility of the practitioner.

The authors, editors, and publisher have exerted every effort to
ensure that drug selection and dosage set forth in this text are in
accordance with current recommendations and practice at the time
of publication. However, in view of ongoing research, changes in
government regulations, and the constant flow of information relat-
ing to drug therapy and drug reactions, the reader is urged to check
the package insert for each drug for any change in indications and
dosage and for added warnings and precautions. This is particularly
important when the recommended agent is a new or infrequently
employed drug.

Some drugs and medical devices presented in this publication have
Food and Drug Administration (FDA) clearance for limited use in
restricted research settings. It is the responsibility of the health care
provider to ascertain the FDA status of each drug or device planned
for use in their clinical practice.

10 9 8 7 6 5 4 3 2 1

Contents

III. Perioperative Issues

Appendix

Preface

The sixth edition of *Clinical Anesthesia Procedures of the Massachusetts General Hospital* was written by residents, fellows, staff, and alumni of the Department of Anesthesia and Critical Care at the Massachusetts General Hospital. This manual continues to emphasize the clinical fundamentals involved in the safe administration of anesthesia, perioperative care, and pain management. The suggestions reflect current clinical practices at our hospital; other methods may be equally effective.

This handbook complements readings in textbooks and journals and assumes some prior knowledge of anesthesia and critical care. It is designed to be an accessible and accurate source of information for practicing anesthesiologists, anesthesia residents, nurse anesthetists, medical students, medical and surgical residents, nurses, respiratory therapists, and other health care professionals involved in perioperative care. The manual is not intended to replace experienced clinical teaching or substitute for detailed study. Each chapter contains a reading list for those who desire additional information on a topic.

Clinical Anesthesia Procedures of the Massachusetts General Hospital has been repetitively edited, revised, and relied upon as a clinical reference for over twenty years. Over one hundred and fifty individuals have contributed to the manual during this time. While constantly adding new information, each new edition is built upon the foundation of previous versions. Source material from prior editions has been included verbatim when appropriate. We acknowledge the guidance and support given to early editions by Richard J. Kitz, M.D. and the continuing support of Warren M. Zapol, M.D. We thank Ms. Rita M. Prevoznik for administrative and editorial assistance. The integral contributions of the editors and authors of earlier editions of this handbook are gratefully acknowledged below:

Editors of Previous Editions: First Edition (1978): Philip W. Zaidan, Robert Lebowitz, John L. Clark, Daniel F. Dedrick, Jarowitz, Leslie A. Newberg, Michael T. Gilette; Third Edition (1982): Philip W. Crone; Second Edition (1982): Philip W.J.: Leonard L. Firestone, Philip W. Lebowitz, Charles Enael T. Bailin, J. Kenneth Davison, neth Davison, William F. Sow. Deniz A. Perese; Fifth Edition (1997): William Paul H. Alfille, James K. Alifimoff, Rae M. Allain, Kenneth L. Jo, Michael Bailin, Keith H. Baker, Jane C. Ballantyne, James M. Barton, Salvatore J. Basta, Wayne H. Bellows, Bierman, Luca M. Bigatello, Janice Bitetti, Kenneth Blazier, Bloomstone, David Borsook, Ronald J. Botelho, Jeffrey B. Brand, James G. Cain, William H. Campbell, Bryn T. Carpenter, Daniel B. Carr, Christopher Carter, Bobby Su-Pen Chang, John L. Clark, David Clement, Lydia Conlay, Charles E. Cook, Jeffrey B. Cooper, Benjamin G. Covino, Garland A. Cowan, Robert K. Crone, Marianna Crowley, Deborah J. Culley, Alberto deArmendi, Daniel F. Dedrick, Mark Dershwitz, John V. Donlon, Richard P. Dutton, William Dylewsky, Clifton W. Emerson, Paul L. Epstein, Leonard L. Firestone, Susan Firestone, Stuart A. Forman, Robert Gaiser, Margaret Gargarian, Clifford M. Gevirtz, Noel Gibney, Michael T. Gilette, Kenneth Giuffre, Randall S. Glidden, Takahisa Goto, Heath Gulden, Douglas M. Hansell, Jane Hardiman, Timothy J. Herbst, J. Fredrik Hesselvik, Randall S. Hickle, Thomas L. Higgins, Thomas Hill, Allen J. Hinkle, Vincent L. Hoellerich, Robert Hunsaker, William E. Hurford, Mansoor Husain, Gloria Hwang, D. Jay Iaconetti, Charles C. Jeffrey, Andrew A. Jeon, Lisa A. Keglovitz, William Kimball, David Kliewer, David Koehler, W. Andrew Kofke, James L. Konigsberg, Peter G. Kovatsis, Mary Kraft, William B. Latta, Charles E. Laurito, Philip W. Lebowitz, Betty Lee, Stephanie Lee, Paul Lennon, Rebecca Leong, David Lerdahl, Jerrold H. Levy, Michael C. Long, Thomas J. Long, James C. Loomis, John J. Marota, Piotr Michalowski, Thomas A. Mickler, Richard A. Miller, Alex Mills, Rowan Molnar, Holly Ann H. Morgan, Brian P. Murray, Michael Natale, Leslie A. Newberg, Ronald S. Newbower, Phillippa Newfield, Ervant Nishanian, Daniel L. Nozik, Conor O'Neill, Vilma E. Ortiz, Charles W. Otto, Onofrio Patafio, Blake M. Paterson, John Pawlowski, Robert A. Peterfreund, May C.M. Pian-Smith, Michael Pilla, Richard M. Pino, Marie Csete Prager, Douglas E. Raines, Frederic M. Ramsey, James T. Roberts, Jesse D. Roberts, Jr., Peter Rosenbaum, Carl Rosow, Fred A. Rotenberg, Peter Rothstein, Steve Rotter, Barbara A. Ryan, Adam Sapirstein, William P. Schecter, Larry B. Scott, Kenneth E. Shepherd, George Shorten, Stephen Small, Aileen Starnbach, David J. Stone, Scott C. Streckenbach, Susan L. Streitz, Veronica C. Swanson, Bobbie-Jean Sweitzer, Michele Szabo, Alfonso A. Tagliavia, Robert E. Tainsh, Frank A. Takacs, Gary D. Thal, Steven Thorup, I. David Todres, Susan A. Vassallo, John S. Wadlington, Samuel Wald, John L. Walsh, James P. Welch, Norman E. Wilson, Julianne S. Wimberly, Lisa Wollman, James R. Zaidan, and Maria M. Zestos.

W. E. Hurford, M.D.

Evaluating the Patient Before Anesthesia

1

Evaluating the Patient Before Anesthesia

Mary Kraft and Richard A. Wiklund

I. Overview

The **preanesthetic evaluation** has specific objectives, which include establishing a doctor–patient relationship, becoming familiar with the surgical illness and coexisting medical conditions, developing a management strategy for perioperative anesthetic care, and obtaining informed consent for the anesthetic plan. The consultation is detailed in the patient's record and concludes with the anesthetic options and their attendant risks and benefits. The overall goals of the preoperative assessment are to reduce perioperative morbidity and mortality and allay patient anxiety.

II. History

Relevant information is obtained by a chart review followed by the patient interview. Knowledge of the patient's history when beginning the interview is reassuring to the anxious patient. When the medical record is not available, the history obtained from the patient may be supplemented by direct discussion with the medical and surgical staff. Although patient age and American Society of Anesthesiologists (ASA) Physical Status Classification are more accurate predictors of adverse outcomes, knowledge of patients' activities of daily living, including maximum activity level, may help predict their overall outcome in the perioperative period.

    A. **The anesthetist** should learn the symptoms of the present surgical illness, the diagnostic studies performed, presumptive diagnosis, initial treatment, and responses. Vital signs should be reviewed and fluid balance estimated.

    B. **Coexisting medical illnesses** may complicate the surgical and anesthetic course. These should be evaluated in a systematic "organ systems" approach with an emphasis on recent changes in symptoms, signs, and treatment (see Chapters 2 through 7). In certain circumstances, preoperative specialty consultation may be advisable. Such consults are most valuable when answering specific questions regarding the interpretation of unusual laboratory tests, unfamiliar drug therapies, or changes from the patient's baseline status. Consultants should not be asked for a general "clearance" for anesthesia because this is the specific responsibility of the anesthesiologist.

    C. **Medications** used to treat present or coexisting illnesses, their dosages, and schedules must be ascertained. Of special importance are antihypertensive, antianginal, antiarrhythmic, anticoagulant, anticonvulsant, and specific endocrine (e.g., insulin) medications. The decision to continue medications during the preanesthetic period depends on the severity of the underlying illness, the potential consequences of discontinuing treatment, the medication's half-life, and the likelihood of deleterious interactions with proposed anesthetic agents. As a general rule, medications can be continued up to the time of surgery.

D.   Allergies and drug reactions. Unusual, unexpected, or unpleasant reactions to perioperative medications and nonallergic adverse reactions, side effects, and drug interactions are relatively common. True allergic reactions are relatively uncommon. The task of determining the exact nature of specific "reactions" may be difficult. Therefore, it is important to obtain a careful description of the "allergic reaction" experience from the patient.

   1.   True allergic reactions. Any drug that (by direct observation, chart documentation, or description by the patient) leads to skin manifestations (pruritus with hives or flushing), facial or oral swelling, shortness of breath, choking, wheezing, or vascular collapse should be considered to have elicited a true allergic reaction.

   a.   Antibiotics, especially sulfonamides, penicillins, and cephalosporin derivatives, are the most common allergens.

   b.   Known allergy to shellfish or seafood is important to document, because allergic cross-reactions with intravenous (IV) contrast dye and the heparin-reversing agent protamine may occur. Known allergy to soybean oil and egg yolk components may preclude the safe use of some preparations of propofol.

   c.   A history of "allergy" to halothane or succinylcholine (in either the patient or any close relative) warrants special attention, because this may represent the occurrence of malignant hyperthermia, halothane hepatitis, or prolonged paralysis caused by an abnormal allele responsible for production of plasma cholinesterase, an enzyme that metabolizes succinylcholine.

   d.   True allergy to the amide-type local anesthetics (e.g., lidocaine) is exceedingly rare, although a syncopal episode, tachycardia, or palpitations in the dentist's chair or before starting an IV with injection of local anesthetic may be falsely labeled as allergic. Ester-type local anesthetics (e.g., procaine) can produce anaphylaxis (see Chapter 15).

   2.   Adverse reactions and side effects. Many perioperative medications can produce memorable unpleasant side effects (e.g., nausea, vomiting, and pruritus after narcotic administration) in a conscious patient.

   3.   Certain rare but important drug interactions must be anticipated because of their life-threatening nature. For example, thiopental may precipitate a fatal episode of acute intermittent porphyria, and meperidine may produce a hypertensive crisis when administered to patients treated with monoamine oxidase inhibitors. Newer antiparkinsonian drugs (anticholinesterases) may prolong paralysis after succinylcholine administration.

E.   Anesthetic history

   1.   Old anesthesia records should be reviewed for the following information:

   a.   Response to sedative/analgesic premedications and anesthetic agents.

   **b.   Ease of mask ventilation, direct laryngoscopy, and the size and type of laryngoscope blade and endotracheal tube used.

c. Vascular access and invasive monitoring used and difficulties encountered.

d. Perianesthetic complications such as adverse drug reactions, cephalgia, intraoperative awareness, dental injury, protracted postoperative nausea and vomiting, cardiorespiratory instability, postoperative myocardial infarction or congestive heart failure, unexpected admission to an intensive care unit (ICU), and prolonged emergence or intubation.

2. Patients should be asked about **prior anesthetics**, including common complaints such as postoperative nausea and hoarseness and specific warnings from previous anesthetists describing prior anesthetic problems.

F. Family history. A history of adverse anesthetic outcomes in family members should be evaluated. This history is perhaps best obtained with open-ended questions, such as "Has anyone in your family experienced unusual or serious reactions to anesthesia?" Patients should be specifically asked about a family history of malignant hyperthermia.

G. Social history

1. Smoking. A history of exercise intolerance or the presence of a productive cough or hemoptysis may indicate a need for further pulmonary evaluation or treatment. Eliminating cigarette use for 2 to 4 weeks before elective surgery may reduce airway hyperreactivity and perioperative pulmonary complications.

2. Drugs and alcohol. Although self-reporting of drug and alcohol intake typically underestimates actual use, it is a helpful starting point to define the drugs used, routes of administration, frequency, and timing of most recent use. **Stimulant abuse** may lead to palpitations, angina, weight loss, and lowered thresholds for serious arrhythmias and seizures. **Acute alcohol intoxication** will decrease anesthetic requirements and predispose to hypothermia and hypoglycemia, whereas **withdrawal from ethanol** may precipitate severe hypertension, tremors, delirium, seizures, and may markedly increase anesthetic requirements. The **routine use of opioids and benzodiazepines** may significantly increase the doses needed to induce and maintain anesthesia or to provide adequate postoperative analgesia.

H. Review of systems. Acute or chronic lung disease, ischemic heart disease, hypertension, and gastroesophageal reflux are examples of commonly encountered coexisting conditions that increase the risk of perioperative morbidity and mortality. A minimum review of systems should seek to elicit history of the following:

1. A recent history of an upper respiratory infection, especially in children, which predisposes patients to pulmonary complications including bronchospasm and laryngospasm during the induction of and emergence from general anesthesia.

2. Asthma, which may be accompanied by airway mucous plugging and acute bronchospasm after the induction of anesthesia or endotracheal intubation.

3. Preexisting coronary artery disease (CAD), which may predispose the patient to myocardial ischemia, ventricular dysfunction, or myocardial infarction with the stress of surgery and anesthesia.

4.   Diabetes, which may predispose the patient to silent ischemia, especially in those with autonomic nervous system dysfunction. Alterations of the autonomic nervous system may also lead to gastroparesis and active reflux. In addition, endotracheal intubation may be difficult in some diabetic patients because of arthritis of the temporomandibular joints and cervical spine, resulting from glycosylation of synovium.

5.   Untreated hypertension, which is frequently associated with blood pressure lability during anesthesia. If associated with left ventricular hypertrophy, hypertension leads to a higher incidence of postoperative complications (e.g., stroke, myocardial infarction). **Diuretic therapy** can produce hypovolemia and electrolyte imbalances, especially in the elderly.

6.   Hiatal hernia with esophageal reflux symptoms, which increases the risk of pulmonary aspiration and may alter the anesthetic plan (e.g., an awake intubation or a "rapid sequence" induction may be chosen).

7.   Likelihood of pregnancy and timing of last menses in women of childbearing age, because premedications and anesthetic agents may adversely influence uteroplacental blood flow, act as teratogens, or lead to spontaneous abortion.

III.   Physical examination

A.   The physical examination should be thorough but focused. Special attention is directed toward evaluation of the airway, heart, lungs, and neurologic examination. When regional anesthetic techniques are to be applied, detailed assessment of the extremities and back is necessary.

B.   As a minimum, the physical examination should include the following:

1.   Vital signs

a.   Height and weight are useful in estimating drug dosages and determining volume requirements and the adequacy of perioperative urine output.

b.   Blood pressure should be recorded in both arms and any disparity between upper extremities noted (significant differences may imply disease of the thoracic aorta or its major branches). Postural signs should be checked in patients suspected of hypovolemia.

c.   Resting pulse is noted for rhythm, perfusion (fullness), and rate. The pulse may be slow in patients receiving β-adrenergic blockade or rapid and bounding in the patient with fever, aortic regurgitation, or sepsis. Anxious or dehydrated patients may have rapid weak pulses.

d.   Respirations are observed for rate, depth, and pattern while at rest.

2.   Head and neck. The details of a thorough head and neck examination are outlined in Chapter 13. During a basic preoperative examination, one should

a.   Note the size of the oral opening as measured by finger breadths and the ability to visualize the posterior pharyngeal structures (Mallampati classification).

b.   Measure thyromental distance.

    c. Document loose or chipped teeth, artificial crowns, dentures, and other dental appliances.

    d. Note the range of cervical spine motion in flexion, extension, and rotation.

    e. Document tracheal deviation, cervical masses, and carotid bruits.

  3. Precordium. Auscultation of the heart may reveal murmurs, gallop rhythms, or a pericardial rub.

  4. Lungs. Auscultation may reveal wheezing, rhonchi, or rales, which should be correlated with observation of the ease of breathing and use of accessory muscles of respiration.

  5. Abdomen. Any evidence of distention, masses, or ascites should be noted, because these might predispose to regurgitation or compromise ventilation.

  6. Extremities. Muscle wasting and weakness should be documented, as well as general distal perfusion, clubbing, cyanosis, and cutaneous infection (especially over sites of planned vascular cannulation or regional nerve block). Ecchymosis or unexplained injuries, especially in children, women, or elderly patients, can be an indication of an abusive relationship.

  7. Back. Note any deformity, bruising, or infection.

  8. Neurologic examination. Document mental status, cranial nerve function, cognition, and peripheral sensorimotor function.

IV. Laboratory studiesRoutine laboratory screening tests are rarely useful. Laboratory tests should be selected based on the patient's medical condition and the proposed surgical procedure. A brief review of current guidelines follows.

  A. Recent hematocrit/hemoglobin level. There is no universally accepted minimum hematocrit level before anesthesia. Hematocrits in the 25% to 30% range are well tolerated by otherwise healthy people but could result in ischemia in patients with CAD. Each case must be evaluated individually for the etiology and duration of anemia. If there is no obvious explanation for anemia, a delay of surgery may be indicated. Healthy patients who are undergoing minimally invasive procedures do not need routine hematocrit screen. A hematocrit screen is recommended for neonates up to 6 months of age, women over 50 years of age, and men over 65 years of age.

  B. Serum chemistry studies are ordered only when specifically indicated by the history and physical examination. For example, blood urea nitrogen and creatinine levels are indicated for patients over 65 years of age or for those with chronic renal disease, diabetes, cardiovascular disease, intracranial disease, hepatic disease, morbid obesity, or in patients using diuretics, digoxin, steroids, or aminoglycosides.

  1. Hypokalemia is common in patients receiving diuretics and is usually readily corrected by preoperative oral potassium supplementation. Most often, mild hypokalemia (2.8 to 3.5 mEq/L) should not preclude elective surgery. Efforts to rapidly correct hypokalemia with IV replacement therapy may lead to arrhythmias and cardiac arrest. In the face of marked hypokalemia with arrhythmias, especially in the setting of digoxin use, a delay in surgery to allow cautious correction is reasonable.

2. Platelet function may be assessed by a history of easy bruising, excessive bleeding from gums or minor cuts, and family history.

3. Coagulation studies are ordered only when clinically indicated (e.g., history of a bleeding diathesis, anticoagulant use, or serious systemic illness) or if postoperative anticoagulation is planned.

C.   An electrocardiogram (ECG) is advisable for men over 40 years of age and women over 50 years of age. Although the resting ECG is not a sensitive test for occult myocardial ischemia, an abnormal ECG mandates correlation with history, physical examination, and prior ECGs and may require further workup and consultation with a cardiologist before surgery.

D.   Chest radiography should be performed only when clinically indicated (e.g., heavy smokers, the elderly, and patients with major organ system disease including malignancy and symptomatic heart disease).

V.   Anesthesiologist–patient relationship

A.   The perioperative period is emotionally stressful for many patients who may have fears about surgery (e.g., cancer, physical disfigurement, postoperative pain, and even death) and anesthesia (e.g., loss of control, fear of not waking up, waking up during surgery, postoperative nausea, confusion, pain, paralysis, and headache). The anesthetist can alleviate many of these fears and foster trust by

1.   Conducting an unhurried organized interview in which you convey to the patient that you are interested and understand his or her fears and concerns.

2.   Reassuring the patient that you will see the patient in the operating room. If the physician performing the assessment will not be the anesthetizing physician, the patient should be advised and reassured that their concerns and needs will be competently relayed and addressed.

3.   Informing the patient of the events of the perioperative period, including:

a.   The time after which the patient must have nothing to eat or drink (nothing by mouth [NPO]).

b.   The estimated time of surgery.

c.   The need for sedative premedications (see section VIII.B.) and whether the patient's daily medications should be continued as usual.

d.   The need for autologous blood donation. This usually is indicated for only a limited number of surgical procedures such as total joint arthroplasty, radical prostatectomy, and extensive spine surgery.

e.   Management of aspirin and nonsteroidal anti-inflammatory drug (NSAID) therapy. Newer NSAIDs that inhibit the cyclooxygenase-2 enzyme do not interfere with platelet function and do not need to be discontinued before surgery.

f.   Tasks to occur on the day of surgery (e.g., placement of IV or arterial catheters, routine monitoring devices, epidural catheters) with reassurance that supplemental IV sedation and analgesia will be provided as necessary during this period.

g.   Postoperative recovery either in the postanesthesia care unit or ICU for closer observation.

h.   Plans for postoperative pain control.
Note: The above discussion should be restricted to those endeavors specific to anesthesia; opinions regarding the surgical diagnosis, prognosis, and issues of surgical technique should be conveyed by the surgeon.

B.   Informed consent involves discussing the anesthetic plan, alternatives, and potential complications in terms understandable to the lay person. It is strongly preferable that this discussion is conducted and any forms written in the patient's native language.

1.   Certain aspects of anesthetic management are outside the realm of common experience and must be explicitly defined and discussed beforehand. Examples include endotracheal intubation, mechanical ventilation, invasive hemodynamic monitoring, regional anesthesia techniques, blood product transfusion, and postoperative ICU care.

2.   Alternatives to the suggested management plan should be presented, because they may become necessary if the planned procedure fails or if there is a change in clinical circumstances.

3.   Risks associated with anesthesia-related procedures should be disclosed in a way that a reasonable person would find helpful in making a decision. In general, disclosure applies to complications that occur with a relatively high frequency, not to all remotely possible risks. The anesthetist should familiarize the patient with the most frequent and severe complications of common procedures, including:

a.   Regional anesthesia: headache, infection, local bleeding, nerve injury, and drug reactions. In patients for whom a regional technique is planned, a discussion of general anesthesia and its attendant risks is suggested, because general anesthesia "backup" may be necessary.

b.   General anesthesia: sore throat, hoarseness, nausea and vomiting, dental injury, allergic drug reactions, and cardiac dysfunction (in patients with known cardiac disease).

c.   Blood transfusion: fever, infectious hepatitis, HIV infection, and hemolytic reactions.

d.   Vascular cannulations: peripheral nerve, tendon, or blood vessel injury; hemothorax; pneumothorax; and infection.
Note: In cases where risk has not been objectively defined, the patient should be so informed.

4.   Extenuating circumstances. Anesthesia procedures may proceed without informed consent (e.g., in dire emergency) or with limited consent (e.g., the Jehovah's Witness patient who agrees to anesthesia with the understanding that blood transfusions will be withheld).

VI.   Anesthesia consultant's note
The preoperative anesthesia note is a medicolegal document in the permanent hospital record. As such, it should contain the following:

A.   A concise legible statement of the date and time of the interview, the planned procedure, and a description of any extraordinary circumstances regarding the anesthesia (e.g., locations outside the operating room).

B.   Relevant positive and negative findings from the history, physical examination, and laboratory studies.

C.   A problem list that delineates all disease processes, their treatments, and current functional limitations; medications and allergies are included.

D.   An overall impression of the complexity of the patient's medical condition, with assignment to one of **ASA Physical Status Classes**:

Class 1. A healthy patient (no physiologic, physical, or psychologic abnormalities).

Class 2. A patient with mild systemic disease without limitation of daily activities.

Class 3. A patient with severe systemic disease that limits activity but is not incapacitating.

Class 4. A patient with an incapacitating systemic disease that is a constant threat to life.

Class 5. A moribund patient not expected to survive 24 hours with or without operation.

Class 6. A declared brain-dead patient whose organs are being removed for donor purposes.

Note: If the procedure is performed as an emergency, an E is added to the previously defined ASA Physical Status.

E.   The anesthesia plan in the hospital record is used to convey a general management strategy (e.g., suggestions for further preoperative evaluation, premedications, intraoperative monitoring, and postoperative care). If the author of the plan is not scheduled to actually administer care on the day of surgery, this person should avoid defining precise details of the anesthetic agents or techniques to be used, because these will be determined by the anesthesia team providing care. In the healthy uncomplicated patient, completion of a preanesthesia form is adequate, but when the history needs to be detailed (i.e., the patient with cardiovascular disease) it should be in a formal legible progress note. If important comorbid problems are present, it is imperative to convey this information directly to the anesthesia team responsible in advance of the surgery.

VII.   Guidelines for NPO status
Generally, adults should not eat solids after midnight of the day before surgery but may have clear fluids up to 2 hours before their procedure. Infants or children may have milk, formula, breast milk, or solid food up to 6 hours before surgery and clear liquids up to 2 hours before surgery (see Chapter 28). More restrictive instructions may be necessary for some patients, such as those with active reflux or those undergoing gastrointestinal tract operations.

VIII.   Premedication

A.   The goals of administering sedatives and analgesics before surgery are to allay the patient's anxiety; prevent pain during vascular cannulation, regional anesthesia procedures, or positioning; and facilitate a smooth induction of anesthesia. It has been shown that the requirement for these drugs is reduced after a thorough preoperative visit by an anesthesiologist.

1.   In elderly, debilitated, or acutely intoxicated patients and in those with upper airway obstruction or trauma, central apnea, neurologic deterioration, or severe pulmonary or valvular heart disease, doses of sedatives and analgesics should be reduced or withheld.

2.   Patients addicted to opioids and barbiturates should be premedicated sufficiently to prevent withdrawal during or shortly after surgery.

B.   Sedatives may be given to calm the anxious patient and help provide a restful night of sleep before surgery.

  1.   Benzodiazepines

  a.   Diazepam (Valium) rarely produces significant cardiovascular or respiratory depression at recommended doses. A dose of 5 to 10 mg orally (PO) 1 to 2 hours before surgery usually suffices. Diazepam should not be given intramuscularly (IM) because injection is painful and absorption unpredictable.

  b.   Lorazepam (Ativan) may be used (1 to 2 mg PO) but usually causes more intense amnesia and prolonged postoperative sedation.

  c.   Midazolam (Versed), 1 to 3 mg IV or IM, is most frequently used in the induction area as a supplemental premedicant and provides excellent amnesia and sedation.

  2.   Barbiturates such as pentobarbital (Nembutal) are rarely used for preoperative sedation, although they are occasionally used by nonanesthetists for sedation during diagnostic procedures (e.g., endoscopy, magnetic resonance imaging, and computed tomography).

  3.   Droperidol (Inapsine) is a butyrophenone that produces long-acting sedation at doses of 0.03 to 0.14 mg/kg IM or IV. At low doses (0.625 to 2.5 mg IV), it is a useful antiemetic. The use of droperidol has been related to cases of QT prolongation and/or torsades de pointes even at doses at or below the recommended range; some cases have been fatal. Droperidol is contraindicated in patients with known or suspected QT prolongation. Use of droperidol should be reserved for patients failing other therapies, and only after it is determined that QT prolongation does not exist. Electrocardiographic monitoring is recommended prior to treatment and for 2 to 3 hours after treatment to monitor for arrhythmias.

C.   Opioids are most frequently given in the preoperative setting to relieve pain (e.g., patient with a painful hip fracture) and occasionally when the placement of extensive invasive monitoring devices is planned. **Morphine** is the primary opioid used, because it has both analgesic and sedative properties. Usual adult doses are 5 to 10 mg IM, 60 to 90 minutes before coming to the operating room.

D.   Anticholinergics are seldom used preoperatively. Occasionally useful agents include the following

  1.   Glycopyrrolate (0.2 to 0.4 mg IV for adults and 10 to 20 µg/kg for pediatric patients) or **atropine** (0.4 to 0.6 mg IV for adults and 0.02 mg/kg for pediatric patients) is given IV during ketamine induction and during oral/dental surgery as an antisialagogue.

  2.   Scopolamine may be given in combination with morphine IM before cardiac surgery to provide additional amnesia and sedation. The adult dose is 0.3 to 0.4 mg IM.

E.   Guidelines for prophylaxis for pulmonary aspiration have been recommended by the ASA and may be beneficial for patients at high risk for aspiration pneumonitis, including the parturient and those with a hiatal hernia and reflux symptoms, a difficult airway, ileus, obesity, or central nervous system depression.

1. **Histamine (H$_2$) antagonists** produce a dose-related decrease in gastric acid production. **Cimetidine** (Tagamet), 200 to 400 mg PO, IM, or IV, and **ranitidine** (Zantac), 150 to 300 mg PO or 50 to 100 mg IV or IM, significantly reduce both the volume and acidity of gastric secretions. Multidose regimens (i.e., the night before and morning of surgery) are the most effective, although parenteral administration may be used to achieve a rapid (<1 hour) onset. Cimetidine has been shown to prolong the elimination of many drugs, including theophylline, diazepam, propranolol, and lidocaine, potentially increasing the toxicity of these agents. Ranitidine has not been associated with such side effects.

2. **Nonparticulate antacids.** Colloidal antacid suspensions effectively neutralize stomach acid but can produce serious pneumonitis if aspirated. Nonsuspension antacids, such as citric acid solutions (Bicitra, 30 to 60 mL, 30 minutes before induction), may be less effective in increasing gastric pH, but their aspiration is less harmful.

3. **Metoclopramide** (Reglan) is a dopamine antagonist that enhances gastric emptying by increasing lower esophageal sphincter tone while simultaneously relaxing the pylorus. An oral dose of 10 mg is given 1 to 2 hours before anesthesia or intravenously in the induction area as soon as the IV is inserted. When administered intravenously, it should be given slowly to avoid abdominal cramping. Metoclopramide also has an antiemetic effect. Metoclopramide can precipitate a dystonic reaction, which can be treated with diphenhydramine, 25 to 50 mg IV. Metoclopramide is contraindicated in the presence of bowel obstruction, where it may increase retrograde peristalsis.

SUGGESTED READING

ACC/AHA task force report. Special report: guidelines for perioperative cardiovascular evaluation for noncardiac surgery. Report of the American College of Cardiology/American Heart Association Task Force on practice guidelines (Committee on Perioperative Cardiovascular Evaluation for Noncardiac Surgery). *J Cardiothorac Vasc Anesth* 1996;10: 540–552.

American Society of Anesthesiologists. Practice guidelines for preoperative fasting and the use of pharmacologic agents to reduce the risk of pulmonary aspiration: application to healthy patients undergoing elective procedures. A Report by the Task Force on Preoperative Fasting and the Use of Pharmacologic Agents to Reduce the Risk of Pulmonary Aspiration. *http://www.asahq.org/practice/npo/npoguide.html* accessed May 1, 2001.

American Society of Regional Anesthesia. Recommendations for Neuraxial Anesthesia and Anticoagulation. *http://www.asra.com/items__of__interest/consensus__statements/* accessed May 1, 2001.

Eagle KA. Surgical patients with heart disease: summary of the ACC/AHA guidelines. American College of Cardiology/American Heart Association. *Am Fam Physician* 1997;56:811–818.

Egbert LD, Battit GE, Turndorf H, et al. The value of the preoperative visit by an anesthetist. A study of doctor-patient rapport. *JAMA* 1963; 185:553–555.

Fleisher LA. Risk of anesthesia. In: Miller RD, ed. *Anesthesia*, 5th ed. New York: Churchill Livingstone, 2000:795–824.

Fleisher LA, Barash PG. Preoperative cardiac evaluation for noncardiac surgery: a functional approach. *Anesth Analg* 1992;74:586–598.

Olsson GL, Hallen B, Hambraeus-Jonzon K. Aspiration during anaesthesia: a computer-aided study of 185,358 anaesthetics. *Acta Anaesthesiol Scand* 1986;30:84–92.

Roizen MF, Foss JF, Fischer SP. Preoperative evaluation. In: Miller RD, ed. *Anesthesia*, 5th ed. New York: Churchill Livingstone, 2000:824–884.

Velanovich V. The value of routine preoperative laboratory testing in predicting postoperative complications: a multivariate analysis. *Surgery* 1991;109:236–243.

White PF. Pharmacologic and clinical aspects of preoperative medication. *Anesth Analg* 1986;65:963–974.

Wiklund RA, McGoldrick KE. Preoperative evaluation of preparation of patients for vitreoretinal surgery. In: Scheppens CL, Hartnett ME, Hirose T, eds. *Scheppens' retinal detachment and allied diseases*, 2nd ed. Boston: Butterworth Heinemann, 2000:221–234.

Specific Considerations with Cardiac Disease

James G. Cain

I. Ischemic heart disease. Coronary artery disease (CAD) afflicts approximately 10 million Americans. CAD increases in prevalence with age: 4 in 1,000 for ages 15 to 44, 48 in 1,000 for ages 45 to 65, and 80 in 1,000 for those over age 65. Nearly 10 million noncardiac surgical patients are at risk annually for perioperative morbidity and mortality from ischemic cardiac events. These include 1 million with diagnosed CAD (angina or Q waves on electrocardiogram [ECG]), 2 to 3 million with two or more coronary risk factors, and 4 million older than age 65. Perioperative cardiac events, including myocardial infarction (MI), unstable angina, congestive heart failure (CHF), and serious arrhythmias, are the leading cause of perioperative deaths.

  A. Physiology

   1. Oxygen supply–demand balance. Myocardial ischemia occurs when oxygen demand exceeds delivery.

   a. Supply. The myocardium is perfused via coronary arteries. The **left coronary artery** branches into the **left anterior descending** and the **circumflex** to supply most of the left ventricle (LV), interventricular septum (including atrioventricular [AV] bundles), and left atrium. The **right coronary artery** supplies the interventricular septum, including the sinoatrial and AV nodes. Coronary arteries are end arteries with minimal collateralization. **Myocardial oxygen supply** depends on coronary artery diameter, LV diastolic pressure, aortic diastolic pressure, and arterial oxygen content.

   (1) Coronary blood flow is dependent on the aortic root to downstream coronary pressure gradient. Most coronary blood flow occurs during diastole. Coronary artery blood flow in normal individuals is primarily controlled through local mediators. Patients with significant coronary diseases may be maximally dilated at rest.

   (2) Heart rate is inversely proportional to the length of diastole. Faster heart rates decrease the duration of maximal coronary perfusion.

   (3) Blood oxygen content is determined by hemoglobin concentration, oxygen saturation, and dissolved oxygen. Increasing inspired oxygen fraction and/or hemoglobin concentration increases blood oxygen content.

   b. Demand. Myocardial oxygen consumption ($M\dot{V}_{O_2}$) increases most by increasing ventricular wall tension and heart rate (velocity of shortening) and, to a lesser degree, contractility.

   (1) Ventricular wall tension is modeled by Laplace's law: wall tension equals transmural ventricular pressure

multiplied by the cardiac radius divided by twice wall thickness. Changes in these parameters affect oxygen demand.
(2) Heart rate. Tachycardia is well tolerated in normal hearts. Atherosclerotic coronary arteries may not adequately dilate to meet increased demands of faster heart rates.
(3) Contractility increases with the increased chronotropy, myocardial stretch, calcium, and catecholamines. Increasing contractility increases oxygen consumption.
c. Supply and demand balance. Atherosclerosis is the most common etiology for supply–demand imbalances. Conditions such as aortic stenosis, systemic hypertension, and hypertrophic cardiomyopathy, which are characterized by marked ventricular hypertrophy and high intraventricular pressures, may also increase MVo_2 and create imbalances, even in the setting of normal coronary arteries. The goal of treatment is to improve the supply–demand balance.
(1) Increase supply
(a) Increase coronary perfusion pressure with administration of volume or α-adrenergic agonists to increase aortic diastolic pressure.
(b) Increase coronary blood flow with nitrates and calcium channel antagonists to dilate coronary arteries.
(c) Increase oxygen content by raising hemoglobin concentration or oxygen partial pressure.
(2) Decrease demand
(a) Decrease heart rate either directly with β-adrenergic antagonists or indirectly by decreasing sympathetic tone with opioids and anxiolytics.
(b) Decrease ventricular size (decrease wall tension) by decreasing preload with nitrates, calcium channel antagonists, or diuretics. Occasionally, increasing inotropy may decrease demand by decreasing ventricular size and wall tension.
(c) Decreasing contractility may decrease $M\dot{V}o_2$ if ventricular size and wall tension do not increase excessively. Calcium channel blockers and volatile anesthetics may decrease contractility.
(d) Intraaortic balloon counter pulsation increases coronary perfusion pressure by augmenting diastolic pressure. It also reduces resistance to LV ejection, thereby reducing LV size and wall tension.
B. Preoperative predictors of cardiac morbidity
Primary risk factors associated with CAD directly influence onset, duration, severity of heart disease, and risk of cardiac morbidity. Secondary risk factors are associated with and influenced by primary risk factors.
1. Primary risk factors
a. CHF may be an important predictor of perioperative morbidity. A large number of patients with CHF die suddenly, often from arrhythmias. Without a treatable precipitating etiology, life expectancy may be from 6 months to 4 years.
b. Angina is classified as stable or unstable. **Stable angina** is induced by exercise or stress, resolves with rest, and can be controlled with medication. **Unstable angina** occurs at

rest or is characterized by increasing severity or number of anginal episodes. Unstable angina may be difficult to control medically. Myocardial ischemia may also be evidenced by fatigue, dyspnea, arrhythmia, and/or CHF. Most ischemia, however, is asymptomatic or "silent."

c. Previous MI. The nature of the previous MI (e.g., age, anatomic location, current cardiac function, remaining myocardium at risk, and current activity level) contributes to the relative risk for future cardiac events. It has been suggested that the reinfarction risk with anesthesia is increased for 6 months after MI. More recent data have not supported this concept. Post-MI myocardial healing occurs primarily over the first 4 to 6 weeks. The risk of perioperative MI in the general population is about 0.7%, with CAD 1%, with prior MI 6%, and with recent MI 6% to 37%.

d. Hypertension is a risk factor for ischemic heart disease, CHF, and stroke but is not independently associated with increased risk of perioperative MI.

e. Arrhythmias. Ventricular arrhythmias may indicate underlying myocardial disease (e.g., CAD or dilated cardiomyopathy) and may predict increased risk. Isolated premature ventricular contractions without evidence of underlying cardiac pathology are not associated with increased cardiac risk. Supraventricular arrhythmias are often associated with underlying pathology and may indicate increased cardiac risk. There appears to be little benefit to preoperatively converting or aggressively treating asymptomatic or well-controlled ventricular or supraventricular arrhythmias. If rate control and conversion of atrial fibrillation is desired, β-adrenergic blockade appears to be more efficacious than either calcium channel blockers or digoxin.

f. Prior cardiac surgery. Medical records should be reviewed to determine the nature of surgery, adequacy of repair, cardiac anatomy, and need for anticoagulation therapy and/or antibiotic prophylaxis. Although percutaneous transluminal coronary angioplasty has not been shown to decrease subsequent cardiac risk for noncardiac surgery, coronary artery bypass grafting has been shown to decrease future risk.

2. Secondary risk factors

a. Diabetes mellitus is a risk factor for CAD. Morbidity and mortality are greater in diabetic patients who suffer an MI. The incidence of "silent" ischemia is no higher in diabetic patients than in nondiabetic patients.

b. Cigarette smoking and dyslipidemia are major modifiable risk factors for CAD. Smoking may double the risk of CAD.

c. Obesity, defined as patient weight greater than 20% above ideal body weight, adversely affects both health and longevity and has a direct relation with most other risk factors.

d. Age. The incidence of CAD and perioperative MI increases with age. Also, as age increases the LV becomes stiffer, LV relaxation is delayed, atrial contribution to stroke volume increases, and ejection fraction (EF) may be reduced.

e. Genetics. A family history of significant cardiac morbidity and mortality is an important risk factor.

f. Vascular disease. Forty percent to 70% of patients undergoing vascular surgery have angiographic evidence of CAD. Vascular surgery patients have an increased incidence of perioperative MI (1% to 15%) compared with the general population (0.7%).

C. Preoperative evaluation

1. Important historical information includes current lifestyle, activity level, exercise limitations, anginal symptoms, CHF, arrhythmias, details of past hospitalization and diagnostic testings, and current and past medications. Ability to perform moderate physical exercise, such as carrying a bag of groceries up a flight of stairs or walking more than 3 miles per hour without symptoms, generally infers a low perioperative for the patient. Recent changes in the patient's history should be noted.

2. Physical examination should be completed as discussed in Chapter 1 with close attention to the following:

a. Evidence of **jugular venous distension** and **carotid bruits**.

b. Chest examination should evaluate evidence of rhonchi, rales, wheezing, and effusions.

c. Cardiac examination should evaluate evidence of heaves, thrills, murmurs, rubs, and gallops.

d. Abdominal examination may reveal evidence of aortic aneurysm (pulsatile mass or bruits) or cardiac dysfunction, (pulsatile liver, hepatomegaly, and/or hepatojugular reflux).

e. Extremities and **peripheral pulses** should be examined. Blood pressure should be measured in both arms. Cyanosis, clubbing, and edema should be noted.

3. Laboratory studies should be tailored to the patient and the specifics of the surgery. Guidelines are under continual discussion. It is suggested that patients with known cardiovascular disease obtain blood urea nitrogen and creatinine levels, chest radiograph, and ECG. It is suggested that preoperative ECGs should be obtained for men over 40 and women over 50 years of age. Perioperative isolated T-wave inversions occur frequently and without other evidence of significant CAD or ischemia/infarct, such as ST depression/elevation, arrhythmias, angina, or hemodynamic instability. They are not in themselves indicative of perioperative ischemia and usually do not warrant further cardiac workup. A hemoglobin level should be obtained for males over 65, females of any age, or if significant blood loss is expected.

4. Noninvasive studies. No absolute recommendations can be made. Specific situations may warrant one or more of the following:

a. Exercise stress testing gives an estimate of functional capacity along with the ability to detect ECG changes and hemodynamic response. Exercise stress tests are highly predictive when ST segment changes are characteristic of ischemia (greater than 2 mm, immediate, sustained into recovery, and/or associated with hypotension).

b. Radionuclide imaging is a safe and effective method to assess myocardial perfusion, infarction, and function.

(1) Thallium 201 is a radioactive tracer that is injected intravenously and avidly extracted as a potassium analogue by cardiac muscle. Myocardial distribution of thallium is closely related to regional myocardial blood flow. Areas of thallium redistribution upon delayed imaging are considered to represent myocardium at risk. A fixed defect (unchanged distribution with time) is believed to represent scar tissue (an old MI). Coronary stenoses of greater then 90% likely produce perfusion abnormalities at rest, whereas stenoses of 50% or greater may only be detected with increased stress or exercise.

(2)   **Dipyridamole-thallium or technetium-99m sestamibi** imaging may be useful in patients who are unable to complete an exercise-based test. The presence of areas of redistribution correlates well with increased perioperative cardiac risk. Specificity is reduced when the test is used as a general screening examination.

(3)   **Technetium-99m sestamibi** is injected intravenously and accumulated in myocardium in proportion to blood flow. Using a first-pass technique, multiple ventricular images synchronized to the cardiac cycle are acquired at rest and during exercise. The occurrence of regional wall motion abnormalities and the inability to increase LV EF during exercise are suggestive of myocardial ischemia.

c.   **Echocardiography** is used to evaluate global and regional ventricular function, pericardial effusions, and congenital abnormalities. Transthoracic and/or transesophageal views may be obtained. Transesophageal echocardiography may provide a better view of valvular function, mural or atrial thrombi, and aortic aneurysms and is often used intraoperatively to evaluate valve function (e.g., during mitral valve reconstruction) and wall motion. Stress echocardiography may be useful if a prior stress ECG is nondiagnostic, there is an abnormal baseline ECG, or atypical symptoms are present. Contrast echocardiography may be useful in quantifying regional myocardial perfusion patterns.

d.   **Continuous ECG monitoring** may be useful for detecting arrhythmias or periods of ischemia and correlating the findings with symptoms.

5.   **Cardiac catheterization** is considered the "gold standard" for evaluating cardiac disease. Information obtained includes anatomy with visualization of direction and distribution of flow, hemodynamics, and overall function of the heart (see Chapter 23).

6.   **Cardiac consultation** may be helpful in identifying patients at risk. The consultant should provide guidance in deciding which tests will be useful and can expedite the process and interpret the results. The consultant can evaluate the patient's perioperative medical therapy and provide follow-up in the postoperative period. Such follow-up is crucial with the initiation of new drug therapies and after pacemaker placement and automatic internal cardioverter/defibrillator (ICD) implantation.

D.   **Preanesthetic considerations**

1.   Patients are likely to be anxious. Reassurance during the preoperative visit has been shown to be useful in decreasing anxiety. **Anxiolytics** may blunt rises in sympathetic tone and may be invaluable.

2.   **Cardiac medications** are usually continued preopera-

tively. Possible exceptions include angiotensin-converting enzyme inhibitors (due to prolonged vasodilation), slow-release or long-acting medications, diuretics, and, rarely, digoxin.

    a. **β-Adrenergic blockers** decrease the risk of perioperative ischemia and infarction, conferring decreased risk for as long as 2 years. Patients receiving β-adrenergic blockers should continue to receive them. Consider initiating perioperative β-adrenergic blockers for patients with increased risk of cardiac events.

    b. **Clonidine.**Small preoperative doses of clonidine may confer cardioprotective effects.

3. **Supplemental oxygen** should be provided to all patients with significant ischemia, especially when sedation is being ordered preoperatively.

4. **Monitoring** is discussed in Chapter 10.

5. **Perioperative issues**

    a. **General versus regional anesthesia.** No convincing outcome data support the superiority of either general or regional anesthesia with regard to cardiac outcome. Reasons other than the cardiac issues should guide the choice of anesthetic technique.

    b. **Site of surgery** may predict perioperative cardiac morbidity. Patients undergoing thoracic, upper abdominal, and major vascular surgery have a severalfold increased risk of cardiac and other perioperative complications.

II. **Noncoronary cardiac disease**

A. **Bacterial endocarditis prophylaxis.** Transient bacteremia after surgical and dental procedures may cause endocarditis. Blood-borne bacteria can lodge on damaged or abnormal valves or tissues. Antibiotic prophylaxis is recommended for patients with prosthetic cardiac valves, previous history of endocarditis, most congenital malformations, rheumatic valvular disease, hypertrophic cardiomyopathy, and mitral valve regurgitation. See Chapter 7 (section VI.B.) for discussion of appropriate prophylactic antibiotic choices. Prophylaxis is not recommended for patients with permanent pacemakers, implantable defibrillators, and mitral valve prolapse without regurgitation. Patients with subacute bacterial endocarditis may experience arrhythmias secondary to nodal abscesses and inflammation; pacing capabilities should be considered preoperatively.

B. **Aortic stenosis**

1. **The etiology** is usually progressive calcification and narrowing of a normal or bicuspid valve. A valve area of 0.6 to 0.8 cm^2 defines severe stenosis and markedly increases obstruction to LV ejection and increases wall tension.

2. **Symptoms** appear late in the disease process. Life expectancy without surgical intervention is 5 years after the onset of angina and 2 years after the appearance of CHF.

3. The **ventricle** becomes **hypertrophied** and stiff in response to the increased load. Atrial contraction becomes critical to maintaining adequate ventricular filling and stroke volume. The ventricle is susceptible to ischemia due to increased intraventricular pressure and muscle mass with decreased coronary perfusion pressure.

4. **Anesthetic considerations.** Aortic stenosis is the only val-

vular lesion directly associated with increased risk of perioperative ischemia, MI, and death.

    a.   Normal sinus rhythm and adequate **volume status**
should be maintained. Hypotension, tachycardia (decreasing
filling and increasing oxygen demands), and severe bradycardia (decreasing cardiac output) are poorly tolerated and
should be aggressively treated to maintain coronary perfusion
pressure.

    b.   Pacing capabilities should be considered to treat brady-
cardia and arrhythmias.

    c.   Pulmonary artery catheters may be useful to assess
baseline filling pressures, ventricular function, and response
to pharmacologic interventions, fluid therapy, and changes of
heart rate and rhythm.

    d.   Nitrates and **peripheral vasodilators** should be admin-
istered with extreme caution because small reductions of ventricular volume can markedly reduce cardiac output.

    e.   The **treatment of ischemia** in these patients is directed
at increasing oxygen delivery by raising coronary perfusion
pressure and decreasing oxygen consumption (usually by
lowering heart rate).

C.   Idiopathic hypertrophic subaortic stenosis results from
asymmetric hypertrophy of the interventricular septum, which
produces outflow obstruction during ejection. The anterior leaflet
of the mitral valve opposes the septal movement and increases
the amount of outflow obstruction.

    1.   Factors that **worsen the outflow obstruction** include de-
creased arterial pressure, decreased intraventricular volume, increased contractility, and increased heart rate.

    2.   Clinical implications and treatment are similar to those
for aortic stenosis.

    3.   Anesthetic considerations include the following:

        a.   Maintain normal sinus rhythm.

        b.   Consider cardioversion for supraventricular tachycardia.

        c.   Continue β-adrenergic and calcium channel blocker
therapy.

        d.   Maintain normal volume status.

        e.   Correct vasodilation with α-adrenergic agonists to avoid
tachycardia and marked changes in contractility.

        f.   Use inotropes with caution because they may exacerbate
the outflow obstruction.

        g.   Use nitrates and peripheral dilators only with extreme
caution.

D.   Aortic regurgitation

    1.   Etiologies include rheumatic heart disease, endocarditis,
trauma, collagen vascular diseases, and processes that dilate
the aortic root (e.g., aneurysm, Marfan disease, and syphilis).

    2.   Pathophysiology

        a.   Acute aortic regurgitation may cause sudden LV volume
overload with increased left ventricular end-diastolic pressure and pulmonary capillary occlusion pressure. Manifestations include decreased cardiac output, CHF, tachycardia, and
vasoconstriction.

        b.   Chronic aortic regurgitation causes concentric ventricu-
lar hypertrophy with an increased LV volume and slightly in-

creased LV pressure. Symptoms may be minimal until late in the disease process when left heart failure occurs.

3. **Anesthetic considerations**

   a. Maintain a normal to slightly increased heart rate to minimize regurgitation and maintain aortic diastolic and coronary artery perfusion pressure.

   b. Maintain adequate volume status.

   c. Improve forward flow, decrease LV end-diastolic pressure and myocardial wall tension with vasodilators.

   d. Avoid peripheral arterial constrictors. They may worsen regurgitation.

   e. Consider pacing. These patients have an increased frequency of conduction abnormalities.

E. **Mitral stenosis**

   1. **The etiology** is almost always rheumatic.

   2. **Pathophysiology**

      a. Increased left atrial pressure and volume overload increases left atrial size and may produce **atrial fibrillation**.

      b. **Elevated left atrial pressure** increases pulmonary venous pressure and pulmonary vascular resistance. In turn, right ventricular (RV) pressure is increased for a given cardiac output. Chronic pulmonary hypertension produces pulmonary vascular remodeling.

      c. **Pulmonary hypertension** may lead to tricuspid regurgitation, RV failure, and decreased cardiac output.

      d. **Tachycardia** is poorly tolerated because it decreases diastolic filling time, decreases cardiac output, and increases left atrial pressure.

   3. **Anesthetic considerations**

      a. **Avoid tachycardia**. Control ventricular response pharmacologically or consider cardioversion for patients with atrial fibrillation. Continue digoxin, calcium channel blockers, and β-adrenergic blockers perioperatively.

      b. **Avoid pulmonary hypertension**. Hypoxia, hypercarbia, acidosis, atelectasis, and sympathomimetics increase pulmonary vascular resistance. Oxygen, hypocarbia, alkalosis, nitrates, prostaglandin E_1, and inhaled nitric oxide decrease pulmonary vascular resistance.

      c. **Hypotension** may be caused by hypovolemia; however, one must have a high suspicion for RV failure. Inotropes and agents that decrease pulmonary hypertension may be useful (e.g., dopamine, dobutamine, milrinone, amrinone, nitrates, prostaglandin E_1, and inhaled nitric oxide).

      d. A **pulmonary artery catheter** may assist perioperative evaluation of volume status, intracardiac pressures, and cardiac output.

      e. **Premedication** should be adequate to prevent anxiety and tachycardia. Exercise caution in patients with hypotension, pulmonary hypertension, or low cardiac output.

F. **Mitral regurgitation**

   1. **Etiologies** include mitral valve prolapse, ischemic heart disease, endocarditis, and post-MI papillary muscle rupture. Mitral regurgitation allows blood to be ejected into the left atrium during systole. The amount of regurgitant flow depends on the

ventricular–atrial pressure gradient, size of the mitral orifice, and duration of systole.

2. **Pathophysiology**

   a. **Acute mitral regurgitation** usually occurs in the setting of MI. Acute volume overload of the left heart leads to LV dysfunction with increased wall tension.

   b. **Chronic mitral regurgitation** causes gradual left atrial and LV overload and dilation with compensatory hypertrophy.

   c. **Measurement of EF** does not quantify forward versus backward flow, because the incompetent valve permits immediate bidirectional ejection with systole.

3. **Anesthetic considerations**

   a. **Relative tachycardia** is desirable to decrease ventricular filling time and ventricular volume. Bradycardia is associated with increased LV volume and regurgitation.

   b. **Afterload reduction** is beneficial. Intraaortic balloon counterpulsation may be life saving. Increased systemic vascular resistance will increase regurgitation.

   c. **Maintain preload**.

   d. **Careful titration** of myocardial depressants is indicated.

G. **Mitral valve prolapse** has a prevalence of 5% to 10%.

1. **Clinical features** include atypical chest pain, a midsystolic click, palpitations, anxiety, dyspnea, and nonspecific ECG changes. Associated pathologic conditions include conduction abnormalities, supraventricular arrhythmias, mitral regurgitation, and endocarditis.

2. **Diagnosis** is confirmed by echocardiography.

3. **Subacute bacterial endocarditis** prophylaxis is recommended if mitral regurgitation is present (see section II.A. and Chapter 7, section VI.B.).

4. **Anesthetic considerations** are those appropriate for the patient's coexisting diseases.

III. **Congenital heart disease (CHD)**. Patients with CHD are either unrepaired or have had surgical intervention and may be considered "cured," "corrected," or "palliated," depending on the nature of the lesion and type of procedure. Outcomes continue to improve. Anesthesiologists are increasingly caring for these patients in noncardiac surgical settings. Additional preoperative information may be obtained from the pediatrician, internist, or cardiologist managing the patient. Review of old medical records is essential.

A. **General considerations**

1. **Systemic air emboli** are a constant danger, particularly due to the dynamic nature of shunting. Intravenous lines must be purged of air bubbles, and bubble filters should be considered.

2. **Cyanotic patients** are often polycythemic and at risk for stroke and thrombosis. Intravenous hydration is important. Hemodilution may be considered with preoperative hematocrits greater than 60% to 70%.

3. **Abnormal hemostasis**, usually mild in severity, has been noted in patients with cyanotic CHD. These include abnormalities of the extrinsic and intrinsic coagulation pathways and platelet function.

4. **Bacterial endocarditis prophylaxis** is mandatory (see section II.A. and Chapter 7, section VI.B.).

B. Unrepaired congenital defects may produce worsening hemodynamic derangements in adulthood.

　1. Atrial septal defect (ASD) is the most commonly diagnosed congenital lesion in adults.

　2. Left-to-right shunts produce RV overload, increased pulmonary blood flow, and pulmonary hypertension.

　3. Patients often present with a flow murmur, arrhythmias, atrial fibrillation, or CHF. Although these findings may resolve after correction, increased pulmonary vascular resistance may persist. Conduction defects, supraventricular arrhythmias, and ventricular arrhythmias may follow corrective surgery.

C. True corrections include the following:

　1. Patent ductus arteriosus, once ligated, rarely has long-term sequelae.

　2. ASD. Repair of secundum-type defects early in life results in normal physiology and function. Repair of primum-type ASDs with mitral valve venosus defect and partial anomalous pulmonary venous drainage may lead to residual mitral regurgitation. Conduction defects, supraventricular arrhythmias, and ventricular arrhythmias may be present.

D. Corrected lesions result in markedly prolonged life expectancy. Some degree of residual cardiovascular impairment remains.

　1. Coarctation of the aorta. Labile blood pressure may occur even after successful repair.

　　a. Residual coarctation occurs in 10% of patients.

　　b. Left arm blood pressure may not equal right arm pressure if a subclavian flap was used in the original repair.

　　c. Hypertension is a late complication developing in 65% of patients after repair.

　　d. Occult aortic valve disease should be considered in patients after repair.

　2. Transposition of the great arteries was historically corrected with an intraatrial baffle rerouting blood to appropriate vessels (e.g., Mustard or Senning procedure). Long-term postoperative derangements include residual ASD, RV dysfunction, conduction disturbances, supraventricular tachyarrhythmias, caval or pulmonary venous obstruction, and tricuspid regurgitation. Because the RV functions as the systemic ventricle, the cardiovascular response to exercise is markedly abnormal. The **atrial switch procedure** (Jatene repair) is now most common, allowing the LV to serve the systemic circulation. Postoperative complications include LV dysfunction, biventricular outflow tract obstruction, aortic regurgitation, and coronary insufficiency.

　3. Ventricular septal defects (VSDs), even after repair, may exhibit residual pulmonary hypertension, RV dysfunction, and CHF.

　　a. Residual VSD, tricuspid regurgitation, elevated pulmonary vascular resistance, and respiratory insufficiency may occur in the early postrepair period.

　　b. Injuries to the bundle of His may produce complete heart block.

　　c. Percutaneous transcatheter umbrella closure of VSDs offers a less invasive option.

4.   Tetralogy of Fallot usually shows normalization of the RV/pulmonary artery systolic gradient.

    a.   Most patients have **residual RV dysfunction** and **right bundle branch block** but still respond to exercise with increased cardiac output. Some show **residual RV outflow obstruction** or **peripheral pulmonic stenosis**, which may lead to RV failure and ventricular arrhythmias.

    b.   **Persistent pulmonary vascular hyperreactivity** may result in shunting, which is usually mild and does not alter arterial oxygen saturation.

    c.   **Pulmonic regurgitation** is common but usually does not affect cardiac output.

    d.   A few patients have residual VSDs or LV dysfunction.

    e.   There is an increased incidence of ventricular tachyarrhythmias and sudden death.

E.   Palliative procedures extend life expectancy, but with markedly abnormal cardiovascular function. Palliative procedures include the following:

    1.   Cardiac transplantation for hypoplastic left heart.

    2.   Pulmonary atresia. Systemic-to-pulmonary shunts were performed in the past (e.g., Blalock-Taussig, Potts, Waterson). Currently, synthetic grafts are used to shunt blood between either the ascending aorta to the main pulmonary artery or subclavian artery to right or left pulmonary artery. The purpose of the shunts is to increase pulmonary blood flow and unload the RV. Late complications include CHF and progressive pulmonary hypertension.

    3.   The **fenestrated Fontan procedure** is commonly used to treat aortic atresia, mitral, or tricuspid atresia and all types of "single functioning ventricle" defects. Right atrial or vena caval blood flow is directed to the pulmonary artery with a fenestrated atrial baffle. **Late complications** include:

        a.   Persistent pericardial and pleural effusions (markedly decreased with fenestrated Fontan vs. original Fontan procedure).

        b.   Limited cardiac reserve with exercise or stress.

        c.   Hemodynamic instability with hypovolemia or arrhythmias.

IV.   Cardiac transplant patient

A.   More than 2,500 cardiac transplants, including 225 pediatric transplants, are performed each year with a 90% 1-year survival rate and a 75% 5-year survival. Increasingly, these patients present for noncardiac surgery.

B.   Postcardiac transplant patients typically require surgery related to underlying vascular disease or complications of chronic steroid or immunosuppressive therapy.

C.   Physiology of cardiac transplantation

    1.   Sympathetic reinnervation may occur over time. Parasympathetic reinnervation does not occur.

    2.   Transplanted hearts exhibit accelerated graft atherosclerosis and are at increased risk for myocardial ischemia.

    3.   Hemodynamics of the transplanted heart

        a.   Cardiac impulse formation and conduction are normal, although the resting heart rate is increased.

        b.   The Frank-Starling mechanism remains intact. Transplanted hearts respond normally to circulating catecholamines.

   c.   Metabolic control of coronary blood flow is intact.
   d.   The transplant patient meets demand for increased cardiac output by increasing stroke volume by the Frank-Starling mechanism and subsequently by increasing heart rate in response to circulating catecholamines.
   4.   Drug effects
   a.   Drugs that act via the autonomic system (e.g., atropine and digoxin) are ineffective.
   b.   Direct-acting agents are effective. Isoproterenol may be used to increase heart rate. Norepinephrine or phenylephrine may be used to increase blood pressure.
   c.   β-adrenergic receptors are intact and may be present in increased density.
 D.   Anesthetic considerations
   1.   The patient's activity level and exercise capacity should be determined. A cardiology consultant may provide data concerning cardiac function and anatomy as measured by echocardiography and catheterization.
   2.   Underlying CAD may be asymptomatic. Evidence of ischemia may include a history of dyspnea, signs of reduced cardiac function, and arrhythmias.
   3.   A baseline 12-lead ECG should be obtained and may demonstrate multiple P waves and right bundle branch block.
   4.   A chest radiograph may be useful.
   5.   To assess the effect of immunosuppression and concomitant drug therapy, baseline laboratory studies should include complete blood count, electrolytes, blood urea nitrogen, creatinine, glucose, and liver function tests.
   6.   Strict aseptic technique is required for all interventions (e.g., intravenous access, intubation), because the patient may be receiving long-term immunosuppression.
   7.   Monitoring. Invasive monitoring is used when indicated by the patient's cardiopulmonary status and the proposed surgical procedure. The right internal jugular vein is often the access site for repetitive endocardial biopsies and may need to be reserved for this purpose.
   8.   Anesthesia
   a.   General, regional, and spinal anesthesia have been administered to cardiac transplant patients. Selection of anesthesia may be guided by issues other than the history of cardiac transplant.
   b.   Hemodynamic goals
   (1)   Maintain preload.
   (2)   Avoid sudden vasodilation. Compensatory changes are dependent on Frank-Starling mechanism initially with a delayed heart rate response.
   (3)   If sudden hypotension occurs, administer volume and direct-acting vasopressors such as phenylephrine or norepinephrine.
V.   Pacemakers
 A.   Definitions
   1.   Unipolar pacing is accomplished by placing a negative stimulating electrode within the atrium or ventricle and a positive ground distant from the heart.
   2.   Bipolar pacing places both positive and negative electrodes in the chamber paced or sensed.

3.   Asynchronous generators are simple pacers that only produce electrical impulses. They have no sensing functions.
4.   Synchronous generators have circuits for impulse formation and sensing functions.
5.   Nomenclature. A five-letter code describes pacemakers:
   a.   The first position designates the **chamber paced** (A denotes atrium; V, ventricle; and D, double [both atrium and ventricle]).
   b.   The second position describes the **chamber sensed** (same abbreviations, and O denotes none).
   c.   The third position defines the **pacemaker's response** to sensed events (I, inhibited; T, triggered; D, double; O, none; and R, reverse [paces when tachycardia sensed]).
   d.   The fourth position details **programmability** (P, rate programmable; M, multiprogrammable; C, communicating; and O, none).
   e.   The fifth position signifies **tachyarrhythmia responses** (B, bursts; N, normal rate competition; S, scanning, and E, external).
   f.   For example, a VVI pacemaker will sense and pace the ventricle yet will be inhibited and not fire if an R wave is detected. A DDD pacemaker is known as a universal, with ability to sense and pace both atrium and ventricle.
B.   Indications
   1.   Permanent
      a.   Sinus node dysfunction
         (1)   Symptomatic bradycardia refractory to drug therapy.
         (2)   Sick sinus syndrome.
      b.   AV block
         (1)   Complete heart block.
         (2)   Type 2 second-degree AV block.
      c.   Fascicular block
         (1)   Symptomatic bifascicular block.
         (2)   Trifascicular block.
   2.   Temporary. Similar indications as for permanent. Additional indications may include:
      a.   Bifascicular block and/or second degree AV block.
      b.   Malfunctioning permanent pacemaker.
      c.   Patient with severe valvular disease dependent on maintaining heart rate.
C.   Physiology
   1.   Atrial versus ventricular pacing. Advantages of atrial pacing include:
      a.   Maintenance of atrial contraction, especially in patients with decreased LV compliance.
      b.   Improved mitral and tricuspid valve function.
      c.   Normal sequence of electrical and mechanical activation.
      d.   Suppression of atrial and ventricular ectopy.
   2.   Rate responsive pacemakers alter pacing rate to adjust cardiac output to meet demands of increased activity. Pacemakers adjust rate based on increased physical activity, increased minute ventilation, pH changes, or other variables.
D.   Preoperative evaluation of patients with permanent pacemakers
   1.   Define the indications requiring the pacemaker.

2. Determine the type of pacemaker (e.g., model, date of insertion, baseline pacing rate). If the information is not readily available, the manufacturer and model number may be obtained from a radiograph of the generator.

3. Outline current symptoms and cardiac status.

4. Determine pacemaker dependence.

5. Determine pacemaker function. Formal interrogation of the pacemaker is not routinely required before surgical procedures.

6. Determine the location the pulse generator. Most are currently placed in the upper chest. Older models may be located in the abdomen.

7. If central access is required, consider placement under fluoroscopic guidance to avoid dislodging a lead if the pacemaker has been placed within 6 weeks.

E. **Intraoperative management**

1. **Modern pacemakers** are extremely resistant to electromagnetic interference (EMI) associated with the use of electrocautery. If interference does occur, the pacemaker output may be inhibited or the pacemaker may be reset to a committed pacing mode (i.e., DOO or VOO).

2. Applying a common donut **magnet** to the pacemaker will cause any pacemaker to function temporarily in the magnet mode, which is a committed mode. This will prevent pacemaker output inhibition by EMI associated with electrocautery use. Normal pacemaker function is restored upon removal of the magnet. Use of a magnet during surgical procedures is necessary only if inhibition of pacemaker output is noted coincident with EMI. This is rarely necessary, because most permanent pacemakers will spontaneously convert to a asynchronous mode during prolonged periods of EMI. If used, the magnet should be placed directly over the pacemaker. It is best to tape the magnet in place to avoid inadvertent dislodgment.

3. **Resetting of pacemakers** by EMI will produce asynchronous (i.e., "competitive") pacing that can be noted on the ECG.

4. The **dispersal electrode (grounding pad)** for the electrocautery should be placed as far away from pulse generator as possible. Interference from electrocautery is less common with chest wall placement of the generator because there is less likelihood for the cautery current to cross the pacer leads. Consider inactivating rate responsive features during the procedure.

5. **Monitor heart rate** during electrocautery with a precordial or esophageal stethoscope, pulse oximeter, arterial line, or a finger on the pulse.

6. **Postoperative evaluation of pacemaker function** is recommended after surgical procedures when there is evidence that the pacemaker has been reset (i.e., asynchronous pacing is present) on the postoperative ECG. Routine postoperative interrogation of the pacemaker is not necessary.

F. **Perioperative pacing options**

1. **Transcutaneous.** External pacing can be performed via large pads placed on the anterior and posterior thorax. This is an easy and inexpensive method of ventricular pacing.

2. **Transvenous**

   a. A temporary pacing electrode can be inserted via a central vein into the heart.

      b. Various pulmonary artery catheters exist that have pacing options. (see Chapter 10).
    3. **Transesophageal.** The left atrium is easily paced with a pacing probe placed in the esophagus.

VI. **The automatic ICD** has dramatically changed the treatment of patients at high risk for sudden death. Currently, more than 50,000 are placed each year in the United States.

    A. Electrical countershock is the only reliable treatment for ventricular fibrillation.

    B. The ICD is implanted in the abdominal or chest wall and connected to two defibrillating electrodes (patches) or transvenous leads. A separate electrode is used for pacing and sensing. This electrode can sense ventricular tachycardia or fibrillation and deliver a counter shock of 20 to 30 joules for up to four consecutive attempts.

    C. All ICDS are exquisitely sensitive to EMI associated with electrocautery. EMI is detected by the ICD as ventricular fibrillation and may result in spurious shocks.

    D. All ICDs are specifically designed to suspend detection in response to a magnet application. Magnet application will therefore prevent misinterpretation of EMI as ventricular fibrillation. Magnet application does not affect the pacing functions of the ICD.

    E. Intraoperative magnet application, rather than deactivation of the ICD, is preferred: If ventricular tachycardia or ventricular fibrillation occurs intraoperatively, simply removing the magnet will cause the ICD to resume detection and deliver therapy, typically in less than 10 seconds. This is more certain and faster than any possible human response (such as external defibrillation).

    F. ICD failure during anesthesia may occur, because defibrillation thresholds change. An external defibrillator should be available, and some advocate the placement of external defibrillator pads preoperatively.

    G. Patients with an ICD should not enter a room with a magnetic resonance imaging machine because of the potential for ICD dysfunction.

    H. One must be aware of potential pacemaker–ICD interactions in presence of tachyarrhythmias. When evaluating such patients, the source for arrhythmia, such as a markedly reduced EF or congenital cardiac malformation, should be noted.

    I. **The atrial defibrillator** is a new device used in the treatment of paroxysmal atrial fibrillation. It is placed in similar fashion as the ICD. Similar anesthesia considerations and precautions should be exercised.

SUGGESTED READING

American College of Cardiology/American Heart Association Task Force on Practice Guidelines. Guidelines for perioperative cardiovascular evaluation for noncardiac surgery. *J Cardiothorac Vasc Anesth* 1996; 10:540–552.

Appleton CP, Hatle LK. The natural history of left ventricular filling abnormalities: assessment of two-dimensional and Doppler echocardiography. *Echocardiography* 1992;9:437–456.

Appleton CP, Hatle LK. The natural history of left ventricular filling abnormalities: assessment of two-dimensional and Doppler echocardiography. *Echocardiography* 1992;9:437–456.

Ballal RS, Kapadia S, Secknus MA, et al. Prognosis of patients with vascular disease after clinical evaluation and dobutamine stress echocardiography. *Am Heart J* 1999;137:469–475.

Bode RH, Lewis KP, Zarich SW, et al. Cardiac outcome after peripheral surgery: comparison of general and regional anesthesia. *Anesthesiology* 1996;84:3–13.

Breslow MJ, Miller CF, Parker SD, et al. Changes in T-wave morphology following anesthesia and surgery: a common recovery-room phenomenon. *Anesthesiology* 1986;64:398–402.

Child JS. Stress echocardiographic techniques. *Echocardiography* 1992; 9:77–84.

Coley CM, Field TS, Abraham SA, et al. Usefulness of dipyrimidole-thallium scanning for preoperative evaluation of cardiac risk for nonvascular surgery. *Am J Cardiol* 1992;69:1280–1285.

Danjani AS, Bisno AL, Chung KJ, et al. Prevention of bacterial endocarditis. Recommendations of the American Heart Association. *JAMA* 1990; 264:2919–2922.

Dawood MM, Gupta DK, Southern J, et al. Pathology of fatal perioperative myocardial infarction: implications regarding pathophysiology and prevention. *Int J Cardiol* 1996;57:37–44.

Deutch N, Hantler CB, Morady F, Kirsch M. Perioperative management of the patient undergoing automatic internal cardioverter defibrillator implantation. *J Cardiothorac Anesth* 1990;4:236–244.

Eagle KA, Berger PB, Calkins H, et al. ACC/AHA guideline update for perioperative cardiovascular evaluation for noncardiac surgery—executive summary. A report of the American College of Cardiology/American Heart Association Task Force on Practice Guidelines (Committee to update the 1996 Guidelines on Perioperative Cardiovascular Evaluation for Noncardiac Surgery). *Circulation* 2002;105:1257–1267.

Go AS, Browner WS. Cardiac outcomes after regional or general anesthesia. *Anesthesiology* 1996;84:1–2.

Mangano D, Goldman L. Preoperative assessment of patients with known or suspected coronary disease. *N Engl J Med* 1995;333:1750–1756.

Mangano DT. Perioperative cardiac morbidity. *Anesthesiology* 1990;72: 153–184.

Palda VA, Detsky AS. Perioperative assessment and management of risk from coronary artery disease. *Ann Intern Med* 1997;127:313–328.

Perloff JK. Congenital disease in adults. *Circulation* 1991;84:1881–1890.

Poldermans D, Boersma E, Bax JJ, et al. The effect of bisoprolol on perioperative mortality and myocardial infarction in high risk patients undergoing vascular surgery. Dutch Echocardiographic Cardiac Risk Evaluation Applying Stress Echocardiography Study Group. *N Engl J Med* 1999;341:1789–1794.

Roizen MF. Cost effective preoperative laboratory testing. *JAMA* 1994; 271:319–320.

Simon AB. Perioperative management of the pacemaker patient. *Anesthesiology* 1997;46:127–131.

Wallace A, Layug B, Tateo I, et al., for the McSPI Research Group. Prophylactic atenolol reduces postoperative myocardial ischemia. *Anesthesiology* 1998;88:7–17.

Wirthlin, DJ, Cambria RP. Surgery-specific considerations in the cardiac patient undergoing noncardiac surgery. *Prog Cardiovasc Dis* 1998;40: 453–468.

Zelzman CH, Miller SA, Zimmerman MA, et al. The case for beta-adrenergic blockade as prophylaxis against perioperative cardiovascular morbidity and mortality. *Arch Surg* 2001;136:286–290.

3

Specific Considerations with Pulmonary Disease

Kevin C. Dennehy and Kenneth E. Shepherd

I. **General considerations**. The incidence of postoperative pulmonary complications is second only to cardiovascular complications as a cause of perioperative mortality. These complications are related to the type and severity of respiratory disease; the site, duration, and magnitude of the surgical procedure; and coexisting extrapulmonary diseases.

A. Patients with significant chronic pulmonary disease are at greater risk for postoperative respiratory failure than the general population, because anesthesia and surgery more easily produce hypoventilation, hypoxemia, and retention of secretions in such patients.

B. Patients with moderate to severe chronic lung disease and those having thoracic and upper abdominal operations have an increased morbidity and mortality rate.

C. Postoperative morbidity and mortality can be reduced by identifying patients at risk for perioperative respiratory complications, optimizing their medical therapy, and instituting a program of chest physiotherapy before and after surgery.

II. **Classification of pulmonary disease**

A. **Obstructive airway diseases** are characterized by abnormal expiratory gas flow rates. The **airflow limitation** can be structural or functional.

   1. **Chronic obstructive pulmonary disease** (COPD) is airflow obstruction attributable to emphysema ("pink puffer") or chronic bronchitis ("blue bloater").

      a. **Emphysema** is due to abnormal permanent enlargement of the airspaces distal to the terminal bronchioles, accompanied by destructive changes of the alveolar wall. This leads to loss of the normal elastic recoil of the lung with subsequent premature airway closure at higher than normal lung volumes during exhalation.

      b. **Chronic bronchitis** is defined as the presence of productive cough for at least 3 months in each of 2 successive years in a person in whom the excessive secretions are not due to other diseases. The most common precipitant is cigarette smoking.

   2. **Asthma** is defined as episodic variable airflow obstruction. Asthma is an inflammatory disease in which a complex cascade of cellular and chemical mediators leads to increased airway tone, edema, mucus secretions, and increased airway responsiveness to a variety of stimuli that includes cooling and drying of the airways, infection, medications, and occupational exposure.

   3. **Cystic fibrosis** leads to the secretion of highly viscous

mucus. This results in airway obstruction, fibrosis, cachexia, and chronic pulmonary infection. Late changes include bronchiectasis with hypoxemia, carbon dioxide retention, and respiratory failure.

4. **The mechanism of hypoxemia** in obstructive disease is primarily through regional mismatching of ventilation and perfusion (**$\dot{V}/\dot{Q}$ mismatch**). **Dyspnea**, a major symptom, is multifactorial in origin but is in large part related to loading of the respiratory muscles.

B. **Restrictive pulmonary disease** is characterized by a decrease in lung compliance and may be intrinsic or extrinsic. Airway resistance is usually normal, whereas lung volumes and diffusing capacity are reduced.

1. **Intrinsic**

   a. **Pulmonary edema** occurs when fluid accumulates in the interstitium and alveoli by hydrostatic, cardiogenic (e.g., congestive heart failure [CHF]), or "noncardiogenic" (e.g., acute respiratory distress syndrome [ARDS]) mechanisms.

   b. **Pulmonary interstitial disease** causes inflammation/fibrosis of interstitium, alveoli, or vascular beds. The latter may lead to pulmonary hypertension and cor pulmonale. Examples include sarcoidosis, chronic hypersensitivity pneumonitis, and radiation fibrosis.

2. **Extrinsic**

   a. **Pleural disease**, either fibrosis or effusion.

   b. **Chest wall deformity**, such as kyphoscoliosis, pectus excavatum, trauma, or burns.

   c. **Diaphragmatic compression** by obesity, ascites, pregnancy, or from retraction during abdominal surgery.

3. As in obstructive disease, the primary cause of hypoxemia in restrictive states is $\dot{V}/\dot{Q}$ mismatch. Often patients have multiple reasons for pulmonary dysfunction, as well as mixed obstructive and restrictive defects. Proper diagnosis requires a careful history and physical examination. Pulmonary function testing may be required to differentiate obstructive from restrictive defects and can be used to assess a patient's response to therapy.

C. **Pulmonary hypertension** is characterized by a mean pulmonary pressure of more than 25 mm Hg that results in right ventricular dilatation, hypertrophy, and failure.

1. **Primary pulmonary hypertension** occurs due to idiopathic fibrin deposition in the pulmonary capillaries and arterioles accompanied by increased thrombogenesis. The total cross-sectional area of the pulmonary vasculature may be markedly decreased.

2. **Secondary pulmonary hypertension** occurs due to any disease process that

   a. **Increases capillary or pulmonary venous pressures** (e.g., mitral regurgitation);

   b. **Increases pulmonary artery blood flow** (e.g., patent ductus arteriosus); or

   c. **Decreases the cross-sectional area of the pulmonary vasculature** (e.g., acute causes such as pulmonary embolus or chronic causes such as pulmonary fibrosis).

3. **Cor pulmonale** is right ventricular failure secondary to

conditions that reduce cross-sectional area of the pulmonary vasculature. Polycythemia, $\dot{V}/\dot{Q}$ mismatch, and right ventricular failure with displacement of the interventricular septum to the left occur with advanced disease.

III.   Identification of the patient at risk

A.   History

1.   Symptoms of respiratory disease such as cough, expectoration, hemoptysis, wheezing, dyspnea, and chest pain should be elicited. Preexisting lung and systemic diseases, occupational exposures, symptoms of disordered breathing during sleep, medications, and recent changes in clinical status should be defined.

2.   **Chronic cough** may suggest bronchitis or asthma. If cough is productive, sputum should be examined for evidence of infection and, if appropriate, sent for Gram and/or Wright stain, culture, or cytology.

3.   **Smoking history** should be quantified in pack-years (number of packs smoked per day multiplied by the number of years smoked). The risks of malignancy, COPD, and postoperative pulmonary complications are directly proportional to the smoking history.

4.   **Dyspnea** is an uncomfortable sensation of breathing. The activity level should be defined; severe dyspnea (occurring at minimal activity or at rest) may be a predictor of both poor ventilatory reserve and the need for postoperative ventilatory support.

B.   Physical findings

1.   **Body habitus** and general appearance.

a.   **Obesity, pregnancy, and kyphoscoliosis** reduce lung volumes (functional residual capacity [FRC], total lung capacity) and pulmonary compliance and predispose to atelectasis and hypoxemia.

b.   **Cachectic malnourished patients** have blunted respiratory drive and decreased muscle strength and are predisposed to pneumonia.

c.   **Cyanosis** requires a reduced hemoglobin concentration of 5 g/dL. The appearance of cyanosis depends on many factors, including cardiac output, of cyanosis depends on tissue, and hemoglobin concentration. Oxygen uptake by the ble sign of hypoxemia. is an unreliable sign of hypoxemia.

2.   **Respiratory signs**. Respiratory rate and pattern, thoracic coordination, and the use of accessory muscles should be assessed.

a.   **Tachypnea**, a respiratory rate greater than 25 breaths/min, is usually the earliest sign of respiratory distress.

b.   **Respiratory pattern**

(1)   **Pursed-lip breathing** and visible expiratory effort may indicate airway obstruction.

(2)   **Accessory muscle use** increases with load and dysfunction of the diaphragm and intercostal muscles.

(3)   **Asymmetry of chest wall expansion** may result from unilateral bronchial obstruction, pneumothorax, pleural effusion, lung consolidation, or unilateral phrenic nerve injury (causing an elevated hemidiaphragm).

(4)   **Tracheal deviation** may suggest pneumothorax or

mediastinal disease with tracheal compression. This may cause difficulty during intubation or airway obstruction during induction of general anesthesia.

(5) **Inspiratory paradox**. Normally the abdominal wall should move outward with the chest wall during inspiration. Inspiratory paradox occurs when the abdomen collapses as the chest wall expands during inspiration and suggests paralysis or severe dysfunction of the diaphragm.

   c. **Auscultation**

   (1) **Diminished breath sounds** may indicate local consolidation or pleural effusion.

   (2) **Rales**, usually in dependent portions, may indicate atelectasis or CHF.

   (3) **Wheezing** may indicate obstructive airway disease.

   (4) **Stridor** may indicate upper airway narrowing.

3. **Cardiovascular signs**

   a. **Pulsus paradoxus** is defined as a fall in systolic blood pressure of greater than 10 mm Hg during inspiration. Its physiologic basis is not clear, but it is probably due to selective impairment of left ventricular filling and ejection during inspiration. It can be seen in asthma, pericardial tamponade, and hypovolemia during positive pressure ventilation.

   b. **Pulmonary hypertension** occurs as a result of elevated pulmonary vascular resistance.

   (1) **Physical signs** include splitting of the second heart sound with an accentuated pulmonic component, jugular venous distention, hepatomegaly, hepatojugular reflux, and peripheral edema.

   (2) **Factors that may increase pulmonary vascular resistance** include hypoxia, hypercarbia, acidosis, ARDS, and application of high levels of positive end-expiratory pressure (PEEP).

C. **Laboratory studies**

1. **Chest radiograph**

   a. **Hyperinflation** and decreased vascular markings are characteristic of COPD.

   b. **Pleural effusion, pulmonary fibrosis, and skeletal abnormalities** (kyphoscoliosis, rib fractures) may predict restrictive disease states.

   c. **Air space disease**, including CHF, consolidation, atelectasis, lobar collapse (bronchial obstruction), or pneumothorax, is an important predictor of $\dot{V}/\dot{Q}$ mismatch and hypoxemia.

   d. **Specific lesions**, including pneumothorax, emphysematous blebs, and cysts, may preclude the use of nitrous oxide.

   e. **Tracheal narrowing or deviation** may occur as a result of mediastinal compression or masses. Further workup with computed tomography, tomography, or magnetic resonance imaging may be of value in detailing the precise location and degree of obstruction of tracheal and bronchial lesions.

2. **Electrocardiogram**. Electrocardiographic signs of significant pulmonary dysfunction include the following:

   a. **Low voltage and poor R-wave progression** attributable to hyperinflation.

   b.   Signs of pulmonary hypertension and cor pulmonale, such as
   (1)   Right-axis deviation.
   (2)   P pulmonale (P waves greater than 2.5 mm in height in lead II).
   (3)   Right ventricular hypertrophy (R/S ratio > 1 in lead V_1).
   (4)   Right bundle branch block.
3.   **Arterial blood gas tensions**
   a.   **Partial pressure of oxygen (Pao_2). Hypoxemia** is considered severe when Pao_2 is less than 55 mm Hg. Patients with severe hypoxemia have significant pulmonary dysfunction and are at increased risk for postoperative pulmonary complications.
   b.   **Partial pressure of carbon dioxide ($Paco_2$). Hypercarbia** occurs when $Paco_2$ is greater than 45 mm Hg. Patients who chronically retain carbon dioxide often have end-stage lung disease with little or no reserve and are at increased risk for postoperative pulmonary complications.
   c.   **Measurement of pH** in conjunction with $Paco_2$ allows determination of acid-base disturbances.
4.   **Pulmonary function tests** (PFTs) measure pulmonary mechanics and functional reserve and provide an objective assessment of lung function. PFTs have been shown to help make decisions on management of lung resection candidates. In this context, they are used to estimate residual lung function after pulmonary resection, as measured by split-function studies (which quantify dysfunction in each lung). The impact of preoperative PFTs in predicting the risk of clinically important postoperative pulmonary complications in other surgical procedures is not as clear. The use of preoperative PFTs in evaluating these patients must be individualized.

   Briefly, PFTs can be interpreted by knowing a few key items. These are total lung capacity, which for a 70-kg adult is approximately 5.5 L; vital capacity, 4 L; FRC, 2.5 L; residual volume, 1.5 L; and forced expiratory volume in the first second (FEV_1), 80% of vital capacity (3.2 L). For example, obstructive defects are characterized by elevated total lung capacity, FRC, and residual volume with reduced FEV_1 ($<80\%$). Restrictive defects are characterized by proportional decreases in all lung volumes with a normal or increased FEV_1/FVC ratio.
IV.   **Effects of anesthesia and surgery on pulmonary function.** General anesthesia decreases lung volumes and promotes $\dot{V}/\dot{Q}$ mismatch. Many anesthetic drugs blunt the ventilatory response to hypercarbia and hypoxia. Postoperatively, atelectasis and hypoxemia commonly result, especially in patients with preexisting pulmonary disease. Pulmonary function is further compromised by postoperative pain, which can limit coughing and lung expansion.
   A.   **Respiratory mechanics and gas exchange**
   1.   **General anesthesia and the supine position decrease FRC**. Atelectasis occurs when lung volumes during tidal breathing fall below the volume at which airway closure occurs (closing capacity). Positive-pressure ventilation and PEEP can minimize this effect.
   2.   **Positive-pressure ventilation compared with sponta-**

neous breathing leads to $\dot{V}/\dot{Q}$ mismatching. During positive-pressure ventilation, nondependent portions of the lung receive a greater proportion of ventilation than do dependent portions. Pulmonary blood flow tends to be increased in dependent portions of the lung; its distribution is affected by gravity and the anatomical distribution of pulmonary vessels. The result is a variable increase in both physiologic dead space and shunt compared with spontaneous ventilation.

3. Respiratory muscle and chest wall changes. In the supine position, the diaphragm is displaced cephalad by abdominal contents. The addition of general anesthesia, muscle paralysis, and positive-pressure ventilation changes the pattern of respiratory muscle use and chest wall motion. These changes may further alter the distribution of ventilation and perfusion within the lungs.

B. Regulation of breathing

1. The ventilatory response to hypercarbia is reduced by inhalation anesthetics, propofol, barbiturates, and opioids. $Paco_2$ is elevated with spontaneous ventilation during general anesthesia, as is the **apneic threshold** (the $Paco_2$ at which patients who have had hyperventilation to apnea resume spontaneous ventilation).

2. The ventilatory response to hypoxia may also be blunted by inhalation anesthetics, propofol, barbiturates, and opioids. This effect may be particularly important in patients with severe chronic lung disease who normally retain carbon dioxide and depend on hypoxic drive to increase ventilation.

C. Effect of surgery. Postoperative pulmonary function is affected by the site of surgery. The ability to cough is reduced after abdominal operations compared with peripheral procedures and appears to be related to the pain produced by coughing. Vital capacity is reduced by 75% after upper abdominal procedures and by approximately 50% after lower abdominal or thoracic operations. Recovery of normal pulmonary function may take several weeks. Peripheral procedures have little impact on vital capacity or the ability to clear secretions.

D. Effect on ciliary function. The upper respiratory tract normally warms and humidifies inspired air, providing an ideal environment for normal function of respiratory tract cilia and mucus. General anesthesia, often conducted with unhumidified gases at high flow rates, dries secretions and can easily damage respiratory epithelium. Endotracheal intubation exacerbates this problem by bypassing the nasopharynx. Secretions become thickened, ciliary function is reduced, and the patient's resistance to pulmonary infections is decreased. These problems may be partially prevented by ensuring adequate warmth and humidity in the anesthesia circuit, and employing low fresh gas flow rates.

V. Preoperative treatment in pulmonary disease. The goals of preoperative treatment are to improve aspects of disease that may be reversible.

A. Cessation of smoking for 12 hours before surgery may reduce nicotine and carboxyhemoglobin levels, promoting better tissue oxygen transport. Cessation of smoking for longer periods (at least several weeks) may reduce the risk of postoperative pulmonary complications by improving ciliary function and reducing airway secretions and irritability.

B.   Acute bacterial infection should be treated before elective surgery. Therapy is guided by sputum Gram stain and culture. Recent viral respiratory infections, especially in children, may predispose the patient to bronchospasm or laryngospasm.

C.   Hydration and humidification of inspired gases aid clearance of bronchial secretions.

D.   Chest physiotherapy (voluntary deep breathing, coughing, incentive spirometry, and chest percussion and vibration combined with postural drainage) improves mobilization of secretions and increases lung volumes, reducing the incidence of postoperative pulmonary complications.

E.   Medical treatment

1.   Sympathomimetics, or β-adrenergic agonist drugs, cause bronchodilation via cyclic AMP-mediated relaxation of bronchial smooth muscle.

a.   Drugs with β_2-adrenergic selectivity may be selected. These are less prone to causing β_1-adrenergic mediated cardiac effects and are most commonly administered by inhalation.

(1)   Albuterol (Proventil or Ventolin), two or more puffs by metered-dose inhaler (MDI) every 3 to 4 hours or by nebulizer with 0.5 mL/2 mL of saline every 4 to 6 hours, is a relatively selective β_2-adrenergic agonist.

(2)   Metaproterenol (Alupent), two or more puffs by MDI every 3 to 4 hours or by nebulizer with 0.5 mL/2 mL of saline every 4 to 6 hours, is less selective than albuterol.

(3)   Salmeterol (Serevent), two puffs by MDI every 12 hours, is a selective β_2-adrenergic agonist with a long duration of action that can be used for maintenance therapy in patients with asthma and COPD. It is not indicated for acute exacerbations of bronchoconstriction.

b.   Drugs with mixed β_1- and β_2-adrenergic effects include **epinephrine** (Adrenalin) and **isoproterenol** (Isuprel). The chronotropic and arrhythmogenic potential of these drugs is of concern in patients with cardiac disease. The intravenous (IV) use of low doses of epinephrine (<1 µg/min) may be considered for severe medically refractory bronchospasm. At low doses (0.25 to 1.0 µg/min), β_2-adrenergic agonist effects predominate, with an increase in heart rate attributable to β_1-adrenergic stimulation. At higher doses of epinephrine, α-adrenergic effects become predominant, with increases in systolic blood pressure.

c.   Terbutaline sulfate (0.25 mg subcutaneously, which may be repeated in 15 minutes but to no more than a total of 0.5 mg in a 4-hour period) is a relatively selective β_2-adrenergic agonist, although it may produce tachycardia in some patients.

2.   Parasympatholytics. Anticholinergics have a direct bronchodilating effect by blocking formation of cyclic guanine monophosphate and may improve FEV_1 in patients with COPD when administered by inhalation. Specific agents include

a.   Ipratropium bromide (Atrovent) by MDI or by nebulizer (0.5 mg).

    b. Glycopyrrolate (Robinul) 0.2 to 0.8 mg by nebulizer.

    c. Atropine sulfate, which has considerable systemic absorption, may cause tachycardia and thus has limited usefulness.

3. Methylxanthines (e.g., aminophylline and theophylline).

    a. These cause bronchodilation by multiple mechanisms, including blocking adenosine receptors, releasing endogenous catecholamines, and increasing the intracellular concentration of cAMP through nonspecific inhibition of phosphodiesterase enzymes.

    b. Many patients with bronchial asthma or COPD receive chronic therapy with oral **theophylline**. Serum theophylline levels should be checked and the dosage adjusted to keep levels 10 to 20 μg/mL. These medications should be continued to the morning of surgery. The use of methylxanthines in patients that have an acute exacerbation should be individualized. For patients not currently taking theophylline, a loading dose of 5 to 6 mg/kg IV may be given over 20 minutes followed by infusion rates of 0.5 to 0.9 mg/kg per hour. Smokers and adolescents may require higher doses, reflecting rapid metabolism. Patients who are elderly, have CHF or liver disease, or are taking cimetidine, propranolol, or erythromycin should receive reduced doses, reflecting slower drug metabolism.

    c. Continuation of methylxanthines during general anesthesia is rarely indicated. Bronchodilation can be achieved more safely and predictably with volatile anesthetics or β_2-adrenergic agonists. Oral theophylline preparations can be restarted once enteral intake of medications is tolerated.

    d. Patients who will remain on "nothing by mouth" status for an extended period may receive IV theophylline or aminophylline (a soluble ethylene diamine salt containing 85% theophylline by weight). For such patients who are already taking theophylline, an infusion rate may be estimated based on the patient's total daily requirement, divided by 24 (divided again by 0.85 if aminophylline is used, because theophylline dose = 0.85 × aminophylline dose).

    e. Toxicity occurs frequently when drug levels exceed 20 μg/mL; symptoms and signs include nausea, vomiting, headache, anxiety, tachycardia, arrhythmias, and seizures.

4. Corticosteroids are often used in patients not responding to bronchodilators. Their clinical effect may take several hours. Although their mechanisms of action are complex and incompletely understood, they reduce airway inflammation and responsiveness, edema, mucus secretion, and smooth muscle constriction.

    a. Steroids are preferably administered by inhalation (e.g., Beclomethasone [Vanceril] by MDI, two puffs every 6 hours) because of decreased systemic side effects.

    b. Commonly used intravenous steroids include **hydrocortisone** (Solu-Cortef), 100 mg IV every 8 hours, and **methylprednisolone** (Solu-Medrol), up to 0.5 mg/kg IV every 6 hours in asthmatic bronchitis and often higher doses in an exacerbation of asthma. Perioperative regimens are usually tapered in dose, frequency, and route of administration as dictated by clinical response.

   c. **"Stress dose"** replacement may be needed in patients currently or recently taking corticosteroids (see Chapter 6).

  5. **Cromolyn** and nedocromil sodium are inhaled medications used as prophylactic therapy for asthma. Their precise mechanisms of action remain unknown, but both appear to act by stabilizing mast cell membranes and blunting the acute release of preformed bronchoactive mediators. They are of no utility in the acute treatment of bronchospasm.

  6. **Mucolytics**

    a. **Acetylcysteine** (Mucomyst), administered by nebulizer, can decrease the viscosity of mucus by breaking the disulfide bonds in mucoproteins.

    b. **Hypertonic saline** is sometimes used to decrease mucus viscosity. When it is given by nebulizer, an osmotic shift of water to mucus enhances mucus volume and promotes clearance. Hypertonic saline, like acetylcysteine—and even occasionally β-adrenergic agonists, anticholinergics, and steroid preparations—may produce increases in airway resistance.

    c. **Recombinant deoxyribonuclease** (DNase or Pulmozyme), 10 to 40 mg inhaled daily, is used in some patients with cystic fibrosis to decrease the viscosity of bronchial secretions by cleaving DNA strands in sputum. This improves airway clearance and pulmonary function by 5% to 20% in many patients with cystic fibrosis.

  7. **Leukotriene (LT) modifying drugs** have anti-inflammatory effects acting by either blocking LT receptors (Zafirlukast and Montelukast) or inhibiting LT synthesis (Zileuton). These are approved currently for prophylaxis and maintenance therapy of chronic asthma. A specific benefit in the perioperative period has not yet been determined. Potential adverse reactions include liver function abnormalities and eosinophilic vasculitis (Churg-Strauss syndrome).

VI. **Premedication.** The goals of premedication are to allay anxiety and to facilitate smooth induction of anesthesia.

A. **Oxygen therapy**, if required preoperatively, should be continued during transport to the operating room and clearly written as a preoperative "order."

B. **If the patient is taking inhaled β-adrenergic agonists or anticholinergics**, these should accompany the patient to the operating room; their preoperative use may decrease airway responsiveness.

C. **Anticholinergics** are often indicated and can prevent bronchospasm secondary to vagal stimulation caused by airway manipulations such as laryngoscopy and endotracheal intubation. Parenteral administration may cause drying of secretions, increasing viscosity of mucus.

D. **Histamine (H_2) antagonists** (cimetidine, ranitidine) may exacerbate bronchospasm in patients with asthma, because blockage of H_2 receptors may result in unopposed H_1-mediated bronchoconstriction. Coadministration of an H_1 blocking agent (diphenhydramine, 25 to 50 mg IV) should be considered.

E. **Benzodiazepines** are effective anxiolytics but may cause excessive sedation and respiratory depression in compromised patients, especially when used with opioids.

F. **Opioids** provide analgesia and sedation but must be carefully titrated to avoid respiratory depression, especially in patients with severe pulmonary dysfunction.

VII. Anesthetic technique

A. Peripheral nerve blockade or local anesthesia may be the best choice of anesthetic for patients with pulmonary disease when the site of operation is peripheral, such as eye or extremity procedures.

B. Spinal or epidural anesthesia is a reasonable choice for lower extremity surgery. Patients with severe COPD depend on accessory muscle use, including intercostals for inspiration and abdominal muscles for forced exhalation. Spinal anesthesia may be deleterious if motor blockade decreases FRC, reduces a patient's ability to cough and clear secretions, or precipitates respiratory insufficiency or failure. **Combined epidural and general anesthetic techniques** ensure airway control, provide adequate ventilation, and prevent hypoxemia and atelectasis. Prolonged peripheral procedures are probably best performed with a general anesthetic or a combined technique.

C. General anesthesia, often in combination with epidural anesthesia, is indicated for upper abdominal and thoracic procedures. Volatile agents provide bronchodilation and an adequate depth of anesthesia to decrease the hyperreactivity of sensitive airways.

VIII. Postoperative care. Chest physiotherapy and suctioning should be immediately available to all patients who are identified as high risk. The possibility of ventilatory support should be anticipated and discussed with the patient. Postoperative pain management is critical to decreasing respiratory complications.

SUGGESTED READING

Anonymous. Drugs for asthma. *Med Lett Drugs Ther* 2000;42:19–24.

Anonymous. Pretreatment evaluation of non-small-cell lung cancer. The American Thoracic Society and European Respiratory Society. *Am J Respir Crit Care Med* 1997;156:320–332.

Barnes PJ. Chronic obstructive pulmonary disease. *N Engl J Med* 2000; 343:269–280.

Drazen JM, Israel E, O'Byrne PM. Treatment of asthma with drugs modifying the leukotriene pathway. *N Engl J Med* 1999;340:197–206.

Kimball WR. The role of spirometry in predicting pulmonary complications after abdominal surgery. *Anesthesiology* 1999;90:356–357.

Pauwels RA, Buist AS, Calverly PM, et al. Global strategy for the diagnosis, management, and prevention of chronic obstructive pulmonary disease. *Am J Respir Crit Care Med* 2001;163:1256–1276.

Rooke GA, Choi J, Bishop MJ. The effect of isoflurane, halothane, sevoflurane, and thiopental/nitrous oxide on respiratory system resistance after tracheal intubation. *Anesthesiology* 1997;86:1294–1299.

Rubin LJ. Primary pulmonary hypertension. *N Engl J Med* 1997;336: 111–117.

Salvaterra CG, Rubin LJ. Investigation and management of pulmonary hypertension in chronic obstructive pulmonary disease. *Am Rev Respir Dis* 1993;148:1414–1417.

Shepherd KE, Hurford WE. Preoperative evaluation of the patient with pulmonary disease. In: Sweitzer BJ, ed. *Handbook of preoperative assessment and management*. Philadelphia: Lippincott, Williams & Wilkins, 2000:97–125.

Smetana GW. Preoperative pulmonary evaluation. *N Engl J Med* 1999; 340:937–944.

Warner DO. Preventing postoperative pulmonary complications. *Anesthesiology* 2000;92:1467–1472.

Warner DO, Warner MA, Barnes RD, et al. Perioperative respiratory complications in patients with asthma. *Anesthesiology* 1996;85:460–467.

4

Specific Considerations with Renal Disease

Adam Sapirstein

I. **General considerations**. Five percent of the adult American population has renal disease that could contribute to perioperative morbidity. In addition to coexisting renal disease, the risk of acute renal failure (ARF) is increased by certain patient characteristics and procedures independent of renal function. Perioperative morbidity and mortality may be reduced by understanding the underlying disease, identifying patients at risk, and optimizing anesthetic and surgical management to prevent further decompensation.

II. **Normal renal physiology**

The kidney represents only 0.5% of total body weight but receives about 20% of the cardiac output. Renal blood flow is autoregulated between mean arterial pressures of 60 to 150 mm Hg by intrinsic mechanisms (e.g., afferent arteriolar tone). Autoregulation, however, does not preclude changes in renal blood flow because of extrinsic mechanisms (e.g., sympathetic vasoconstrictor innervation, the dopaminergic receptors, and the renin-angiotensin system).

A. **The principal roles of the kidney** are to excrete end products of metabolism (e.g., urea, hydrogen ion), retain nutrients (amino acids, glucose), and maintain the volume and composition of body fluids. This is accomplished by the following:

1. **Renin-angiotensin-aldosterone system**.

a. **The juxtaglomerular apparatus** of the kidney secretes renin in response to renal hypoperfusion, decreased Na^+ delivery, and increased sympathetic activity. Renin cleaves angiotensinogen to form angiotensin I, which is then converted to angiotensin II by angiotensin-converting enzyme in the lung.

b. **Angiotensin II** produces arteriolar vasoconstriction and stimulates aldosterone release.

c. **Aldosterone** is a mineralocorticoid released by the adrenal cortex in response to angiotensin II, increased K^+ levels, decreased Na^+ content, and adrenocorticotropic hormone. Aldosterone acts on the distal tubule to increase the resorption of Na^+ in exchange for K^+ and H^+.

2. **Arginine vasopressin (AVP)** is released by the posterior pituitary gland in response to increased osmolality, decreased extracellular volume, positive-pressure ventilation, or surgical stimuli. AVP increases the permeability of the collecting duct to water. Thus, AVP conserves water and concentrates the urine. It is also known as antidiuretic hormone.

3. **Atrial natriuretic peptide (ANP)** is released by specialized atrial cells in response to atrial distention (i.e., increased intravascular volume). ANP increases glomerular filtration rate

(GFR), produces a diuresis, and generally counteracts the renin-angiotensin-aldosterone system.

4. Kinins are converted from kininogens by kallikreins and are regulated by salt intake, renin release, and hormone levels. They cause renal vasodilatation and natriuresis.

5. Prostaglandins (PGE_2, PGI_2) and **thromboxane A_2** production is stimulated by the kinins and inflammation. They regulate renal hemodynamic balance and their production is blocked by cyclooxygenase inhibitors (nonsteroidal antiinflammatory drugs [NSAIDs]).

B. Secondary roles of the kidney include extrarenal regulatory and metabolic functions.

1. Erythropoietin is produced to stimulate red blood cell production. Treatment of patients with exogenous recombinant erythropoietin can prevent the anemia of chronic renal failure (CRF) and its sequelae.

2. Vitamin D is converted to its most active form, 1,25-dihydroxy vitamin D.

3. Parathyroid hormone acts on the kidney to conserve Ca^{2+}, inhibits PO_4^{2-} resorption, and increases conversion of vitamin D by the kidney.

4. Peptides and protein hormones such as insulin are metabolized, accounting for the generally decreased insulin requirements as renal failure progresses.

III. Fluids and electrolytes

A. Fluid compartments

1. Total body water (TBW) equals 60% of body weight.

    a. Two-thirds of TBW is intracellular fluid.

    b. One-third of TBW is extracellular fluid. Approximately two-thirds of extracellular fluid is interstitial and one-third is intravascular.

2. Estimated adult blood volume = 75 mL/kg, estimated plasma volume = 50 mL/kg.

B. Normal fluid balance

1. Daily adult water intake is approximately 2,600 mL: 1,400 mL in liquids, 800 mL in solid food, and 400 mL from metabolism. The minimum intake to excrete solute load is about 600 mL/day.

2. Daily water loss normally equals intake: 1,500 mL in urine, 400 mL from respiration, 500 mL from skin evaporation, and 200 mL in stool.

3. Insensible losses will be increased by fever (about 500 mL/°C/day), perspiration, and low humidity. Measurable loss will be increased by solute diuresis (as with hyperglycemia and contrast dyes), drug therapy, bowel preparations, and adrenal disease.

C. Serum osmolality

1. Osmolality (mOsm/kg) $\cong$ $2[Na^+]$ + [BUN]/2.8 + [glucose]/18, where

$[Na^+]$ = sodium concentration, mEq/L
[BUN] = blood urea nitrogen, mg/dL
[glucose] = glucose concentration, mg/dL
Normal Osm = 290 mOsm/kg

2. Osmolal gap = Osm (measured) − Osm (calculated). Normal < 10. The osmolal gap is increased when the serum contains a large amount of unmeasured osmotically active substances (e.g., ethanol, sorbitol, mannitol, methanol).

D. Disorders of sodium homeostasis

1. Hyponatremia: plasma sodium concentration less than 134 mEq/L.

a. TBW may be high, low, or normal (usually a sign of free water excess).

b. Hyponatremia often results in **reduced plasma osmolality**.

c. Clinical features vary with the degree of hyponatremia and the rapidity of onset. Symptoms generally do not appear until the sodium concentration falls below 125 mEq/L.

(1) Moderate hyponatremia or gradual onset: confusion, muscle cramps, lethargy, anorexia, and nausea.

(2) Severe hyponatremia or rapid onset: seizures, coma.

d. Treatment depends on the volume status of the patient. Generally, acute normalization of the serum [Na^+] is not necessary. It should be corrected at a rate of 0.5 mEq/L per hour until 120 mEq/L is reached to prevent complications from rapid correction (e.g., cerebral edema, central pontine myelinolysis, seizures). At this point, the patient should be out of danger, and the Na^+ concentration should be normalized slowly over a period of days.

(1) Hypervolemic hyponatremia due to renal failure, congestive heart failure, cirrhosis, or nephrotic syndrome is treated by sodium and water restriction and possibly with diuresis.

(2) Hypovolemic hyponatremia from diuretics, vomiting, or bowel preparations is treated with normal saline. For severe hypovolemic hyponatremia, the Na^+ concentration may be partially corrected to 125 mEq/L or a serum osmolality of 250 mmol/L over a 6- to 8-hour period with 3.5% hypertonic saline. Hypertonic saline is dangerous in volume-expanded salt-retaining states such as congestive heart failure.

(3) Normovolemic hyponatremia from syndrome of inappropriate AVP secretion, hypothyroidism, drugs that impair renal water excretion, or water intoxication is treated by fluid restriction.

2. Hypernatremia: plasma sodium concentration greater than 144 mEq/L. Usually caused by impairment of thirst or the ability to obtain water.

a. TBW may be high, low, or normal (usually a sign of free water deficit).

b. Clinical features vary with degree of hypernatremia and rapidity of onset, ranging from tremulousness, weakness, irritability, and mental confusion to seizures and coma.

c. Treatment depends on determining the volume status of the patient. Rapid correction can induce cerebral edema, seizures, permanent neurologic damage, and death. Plasma [Na^+] should be corrected at a maximum rate of 0.5 mEq/L per hour. The water deficit, if present, can be calculated as follows:

Normal TBW (L) = 0.6 × body weight (kg)

(Normal serum $[Na^+]$/current serum $[Na^+]$) × TBW

= current TBW

H_2O deficit = normal TBW − current TBW

(1) Hypervolemic hypernatremia secondary to Na^+ overload from mineralocorticoid excess, dialysis with hypertonic solutions, or treatment with hypertonic saline or sodium bicarbonate ($NaHCO_3$).

(a) The excess total body Na^+ (i.e., volume) may be removed by dialysis or with diuretic therapy and the water loss replaced with 5% dextrose in water (D5W).

(2) Hypovolemic hypernatremia secondary to water loss exceeding Na^+ loss (e.g., diarrhea, vomiting, osmotic diuresis) or inadequate water intake (e.g., impaired thirst mechanism, altered mental status).

(a) If hemodynamic instability or evidence of hypoperfusion is present, initial volume therapy should consist of 0.45% or even 0.9% NaCl.

(b) After volume replenishment, the remaining free water deficit should be replaced with D5W until the Na^+ concentration decreases. Then, 0.45% saline may be substituted.

(3) Normovolemic hypernatremia is typically the result of diabetes insipidus in patients with a normal thirst response. Therapy consists of treating the underlying etiology, correction of free water deficit with D5W, and the use of exogenous vasopressin in neurogenic diabetes insipidus (see Chapter 6).

E. Disorders of potassium homeostasis

1. Hypokalemia: plasma $[K^+]$ less than 3.3 mEq/L.

a. Etiologies

(1) Total body K^+ deficit.

(2) Shifts in the distribution of K^+ (extracellular to intracellular).

b. Serum K^+ is a poor index of total body potassium stores, because 98% of body potassium is located intracellularly. Thus, large K^+ deficits must be present before seeing a decrease in serum $[K^+]$. In a 70-kg man with normal pH, a fall in serum $[K^+]$ from 4 to 3 mEq/L reflects a deficit of 100 to 200 mEq. Below 3 mEq/L, each fall of 1 mEq/L reflects an additional deficit of 200 to 400 mEq.

c. K^+ loss may be from:

(1) Gastrointestinal tract (e.g., vomiting, diarrhea, or obstructed ileal loops).

(2) Kidney (e.g., diuretics, mineralocorticoid and glucocorticoid excess, renal tubular acidosis).

d. Changes in K^+ distribution occur with alkalosis (H^+ shifts to the extracellular fluid and K^+ moves intracellularly). Thus, rapid correction of acidosis, by hyperventilation or $NaHCO_3$ administration, may produce undesirable hypokalemia.

e. Clinical features rarely appear unless $[K^+]$ is less than 3 mEq/L or the rate of fall is rapid.

(**1**) **Signs** include weakness, augmentation of neuromuscular block, ileus, and disturbances of cardiac contractility.

(**2**) **Electrocardiographic (ECG) changes** include flattened T waves, U waves, increased PR and QT intervals, ST segment depression, and atrial and ventricular arrhythmias. Ventricular ectopy is more likely with concomitant digitalis therapy.

(**3**) Serum $[K^+]$ less than 2.0 mEq/L is associated with vasoconstriction and rhabdomyolysis.

f. Treatment: Rapid replacement of K^+ may cause more problems than hypokalemia itself. There is no need to correct chronic hypokalemia ($[K^+] \geq 2.5$ mEq/L) before induction of anesthesia. Hypokalemia-induced conduction disturbances or diminished contractility can be treated with K^+ (0.5 to 1.0 mEq IV every 3 to 5 minutes) until resolution. Serum $[K^+]$ must be closely followed during correction.

2. Hyperkalemia: plasma $[K^+]$ greater than 4.9 mEq/L.

a. Etiologies

(**1**) Decreased excretion (e.g., renal failure, hypoaldosteronism).

(**2**) Extracellular shift (e.g., acidosis, ischemia, rhabdomyolysis, tumor lysis syndrome and drugs such as **succinylcholine**).

(**3**) Administration of blood, potassium penicillins, and salt substitutes to renal failure patients.

(**4**) Pseudohyperkalemia from a hemolyzed specimen.

b. Clinical features are more likely with acute changes than with chronic elevation.

(**1**) **Signs and symptoms** include muscle weakness, paresthesias, and cardiac conduction abnormalities, which become dangerous as K^+ levels approach 7 mEq/L. Bradycardia, ventricular fibrillation, and cardiac arrest may result.

(**2**) **ECG findings** include high peaked T waves, ST segment depression, prolonged PR interval, loss of the P wave, diminished R-wave amplitude, QRS widening, and prolongation of the QT interval that progresses to a sine wave morphology.

c. Treatment depends on the nature of ECG changes and serum levels.

(**1**) ECG changes are treated with slow IV administration of 0.5 to 1.0 g of calcium chloride ($CaCl_2$). The dose may be repeated in 5 minutes if changes persist.

(**2**) Hyperventilation and $NaHCO_3$ administration shifts K^+ intracellularly. $NaHCO_3$ 50 mEq of may be given IV over 5 minutes, with a repeated dose in 10 to 15 minutes.

(**3**) Glucose and insulin also shift K^+ intracellularly. Regular insulin (10 units) is given IV simultaneously with 25 g of glucose (one ampule of a 50% solution) over 5 minutes.

(**4**) The above therapies are short-term measures to decrease $[K^+]$ via cellular shifts. Cation exchange resins (sodium polystyrene sulfonate [Kayexalate], 20 to 50 g with sorbitol) will slowly remove K^+ from the body and should be used as soon as possible. Serum $[K^+]$ can also be lowered by dialysis.

Table 4-1. Urine and serum diagnostic indexes

	Prerenal	Renal	Postrenal
Urine (Na)	<10 mEq/L	>20 mEq/L	>20 mEq/L
Urine (Cl)	<10 mEq/L	>20 mEq/L	
FE_{Na}	<1%	>2%	>2%
Urine osmolarity	>500	<350	<350
Urine/serum (creatinine)	>40	<20	<20
Renal failure index	<1%	>2%	>2%
Urine/serum (urea)	>8	<3	<3
Serum (BUN)/ creatinine	>20	=10	=10

BUN, Blood urea nitrogen; FE_{Na}, fractional excretion of sodium.

IV. Renal failure

   A. ARF is a sudden decrease in renal function that may occur in anuric, oliguric (<20 mL/h), or nonoliguric states. Mortality in ARF is significant, being greater than 30% in surgical and trauma patients.
   1. Etiologies (see Table 4-1)
      a. Prerenal (e.g., volume contraction, low cardiac output). Early correction of the underlying cause usually results in rapid reversal of renal dysfunction, but continued renal hypoperfusion may result in intrinsic renal damage.
      b. Intrarenal (e.g., acute tubular necrosis) secondary to prolonged prerenal failure, toxins, acute glomerulonephritis, or acute interstitial nephritis.
      c. Postrenal (e.g., obstructive uropathy) due to renal calculi, neurogenic bladder, or prostatic disease.
   2. Clinical features
      a. Hypervolemia due to impaired ability to excrete water and Na^+ with resultant hypertension and peripheral edema.
      b. Potential hypovolemia due to lack of urine concentrating ability.
      c. Potassium retention.
      d. Impaired excretion of drugs and toxins.
      e. Potential progression to CRF.
   B. CRF is characterized by a permanent decrease in GFR with a rise in serum creatinine and azotemia. Patients may be well compensated until late in the course of CRF.
   1. Etiologies. Common causes include hypertension, diabetes mellitus, chronic glomerulonephritis, tubulointerstitial disease, renovascular disease, and polycystic kidney disease.
   2. Clinical features
      a. Hypervolemia and **hypertension**, sometimes resulting in CHF and edema.
      b. Accelerated atherosclerosis, which may increase the risk of coronary artery disease.

c. Uremic pericarditis and **pericardial effusions**, which may cause cardiac tamponade.

d. Hyperkalemia, hypermagnesemia, and **hyponatremia** may occur.

e. Hypocalcemia and **hyperphosphatemia** due to elevated parathyroid hormone, resulting in renal osteodystrophy.

f. Metabolic acidosis because of inability to excrete products of metabolism.

g. Chronic anemia secondary to decreased erythropoietin production and decreased red blood cell survival (see section II.B.1).

h. Platelet dysfunction can be temporarily treated with **desmopressin acetate (DDAVP)**.

i. Increased gastric volume, acid production, and **delayed gastric emptying** resulting in increased incidence of nausea, vomiting, and peptic ulceration.

j. Increased susceptibility to infection.

k. Central nervous system (CNS) changes range from mild changes in mentation to severe encephalopathy and coma. Peripheral and autonomic neuropathies are common.

l. Glucose intolerance, type IV hyperlipidemia, and abnormal thyroid function tests.

m. Altered pharmacodynamics of most drugs, because of changes in compartment volumes, electrolytes, pH, total protein, and rates of excretion.

C. Dialysis is indicated in ARF and CRF for hyperkalemia, acidosis, volume overload, uremic complications (pericarditis, tamponade, encephalopathy), and severe azotemia.

1. Hemodialysis uses an artificial semipermeable membrane that separates the patient's blood from dialysate and allows the exchange of solutes by diffusion. Vascular access (via central venous catheters or a surgically created arteriovenous fistula) and systemic or regional anticoagulation is required. Hemodialysis typically is performed two or three times a week, and serum electrolyte and volume abnormalities are corrected by adjusting the dialysis bath fluid. Blood samples taken immediately after dialysis will be inaccurate, because redistribution of fluid and electrolytes takes about 6 hours. Continuous arteriovenous or venovenous hemodialysis may also be performed. Complications include arteriovenous fistula infection or thrombosis, dialysis disequilibrium or dementia, hypotension, pericarditis, and hypoxemia.

2. Ultrafiltration and hemofiltration allow for the removal of volume with minimal removal of waste products. These techniques are useful in volume-overloaded patients. As with standard hemodialysis, anticoagulation is required.

a. Ultrafiltration uses hemodialysis equipment to create a hydrostatic driving force across the membrane without a dialysate on the opposing side. Thus, an ultrafiltrate of serum is removed and this volume is not replaced. If large volumes of fluid are removed rapidly, hypotension may ensue.

b. Hemofiltration uses the same principle as ultrafiltration; however, replacement fluid is given to the patient either before or after the membrane filter. Volume shifts are minimized so that patients can tolerate longer periods of continuous filtration.

3. Peritoneal dialysis uses the capillaries of the peritoneum as a semipermeable exchange membrane with the dialysate infused into the peritoneal cavity via an indwelling peritoneal catheter. Advantages over hemodialysis include less hypotension or disequilibrium and no need for heparinization. However, peritoneal dialysis is less efficient and limited in catabolic states when compared with hemodialysis. Complications include infection, hyperglycemia from the dextran in the dialysate, and increased protein loss into the dialysate.

D. Specific causes of renal failure

1. Acute tubular necrosis may be produced by ischemic or toxin injuries and is the major intrinsic form of ARF. Acute tubular necrosis is the most common cause of perioperative renal failure, and its development is associated with a high mortality. The major risk factors for acute tubular necrosis are a history of preexisting renal insufficiency, administration of radiocontrast agents or aminoglycosides, and advanced age. Anesthetic treatment of patients who are at risk for developing acute tubular necrosis includes meticulous management of fluids and hemodynamics with the goal of maintaining euvolemia, normal renal blood flow, and urinary output. No specific therapies have proved consistently beneficial in the prevention or treatment of perioperative acute tubular necrosis.

2. Glomerulonephropathies are a diverse disease family that may present insidiously or more acutely with fulminant renal failure. Nephrotic syndrome may be the initial presentation with severe proteinuria (>3.5 g/day), hypoalbuminemia, hyperlipidemia, and edema. Anesthetic concerns include depleted intravascular volume and protein, accelerated atherosclerotic disease, and increased infection risk. Glomerulonephropathy may be secondary to autoimmune diseases such as systemic lupus erythematosus or vasculitides such as Wegener granulomatosis. Therapy may include glucocorticoids and cytotoxic agents.

3. Hypertensive nephrosclerosis is a major etiologic factor in the development of end-stage renal disease (ESRD) and may account for as many as 30% of patients beginning dialysis. Treatment of diastolic hypertension reduces disease progression and the associated morbidity and mortality.

4. Diabetic nephropathy is the single largest cause of ESRD in the United States. One-half of all adult insulin-dependent diabetics will develop a nephropathy that begins with proteinuria and a progressive decline in renal function 10 to 30 years after initial diagnosis. Diabetic nephropathy often manifests as a type IV renal tubular acidosis (hyporeninemic hypoaldosteronism) or as papillary necrosis. There is a high correlation between renal dysfunction and diabetic retinopathy. Aggressive control of blood glucose and blood pressure may forestall the development and prevent progression of nephropathy.

5. Tubulointerstitial diseases primarily affect the renal tubules and interstitium and include acute and chronic forms of interstitial nephritis.

a. Acute interstitial nephritis, in the adult population, is most commonly caused by drugs, including penicillins, cephalosporins, sulfonamides, rifampin, and NSAIDs. Systemic infections are the most likely etiology in children. Acute interstitial nephritis usually presents as oliguric renal failure with a variable degree of proteinuria. Symptoms of an inflammatory response, such as fever, rash, eosinophilia, and eosinophiluria, are suggestive of the diagnosis of acute interstitial nephritis. Treatment includes discontinuation of suspect drugs.

b. Chronic interstitial nephritis is most commonly due to urinary obstruction or reflux, analgesic abuse, or heavy metal intoxications. Early in the disease patients lose urine concentrating ability and have polyuria and nocturia. With disease progression, manifestations depend on specific anatomic lesions. Involvement of the proximal convoluted tubule results in a Fanconi-like syndrome (HCO_3^- wasting and renal tubular acidosis with glucose, phosphate, and amino acid wasting). Involvement of the distal convoluted tubule and collecting ducts will cause loss of acid secretion, acidemia, and salt wasting with resultant hyperkalemia. Treatment of the underlying cause is the only specific therapy for chronic interstitial nephritis.

c. Polycystic kidney diseases are autosomal dominant diseases responsible for 5% to 8% of adult ESRD. Approximately 25% of patients at age 50 years and 50% of patients at age 75 years will manifest ESRD. Cystic disease may also occur in the liver, and there is an association with intracranial and aortic aneurysms. Tuberous sclerosis and von Hippel-Lindau disease may also present as cystic renal disease.

V. Pharmacology and the kidney

A. Diuretics are used to increase urine output (Table 4-2), treat hypertension, and manage electrolyte, fluid, and acid-base disturbances.

B. Dopamine and fenoldopam dilate renal arterioles, increase renal blood flow, and augment natriuresis and the GFR. Low dose dopamine (0.5 to 3 μg/kg/min) has been proposed to prevent and treat ARF, but efficacy has never been demonstrated. Low dose fenoldapam, a specific dopamine-1 receptor agonist, may preserve renal function without the toxicity of dopamine.

C. Anesthetic effects on the kidney. Patients with normal kidneys experience transient postanesthetic alterations in renal function. These alterations may occur despite insignificant changes in blood pressure and cardiac output, suggesting that changes in intrarenal distribution of blood flow are responsible.

1. Indirect effects. All inhalational agents and many induction agents cause myocardial depression, hypotension, and a mild to moderate increase in renal vascular resistance, leading to decreased renal blood flow and GFR. Compensatory catecholamine secretion causes redistribution of renal cortical blood flow. AVP levels do not change during halothane or morphine anesthesia but increase with the onset of surgical stimulation. Hydration before the induction of anesthesia attenuates the rise in AVP produced by painful stimuli. Spinal and epidural anesthesia produce decreases in renal blood flow, GFR, and urine output.

Table 4-2. Diuretics

	Primary Site of Action	Primary Effect	Side Effects	Comments
Nonosmotic				
Loop (furosemide, edecrin, bumetanide)	Thick ascending loop of Henle, active Na^+Cl pump	Moderate to severe natriuresis, chloruresis	Hypokalemia, alkalosis, volume contraction	Interferes with both urinary concentration and dilution
Thiazides (chlorothiazide, dyazide, metolazone)	Distal tubules (Na^+-H^+, Na^+-K^+ exchange)	Mild to moderate natriuresis	Hyponatremia, hypokalemia, alkalosis, volume contraction	Interferes with urinary dilution, tends to be ineffective in renal failure and CHF
Carbonic anhydrase inhibitors (acetazolamide)	Proximal tubule Na^+-H^+ exchange)	Mild natriuresis	Hyperchloremia, hypokalemia	Used primarily for ophthalmology; self-limiting renal effect
Potassium sparing (aldactone, triamterene, amiloride)	Collecting duct, Na^+-K^+, Na^+-H^+ exchange	Mild to moderate natriuresis	Hyperkalemia	Used in conjunction with K^+ losing diuretics or in hyperaldosterone states
Osmotic				
Mannitol	Intratubular osmotic load	Moderate to severe diuresis	Early: vasodilation, volume expansion; Late: hyperosmolality, volume contraction	Draws intracellular fluid into intravascular space

CHF, congestive heart failure.

2. Direct effects. The direct toxicity of fluorinated agents is of concern, because fluoride (F^-) inhibits metabolic processes, affects urine concentrating ability, and can cause proximal tubular swelling and necrosis. The magnitude of serum F^- elevation is concentration and duration dependent.

a. Isoflurane and **desflurane** are not associated with significant release of F^-.

b. Only 2% of absorbed **enflurane** is metabolized to fluoride ion, thus producing low levels of F^- (typically < 15 μM/L). There is a theoretical concern that use of enflurane in patients with renal dysfunction may lead to F^- accumulation and additional nephrotoxicity.

c. Sevoflurane is also metabolized to F^-. Strong bases that accumulate in CO_2 absorbent at low gas flows can degrade sevoflurane to a nephrotoxic byproduct. Nephrotoxicity has been observed in rats. The Food and Drug Administration warns against using low inspired gas flows, and some have warned against use in patients with preexisting renal disease.

d. Halothane metabolism results in very low F^- levels.

3. With brief anesthesia, changes in renal function are reversible (renal blood flow and GFR return to normal within a few hours). With extensive surgery and prolonged anesthesia, impaired ability to excrete a water load or concentrate urine may last for several days.

VI. Pharmacology and renal failure

A. Alterations in drug action seen in renal failure may be due to the following:

1. Changes in volume of distribution.

2. Decreased serum protein concentration resulting in increased bioavailability of protein-bound drugs.

3. Acidemia resulting in a higher percentage of non-ionized drug.

4. Electrolyte abnormalities.

5. Impaired biotransformation.

6. Decreased renal elimination.

7. Uremia, which may be associated with CNS depression and may reduce the requirement for sedation by up to 50%.

B. Lipid-soluble drugs generally are poorly ionized and must undergo metabolism by the liver to water-soluble forms before elimination by the kidney. With few exceptions, the metabolites have little biologic activity.

1. Benzodiazepines and **butyrophenones** are metabolized in the liver to both active and inactive compounds, which are then eliminated by the kidney. Benzodiazepines are 90% to 95% protein bound. Great care must be used with diazepam because of its long half-life and its active metabolites. Accumulation of benzodiazepines and their metabolites may occur in severe renal failure. Benzodiazepines are not appreciably removed by dialysis.

2. Barbiturates, etomidate, and **propofol** are highly protein bound, and in hypoalbuminemic patients a much greater proportion will be available to reach receptor sites. Acidosis and changes in the blood–brain barrier will further reduce induction requirements. Lower initial doses are recommended in renal failure.

3.   Opioids are metabolized in the liver but may have a more intense and prolonged effect in patients with renal failure, particularly in hypoalbuminemic patients, in whom protein binding will be reduced. Active metabolites of morphine and meperidine may prolong their actions and accumulation of normeperidine may cause seizures. The pharmacokinetics of fentanyl, sufentanil, alfentanil, and remifentanil are unchanged in renal failure.

C.   Ionized drugs. Drugs that are highly ionized at physiologic pH tend to be eliminated unchanged by the kidney, and their duration of action may be prolonged by renal dysfunction.

  1.   Muscle relaxants (see Chapter 12).

  2.   Cholinesterase inhibitors (see Chapter 12). With impaired renal function, the elimination of the reversal drugs is decreased and their half-lives are prolonged. Prolongation is similar or greater than the duration of blockade from pancuronium or d-tubocurarine, so that the return of muscle relaxation after adequate reversal (recurarization) is rarely seen.

  3.   Vasoactive agents

    a.   Catecholamines with α-adrenergic effects (norepinephrine, epinephrine, phenylephrine, ephedrine) constrict the renal vasculature and may reduce renal blood flow.

    b.   Isoproterenol also reduces renal blood flow but to a lesser extent.

    c.   Dopamine and **fenoldopam** (see section V.B.).

    d.   Sodium nitroprusside contains cyanide and is metabolized by the kidney and excreted as thiocyanate. Toxicity, primarily neurologic, from excessive accumulation of thiocyanate is thus more likely in renal failure patients.

  4.   Digoxin is excreted in the urine and patients with renal failure are at increased risk of digitalis toxicity.

VII.   Anesthetic management of patients with renal disease

A.   Preoperative assessment. The etiology of renal disease should be elucidated (e.g., diabetes mellitus, glomerulonephritis, polycystic kidney disease). Elective surgery should be postponed pending resolution of acute disease processes. The degree of residual renal function (best estimated by the creatinine clearance; see below) is the most important consideration for anesthetic management.

  1.   History

    a.   Signs and symptoms of polyuria, polydipsia, dysuria, edema, and dyspnea should be sought.

    b.   Relevant medications should be detailed: Diuretics, antihypertensives, K^+ supplements, digitalis, and nephrotoxic agents (NSAIDs, aminoglycosides, exposure to heavy metals, and recent radiographic dye).

    c.   Patients on hemodialysis should be dialyzed before surgery, allowing time between dialysis and surgery to permit equilibration of fluids and electrolytes. The patient's dialysis schedule, pre- and postdialysis weights, and any problems during dialysis should be determined.

  2.   Physical examination

    a.   Patients should be thoroughly examined for stigmata of renal failure as described in section IV.B.2.

    b.   Arteriovenous fistula should be evaluated for patency (by the presence of a thrill or a bruit). IV access and blood pressure determinations should be performed on the opposite limb.

3. **Laboratory studies**

a. **Urinalysis** provides a qualitative assessment of general renal function.

(1) Positive findings include abnormal pH, proteinuria, pyuria, and casts.

(2) The kidney's ability to concentrate urine is often lost before other changes become apparent. A specific gravity of 1.018 or greater after an overnight fast suggests that concentrating ability is intact. However, radiographic dye and osmotic agents will elevate specific gravity and invalidate this test.

b. **Urine electrolytes, osmolality**, and **urine creatinine** will help in determining volume status and concentrating ability and are used to help differentiate between prerenal and intrarenal disease (Table 4-1).

c. **Blood urea nitrogen** is an insensitive measure of GFR, because it is influenced by volume status, cardiac output, diet, and body habitus. The ratio of blood urea nitrogen to creatinine is normally 10 to 20 to 1; disproportionate elevation of the blood urea nitrogen may reflect hypovolemia, low cardiac output, or gastrointestinal bleeding.

d. **Serum creatinine** normally is 0.6 to 1.2 mg/dL but is affected by the patient's skeletal muscle mass and activity level. Creatinine concentration is inversely proportional to GFR such that a doubling of the creatinine generally corresponds to a 50% reduction in GFR.

e. **Creatinine clearance**, normally 80 to 120 mL/min, provides the best estimate of renal reserve. Creatinine clearance can be estimated as follows:

Creatinine clearance

$$= [(140 - \text{age}) \times \text{weight (kg)}]/72 \times \text{creatinine}$$

Multiply by 0.85 for women. This formula is invalid in the presence of gross renal insufficiency or changing renal function. Mild dysfunction occurs with values between 50 and 80 mL/min.

f. **Serum Na^+, K^+, Cl^-**, and **HCO_3^-** concentrations usually will be normal until renal failure is advanced. Careful consideration of the risk and benefit of proceeding with elective surgery should be made if $[Na^+]$ is less than 131 or greater than 150 mEq/L or $[K^+]$ is less than 2.5 or greater than 5.9 mEq/L, because these abnormalities may exacerbate arrhythmias and compromise cardiac function.

g. **Serum Ca^{2+}, PO_4^-**, and **Mg^{2+}** concentrations are altered as outlined in sections IV.B.2.d and e.

h. **Hematologic studies** should assess anemia and coagulation abnormalities.

i. **ECG** may reveal myocardial ischemia or infarction, pericarditis, and the effects of electrolyte abnormalities (see sections III.E.1.e and 2.b).

j. **Chest radiographs** may reveal evidence of fluid over-

load, pericardial effusion, infection, uremic pneumonitis, or
cardiomegaly.
**B. Identification of patients at high risk for perioperative
ARF**
   1. Elderly patients, because renal reserve and GFR decrease
   with advancing age.
   2. Coexisting renal disease.
   3. Congestive heart failure.
   4. High risk surgery such as renal artery surgery, thoracic
   or abdominal aortic surgery, and cardiopulmonary bypass.
   5. Major trauma and **extensive burns**. Intravenous hydration, mannitol, and HCO_3 may be helpful.
   6. Prolonged renal hypoperfusion resulting from shock,
   sepsis, nephrotic syndrome, and cirrhosis.
   7. Angiographic procedures. Aggressive saline hydration before and after procedures can help to preserve renal function.
C. Premedication should be administered carefully, because
renal failure patients have increased sensitivity to CNS depressants. Because of increased gastric volume and delayed emptying,
a combination of antacids, H_2 blockers, and antiemetics should
be considered.
D. Anesthetic technique. Either general or regional anesthesia
is acceptable. Before proceeding with regional anesthesia, the current coagulation status should be determined and the presence of
uremic neuropathy documented.
E. Intraoperative management
   1. Routine monitoring as described in Chapter 10 should be
   used. The need for invasive hemodynamic monitoring should
   be based on concomitant disease, clinical status, and anticipated
   volume shifts during surgery.
   2. Positioning should be done carefully, because these patients are prone to fractures secondary to renal osteodystrophy.
   3. Induction. The dose of induction agents may need to be
   reduced and their rate of administration slowed to avoid hypotension. Serum potassium should be checked before the administration of succinylcholine.
      a. The airway should be protected with a cuffed endotra-
      cheal tube because of the increased risk of aspiration in these
      patients (see section IV.B.2.i). The need for a rapid sequence
      induction must be evaluated on an individual basis.
   4. Anesthesia is typically maintained with nitrous oxide, oxygen, and isoflurane. **Opioids** should be administered carefully
   because of active metabolites and a prolonged duration of action. Cisatracurium is a useful muscle relaxant for patients with
   significant renal failure. The pharmacokinetics and pharmacodynamics of atracurium and cisatracurium are preserved in patients with renal failure. Rocuronium clearance is unchanged in
   renal failure. Mivacurium has an increased duration of action
   and repeated bolus doses of vecuronium may result in prolonged
   blockade.
   5. Fluid administration should proceed cautiously. Avoid
   K^+ containing fluids in anuric patients.
      a. For brief noninvasive procedures insensible losses
      should be replaced with D5W.
      b. For more extensive procedures, a central venous pres-

sure or pulmonary artery catheter may help guide fluid management.

6. Hypertension is a common postoperative problem aggravated by fluid overload. For those not on dialysis, diuretics and short-acting antihypertensives are effective. For those on dialysis, postoperative dialysis may be required.

SUGGESTED READING

Bellomo R, Chapman M, Finfer S, et al. Low-dose dopamine in patients with early renal dysfunction: a placebo-controlled randomised trial. Australian and New Zealand Intensive Care Society (ANZICS) Clinical Trials Group. *Lancet* 2000;356:2139–2143.

Byrick RJ. Anesthesia and end stage renal failure: is TIVA an advance? *Can J Anaesth* 1999;46:621–622.

Cronnelly R, Stanski DR, Miller RD, et al. Renal function and the pharmacokinetics of neostigmine in anesthetized man. *Anesthesiology* 1979; 51:222–226.

Galley HF. Renal-dose dopamine: will the message now get through? *Lancet* 2000;356:2112–2113.

Gilbert PL, Stein R. Preoperative evaluation of the patient with chronic renal disease. *Mt Sinai J Med* 1991;58:69–74.

Hoke JF, Shlugman D, Dershwitz M, et al. Pharmacokinetics and pharmacodynamics of remifentanil in persons with renal failure compared with healthy volunteers. *Anesthesiology* 1997;87:533–541.

Hunter JM. Muscle relaxants in renal disease. *Acta Anaesthesiol Scand Suppl* 1994;102:2–5.

Mazze RI, Jamison RL. Low-flow (1 L/min) sevoflurane: is it safe? *Anesthesiology* 1997;86:1225–1227.

Nancarrow C, Mather LE. Pharmacokinetics in renal failure. *Anaesth Intensive Care* 1983;11:350–360.

Rose BD, Post T, Narins R. *Clinical physiology of acid-base and electrolyte disorders.* New York: McGraw-Hill Professional Book Group, 2000.

Schrier RW. *Renal and electrolyte disorders*, 5th ed. Philadelphia: Lippincott Williams & Wilkins, 1997.

Sladen RN. Anesthetic considerations for the patient with renal failure. *Anesthesiol Clin North America* 2000;18:863–882.

Sladen RN. Will this magic bullet fly true? *Crit Care Med* 2001;29:911–913.

Thadhani R, Pascual M, Bonventre JV. Acute renal failure. *N Engl J Med* 1996;334:1448–1460.

Vitez TS, Soper LE, Wong KC, et al. Chronic hypokalemia and intraoperative dysrhythmias. *Anesthesiology* 1985;63:130–133.

Zaloga GP, Hughes SS. Oliguria in patients with normal renal function. *Anesthesiology* 1990;72:598–602.

5

Specific Considerations with Liver Disease

Robert Peloquin and Michael T. Bailin

I. Hepatic anatomy
A. **Hepatic blood supply**. The liver comprises only 2% of the total body mass yet receives 20% of the cardiac output.
  1. The **hepatic artery** supplies approximately 25% of the total liver blood flow and 50% of the liver's oxygen requirements.
  2. The **portal vein** provides 75% of the hepatic blood flow and 50% of its oxygen supply. The portal vein drains the stomach, spleen, pancreas, and intestine. Portal venous blood has a low oxygen content and contains nutrients (carbohydrates, lipids, amino acids), hormones (insulin, glucagon, gastrin, vasoactive intestinal peptide), drugs, and toxins absorbed from the intestine.
  3. Blood from the liver is drained by the **hepatic veins** into the inferior vena cava.
  4. Total hepatic blood flow depends on venous return from the preportal organs. Flow in the hepatic artery is regulated by sympathetic tone and local adenosine concentration. Hepatic arterial flow can increase in response to diminished portal venous flow. Total hepatic blood flow may be reduced in diseases causing increased hepatic vascular resistance (e.g., cirrhosis, infiltrative disease, Budd-Chiari syndrome).
  5. The liver functions as a reservoir for blood given its large vascular capacity. It normally contains approximately 15% of total blood volume, which may contribute to venous return in periods of hypovolemia or systemic hypotension.
B. **Liver structure** can be described in anatomic (lobule) or functional (acinus) terms.
  1. The **lobule** is best described as a hexagonal prism, with portal triads (terminal portal vein, hepatic artery, bile duct branches) located at the tips of the hexagonal angles and a central (hepatic) vein at the center of each lobule.
  2. The **acinus** is based on a functional concept wherein liver cells are classified depending on their distance from the portal triad. Zone 1 cells are located closest to the triad and receive most of the oxygen and nutrients, whereas zone 3 cells are the farthest away and are more prone to ischemic injury.
II. **Hepatic function**
A. **Synthesis and metabolism**
  1. **Proteins**. With the exception of gamma globulins and hemoglobin in the adult, nearly all plasma proteins are formed by hepatocytes. The liver contributes to protein metabolism through deamination of amino acids and subsequently generates urea to eliminate ammonia. Liver disease patients may lack the

ability to form urea and may rapidly develop increased plasma ammonia levels and hepatic encephalopathy.

a. **Albumin** is manufactured exclusively in the liver. It comprises 50% of all circulating plasma proteins and is the most important drug-binding protein (binding organic acids such as penicillins and barbiturates). Albumin contributes to oncotic pressure and also serves as a carrier for bilirubin and hormones.

b. **α_1-Acid glycoprotein** binds basic drugs, such as amide local anesthetics, propranolol, and opioids. As an "acute-phase reactant," its plasma concentration increases in many acute and chronic illnesses.

c. **Butyrylcholinesterase**, also known as nonspecific cholinesterase or **pseudocholinesterase**, is responsible for the degradation of succinylcholine, mivacurium, and ester type local anesthetics. In the presence of depressed hepatocellular function or a genetically mediated enzyme deficiency, low plasma levels of this enzyme may become clinically relevant.

d. All **clotting factors**, with the exception of factor VIII, are produced in the liver. Synthesis of factors II, VII, IX, X, protein C, and protein S depends on the presence of vitamin K, which is absorbed from the intestine. Intestinal absorption of vitamin K depends on appropriate bile production and release.

2. **Carbohydrates**. Homeostatic regulation of plasma glucose levels depends on normal hepatic function. The liver is responsible for glycogen synthesis and degradation, gluconeogenesis, and formation of many intermediate products of carbohydrate metabolism. The normal liver can store enough glycogen to provide glucose during a fast of approximately 12 hours. After this time glucose is derived by gluconeogenesis from amino acids, glycerol, and lactate. Perioperative release of stress hormones (e.g., epinephrine, norepinephrine, cortisol, and glucagon) promotes gluconeogenesis and hyperglycemia.

3. **Lipids**. Large quantities of carbohydrates and proteins are converted to fats by hepatocytes. Most **lipoproteins** are formed in the liver as well as **cholesterol** and **phospholipids**. Cholesterol is also degraded by the liver, serving as a substrate for production of bile salts, steroid hormones, and cell membranes. The liver participates in lipid metabolism through oxidation of fatty acids that serve as an energy source for other metabolic functions.

4. Because the liver is the major site of **steroid hormone degradation**, hepatic failure results in steroid excess. Elevations of serum aldosterone and cortisol result in enhanced reabsorption of sodium and water (contributing to edema and ascites) and loss of potassium in the urine. Decreased metabolism of estrogens and impaired conversion to androgens cause the clinical stigmata of liver disease, including spider angiomata, gynecomastia, palmar erythema, and testicular atrophy.

5. **Heme and bile**

a. The liver converts **heme** (from hemoglobin, myoglobin, and heme-containing cytochromes) to biliverdin and (free) **bilirubin** in the reticuloendothelial system. Albumin binds and delivers bilirubin to the hepatocytes. Bilirubin then undergoes conjugation with glucuronic acid to form water-soluble complexes. These are excreted with bile into the intestines and transformed into urobilinogen. Urobilinogen enters the enterohepatic cycle and is eliminated in the feces or excreted in the urine.

b. **Bile** contains primary bile salts (manufactured by the liver from cholesterol), secondary bile salts (synthesized from primary bile salts by normal colonic flora), and bilirubin. Bile carries metabolic waste products and drug metabolites released by the liver into the intestine. Bile also acts as a fat emulsifier, facilitating fat absorption by the small intestine. Failure to manufacture or release bile causes jaundice and an inability to absorb fat, resulting in steatorrhea and fat-soluble vitamin (vitamins A, D, E, and K) deficiencies.

6. **Drug metabolism**

   a. **Hepatic extraction ratio** (HER). Although the relationship between metabolism and clearance is complex, the concept of HER aids in the understanding of pharmacokinetics. The HER is defined as the fraction of the drug concentration flowing into the liver that is removed through hepatic elimination or metabolism.

   b. **Hepatic clearance** is the product of the hepatic blood flow rate and the HER. Some drugs, such as propofol, are extensively metabolized by the liver and have an HER close to 1.0. In such cases, hepatic metabolism is predominantly dependent on flow. Because the metabolic capacity is so extensive, moderate changes in hepatic metabolic function such as disease or enzyme induction have little effect on clearance. Other drugs, such as alfentanil, have a HER much less than 1, and clearance depends heavily on hepatic metabolic capacity. Here, changes in hepatic blood flow have little effect on hepatic clearance.

   c. **Protein binding**. Only the free (unbound) drug fraction is pharmacologically active and available for conversion by the hepatocyte to a less active form. The degree of protein binding is dependent on the drug's **protein binding affinity** and the **protein concentration**. Reduced concentrations of plasma proteins associated with hepatic disease will result in a greater proportion of unbound drug. This may result in a higher apparent potency, and the hemodynamic effects of bolus doses may be exaggerated. The larger the unbound fraction of a drug, the more rapid is its hepatic elimination.

   d. Two steps are involved in **drug elimination**.

   (1) **Phase I** reactions change the compound's structure, mainly via the action of the mixed function oxidases (**cytochrome P450**) family of enzymes. Oxidation, reduction, and hydrolysis can occur in this phase. The products of this phase may retain the activity of the parent drug. Some metabolites are more active (prednisolone > prednisone) or have longer half-lives (desmethyldiazepam > diazepam) than the original drug. If two substances are metabolized simultaneously, the speed of elimination depends on their relative affinity to P450 binding sites. Cimetidine has a strong affinity to the P450 complex and may decrease metabolism of concurrently administered drugs.

Table 5-1.   Minimum alveolar concentration (MAC) values and the extent of metabolism for various volatile anesthetics

	MAC with oxygen	% Metabolized
Halothane	0.74	20
Enflurane	1.68	2
Isoflurane	1.15	0.2
Desflurane	6.0	0.02–0.2
Sevoflurane	2.05	2–5

(2) **Phase II** reactions are enzymatically enhanced **conjugations**, increasing the water solubility of the metabolite. Conjugations with sulfate, glucuronic acid, acetate, and amino acids facilitate excretion into bile and urine.

c. **Enzyme induction.** Certain drugs (e.g., barbiturates, benzodiazepines, corticosteroids, antihistamines, ethanol, phenytoin, and chloral hydrate), when administered in increasing concentrations, can stimulate microsomal enzyme activity. Enzyme induction is nonspecific, and accelerated drug metabolism may affect any drug biotransformed by the mixed function oxidases.

III. **Metabolism of anesthetics**

A. **Volatile anesthetics** are metabolized in the liver by the cytochrome P450 system. **Cytochrome P450 2E1** metabolizes halothane, methoxyflurane, enflurane, isoflurane, sevoflurane, and probably desflurane.

1. Varying amounts of **inorganic fluoride** ions (F^-) with potential for nephrotoxicity are produced by metabolism of volatile anesthetics. Only 0.2% of absorbed isoflurane undergoes hepatic metabolism, generating insufficient amounts of F^- to cause nephrotoxicity. Metabolism of sevoflurane may yield a high serum F^- concentration, but clinical nephrotoxicity has not been reported.

2. Metabolism of both halothane and desflurane may lead to formation of **neoantigens** with rare development of immune hepatitis (see section VII.C.3.b). Neoantigens produced in the metabolism of enflurane and isoflurane may cross-react with anti-halothane antibodies, leading to cross-sensitization between these anesthetics. Because the extent of metabolism of enflurane, isoflurane, and desflurane is much lower than that of halothane (Table 5-1), the risk of developing hepatitis is extremely remote with these three agents. Metabolites of sevoflurane do not form antigens.

B. **Intravenous induction agents**

1. **Propofol** is metabolized by the liver to water-soluble compounds through conjugation to glucuronide and sulfate. These metabolites are excreted by the kidneys and appear to have no hypnotic activity. Because the clearance of propofol exceeds total hepatic blood flow, extrahepatic metabolism must contribute to total propofol clearance. Propofol results in a concentra-

tion-dependent inhibition of the cytochrome P450 system. Liver disease results in a prolonged propofol elimination half-life, but clearance appears to be unaffected.

2.   Barbiturates. Long- and intermediate-acting barbiturates (e.g., phenobarbital, pentobarbital, secobarbital), whose durations of action are determined by metabolism, have prolonged effects in liver failure. Short-acting barbiturates (e.g., thiopental, thiamylal, and methohexital) have a duration of action determined by redistribution. All barbiturates should be cautiously titrated in liver disease, because preexisting hypoalbuminemia will reduce the degree of protein binding and increase the active free fraction. Generally, bolus doses should be reduced.

3.   Etomidate is metabolized by the liver through ester hydrolysis and *N*-dealkylation to inactive metabolites. With a high HER, its terminal half-life should be decreased by drugs or conditions that reduce hepatic blood flow. Recovery from an initial induction dose results from a rapid redistribution phase. Cirrhotic patients have an increased volume of distribution with a relatively normal hepatic clearance for etomidate. Etomidate is 75% protein bound, however, and may exhibit an exaggerated pharmacologic response with hypoalbuminemia. It should be carefully titrated with reduced bolus doses.

4.   Ketamine is metabolized by the hepatic microsomal enzyme system primarily through demethylation to norketamine. Norketamine has approximately 30% of the pharmacologic activity of ketamine. Ketamine has an HER near 1.0, and clearance approximates hepatic blood flow. Few data exist concerning the use of ketamine in liver disease.

C.   Benzodiazepines metabolized primarily by oxidative mechanisms (e.g., diazepam, midazolam) have significantly increased half-lives in patients with hepatic insufficiency. Benzodiazepines cleared predominantly by glucuronidation (e.g., lorazepam), have normal half-lives.

D.   Opioids may worsen hepatic encephalopathy and should be titrated carefully. Narcotic-induced respiratory depression may be more pronounced in liver failure. Elimination may be prolonged. Meperidine clearance is significantly reduced in liver disease, whereas clearance of morphine and fentanyl is less impaired. The elimination half-life of remifentanil is totally independent of liver function.

E.   Nondepolarizing neuromuscular blocking drugs. Patients with liver disease often demonstrate resistance to these drugs and require higher doses to achieve adequate neuromuscular blockade. This is probably caused by an increase in the volume of distribution, inhibitors, or increases in neuromuscular receptors. In turn, slower elimination may lead to a lower requirement for maintenance doses.

1.   Long-acting neuromuscular blocking drugs (e.g., doxacurium, d-tubocurarine, pancuronium) are predominantly excreted in the urine. **Doxacurium** undergoes no hepatobiliary uptake, and its metabolism should be unaffected by liver disease. Only 10% to 20% of **d-tubocurarine** is eliminated through hepatic uptake. Approximately 30% of **pancuronium** is eliminated through hepatobiliary mechanisms, and its effect may be prolonged in patients with biliary obstruction or cirrhosis.

2. Intermediate-acting neuromuscular blocking drugs. **Vecuronium** and **rocuronium** are highly dependent on hepatobiliary excretion and metabolism. These drugs demonstrate a decreased clearance and prolonged effect in patients with liver disease. **Atracurium** and **cisatracurium** are degraded via Hofmann elimination and by plasma esterases. Their metabolism is practically independent of hepatic functional status.

3. Short-acting neuromuscular blocking drugs. Mivacurium, like succinylcholine, is completely metabolized in the plasma by butyrylcholinesterase. Cholinesterase production may be depressed in severe liver disease, and mivacurium may act more potently and with a prolonged effect in patients with liver disease.

IV. **Liver disease**

   A. Liver diseases can be classified according to **etiology**, **time course** (acute versus chronic), and **severity** (as measured by liver function tests).

      1. **Parenchymal liver disease**

         a. **Acute hepatocellular injury** may be caused by viral infection (hepatitis A, B, C, D, E, Epstein-Barr virus, cytomegalovirus, herpes simplex, Echo virus, and Coxsackie virus), various drugs, chemicals and poisons (including alcohol, halothane, phenytoin, propylthiouracil, isoniazid, tetracycline and acetaminophen), and inborn metabolic defects (e.g., Wilson disease and α_1-antitrypsin deficiency). Some patients progress to fulminant hepatic failure and rapid development of encephalopathy.

         b. **Chronic parenchymal disease** may be associated with varying degrees of functional impairment. **Cirrhosis** may result from chronic active hepatitis, alcoholism, hemochromatosis, primary biliary cirrhosis, or congenital disorders. End-stage hepatic fibrosis causes significant resistance to portal blood flow. This in turn increases portal venous pressure, resulting in portal hypertension and esophageal varices. Complication resulting from the combination of portal hypertension and decreased hepatic synthetic and metabolic function include ascites, coagulopathy, gastrointestinal bleeding, and encephalopathy. Such patients will present for procedures aimed at reducing the manifestations of portal hypertension, including splenorenal shunt, transjugular intrahepatic portasystemic shunt, LeVeen shunt, and orthotopic liver transplantation.

      2. **Cholestasis** occurs most frequently in cholelithiasis and acute or chronic cholecystitis. Primary biliary cirrhosis and primary sclerosing cholangitis also begin as cholestatic diseases, ultimately leading to parenchymal damage and liver failure. **Hyperbilirubinemia** is an important marker for hepatobiliary disease. **Unconjugated hyperbilirubinemia** is due to excess bilirubin production (e.g., massive transfusion, absorption of large hematomas, or hemolysis) or impaired uptake of unconjugated bilirubin by the hepatocyte (e.g., Gilbert syndrome). **Conjugated hyperbilirubinemia** generally occurs with hepatocellular disease (e.g., alcoholic or viral hepatitis, cirrhosis), disease of the small bile ducts (e.g., primary biliary cirrhosis, Dubin-Johnson syndrome), or obstruction of the extrahepatic bile

Table 5-2. Modified Child-Pugh Score

Parameter	Points		
	1	2	3
Albumin (g/dL)	>3.5	2.8–3.5	<2.8
Bilirubin (mg/dl)[a]	<2.0	2.0–3.0	>3.0
Ascites	Absent	Slight	Moderate
Encephalopathy	Absent	Grades I and II	Grades III and IV
PT prolongation (s)	<4.0	4.0–6.0	>6.0

Class A, 5 to 6 points; class B, 7 to 9 points; class C; 10 to 15 points; PT, prothrombin time.
[a] For primary biliary cirrhosis: one point for bilirubin < 4.0 mg/dl, two points for bilirubin 4–10 mg/dL, and three points for bilirubin > 10 mg/dL.

ducts (e.g., pancreatic carcinoma, cholangiocarcinoma, gallstones).

3. **Severity** of liver disease can be estimated by laboratory analysis of synthetic function (e.g., albumin concentration and prothrombin time prolongation). The **modified Child-Pugh score** (Table 5-2) incorporates these indices and frequently is used to stratify perioperative risk. The composite score ranges from 5 to 15 and is used to assign the patient to class A (scores of 5 to 6; low risk), class B (scores of 7 to 9; moderate risk), or class C (scores > 9; high risk).

B. **Manifestations of liver disease**

1. **Central nervous system**. Hepatic dysfunction leads to **encephalopathy**. Signs may vary from sleep disturbances and the presence of asterixis to coma. Impaired neurotransmission, presence of intrinsic γ-aminobutyric acid-ergic substances, and altered cerebral metabolism may be involved in its pathogenesis. **Ammonia levels** often are elevated in encephalopathic patients but do not correlate with outcome or the severity of encephalopathy. Patients with severe acute liver failure often present with a rapidly progressive encephalopathy complicated by **cerebral edema**. Elevated intracranial pressure must be aggressively managed to prevent cerebral ischemia. Extreme hyponatremia or its overly aggressive treatment may lead to fatal **central pontine myelinolysis** (see Chapter 6). Changes in mental status and increased sensitivity to sedatives mandates caution with premedication.

2. **Cardiovascular system**

a. Patients with advanced liver disease exhibit a **hyperdynamic circulatory state** with an elevated **cardiac output**, resting tachycardia, and **decreased systemic vascular resistance**. Elevated levels of nitric oxide, glucagon, and prostaglandins are thought to be responsible for arteriolar vasodilation. Multiple **arteriovenous shunts**, such as spider angiomata in the skin, may be present in almost all vascular beds.

b. Shunting and arterial vasodilation result in a decreased **effective intravascular volume**. Hypoalbuminemia, increased levels of aldosterone, and inappropriate secretion of antidiuretic hormone all lead to increased **total body fluid volume** (e.g., ascites, edema).

c. **Alcoholic cardiomyopathy** should always be considered in patients with a history of alcohol abuse.

3. Respiratory system

a. **Airway protection** is of primary in concern in patients with altered mental status or a "full stomach." Presence of ascites may increase intraabdominal pressure and the risk of aspiration. Definitive airway protection with rapid sequence induction and intubation is frequently advisable when general anesthesia is required.

b. Gas exchange may be impaired in the presence of **hepatopulmonary syndrome**. Massive ascites (decreased diaphragmatic excursions), pleural effusions, diminished hypoxic pulmonary vasoconstriction producing mismatch of ventilation to perfusion, and development of pleural arteriovenous fistulas can produce severe hypoxemia. Pulmonary hypertension can coexist with portal hypertension, and can produce right heart failure.

4. Gastrointestinal system

a. The increased resistance to portal blood flow results in **portal hypertension**, splenomegaly, and splanchnic venous congestion. Portosystemic collateral channels are manifested as hemorrhoids, esophageal varices, and dilated abdominal wall veins (caput medusae).

b. **Variceal bleeding** can progress rapidly to hemorrhagic shock. After volume resuscitation, treatment consists of vasopressin, somatostatin, β-adrenergic blockade, sclerotherapy, or endoscopic ligation. Balloon tamponade with a **Blakemore tube** may achieve temporary hemostasis.

5. Renal system

a. Intravascular volume depletion may produce **prerenal azotemia**. The blood urea nitrogen level may be deceptively low because of the liver's inability to synthesize urea from ammonia.

b. **Water and electrolyte balance** is complicated by frequent use of diuretics. In general, patients with hepatic insufficiency are hyponatremic (despite total body sodium overload), hypokalemic, and have a metabolic alkalosis.

c. **Hepatorenal syndrome** is characterized by increased renal vascular resistance, oliguria, and renal failure in the presence of hepatic failure. Intrarenal blood flow diminishes, especially to the renal cortex, producing sodium retention. Abnormal prostaglandin metabolism may contribute to this syndrome and may explain the increased sensitivity of these patients to renal insufficiency induced by nonsteroidal antiinflammatory drugs. Normal renal function may return if liver failure resolves.

6. Coagulopathy is caused by several factors.

a. **Synthesis of clotting factors** is impaired in liver failure.

b.   Cholestasis leads to impaired absorption of fat and fat-soluble vitamins (A, D, E, K). **Vitamin K** is an important cofactor in the synthesis of factors II, VII, IX, and X.

c.   Thrombocytopenia, secondary to hypersplenism, alcohol-induced bone marrow failure, and consumption, impairs clot formation.

d.   Preoperative correction of clotting abnormalities with fresh frozen plasma or vitamin K should be performed as necessary. Regional anesthesia may not be appropriate. Invasive monitoring may help guide volume replacement, and blood bank support is necessary. The importance of adequate venous access for intraoperative transfusion cannot be underestimated.

7.   Hypoglycemia may occur in end-stage hepatic insufficiency; blood glucose determinations should be performed and glucose-containing solutions administered as necessary.

a.   Glycogen stores are diminished, requiring gluconeogenesis to maintain normoglycemia.

b.   Gluconeogenesis is impaired in severe liver disease and alcoholism.

V.   Surgical risk in patients with liver disease

A.   The presence of hepatic disease carries a significant **risk of perioperative morbidity and mortality** that depends on the severity and type of liver disease and the type of proposed surgery. Patients with liver disease undergoing cholecystectomy demonstrate an odds ratio of 8.47 for perioperative mortality compared with patients without liver disease. The most common causes of perioperative mortality include hemorrhage, sepsis, liver failure, and hepatorenal syndrome.

1.   Acute symptomatic hepatitis carries the worst prognosis; surgery should be delayed until after recovery, if possible, in these patients. In patients with acute viral hepatitis undergoing laparotomy, a 10% mortality rate has been reported; in patients with acute alcoholic hepatitis, mortality was 60%. Some series have reported an operative mortality of 100% in patients with acute alcoholic hepatitis.

2.   Mortality in patients with **cirrhosis** has been correlated with the Child classification. Studies of cirrhotics undergoing portacaval shunt surgery have reported mortality rates of 0 to 10% for Child class A, 4% to 31% for class B, and 19% to 76% for Child class C. Cholecystectomy in patients with cirrhosis and coagulopathy has an extremely high mortality rate.

3.   Patients with cirrhosis undergoing emergency surgery have a greater risk of morbidity and mortality than similar patients undergoing elective surgery.

B.   Careful **preoperative assessment** of liver function and assessment of risk should be performed.

1.   Screening liver function tests in general surgical populations are not useful.

2.   History of jaundice, pruritus, malaise, anorexia, and exposure to halothane, drugs, alcohol, and other toxins should be sought. On **physical examination**, stigmata of liver disease should be sought: hepatosplenomegaly, ascites, peripheral edema, spider angiomata, testicular atrophy, caput medusae, hemorrhoids, asterixis, gynecomastia, and temporal wasting.

3. If liver disease is suspected, **laboratory tests**, including bilirubin, transaminases, alkaline phosphatase, albumin, total protein, prothrombin time, and hepatitis serologies, should be considered.

4. Duration and severity of liver disease have prognostic implications and **percutaneous liver biopsy** may be indicated to establish a diagnosis before elective surgery. For example, there is no evidence that a patient with liver function test abnormalities because of fatty infiltration of the liver has an increased perioperative risk.

5. Every effort should be taken to **correct abnormalities before surgery**, including coagulopathy, poorly controlled ascites, volume and electrolyte imbalances, renal function, encephalopathy, and nutritional status.

VI. Anesthesia in patients with liver disease

A. Anesthetic agents generally reduce hepatic blood flow, and meticulous attention must be paid to **maintain adequate hepatic perfusion** and oxygen delivery. Episodes of perioperative ischemia can exacerbate preexisting liver disease when hypoxemia, hypotension, hemorrhage, and vasopressors have compromised hepatic oxygenation. Planning the anesthetic must take into account the type and severity of liver disease (see section IV.B).

1. Regional anesthesia may be contraindicated because of an increased risk of bleeding and hematoma formation. In a patient with well-compensated liver disease and a reasonably normal coagulation profile and platelet count, regional anesthesia may be appropriate.

2. Sufficient **venous access** is of paramount importance, especially in surgery involving the liver parenchyma.

    a. Large-bore peripheral intravenous cannulas are inserted before or after induction of anesthesia for major surgery. Often, 12-gauge or larger infusion catheters are required.

    b. In patients with insufficient peripheral access, **large-bore central venous catheters** (8.5 to 9.5 French single-lumen or 12 French double-lumen catheters) can be inserted.

    c. Placement of central venous catheters is indicated for pressure monitoring and rapid drug administration into the central circulation. Pulmonary artery catheters may help guide therapy in some patients. Skillful line placement is important in coagulopathic patients, and ultrasonic visualization of the vein before cannulation may be helpful.

3. An **arterial catheter** facilitates blood sampling and arterial blood pressure measurement and is routine in major surgery for patients with end-stage liver disease.

B. A low threshold for performing a **rapid sequence induction** should exist.

C. Consideration should be given to choice of maintenance agent and timing of postoperative extubation.

1. Anesthetic agents with appropriate pharmacokinetic and pharmacodynamic profiles should be selected (see section III.B).

2. Hepatic dysfunction causes inconsistent changes in drug disposition and "titration to effect" is recommended for induction and maintenance.

3. **The cirrhotic liver is vulnerable to hypoxic damage.**
   a. General or regional anesthesia can decrease total hepatic blood flow. Additional factors reducing blood flow include hypovolemia, hypocapnia, positive pressure ventilation, surgical traction, β-adrenergic agonists, and patient position.
   b. **Isoflurane** and **sevoflurane** in concentrations up to 2 times the minimum alveolar concentration have minimal effects on hepatic blood flow in experimental animals.
   c. **Hyperventilation** should be avoided because hypocarbia and positive pressure ventilation can independently reduce hepatic blood flow.
D. Physiologic variables, including urine output, body temperature, blood sugar levels, and coagulation status, should be carefully monitored.

VII. **Postoperative liver dysfunction.** Liver dysfunction after surgery and anesthesia is not rare and can range from mild enzyme elevations to fulminant hepatic failure. Etiologies for postoperative hepatic dysfunction include the following:

A. **Surgical interventions** that impair hepatic blood flow or obstruct the biliary system (clamped vessels, retraction, or direct injury). Postoperative elevations of hepatocellular enzymes or bilirubin also can be caused by increased bilirubin loads after massive transfusion, resorption of hematoma, or hemolysis. A picture of "benign postoperative intrahepatic cholestasis" may be a marker of a systemic process (e.g., sepsis) rather than intrinsic hepatic dysfunction. Overt hepatic failure can occur during or after shock of any etiology.

B. **Nonsurgical causes.** Hepatic dysfunction from common entities such as viral hepatitis, alcoholism, and cholelithiasis can exist preoperatively (and can be undetected) or can occur postoperatively as mere coincidence. The stress of surgery can convert nonicteric illness into frank jaundice. Drug therapy in the perioperative period must also be evaluated as a cause of jaundice.

C. **Halothane-associated hepatitis** is clinically indistinguishable from viral hepatitis. The diagnosis is one of exclusion. The availability of enflurane, isoflurane, and sevoflurane generally eliminates the need for halothane administration to adults.
   1. The **presentation** is variable and may include an asymptomatic elevation in serum transaminases, fever of unknown origin, clinical jaundice, or, very rarely, massive hepatic necrosis and death. Predisposing factors include previous halothane exposure, obesity, advanced age, and female gender. The problem is rare in pediatric patients.
   2. **The United States National Halothane Study** found that otherwise unexplained massive hepatic necrosis after halothane exposure was an exceedingly rare complication and occurred in only 1 in 35,000 exposures. Risks were highest in adults who received multiple halothane exposures and in those who underwent procedures that carried an intrinsically higher mortality rate.
   3. **Possible mechanisms.** It is now recognized that two types of halothane-induced hepatic dysfunction exist.
      a. One is caused by **hepatotoxic lipoperoxidases** generated during reductive metabolism of halothane in a hypoxic environment.

b. The more fulminant form is due to an **immunologic phenomenon** whereby an oxidative metabolite of halothane, **trifluoroacetyl chloride**, binds to hepatocytes, creating a neoantigenic structure to which antibodies may be generated. Hepatocellular damage occurs on subsequent exposure to halothane.

4. The Massachusetts General Hospital has established restrictive guidelines for the use of halothane in adults. There are no restrictions on the use of halothane in pediatric patients. Halothane use in adults may be considered in patients with severe airway compromise or bronchospasm, but sevoflurane appears to be an acceptable alternative. If halothane use is anticipated, the informed consent should specifically include the indications for its use and the possible risks.

SUGGESTED READING

Badalamenti S, Graziani G, Salerno F, et al. Hepatorenal syndrome. New perspectives in pathogenesis and treatment. *Arch Intern Med* 1993; 153:1957–1967.

Carton EG, Plevak DJ, Kranner PW, et al. Perioperative care of the liver transplant patient. Part 2. *Anesth Analg* 1994;78:382–399.

Carton EG, Rettke SR, Plevak DJ, et al. Perioperative care of the liver transplant patient. Part 1. *Anesth Analg* 1994;78:120–133.

Child CG, Turcotte JG. Surgery and portal hypertension. *Major Probl Clin Surg* 1964;1:1–85.

Cook RC. Pharmacokinetics and pharmacodynamics of nondepolarizing muscle relaxants. In: Park GR, Kang Y, eds. *Anesthesia and intensive care for patients with liver disease.* New York: Butterworth-Heinemann, 1995:79–88.

Dershwitz M, Hoke JF, Rosow CE, et al. Pharmacokinetics and pharmacodynamics of remifentanil in volunteer subjects with severe liver disease. *Anesthesiology* 1996;84:812–820.

Kamath PS. Clinical approach to the patient with abnormal liver test results. *Mayo Clin Proc* 1996;71:1089–1095.

Parks DA, et al. Hepatic physiology. In: Miller RD, ed. *Anesthesia*, 5th ed. New York: Churchhill Livingstone, 2000:647–662.

Patel T. Surgery in the patient with liver disease. *Mayo Clin Proc* 1999; 74:593–599.

Scott VL, Dodson SF, Kang Y. The hepatopulmonary syndrome. *Surg Clin North Am* 1999;79:23–41.

Specific Considerations with Endocrine Disease

Robert A. Peterfreund and Stephanie L. Lee

I. Diabetes mellitus

A. Diabetes mellitus (DM) is a chronic systemic disease characterized by an absolute or relative lack of insulin. Abnormal blood sugar regulation and end-organ damage resulting from DM contribute to perioperative morbidity and mortality.

B. Physiology of DM. Insulin is synthesized in pancreatic beta cells and stored in granules. Glucose, β-adrenergic agonists, arginine, and acetylcholine stimulate, and α-adrenergic agonists and somatostatin inhibit, insulin secretion. Insulin facilitates glucose and potassium transport across cell membranes, increases glycogen synthesis, and inhibits lipolysis. Low level insulin production continues during fasting periods, which prevents catabolism and ketoacidosis. Peripheral tissues resist the effects of insulin during times of stress (e.g., surgery, infection, and cardiopulmonary bypass). The liver and kidney metabolize insulin. Prolongation of insulin action may be clinically significant in renal insufficiency.

C. DM type 1 (formerly known as juvenile or insulin-dependent diabetes). Patients have autoimmune destruction of beta cells and an absolute insulin deficiency. They generally present at a younger age, are sensitive to small amounts of insulin, and are prone to ketosis but not obesity. Management is with human insulin.

D. DM type 2 (formerly known as non–insulin-dependent or adult-onset diabetes). Patients have peripheral resistance to insulin effects and require high insulin levels to maintain euglycemia. They represent 90% of all diabetics and generally are older, obese, and ketosis resistant, but prone to hyperosmolar complications. They are initially managed with diet and exercise alone. Oral hypoglycemic agents and/or insulin are added as needed.

E. Other causes of absolute or relative insulin insufficiency. Pancreatic insulin hyposecretion is seen with cystic fibrosis, chronic pancreatitis, hemochromatosis, and after pancreatic surgery. Glucose intolerance may result from glucagonoma, pheochromocytoma, thyrotoxicosis, acromegaly, or glucocorticoid excess.

F. Therapy for DM

1. Oral hypoglycemic agents (Table 6-1). A number of new medications have been released for treating DM type 2. The drugs have different mechanisms, durations of action, and side effects. Oral agents have no role in the treatment of DM type 1. **Sulfonylureas** act by increasing pancreatic insulin release. The longest acting forms, such as **glyburide**, can induce hypoglycemia up to 50 hours after administration in the fasting patient. These medications increase the effectiveness of thiazide diuretics, barbiturates, and anticoagulants. A nonsulfonylurea,

Table 6-1. Oral agents used to treat diabetes mellitus

Agent	Onset (h)	Duration (h)
Sulfonylurea[a]		
Tolbutamide (Orinase, Oramide)	1	6–12
Glipizide (Glucotrol)	1	6–12
Glipizide XL	1–4	10–24
Acetoheximide (Dymelor)	1	8–12
Tolazamide (Tolinase)	4–6	10–15
Glyburide (Micronase, Diabeta)	1–4	10–24
Glimepiride (Amaryl)	1	18–24
Chlorpropramide (Diabinase)	1	24–72
α-Glucosidase inhibitor[b,c]		
Acarbose (Precose)	Immediate	<0.3
Miglitol (Glyset)	Immediate	<0.3
Biguanide[c,d]		
Metformin (Glucophage)	1	8–12
Thiazolidinedione[c,d]		
Pioglitazone (Actos)	1	24
Rosiglitazone (Avandia)	1	24
Meglitinide[a,e]		
Repaglinide (Prandin)	≤0.25	6–7
D-Phenylalanine derivative[a,e]		
Netaglinide (Starlix)	<0.25	3–4

[a] Increases insulin secretion.
[b] Nonsystemic. Delays digestion and absorption of complex carbohydrates from the intestine.
[c] When used as the *sole agent* for treatment, hypoglycemia (insulin reaction) is unlikely; may be taken on the morning of surgery.
[d] Increases sensitivity to insulin. No increase in insulin secretion.
[e] Closes ATP-dependent potassium channels, depolarizing pancreatic beta cells leading to calcium channel opening and enhanced insulin release. Nonsulfonylurea. Peak effect at 1 h. Little insulin releases in the absence of food.

repaglinide, acts rapidly to increase insulin release from the pancreas and is given before each meal. The biguanide **metformin** and **thiazolidinedione drugs** such as **pioglitazone** and **rosiglitazone** increase sensitivity to insulin. These do not increase insulin secretion. **Acarbose and miglitol**, α-glucosidase inhibitors, delay digestion and absorption of complex carbohydrates from the intestine. They also prevent postprandial hyperglycemia. Single agent therapy with metformin, pioglitazone, rosiglitazone, miglitol, or acarbose is not associated with hypoglycemia.

 2. **Insulin (Table 6-2)** is available in animal and human preparations. At the present time, most insulin-treated patients take human insulin. It is associated with decreased antigenicity compared with animal insulins. Analogues of insulin that have been synthesized to modify the duration of action are being introduced. **Lispro** and **Insu-**

Table 6-2.   **Insulin preparations for diabetes mellitus therapy**

Agent (SC administration)	Onset (h)	Peak effect (h)	Duration (h)
Lispro (Humalog)	≤0.25	1	3.5–4.5
Insulin Aspart (Novorapid/Novolog)	≤0.25	1–2	3–4
Regular	0.5–1	1–5	5–8
NPH	1–4	4–12	24–28
Lente	1–3	6–15	22–28
Ultralente	2–8	10–30	24–36
Glargine (Lantus)	2–4	No peak	24

SC, subcutaneous.
Note: When regular insulin is administered IV, the onset of action is immediate. The duration is ~1 h. The preparations semilente insulin and protamine zinc insulin are no longer available.

lin Aspart, both fast onset insulins, have short durations of action. They are given with meals to treat postprandial glucose elevations. **Glargine**, a long-acting virtually peakless form of insulin, is given every 24 hours to mimic basal insulin secretion. Infusions of regular insulin, the only insulin preparation for intravenous (IV) administration, are recommended for the intraoperative management of type 1 patients or type 2 patients with difficult to control glucose levels (Table 6-3).

   G.   **Acute complications of diabetes**
      1.   **Diabetic ketoacidosis (DKA)**. Ketoacidosis results from insulin deficiency or resistance to insulin seen during stress (e.g., infection, surgery, and trauma). This occurs almost exclusively in DM type 1.
         a.   **DKA** is associated with depressed myocardial contractility and peripheral tone, hyperglycemia (and concurrent hyperosmolarity), high anion gap acidosis, intracellular dehydration, and an osmotic diuresis that can produce profound hypovolemia.
         b.   **Electrolyte abnormalities** include hyperglycemia (although glucose is usually less than 500 mg/dL), hyperkalemia, and hyponatremia. The total body K^+ is depressed (3 to 10 mEq/kg body weight), but serum levels are elevated because acidosis shifts K^+ out of cells that have insufficient insulin to maintain intracellular K^+ levels. Measured Na^+ concentrations are artifactually lowered 1.6 mEq/L for every 100 mg/dL that the glucose is elevated. Hypophosphatemia and hypomagnesemia may occur.
         c.   **Treatment of DKA**:
            (1)   Regular insulin, bolus (0.1 U/kg IV or 10 U IV push) and then continuous insulin infusion (starting at ~0.1 U/kg/h).
            (2)   Hourly glucose and electrolyte determinations to guide adjustment of insulin dose.

Table 6-3. Guidelines for routine regular insulin infusions

Starting infusion rate (regular insulin, 25 Units/250 mL saline)

Type I DM (female); 0.5 U/h
Type I DM (male); 1.0 U/h
Type II DM (male or female); 1.0 U/h

Adjustment of Regular Insulin Infusion Rate, Units/h

Blood Glucose (mg/dL)	Infusion Change	Other Treatment
<70	Hold 30 min	Administer D50, 15–20 mL. Recheck glucose after 30 min. Repeat glucose administration until serum glucose >70 mg/dL.
70–120	−0.3 U/h	
121–180	No change	
181–240	+0.3 U/h	
241–300	+0.6 U/h	
>300	+1.0 U/h	

DM, diabetes mellitus.
Note: Guidelines assume the patient is fasting and not in diabetic ketoacidosis. Patients should have a source of exogenous carbohydrate available or infusing, such as glucose at 5 g/h. Dosing must be individually titrated based on frequent blood glucose monitoring.

(3) Adjustments to insulin infusion:

(a) If serum glucose, measured hourly, falls less than 10% or if the anion gap and pH are unchanged, double the insulin infusion rate.

(b) Maintain the insulin infusion rate until the glucose is less than 250 mg/dL or serum bicarbonate corrects to greater than 18 mEq/L.

(c) Reduce insulin infusion rate to 2 to 3 U/h and add 5% dextrose when the serum glucose falls below 250 mg/dL. Continue the insulin infusion until the anion gap and serum bicarbonate are normal. Premature cessation of the insulin infusion may result in recrudescence of DKA.

(4) Volume replacement, initially with normal saline and then one-half normal saline.

(5) Electrolyte replacement (K^+, Mg^{2+}, PO_4^{2-}). Potassium and phosphate are essential for insulin action and should be replaced carefully. Verify normal renal function first.

(6) Consider bicarbonate therapy only for severe acidosis (pH < 7), hemodynamic instability, or cardiac rhythm disturbances.

2. Hyperglycemic, hyperosmolar, nonketotic state (HONK) is often triggered by infection, dehydration, an acute cardiovascular event (including silent myocardial infarction), trauma, or surgery in elderly patients with known DM type 2. It may be the initial presentation of DM type 2 in previously undiagnosed patients.

a.   Characteristics of HONK include glucose levels that can exceed 500 mg/dL, hypovolemia from an osmotic diuresis, electrolyte abnormalities, hemoconcentration, and central nervous system (CNS) dysfunction (depressed sensorium, seizure or coma). Insulin levels are sufficient to block lipolysis and ketogenesis, preventing ketoacidosis.

b.   Treatment of HONK

(1)   Vigorous volume replacement with normal saline can reduce plasma glucose load up to 50% over several hours. Typical adult replacement is with one-half normal saline: first hour, 1.5 L; second and third hours, 1 L/h; after 3 hours, 0.5 to 1 L/h.

(2)   Careful monitoring of volume status, especially in elderly patients with cardiovascular or renal disease, is necessary. Consider invasive monitoring.

(3)   Glucose and electrolyte levels should be determined hourly.

(4)   Regular insulin (10 U IV bolus, followed by a continuous insulin infusion starting at ~0.1 U/kg/h IV) should be administered. Double the insulin infusion rate if the glucose concentration is unchanged after 1 to 4 hours. Titrate insulin infusion rates to maintain glucose less than 250 mg/dL until cardiovascular, electrolyte, and metabolic parameters are normal.

(5)   Electrolyte replacement. The absence of acidosis in type 2 DM decreases the likelihood of severe potassium depletion.

H.   Chronic complications of DM

1.   Atherosclerosis. Diabetics have a strong predisposition to all types of vascular disease. Macrovascular disease (coronary artery, cerebrovascular, and peripheral vascular) and microvascular disease (retinopathy and nephropathy) occur more frequently, more extensively, and at an earlier age than in the general population.

2.   Neuropathy. Autonomic neuropathy may result in symptomatically silent cardiac ischemia, postural hypotension, gastroparesis, and bladder atony. There is an increased risk of sudden cardiac death because of autonomic cardiac dysfunction and a diminished central ventilatory response to hypoxia. Peripheral neuropathies may cause pain and/or numbness.

3.   Other manifestations. Infection and poor wound healing are major postoperative complications.

I.   Anesthetic considerations with DM

1.   Ketoacidosis or hyperosmolar coma must be corrected before elective surgery.

2.   Surgical procedures should be planned as the first case in the morning.

3.   Glucose and insulin management ideally should maintain serum glucose levels between 120 and 200 mg/dL.

a.   Ketoacidosis or hyperosmolar coma must be prevented without inducing hypoglycemia.

b.   Sulfonylurea agents should be withheld within 24

hours of surgery. If they have been taken, IV glucose supplementation is necessary during the fasting period.

c. **Metformin (Glucophage), thiazolidinediones (troglitazone, rosiglitazone), and miglitol (Glyset) or acarbose (Precose)** can be administered until the patient is no longer allowed anything by mouth because there is no risk of hypoglycemia with single-agent therapy.

d. **Insulin-treated type 2 diabetics**. For patients having minor procedures of short duration (e.g., in the ambulatory care setting), the morning insulin can be held until the patient is alert postoperatively and able to eat. Glucose may be checked by fingerstick immediately before and after the procedure. For more substantial procedures, patients should receive one-half of their total normal morning dose of intermediate- or long-acting insulin in a subcutaneous dose. Regular or rapid-onset insulins (Lispro insulin, Insulin Aspart) should be held. For hospitalized patients, a glucose-containing infusion should be started simultaneously. Patients admitted to the hospital from home on the day of surgery should also hold the morning dose of regular or fast-onset insulins, but they should take half of the morning dose of intermediate- or long-acting insulin. The blood glucose should be checked promptly upon arrival to the hospital and at frequent intervals thereafter, especially if surgery or placement of an IV with dextrose is delayed. Patients on split-dose insulin regimens preoperatively should receive the usual doses of any long- or intermediate-acting insulin the night before surgery. Frequent (every 2 to 4 hours intraoperatively) monitoring of blood sugar is recommended. **Because of unreliable subcutaneous absorption, IV insulin dosing is preferable during surgery, especially in the presence of hypothermia, hemodynamic instability, or if the patient requires vasopressors.** A guideline for managing intraoperative infusions of regular insulin is presented in Table 6-3.

e. **Type 1 diabetics**. **These patients must always receive some insulin to prevent ketoacidosis**. Simultaneous infusion of a glucose-containing solution may also be necessary to prevent hypoglycemia. Perioperative insulin management for the type 1 diabetic on an insulin pump or patients receiving the newer intensive regimens of three or more daily insulin injections should be discussed with the physician responsible for managing the patient's diabetes. See Table 6-3 for guidelines on managing insulin infusions.

f. **Fixed ratio insulin combinations** (e.g., 70/30 NPH/Regular) are prescribed for the outpatient management of some diabetics. In consultation with the physician managing the diabetes, these patients should be switched to preparations of individual insulins in the immediate preoperative period. An appropriately reduced dose of only the intermediate acting insulin can then be taken on the morning of surgery.

4. **Patients with peripheral neuropathy** are vulnerable to positioning injuries. Document neuropathies before initiating regional anesthesia.

5. Diabetics may have delayed gastric emptying and should receive aspiration prophylaxis. They may be less able to compensate for the sympathectomy of regional anesthesia.

6.   Protamine must be administered cautiously in the diabetic receiving NPH insulin. These patients are at increased risk for protamine reactions.

II.   Hypoglycemia

A.   Etiologies. Although extremely rare, when present hypoglycemia may be due to pancreatic adenoma (insulinoma) or carcinoma, cirrhosis, hypopituitarism, adrenal insufficiency, hepatoma, sarcoma, ethanol ingestion, or sulfonylurea or insulin therapy.

B.   Signs and Symptoms. Adrenergic excess produces tachycardia, diaphoresis, palpitations, and tremulousness. Neuroglycopenia results in headache, confusion, stupor, seizure, and coma. These are masked by general anesthesia. **Hypoglycemic unawareness** is a condition in which patients with long-standing DM under tight control lose the sympathetic response to hypoglycemia.

C.   Anesthetic considerations include providing a continuous glucose infusion and periodically checking the serum glucose.

III.   Thyroid disease

A.   Physiology. Thyroid hormones are the major regulators of cellular metabolic activity. They alter the speed of biochemical reactions, total body oxygen consumption, and heat production. Under the control of thyroid-stimulating hormone (TSH) from the anterior pituitary, iodine is taken up into the thyroid gland and incorporated into tyrosine residues of thyroglobulin, and the hormones triiodothyronine (T_3) and L-thyroxine (T_4) are formed and stored. Peripheral tissues convert T_4 to T_3, which is 20 to 50 times more potent than T_4 but has a shorter half-life. Both forms of thyroid hormone are extensively (>99%) bound to plasma proteins. Only the free (unbound) thyroid hormone is biologically active.

B.   Evaluation and laboratory studies. No single test can exclude all types of thyroid disease in the sick patient. Thyroid function tests must be used in close conjunction with observation of the patient's clinical status. Measurements of serum TSH are currently the best initial screen for determination of thyroid function. TSH levels rise above the normal range in hypothyroidism. Thyrotoxicosis will suppress the TSH level. The TSH level may also be lowered by starvation, glucocorticoids, stress, dopamine, and fever. The free T_4 may aid diagnosis under these conditions. History and physical examination to exclude airway compromise because of goiter are essential.

C.   Thyrotoxicosis

1.   Etiologies of thyrotoxicosis in order of decreasing frequency include Graves disease, toxic multinodular goiter, subacute thyroiditis (acute phase), toxic adenoma, ovarian tumors secreting thyroid hormone (struma ovarii), and (rarely) TSH or β-human chorionic gonadotropin (which weakly stimulates TSH receptors) overproduction due to pituitary or placental tumors. Ingestion of thyroid hormone can also lead to thyrotoxicosis.

2.   Clinical features of thyrotoxicosis

a.   Thyrotoxicosis is a hypermetabolic state. Patients present with nervousness, heat intolerance, muscle weakness, tremors, and weight loss. Cardiovascular signs include

Table 6-4.   Treatment of thyrotoxic crisis

Block sympathetic response
    Propranolol: 1–2 mg IV, repeat as needed or 40–80 mg PO, repeat q6h
    Verapamil: 5–10 mg IV, repeat as needed
Block thyroid hormone synthesis
    Propylthiouracil (PTU): 250 mg PO q4–6h
    Methimazole: 30 mg per rectum q8h
Block thyroid hormone release
    Sodium Iodide (SSKI)[a]:10 drops PO q12h
    Ipodate[a]: 1 g PO qd
    Dexamethasone: 2 mg PO q6h
Block T_4 to T_3 conversion
    Beta-adrenergic blockade, PTU, ipodate, dexamethasone
Supportive therapy[b]
    Fluids
    Cooling
    Electrolyte replacement

[a]Give SSKI or ipodate 1h after PTU or methimazole.
[b]In extreme circumstances consider plasmapheresis.

arrhythmias (e.g., sinus tachycardia, atrial fibrillation), systolic murmurs, and high output or ischemic congestive heart failure. Thyrotoxicosis should be considered as a possible cause of sustained tachycardia. Patients can have leukopenia and thrombocytopenia. Low clotting factor concentrations may indicate increased metabolism or thyrotoxic liver damage; such patients are sensitive to warfarin.

b.   Thyroid storm is a state of physiologic decompensation in severe thyrotoxicosis. Surgical stress may precipitate this condition, but usually thyroid storm manifests 6 to 18 hours postoperatively. Manifestations include diarrhea, vomiting, and hyperpyrexia (38 to 41°C) leading to hypovolemia, irritability, delirium, or coma. Thyroid storm may mimic malignant hyperthermia, neuroleptic malignant syndrome, sepsis, hemorrhage, or transfusion/drug reaction.

3.   Treatment of thyrotoxicosis. Chronic thyroid hormone excess is treated by gland ablation with surgery or radioactive iodine, or with specific antithyroid drugs (e.g., propylthiouracil [PTU] and methimazole) that interfere with thyroid hormone synthesis. Two to 6 weeks of drug therapy may be required to normalize hormone levels. The most serious side effects of antithyroid agents are hepatitis and agranulocytosis. Therapy for thyroid storm (Table 6-4) includes **active** cooling, along with meperidine to attenuate shivering, **hydration**, β-adrenergic blockade, steroids if there is any indication of adrenal insufficiency including cardiovascular collapse, high dose IV iodine to block synthesis and release of hormones, and PTU.

4.   Anesthetic considerations. Only emergency surgery should be performed in thyrotoxic patients. Generous sedative premedication should be considered. Avoid sympathetic stimu-

lation (pain, ketamine, pancuronium, local anesthetics with epinephrine). Regional anesthesia may be beneficial in thyrotoxic
patients, because it blocks sympathetic responses. Hypotension
should be treated with direct-acting agents. The eyes of patients
with Graves disease should be well protected from exposure.
In general, drug metabolism and anesthetic requirements appear
to be increased. However, therapeutic dose requirements for
anticoagulants may be lower. Myasthenia gravis may be seen in
some Graves patients (30-fold increased incidence), so relaxants
should be titrated carefully. Large goiters may displace the trachea and compromise the airway.

D. **Hypothyroidism**

1. **Etiologies of hypothyroidism**. Insufficient synthesis of
thyroid hormone may be congenital, result from ablation (surgery, radioiodine), or follow radiation therapy. Other causes include Hashimoto thyroiditis, iodine deficiency, drug therapy
(lithium or phenylbutazone), and late phase subacute thyroiditis. Hashimoto thyroiditis is the most common cause of hypothyroidism in adults and can be associated with other autoimmune
processes, including systemic lupus, rheumatoid arthritis, primary adrenal insufficiency, pernicious anemia, DM, or Sjögren
syndrome.

2. **Clinical features of hypothyroidism**

a. Patients demonstrate lethargy, cold intolerance, facial
edema with an enlarged tongue, a reversible cardiomyopathy,
pericardial effusion, ascites, anemia, constipation, and an ady-
namic ileus with delayed gastric emptying. There may be adrenal atrophy with decreased cortisol production, dilutional hyponatremia, and decreased water excretion. Cardiac output
decreases. There may also be bradycardia, hypovolemia, and
diminished baroreceptor reflexes.

b. **Myxedema coma** (profound hypothyroidism) is a clinical diagnosis. Surgery, drugs, trauma, or infection initiate this
decompensated state in a severely hypothyroid patient. It is
defined by decreased mental status associated with hypore-
sponsiveness to CO_2, congestive heart failure, hypothermia,
and exaggerated symptoms of hypothyroidism.

3. **Treatment of hypothyroidism**. Chronic treatment involves the oral supplementation of thyroid hormone. T_4 requires
7 to 10 days to have initial effects; 3 to 4 weeks of therapy are
needed to achieve a stable state. T_3 begins to have an effect in
6 hours. Cautious IV or oral thyroid hormone loading will hasten
recovery. T_4 dosing is usually adjusted every 4 to 6 weeks based
on serum TSH levels.

4. **Anesthetic considerations**. Elective surgery should be
postponed in severe hypothyroidism. In moderately hypothyroid
patients, postponing surgery is not necessary. Additional considerations include the following:

a. Preoperative sedative should be administered with caution because of the profound CNS and respiratory sensitivity
to depressants.

b. Cortisol supplementation may be necessary.

c. Hypovolemia may be present.

d. Anemia should be corrected.

e. Airway and respiratory difficulties may be caused by an

enlarged tongue and relaxed oropharyngeal tissues, CO_2 insensitivity, poor gastric emptying, and increased sensitivity to all depressant medications.

f. Thyroid gland dysfunction has no effect on minimum alveolar concentration for inhalational anesthetics.

IV. Calcium metabolism and parathyroid disease

A. Physiology. Parathyroid hormone (PTH) and vitamin D maintain the extracellular calcium concentration within a narrow physiologic range. PTH increases intestinal calcium absorption, decreases renal clearance of calcium, and enhances formation of 1,25-dihydroxy-vitamin D by the kidney. Secretion of PTH is determined by the activity of the intramembranous calcium sensor and levels of ionized calcium and magnesium. Calcitonin from thyroid "C" cells antagonizes PTH by lowering both calcium and phosphorous concentrations. Calcitonin's physiologic role is limited in humans.

B. Calcium is essential for neuromuscular excitability, coagulation, muscle contraction, neurotransmitter and hormone secretion, and hormone action. At normal pH, phosphate, citrate, and other anions complex about 6% of total calcium. The remainder is equally divided between protein bound (primarily to albumin) or unbound (free, ionized). Alterations in total calcium levels can be estimated from albumin levels. Hypoalbuminemia produces a decrease in total calcium of approximately 0.8 mg/dL for each g/dL of albumin below normal (4.0 g/dL). Ionized calcium, the physiologically important form, can be measured easily in whole blood, but improper sample handling can lead to nonreproducible measurements. Acidosis increases, and alkalosis decreases, ionized calcium due to alterations in albumin binding. Thus, signs and symptoms of hypocalcemia may be precipitated by hyperventilation and respiratory alkalosis.

1. Hypercalcemia

a. Etiologies of hypercalcemia include hyperparathyroidism, malignancy, immobilization, granulomatous diseases (sarcoidosis, berylliosis, tuberculosis), vitamin D intoxication, familial hypocalciuric hypercalcemia, thyrotoxicosis, and adrenal insufficiency. **Hyperparathyroidism** is characterized by hypercalcemia and hypophosphatemia with an elevated intact PTH level, usually caused by a parathyroid adenoma. Four-gland parathyroid hyperplasia causes only 10% of cases of hyperparathyroidism. Parathyroid hyperplasia can be associated with medullary thyroid carcinoma and pheochromocytoma in multiple endocrine neoplasia type I. Parathyroid carcinoma is a rare cause of hyperparathyroidism and hypercalcemia. Treatment of a parathyroid adenoma or carcinoma is by removal of the abnormal gland, coupled with intraoperative sampling of blood for immunoreactive PTH to confirm an adequate resection. The remaining glands are evaluated to exclude hyperplasia. Removal of three and a half to four glands, with optional frozen storage or forearm reimplantation, is the treatment for hyperplasia. **Hypercalcemia of malignancy** is due to release of a PTH-like molecule (PTH-related protein) from tumors (lung, breast, gut, urinary tract) and cytokine-mediated or direct bony destruction resulting in resorption of calcium from the skeleton.

   b.   Clinical features of hypercalcemia include anorexia, nausea/vomiting, polyuria, dehydration, constipation, peptic ulcer disease, impaired memory, somnolence, depression, lethargy, nephrolithiasis, polyuria, hypertension, and electrocardiographic changes (e.g., prolonged PR interval with a short QT interval).

   c.   Treatment of hypercalcemia. Hypercalcemia is considered an emergency when (albumin-corrected) values are greater than 15 mg/dL. Treatment includes limiting oral intake of calcium, hydration with normal saline (6 to 10 L/day, IV), and diuresis with furosemide or ethacrynic acid. The patient must be closely observed for fluid overload, hypokalemia, and hypomagnesemia. Administration of oral phosphate (1 to 2 g/day) limits intestinal absorption and increases skeletal reuptake of calcium. Phosphate is effective but poorly tolerated because of diarrhea. Elevations in serum phosphorus (>5 mg/dL) should be avoided. Pamidronate, mithramycin, zoledronic acid, and calcitonin decrease bone resorption and are used in life-threatening cases of hypercalcemia. Mithramycin (25 mg/kg body weight, IV, over 30 minutes) will correct hypercalcemia in 48 hours. A lower dose of mithramycin (5 to 15 mg/kg body weight) may be given in less critical cases. For severe hypercalcemia, the standard treatment is parenteral pamidronate. For serum calcium levels greater than 13.5 mg/dL, pamidronate (90 mg IV) is administered in saline over 4 hours. Patients with renal insufficiency or calcium levels less than 13.5 mg/dL may be treated with 60 mg IV over 4 to 24 hours. Renal failure requires lower doses. Maximal lowering of calcium occurs between 4 and 7 days with a duration of about 2 weeks. Zoledronic acid (Zometa) is a newly approved parenteral treatment for hypercalcemia of malignancy. A 4 mg IV dose will decrease calcium levels more rapidly and for a longer period of time than pamidronate. Hypercalcemia may also respond to salmon calcitonin (4 to 8 IU/kg every 12 hours). Glucocorticoid therapy is effective in some cases of multiple myeloma, although not in other causes of hypercalcemia.

   d.   Anesthetic considerations. Hypercalcemia warrants correction. Intravascular volume and other electrolyte abnormalities should be normalized. Hypercalcemia has an unpredictable effect on neuromuscular blockade so relaxants should be carefully titrated. Careful positioning is required, because these patients can be osteoporotic. Patients with hypercalcemia are predisposed to digitalis toxicity. After thyroid or parathyroid surgery patients may have transient or permanent hypocalcemia requiring supplementation.

2.   **Hypocalcemia**

   a.   Etiologies of hypocalcemia. Hypocalcemia is defined as serum calcium less than 8.5 mg/dL in the absence of hypoalbuminemia or abnormalities in pH. Patients are not usually symptomatic until the total calcium is less than 7.5 mg/dL, especially if calcium concentrations decline slowly. Hypoparathyroidism is due to underproduction of PTH or, rarely, resistance to its effects by end-organ tissues. PTH underproduction may occur after neck surgery with damage to, or excision of, parathyroid glands. Symptoms are usually seen in the immediate postoperative period but occasionally occur days to weeks later. Other causes include radiation therapy, hemosiderosis, infiltrative processes like malignancy or amyloidosis, severe hypomagnesemia, and severe vitamin D deficiency or malabsorption. Extensive burns and pancreatitis cause sequestration of calcium.

b. Clinical features of hypocalcemia. Acute hypocalcemia (c.g., after neck surgery and removal or damage of the parathyroid glands) produces neuromuscular irritability with muscle cramps, and hand, foot, and circumoral paresthesias. Severe hypocalcemia results in stridor, laryngospasm, tetany, apnea, and focal or grand mal seizures unresponsive to conventional therapy. Bedside demonstration of facial nerve irritability to percussion (Chvostek sign) or carpal spasm with tourniquet ischemia for 3 minutes (Trousseau sign) indicates the need for supplementation. However, 10% to 15% of normocalcemic patients will have a positive Chvostek sign.

c. Treatment of hypocalcemia. Symptomatic severe hypocalcemia should be treated with IV calcium. Of note, a 10-mL ampule of calcium gluconate contains only 93 mg of elemental calcium. A 10-mL ampule of calcium chloride contains 273 mg of elemental calcium. For urgent therapy, two ampules of calcium gluconate or one ampule of calcium chloride may be given slowly (10 to 20 minutes) IV. Less urgent situations are treated with IV calcium (15 mg/kg of elemental calcium) infused over 8 to 12 hours. Parenteral therapy must be monitored by serum calcium measurements. Oral supplementation with calcium and vitamin D is the usual therapy for mild to moderate hypocalcemia. Patients require 1.5 to 3 g/day of elemental calcium (3,750 to 7,500 mg of calcium carbonate) in divided doses. In acute symptomatic hypocalcemia treated with oral calcium, 1,25-dihydroxyvitamin D (calcitriol; Rocaltrol, 0.25 to 3.0 µg/day in divided doses) is given to enhance gastrointestinal absorption. For chronic replacement, either calcitriol or the parent vitamin D (ergocalciferol, 50,000 IU, one to three times weekly) is given. Therapeutic goals are a serum calcium near 8 mg/dL and a low urinary calcium level. Phosphorus and magnesium should also be evaluated and corrected if abnormal. Elevated phosphorus levels are treated with oral phosphate binders, whereas low magnesium levels (<1 mg/dL) that suppress PTH secretion are treated with parenteral magnesium sulfate.

d. Anesthetic considerations. Calcium and other electrolyte abnormalities should be corrected. Hypocalcemia can be worsened by respiratory or metabolic alkalosis, rapid infusions of multiple units of blood products (especially in states of hepatic insufficiency), hypothermia, and renal dysfunction. Coagulation status must be followed carefully. Patients may have hypotension with relative insensitivity to β-adrenergic agonists and a prolonged QT interval, as well as advanced atrial-ventricular block.

V. Adrenal cortical disease

A. Physiology. The human adrenal gland consists of an outer cortex that secretes steroid hormones and an inner medulla that secretes catecholamines. These hormones act to maintain homeostasis in states of stress such as fight-or-flight situations, fasting, injuries, or shock. Three types of hormones are produced in the adrenal cortex: glucocorticoids, mineralocorticoids, and androgens.

1.   Glucocorticoids. Cortisol is the principal hormone of this class. It is produced in response to adrenocorticotropic hormone (ACTH) from the anterior pituitary in a diurnal manner and in response to stress. About 30 mg of cortisol is produced daily. It has multiple effects on carbohydrate, protein, and fatty acid metabolism. Cortisol decreases the cellular uptake of glucose and promotes gluconeogenesis and hepatic glycogen synthesis. It is crucial to the conversion of norepinephrine to epinephrine in the adrenal medulla and is required for the production of angiotensin II and adequate vascular tone. It acts as an anti-inflammatory agent. Cortisol is metabolized by the liver and filtered and excreted unchanged by the kidney.

2.   Mineralocorticoids. Adrenal steroids such as deoxycorticosterone and cortisol (at high levels) have some mineralocorticoid activity. Aldosterone is the major regulator of extracellular fluid volume and potassium homeostasis. Its production is regulated by the renin-angiotensin system and, to a lesser extent, by potassium concentration (see Chapter 4). Aldosterone's principal effect causes reabsorption of Na^+ in the distal renal tubule. The resulting excess of cations in the tubule causes a passive transfer of K^+ and H^+ into the tubule for urinary excretion.

3.   Androgens. Abnormal secretion of these sex hormones may indicate abnormalities in biosynthesis of multiple steroids, including cortisol. The most common cause of increased adrenal androgen secretion is congenital adrenal hyperplasia, resulting in hirsutism and menstrual irregularities in women.

B.   Pharmacology. A variety of synthetic steroids is available with varying potencies and ratios of glucocorticoid to mineralocorticoid effects (Table 6-5).

C.   Adrenal cortical hyperfunction

1.   Etiologies. Most cases (80%) are due to adrenal hyperplasia secondary to excess secretion of ACTH (from pituitary tumors, ectopic production by carcinoids, or tumors of the pancreas or lung). Other causes include adrenal adenoma, bilateral adrenal micronodular hyperplasia, or exogenous steroid administration.

2.   Clinical features. Patients can present with truncal obesity, hypertension, hypernatremia, excess intravascular volume, hyperglycemia, hypokalemia, cutaneous striae, poor wound healing, muscle wasting and weakness, osteopenia/osteoporosis, hypercoagulability with thromboembolism, mental status changes and emotional lability, aseptic osteonecrosis, pancreatitis, benign intracranial hypertension, peptic ulceration, glaucoma, or infection.

3.   Anesthetic considerations

a.   Excess intravascular volume can be reduced with diuretics, but potassium must be replaced. Serum glucose must be monitored. Osteoporosis makes careful positioning necessary.

b.   Adrenalectomy. There is no specific anesthetic tech-

Table 6-5. Glucocorticoid and mineralocorticoid hormones

Steroid	Relative Potency		Equivalent dose (mg)	Duration (h)
	Gluco-corticoid	Mineralo-corticoid		
Short acting				
Cortisol	1.0	1.0	20	8–12
Cortisone	0.8	0.8	25	8–12
Aldosterone	0.3	3,000	—	8–12
Intermediate acting				
Prednisone	4.0	0.8	5	12–36
Prednisolone	4.0	0.8	5	12–36
Methylprednisolone	5.0	0.5	4	12–36
Fludrocortisone	10.0	125	—	12–36
Long acting				
Dexamethasone	25–40	0	0.75	>24

nique required for adrenalectomy. Steroid replacement should begin postoperatively for both unilateral and bilateral adrenalectomy. Both glucocorticoid and mineralocorticoid replacement are necessary in bilateral adrenalectomy. In unilateral resection, mineralocorticoid secretion remains normal and glucocorticoid supplementation is necessary until the remaining adrenal cortex produces normal glucocorticoid output after several months.

D. Adrenal cortical hypofunction

    1. Etiologies. Idiopathic changes, autoimmune atrophy, surgical removal, radiation therapy, metastatic destruction, infection (e.g., fungus, tuberculosis, human immunodeficiency virus, cytomegalovirus), hemorrhage (septicemia, Waterhouse-Friderichsen syndrome, anticoagulant therapy), drugs (ketoconazole, rifampin, metyrapone), or loss of ACTH stimulation can produce adrenal cortical hypofunction. Exogenous steroid administration may suppress the pituitary–adrenal axis for 12 or more months after cessation of therapy.

    2. Clinical features

        a. Primary adrenal insufficiency (Addison disease) is associated with both low cortisol and aldosterone levels resulting in weight loss, weakness, fatigue, anorexia, nausea/vomiting, abdominal pain, postural hypotension, diarrhea or constipation, and hyperpigmentation. Lack of glucocorticoids may produce episodic fever, abdominal pain, and hypotension that is difficult to distinguish from an acute surgical abdomen. Mineralocorticoid deficiency will lead to decreased urinary sodium conservation, decreased response to circulating catecholamines, and hyperkalemia.

        b. Secondary adrenal insufficiency, precipitated by abnormalities in ACTH secretion, results in low cortisol levels but normal aldosterone function. If surgery is required, drugs must be titrated carefully, because these patients are exquisitely sensitive to drug-induced myocardial depression.

3. **Treatment**

    a. Acute adrenal insufficiency (addisonian crisis), a medical emergency, presents with hypotension and tachycardia unresponsive to fluids. Fever and abdominal pain may occur. Treatment includes fluids (5% dextrose in normal saline), steroid replacement (hydrocortisone 100 to 150 mg IV or dexamethasone 6 mg IV and then hydrocortisone 30 to 50 mg IV q8h), inotropes as necessary, and electrolyte correction. Precipitating causes must be detected and treated. Hydrocortisone dosage may be decreased by 50% every 1 to 2 days depending on the clinical status. Primary adrenal insufficiency requires both glucocorticoid and mineralocorticoid replacement. Once the hydrocortisone dose is below 75 mg daily, mineralocorticoid therapy is added in the form of fludrocortisone (Florinef) 0.05 to 0.1 mg daily. Under basal conditions the usual hydrocortisone replacement is 30 mg daily (20 mg upon awakening and 10 mg at 4 p.m.) or prednisone 5 to 7.5 mg once daily. During times of stress such as with upper respiratory infection, tooth extraction, and so on, the glucocorticoid dose is doubled for 1 to 2 days.

4. **Anesthetic considerations**

    a. Evaluate and treat volume and electrolyte status as necessary.

    b. Individualize perioperative steroid replacement. Any patient who has received more than a 14-day treatment with supraphysiologic steroids in the past year should receive glucocorticoid supplementation perioperatively (see Table 6-6 for recommendations).

    c. Avoid etomidate in the hypoadrenal patient because of the potential for further adrenal suppression.

    d. Patients with adrenal hypofunction may exhibit marked sensitivity to sedative, anesthetic, or vasoactive drugs. Titrate drug doses carefully to avoid cardiovascular depression.

VI. Adrenal medullary disease

A. Physiology. Preganglionic fibers of the sympathetic nervous system end in the adrenal medulla and stimulate release of catecholamines (norepinephrine 20%, epinephrine 80%). Peripheral effects of these catecholamines include chronotropic and inotropic stimulation of the heart, vasomotor changes, enhanced hepatic glycogenolysis, and inhibition of insulin release. They are biotransformed in the kidney and liver primarily to metanephrine, normetanephrine, and vanillylmandelic acid.

B. Pheochromocytoma

1. **Physiology**. Pheochromocytoma, a tumor of the adrenal medulla, may occur in other locations but usually within sympathetic ganglia (paraganglioma). It is a rare cause of hypertension (0.1%). Most tumors are solitary, but 10% are bilateral and 10% are metastatic in the adult. Also, 10% of pheochromocytomas are familial and may occur as part of multiple endocrine neoplasia syndromes types II and III and can be associated with neurofibromatosis. Most tumors secrete both epinephrine and norepi-

Table 6-6. Perioperative hydrocortisone supplementation guidelines

Anticipated Surgical stress	Preoperative	Intraoperative	Postoperative
Minor[a]	25 mg or 1–2 times usual dose	None, unless complications	Resume usual replacement POD 1
Moderate[b]	50–75 mg or usual steroid dose, whichever is higher	50 mg IV	20 mg IV q8h on POD 1, then resume preoperative replacement dose on POD 2
Major[c]	100–150 mg or usual steroid dose, whichever is higher, within 2 h of start of procedure	50 mg IV q8h after initial dose	50 mg IV q8, or 150 mg continuously over 24 h for 2–3 days, then reduce dose by 50% per day until preoperative regimen is reached

POD, postoperative day.

Note that these guidelines may not meet the requirements of all patients. Perioperative or stress steroid replacement should be individually tailored.

[a]Inguinal herniorrhaphy, minor urologic or gynecologic procedures, oral surgery, plastic surgery.

[b]Total joint replacement, open cholecystectomy, lower extremity revascularization.

[c]Thoracotomy. cardiac surgery, major abdominal surgery.

nephrine, and their release is independent of neurogenic control.

2. Clinical features. Most signs and symptoms are due to excess catecholamine release. The classic symptom complex includes palpitations, headache, and diaphoresis in an episodically hypertensive patient, but 10% of patients are not hypertensive. Other symptoms include pallor followed by flushing, anxiety, tremor, hyperglycemia, hypovolemia-induced orthostatic hypotension, polycythemia, and weight loss. Patients with pheochromocytoma are usually dehydrated and hemoconcentrated. Chronic exposure to high catecholamine concentrations may produce a cardiomyopathy. A 24-hour urine collection for catecholamines and their metabolites is the routine screening procedure.

3. Perioperative considerations

  a. Hypertensive crisis. Treatment options include labetalol, nitroprusside infusion, or phentolamine (bolus 1 to 5 mg IV or as an infusion [10 mg/L in saline]), titrated to blood pressure, along with normal saline for volume expansion. After controlling blood pressure, tachycardia may be treated with beta-adrenergic blockade.

  b. Preoperative preparation. Alpha-receptor blockade is often started with oral phenoxybenzamine, a long-acting α_1- and α_2-adrenergic blocker (starting with 20 to 30 mg/day and increasing to 60 to 250 mg/day until blood pressure is controlled). Achieving adequate alpha-receptor blockade may require 10 to 14 days of therapy. Other clinical endpoints include postural hypotension, nasal stuffiness, and decreased sweating. Adequate volume repletion is reflected by weight gain and decreasing hematocrit. Alternatively, prazosin, a shorter acting alpha-1 blocker, may be preferred. Since prazosin lacks alpha-2 blocking activity, it does not increase sympathetic nerve outflow. Its shorter duration of action allows reversal of alpha blockade soon after resection of the pheochromocytoma. Alternatively, preoperative depletion of catecholamine stores may be accomplished with alpha-methyl-L-tyrosine therapy. **Beta-adrenergic blockade is instituted only after the onset of adequate alpha blockade**.

4. Anesthetic considerations. The goal is to avoid sympathetic outflow that commonly occurs with induction and surgical stimulation. The need for invasive monitoring depends on the patient's underlying medical condition and response to preoperative preparation. A combined technique using a spinal or epidural catheter is effective in ablating sympathetic responses while providing profound muscle relaxation. Intravenous magnesium may be a useful adjunct. Arrhythmias and severe hypertension caused by intubation, surgical incision, or tumor manipulation may require treatment. After the tumor is isolated and its veins ligated, a sudden decrease in blood pressure may occur. Vigorous volume support and treatment with a direct-acting vasopressor such as phenylephrine (especially with spinal- or epidural-induced sympathectomy) is customary. Preoperative normalization of fluid status may help in limiting hypotension after tumor resection. Endogenous catecholamine levels should return to normal within a few days after successful removal of the tumor.

VII. Pituitary disease
A. Anterior pituitary gland
1. **Physiology**. The anterior pituitary regulates the thyroid and adrenal glands, the ovaries and testes, growth, and lactation. The anterior pituitary secretes a variety of hormones. Growth hormone (GH) and prolactin act directly on target tissues, whereas ACTH, TSH, follicle-stimulating hormone, and luteinizing hormone act by stimulating other endocrine glands. Pituitary tumors are usually benign adenomas. Although some adenomas are nonsecreting, others secrete prolactin, GH, ACTH, TSH, or gonadotropins. Secreting adenomas may lead to hormone excess (e.g., prolactin) but rarely cause pituitary insufficiency. Pituitary apoplexy, metastatic tumors, lymphocytic hypophysitis, infiltrative diseases such as sarcoid or histiocytosis, and the rare pituitary carcinoma may cause isolated or complete pituitary insufficiency.
2. **Pituitary hyperfunction**. Most hyperfunctioning adenomas are benign pituitary tumors that do not cause special concerns for the anesthetist. The hyperthyroidism of a TSH-secreting adenoma and the hyperadrenalism of the ACTH-secreting adenoma are treated as described above. The anatomic changes seen in GH-secreting tumors are important for the anesthesiologist and are described in detail below.
   a. **Acromegaly**
      (1) Clinical features. Excess GH secretion in the adult will lead to prognathism, soft-tissue overgrowth of the lips, tongue, epiglottis, and vocal cords, with subglottic narrowing of the trachea. Connective tissue overgrowth can cause recurrent laryngeal nerve paralysis and carpal tunnel syndrome. These patients often develop peripheral neuropathies, glucose intolerance, congestive heart failure, arrhythmias, and an increased incidence of coronary artery disease and colon carcinoma.
      (2) Anesthetic considerations. Conventional face mask airways are often difficult to achieve, and endotracheal intubation can be challenging. Small diameter endotracheal tubes and awake intubation with or without a fiberoptic laryngoscope often is chosen. Serum glucose levels should be carefully maintained and muscle relaxants titrated using a peripheral nerve stimulator in patients with a history of skeletal muscle weakness.
3. **Hyposecretion** (panhypopituitarism)
   a. **Sheehan syndrome** is a condition of pituitary failure in which hemorrhagic shock causes vasospasm and subsequent pituitary necrosis and pituitary insufficiency in postpartum patients. Other causes of pituitary failure include trauma, radiation therapy, pituitary apoplexy, tumors such as metastatic carcinoma or craniopharyngiomas, and surgical hypophysectomy.
   b. **Anesthetic considerations**. Perioperative treatment with glucocorticoids is necessary for patients with a history of adrenal insufficiency. As discussed in section III.D, no special treatment or supplementation of patients with mild to moderate hypothyroidism is necessary. Intraoperative care of the hypothyroid patient requires attention to fluid management

because these patients do not excrete free water normally. Hypothyroid patients have a reduced metabolism and increased sensitivity to anesthetic agents, narcotics, and sedatives. The onset of pituitary insufficiency after pituitary surgery or apoplexy is delayed. Adrenal insufficiency develops over 4 to 14 days after destruction or removal of the pituitary. Glucocorticoid, not mineralocorticoid, replacement is required as discussed above. Because of the long half-life of thyroid hormone (7 to 10 days), symptomatic hypothyroidism does not occur until 3 to 4 weeks after pituitary surgery or apoplexy.

B. Posterior pituitary gland

   1.   Physiology. Antidiuretic hormone (ADH, vasopressin) and oxytocin are stored in the posterior pituitary. ADH regulates plasma osmolarity and extracellular fluid volume. ADH facilitates renal tubular resorption of water, causing urinary osmolarity to increase. Decreases in intravascular volume, pain from trauma or surgery, nausea, and positive airway pressure stimulate ADH secretion.

   2.   Diabetes insipidus (DI)

      a.   Etiologies. DI results from insufficient ADH secretion by the posterior pituitary (central DI) or failure of the renal tubules to respond to ADH (nephrogenic DI). Central DI can be caused by intracranial trauma, hypophysectomy, hypophysitis, metastatic disease to the pituitary or hypothalamus, and infiltrative diseases such as histiocytosis and sarcoidosis. Causes of nephrogenic DI include hypokalemia, hypercalcemia, sickle cell anemia, chronic myeloma, obstructive uropathy, chronic renal insufficiency, lithium therapy, and may be seen in the third trimester of pregnancy.

      b.   Clinical features include polydipsia and polyuria. The urine is inappropriately dilute relative to the high serum osmolarity. After pituitary surgery resulting in central DI, urinary output may follow a triphasic pattern. An immediate increase in urine volume occurs for 4 to 5 days after the acute injury from dysfunction of the ADH neurons. Urine flow then falls abruptly because of retrograde neuronal degeneration and release of ADH. The final phase consists of hypotonic polyuria (DI) from the complete destruction of the ADH neurons.

      c.   Anesthetic considerations. Treatment includes careful monitoring of urine output, plasma volume, and plasma osmolarity. The total body water deficit can be estimated as follows:

Water deficit (L)

$$= \{0.6 \times body\ weight\ (kg)\} \times \{([Na^+] - 140)/140\}$$

Body weight is the initial weight in kilograms before dehydration. In patients who cannot drink, initial therapy should be with isotonic fluids (normal saline) to reverse shock until osmolality is less than 290 mOsm/kg and then hypotonic fluids (half normal saline) are necessary. Mild DI (daily urinary volumes of 2 to 6 L in patients with an adequate thirst mechanism) does not require treatment. Central DI may be treated with the synthetic vasopressin analog desmopressin (DDAVP) at 1 to 2 µg (0.25 to 0.5 mL) subcutaneously or intravenously every 6 to 24 hours as needed. Side effects of DDAVP include hyponatremia, hypotension, and coronary artery vasospasm.

3. Nephrogenic DI. The polyuria of nephrogenic DI is associated with hypotonic urine, normal or high levels of plasma vasopressin, and failure of exogenous vasopressin to reduce urinary volume. Renal tubule insensitivity to vasopressin occurs as a rare X-linked hereditary disorder or a complication of medical treatment such as lithium therapy. There is no specific therapy for nephrogenic DI. Adequate oral or parenteral hydration must be assured. Inhibition of prostaglandin synthesis (by ibuprofen, indomethacin, or aspirin) or mild salt depletion with a thiazide diuretic may reduce urine volume.

4. Syndrome of inappropriate ADH secretion (SIADH). SIADH is persistent secretion of ADH with hyponatremia in the absence of an osmotic stimulus. SIADH can be caused by carcinoma (bronchogenic, duodenal, pancreatic, ureteral, prostatic or bladder), other malignancies (lymphoma, leukemia, thymoma, mesothelioma), CNS disorders (trauma, infections, tumors), pulmonary disorders (tuberculosis, pneumonia, positive pressure ventilation), drugs (nicotine, narcotics, chlorpropamide, clofibrate, vincristine, vinblastine, cyclophosphamide), hypothyroidism, Addison disease, or porphyria. The diagnosis is made by examining simultaneous serum and urine sodium and osmolality values. SIADH is associated with a high urine osmolality (higher than serum value), urine sodium greater than 20 mEq/L, and serum sodium less than 130 mEq/L. If serum sodium falls below 110 mEq/L, cerebral edema and seizures may result. Fluid restriction (800 to 1,000 mL daily) is the primary treatment for the mild hyponatremia of SIADH. Chronic hyponatremia without symptoms has virtually no mortality. Thus, resuscitation using sodium-containing solutions is reserved for symptomatic severe hyponatremia (serum Na^+ less than 120 mEq/L). Hyponatremia should be corrected slowly, no faster than an increase of 0.5 mEq/L/hr, because overly aggressive replacement may produce central pontine myelinolysis, an irreversible neurologic disorder (see Chapter 4).

VIII. Carcinoid

A. Carcinoid tumors. Most carcinoid tumors arise from the embryonic foregut (bronchus, stomach, pancreas), midgut (mid-duodenum to mid-transverse colon), or hindgut (descending colon and rectum). Carcinoid tumors arising from the foregut primarily secrete the serotonin precursor 5-hydroxytryptophan. Carcinoid tumors arising from the embryonic midgut secrete serotonin (5-hydroxytryptamine). Tumors of the hindgut do not secrete large amounts of either 5-hydroxytryptophan or serotonin. The most common location of carcinoid tumors is the appendix, followed by the ileum and rectum. In addition to serotonin, mediators secreted by carcinoid tumors include bradykinin, histamine, prostaglandins, and kallikrein. The biochemical hallmark of carcinoid syndrome is the overproduction of serotonin and/or 5-hydroxytryptophan and increased excretion of the degradation product 5-hydroxyindoleacetic acid in the urine. Stimuli for the release of mediators include catecholamines, histamine, and tumor manipulation.

B.   Carcinoid syndrome. Clinical features of the carcinoid syndrome depend on the tumor's location and extent of liver metastasis. The syndrome includes episodic flushing, bronchoconstriction, gastrointestinal hypermotility, and mild hyperglycemia. Cardiac manifestations include supraventricular tachycardias and right-sided valve cusp distortions that can cause tricuspid regurgitation and pulmonic stenosis. Peripheral vasodilation can produce profound hypotension. Forty percent to 50% of patients with carcinoids located in the small bowel and the proximal colon will have the symptom complex. Symptoms are less frequent with carcinoids of the bronchus, rarely seen with appendiceal carcinoids, and never seen with rectal carcinoid tumors. Compounds released by the tumor are typically metabolized during the first pass through the liver, and symptoms are only seen when there are extensive hepatic metastases, when blood flow from a gut tumor bypasses liver parenchyma, or when a tumor occurs located outside the portal vein system.

C.   Anesthetic considerations

1.   In the symptomatic patient, preoperative and intraoperative treatment with the somatostatin analogue **octreotide** (Sandostatin) prevents the release of serotonin and its precursors and may block the peripheral actions of serotonin, kinins and other mediators.

2.   Paroxysmal bronchoconstriction occurs concurrently with a flushing episode and is associated with release of mediators from the tumor. In addition to the usual treatment of bronchoconstriction, octreotide should be given to decrease release of mediators.

3.   Plaque-like thickenings on the endocardium of the cardiac valve leaflets, atria, and ventricles occurs in 20% of patients with carcinoid and are usually associated with high levels of serotonin. Thickening of the endocardium can produce pulmonic stenosis and tricuspid insufficiency.

4.   If a carcinoid crisis with refractory hypotension and bronchoconstriction does occur, treatment should be initiated with octreotide (50 to 100 μg IV, diluted and infused over 30 to 60 minutes), fluid resuscitation, and a direct-acting vasopressor (e.g., phenylephrine). Catecholamines may further stimulate the release of mediators and exacerbate the crisis.

IX.   Porphyrias

A.   Etiology. The porphyrias result from the abnormal accumulation of porphyrins, the metabolic intermediates formed during the creation of heme. There are a variety of forms, depending on where the exact biochemical aberration occurs in the complex heme biosynthetic pathway. A clinical presentation of porphyria results from an environmental or physiologic trigger that stimulates ALA synthetase, the enzyme initiating heme synthesis from precursors, and the controlling enzyme in the pathway.

B.   Classification of the porphyrias. At least two overlapping classification schemes for the porphyrias exist. One classification is based on the site of the enzymatic defect, which may occur in either the liver or in the erythropoietic system. Another classification scheme categorizes the porphyrias based on their propensity to cause acute symptoms, especially in response to drugs or physiologic perturbations.

1. The acute porphyrias include acute intermittent porphyria, variegate porphyria, hereditary coproporphyria, and the rare plumboporphyria. These are also classified as hepatic porphyrias. Relevant to anesthesia practice (see section IX.D below) is that many drugs commonly encountered in the perioperative period may precipitate an attack. Hallmarks of an acute attack are abdominal pain; autonomic disturbances with sweating, tachycardia, and sustained hypertension; and neurologic manifestations including seizures and neuromuscular weakness.

2. The nonacute porphyrias include porphyria cutanea tarda, which is a hepatic porphyria. Other nonacute porphyrias include congenital erythropoietic porphyria, erythropoietic protoporphyria, and X-linked sideroblastic anemia. Attacks with neurovisceral manifestations precipitated by drugs or physiologic stresses are unlikely.

C. Photosensitivity is a feature of erythropoietic protoporphyria, congenital erythropoietic porphyria P, porphyria cutanea tarda, variegate porphyria, and hereditary coproporphyria. Light at the visible wavelengths 400 to 410 nm and 580 to 650 nm interacts with the heme compounds accumulated in the skin to precipitate cutaneous changes, including blistering and a burning sensation. Clinical equipment may generate light at these wavelengths.

D. Anesthetic implications of the porphyrias include the possible presence of mental status changes, neuropathy and autonomic instability, alterations in fluid and electrolyte status, and reduced respiratory muscle reserve.

1. A number of drugs used in the perioperative period may precipitate acute attacks of porphyria. Recommendations remain largely based on clinical anecdotes, animal or other laboratory studies. **Drugs that are contraindicated** in patients with known or suspected porphyria, particularly the acute porphyrias, include etomidate and the barbiturates, valproic acid, carbamazepine and phenytoin, ergots, and pentazocine. The benzodiazepines chlordiazepoxide and nitrazepam should be avoided. Other benzodiazepines should be used cautiously, if at all.

2. Useful drugs for general anesthesia include propofol, ketamine, muscle relaxants, opioids, and nitrous oxide. Firm data about the safety of volatile anesthetics do not exist. Neuromuscular blockade reversal agents, droperidol and the phenothiazines, and most vasoactive agents (with the possible exception of hydralazine, nifedipine, and phenoxybenzamine) are likely to be safe. Ondansetron, ranitidine, and metoclopramide should be used cautiously. Administer all drugs with caution and with attention to the possible acute presentation of signs and symptoms consistent with an attack of porphyria.

3. Regional anesthesia may be used. Commonly used local anesthetics, with the possible exception of cocaine, mepivacaine, and ropivacaine, are likely to be safe.

SUGGESTED READING

Diabetes

Genuth SM. Diabetic ketoacidosis and hyperglycemic hyperosmolar coma. *Curr Ther Endocrinol Metab* 1997;6:438–447.

Mahler RJ, Adler ML, Clinical review 102. Type 2 diabetes mellitus: update on diagnosis, pathophysiology and treatment. *J Clin Endocrinol Metab* 1999;84:1165–1171.

McAnulty GR, Robertshaw HJ, Hall GM. Anaesthetic management of patients with diabetes mellitus. *Br J Anaesth* 2000;85:80–90.

Milaszkiewicz RM. Diabetes mellitus and anesthesia: what is the problem? *Int Anesthesiol Clin* 1997;35:35–62.

Thyroid

Dabon-Almirante CLM, Surks MI. Clincial and laboratory diagnosis of thyrotoxicosis. *Endocrinol Metab Clin North Am* 1998;27:25–36.

Dillmann WH. Thyroid storm. In: Bardin CW, ed. *Current therapy in endocrinology and metabolism*, 6th ed. New York: Mosby, 1997:81–85.

Farling PA. Thyroid disease. *Br J Anaesth* 2000;85:15–28.

Gomberg-Maitland M, Frishman WH. Thyroid hormone and cardiovascular disease. *Am Heart J* 1998;135:187–196.

Hofbauer LC, Heufelder AE. Coagulation disorders in thyroid diseases. *Eur J Endocrinol* 1997;136:1–7.

Klein I, Ojamaa K. Thyrotoxicosis and the heart. *Endocrinol Metab Clin North Am* 1998;27:51–62.

Pittman CS, Zayed AA. Myxedema coma. In: Bardin CW, ed. *Current therapy in endocrinology and metabolism*, 6th ed. New York: Mosby, 1997:98–101.

Calcium

Adams J, Andersen P, Everts E, et al. Early postoperative calcium levels as predictors of hypocalcemia. *Laryngoscope* 1998;108:1829–1831.

Bushinsky DA, Monk RD. Calcium. *Lancet* 1998;352:306–311.

Marx SJ. Hyperparathyroid and hypoparathyroid disorders. *N Engl J Med* 2000;343:1863–1875.

Adrenals

Barquist E, Kirton O. Adrenal insufficiency in the surgical intensive care unit. *J Trauma* 1997;42:27–31.

Horton R, Nadler JL. Hypoaldosteronism. In: Bardin CW, ed. *Current therapy in endocrinology and metabolism*, 6th ed. New York: Mosby, 1997:164–167.

Lamberts SWJ, Bruining HA, de Jong FH. Corticosteroid therapy in severe illness. *N Engl J Med* 1997;337:1285–1292.

Malchoff CD, Carey RM. Adrenal insufficiency. In: Bardin CW, ed. *Current therapy in endocrinology and metabolism*, 6th ed. New York: Mosby, 1997:142–147.

Napolitano LM, Chernow B. Guidelines for corticosteroid use in anesthetic and surgical stress. *Int Anesthesiol Clin* 1988;26:226–232.

Oelkers W. Adrenal insufficiency. *N Engl J Med* 1996;335:1206–1212.

Salem M, Tainsh RE, Bromberg J, et al. Perioperative glucocorticoid coverage. *Ann Surg* 1994;219:416–425.

Pheochromocytoma

Kenady DE, McGrath PC, Sloan DA, et al. Diagnosis and management of pheochromocytoma. *Curr Opin Oncol* 1997;9:61–67.

O'Riordan JA. Pheochromocytomas and anesthesia. *Int Anesthesiol Clin* 1997;35:99–127.

Prys-Roberts C. Phaeochromocytoma-recent progress in its management. *Br J Anaesth* 2000;85:44–57.

Pituitary

Kumar S, Berl T. Sodium. *Lancet* 1998;353:220–228.

Singer I, Oster JR, Fishman LM. The management of diabetes insipidus in adults. *Arch Intern Med* 1997;157:1293–1301.

Smith M, Hirsch NP. Pituitary disease and anesthesia. *Br J Anaesth* 2000; 85:3–14.

Van den Berghe G, de Zegher F, Bouillon R. Acute and prolonged critical illness as different neuroendocrine paradigms. *J Clin Endocrinol Metab* 1998;83:1827–1834.

Carcinoid

Badola RP. The patient with carcinoid syndrome. In: Frost EAM, ed. *Preanesthetic assessment 3*. Boston: Birkhauser, 1994:12–25.

Kulke MH, Mayer RJ. Carcinoid tumors. *N Engl J Med* 1999;340:858–868.

Vaughan DJA, Brunner MD. Anesthesia for patients with carcinoid syndrome. *Int Anesthesiol Clin* 1997;35:129–142.

Porphyria

James MFM, Hift RJ. Porphyrias. *Br J Anaesth* 2000;85:143–153.

7

Infectious Diseases and Infection Control in Anesthesia

Judith Hellman

I. **General**. Anesthetists play an important role in many aspects of infection control in the operating room (OR).
   A. **Infection control-related responsibilities of anesthetist**
      1. **Prevention of transmission** of infectious agents between patients, between patients and operating personnel, and between OR personnel and patients.
      2. **Prevention of infectious complications** resulting from invasive procedures such as placement of intravenous, intraarterial, and regional anesthetic catheters; nerve blocks; and spinal anesthetics.
      3. **Avoidance of anesthesia-related complications** that can predispose to infection, such as aspiration during induction and intubation.
      4. **Participation in preventing surgical wound infections** by timely and proper administration of perioperative antibiotics.
   B. **Routes of infection transmission in the OR**
      1. **Physical contact** between the host and a contaminated object or a colonized or infected person is the most common mechanism of infection transmission.
      2. **Droplet transmission** results from deposition of large microorganism-containing droplets that are produced by an infected individual by coughing, sneezing, and talking. The droplets travel short distances and are deposited on the mucous membranes of the new host or are deposited on surfaces and then transmitted by direct contact.
      3. **Airborne transmission** results from inhalation of small particles that contain microorganisms and are suspended in the air by coughing, sneezing, and talking. Unlike larger droplets, these particles may remain suspended in the air and can be spread by air currents.
      4. **Blood and body fluids** can be a source of infected material, which can be transmitted through breaks in the host's skin or mucosa when there is contact between the infected body fluid and the host. Routine testing of blood products for some common bloodborne pathogens (human immunodeficiency virus [HIV], hepatitis B virus [HBV], hepatitis C virus [HCV]) has dramatically reduced the incidence of transfusion-related infections.

II. **Infection control in the OR**
   A. **Infection control measures** must be undertaken to prevent transmission of pathogens from patients to OR staff and vice versa, to prevent surgical wound infections, and to prevent introduction of microorganisms during invasive procedures such as placement of central venous, pulmonary artery, and epidural catheters. Adherence to **isolation precaution** guidelines reduces occupational

risk of infectious diseases and decreases transmission of infections in the hospital.

B. Standard precautions are intended to limit transmission of microorganisms by decreasing microbial colonization of surfaces, equipment, clothing, and hands and by preventing occupational exposure to blood and other potentially infected body fluids. Routine **handwashing** is essential to control spread of infection.

> **1. Minimize colonization of OR surfaces and OR equipment**
>> **a. Clean the OR**, including the anesthesia machine and anesthesia monitoring devices with a bactericidal agent between cases.
>> **b. Limit flow of traffic** through OR.
>> **c. Sterilize reusable equipment** (e.g., laryngoscopes, bronchoscopes, surgical instruments).
>> **d. Other** (not always used): laminar flow ventilation, ultraviolet radiation, high-efficiency particulate air filtration.

> **2. Minimize transmission through contact with patients**
>> **a. Wash hands** with antiseptic-containing solutions before and after contact with each patient or after contact with contaminated materials.
>> **b. Wear gloves** when hands are likely to come in contact with blood or other body fluids. Gloves must be changed (and hands washed) before and after contact with each patient.
>> **c. Wear lint-free OR attire**, including cap, mask, suit, and shoe covers or properly and regularly cleansed dedicated OR shoes.

> **3. Minimize likelihood of infections related to anesthesia and anesthetic procedures**
>> **a. Use sterile technique** for placement of catheters, nerve blocks, and spinal anesthesia. Sterile gloves and drapes should be used, and the insertion site should be carefully inspected and cleaned with antiseptic solution. Indwelling catheters should not be placed through areas that appear infected or inflamed. A sterile gown should be worn for placement of central venous and pulmonary artery catheters. Peripheral intravenous catheters may be placed after cleaning the insertion site with 70% isopropyl alcohol or povidone iodine.
>> **b. Cover catheter sites with sterile transparent dressings**. Catheter sites should be regularly inspected postoperatively for signs of infection.
>> **c. Administer drugs** using sterile technique.

> **4. Universal precautions** apply to all patients, regardless of underlying diseases. Barrier precautions are required when there is potential for contact with blood and other bodily secretions and fluids, because these may harbor infectious agents. Barriers include gloves, protective eyewear or face shields, and gowns.

C. Transmission-based precautions. Specialized precautions, including **contact**, **airborne**, and **droplet precautions** apply to patients that are suspected or are known to be infected or colonized with particular microorganisms. Different precautions apply to different microorganisms. When special precautions are in effect, **signs** are placed at the entrance of the patient's room indicating the type of precaution and required procedures to enter and exit the room. These guidelines should be followed in the OR and postanesthesia care unit (PACU), and signs should be placed on the door(s) to the OR and near the patient in the PACU.

1.   Contact precautions apply in many situations, including (but not limited to) colonization or infection with various antibiotic-resistant bacteria, such as methicillin-resistant *Staphylococcus aureus* (MRSA) and vancomycin-resistant enterococcus (VRE), some viral infections, and *Clostridium difficile*.

   a.   Wear gloves when entering the room.

   b.   Wear gowns if there is direct contact with the patient or equipment or surfaces in the patient's room.

   c.   Remove gowns and gloves and wash hands upon exiting the room.

   d.   Medical record. Leave charts and flow sheets outside the room and do not allow them to be in contact with the patient or contaminated bedding (place in plastic bag during transport).

   e.   Placement after PACU. A private room is preferred. A semiprivate room shared with a patient that is colonized or infected with the same microorganisms is acceptable.

2.   Droplet precautions are used to limit spread of infectious agents that are present in larger droplets produced from coughing, sneezing, and talking. *Neisseria meningitidis, Haemophilus influenzae, Mycoplasma pneumoniae*, adenovirus, and rubella virus are examples of infectious agents that are transmitted through droplets.

   a.   Wear a surgical mask when within 3 feet of infected individual. Discard the mask upon exiting the room and wash hands after discarding the mask.

   b.   Transport. The infected patient should wear a surgical mask during transportation.

   c.   Placement after PACU. A private room is preferred. A semiprivate room shared with a patient that is colonized or infected with the same microorganisms is acceptable.

3.   Airborne precautions are used to limit spread of infectious agents in particles that remain suspended in the air. *Mycobacterium tuberculosis* (MTB), varicella zoster virus (VZV), Ebola virus, and rubeola (measles) are examples of microorganisms that are transmitted through airborne particles.

   a.   Specialized masks (respirators) are designed to filter out very small particles.

     (1)   Respirators, and not standard surgical masks, should be worn by:

       (a)   All persons entering rooms of patients that require airborne precautions for tuberculosis.

       (b)   Persons who are not immune to VZV (have not had chickenpox) or rubeola who must enter the room.

     (2)   Personnel using respirators must be **fit-tested** before use to ensure an adequate seal.

   b.   A private room with negative-pressure isolation is required for all patients on airborne precautions.

   c.   Transport. The patient should wear a surgical mask for transport. Intubated patients should be transported with a bacterial filter in place on the endotracheal tube.

4.   The **PACU (or intensive care unit)** and the floor to which the patient will eventually be going should be informed of any special isolation precautions in advance.

D. **Preventing exposure to infected blood and body fluids**

1. **Occupational exposure** to bloodborne pathogens such as HIV, HBV, and HCV are of particular concern to anesthetists who routinely perform procedures that involve needles and blood. Exposure can occur through needlesticks but may also occur as a result of exposure through open cuts, splashes into eyes and other exposed areas, and contact with sharp contaminated objects other than needles (e.g., scalpels, cracked ampules).

2. **Preventive measures**

   a. **Hand washing, gloves, protective eyewear** as above.

   b. **Do no recap used needles or remove used needles from syringes.** Needlestick injuries most often occur during recapping of used needles. Used needles should be discarded without recapping. A number of devices recently have been developed that protect the used needle tip without requiring recapping.

   c. **Dispose of used needles immediately**. All needles should be discarded in special puncture-proof receptacles.

   d. **Administer parenteral drugs using needleless systems**.

   e. **Do not place syringes with attached needles in pockets**.

E. **Management of exposure to infected blood and bloody fluids**

1. **Wash areas of contact**. Use soap and water or sterile saline for skin; flush mucous membranes with water or sterile saline. Washing with caustic agents such as bleach is not recommended.

2. **Immediately report exposure** to hospital occupational/employee health or equivalent service. The Occupational Safety and Health Agency requires that all health care institutions have protocols for assessing and managing occupational exposures that includes:

   a. **Serologic testing** (HIV, HBV, and HCV) of the source (if known) and the health care worker.

   b. Consideration of **postexposure prophylaxis** (PEP) for HIV and HBV exposures.

   c. **Counseling**.

III. **Microorganisms of concern to anesthetists**. The Centers for Disease Control and Prevention (CDC) website (*www.cdc.gov*) contains current reviews of potential pathogens, including all of the microorganisms reviewed here, and their treatment.

A. **Viruses**

1. **HIV**

   a. **Transmission**. HIV is transmitted through percutaneous or mucosal exposure to infected blood or body fluids through needlestick and other sharp injury, blood transfusions, and sexual contact. Perinatal transmission of HIV from an infected mother to the neonate also occurs.

   b. **Occupational risk of HIV**. The risk of occupationally acquired HIV in health care workers is low. Most documented cases of seroconversion have occurred after percutaneous exposure; mucosal exposure is believed to be low risk.

   (1)   The risk of seroconversion is 0.3% after percutaneous exposure to blood from an HIV-infected person.

   (2)   The risk for HIV transmission is increased with:

   (a)   Deep injury

   (b)   Patient blood visible on device causing injury

   (c)   Needle placed in vein or artery of the source patient

   (d)   Patient in terminal stages of HIV infection

   (e)   Possibly larger bore hollow needles

c.   PEP. The CDC has published guidelines for management of HIV-exposed health care workers. Multiple factors are taken into consideration in deciding whether to initiate PEP. Basic and extended regimens may be considered based on the type of exposure, the volume of the exposure source blood or body fluid, the HIV status of the exposure source, and, if known, the sensitivity of the virus to antiretroviral drugs. There have been reports of PEP failures. The **basic regimen** that is currently recommended involves a 4-week course of two drugs, either zidovudine and lamivudine, stavudine and lamivudine, or stavudine and didanosine. In some cases an **extended regimen** is recommended that adds an additional agent to the basic regimen. Persons taking PEP should be monitored for side effects and drug toxicity. The CDC guidelines stress the importance of institutional protocols for early reporting of exposure to HIV, timely administration of PEP, and recommends that practitioners with expertise in antiretroviral therapy be involved in PEP management.

2.   HBV. Acute HBV hepatitis usually resolves without sequelae. Ten percent of infected individuals become chronic HBV carriers and are at risk of developing chronic active hepatitis, cirrhosis, and hepatocellular carcinoma. The severity and chronicity of infection varies among people; those infected with hepatitis B can remain infectious throughout their lifetime. Approximately 250 health care workers die each year from sequelae of occupationally transmitted HBV infection. Vaccination against hepatitis B is an effective and safe means for preventing hepatitis B infection.

   a.   Transmission of HBV is through percutaneous or mucosal exposure to infected blood or body fluids caused by needlestick and other sharp injury, blood transfusions, sexual contact, or during the perinatal period.

   b.   The occupational risk of HBV is approximately 30% after percutaneous exposure to blood from hepatitis B surface antigen (HBsAg) positive individuals.

   c.   Vaccination against HBV. A recombinant HBV vaccine is recommended for all health care workers having contact with blood or bloody body fluids. The vaccine series consists of three vaccinations over a 6-month period that should be completed before potential contact with contaminated blood or body fluids. Standard vaccination is effective at least 90% of the time. Antibody levels should be checked after completion of the vaccination series. Twenty-five percent of initial nonresponders will respond to repeating the vaccination series.

d. **PEP** may be indicated after exposure to blood or body fluids if the source is known to be HBsAg positive or if the HBsAg state of the source is unknown. The decision depends on the immune statues of the exposed individual. PEP usually involves a combination of passive immunization with hepatitis B immune globulin (HBIG) and active immunization against HBsAg (antibody to HBsAg [anti-HBs]). PEP should be administered as early as possible after exposure. According to the CDC guidelines,

(1) **Previously unvaccinated individuals** should begin the vaccine series in any instance of exposure, regardless of the HBsAg state of the source. If the source is known to be HBsAg positive, HBIG is also recommended in a single dose.

(2) **Vaccinated individuals** should be evaluated for adequacy of anti-HBs response.

(a) Nonresponders (anti-HBs < 10 mIU/mL) are treated with HBIG and, in some cases, revaccinated if the source is known to be HBsAg positive or if the HBsAg status is of the source is unknown and they are believed to be high risk.

(b) Responders (anti-HBs ≥ 10 mIU/mL) require no additional treatment.

3. **HCV.** Health care workers with occupational exposure to blood are at risk of contracting HCV. Chronic HCV infection and chronic hepatitis occur in 85% and 75%, respectively, of those infected with HCV.

a. **Transmission in the hospital setting** generally occurs through large volume or repeated percutaneous exposure to blood, although transmission has been reported through blood splashing into the conjunctivae.

b. **Risk of HCV transmission.** The rate of HCV seroconversion after needlestick or other sharp injury involving infected blood has been reported at 0 to 10%.

c. **Postexposure prophylaxis.** There are not yet guidelines for PEP in HCV. Although interferon is approved for treatment of chronic hepatitis C, it has not been extensively studied as a prophylactic agent and is not recommended for PEP.

4. **Herpes simplex viruses (HSV) I and II**

a. **Transmission of HSV** is via direct contact between an infected individual or infected secretions and mucosa or damaged skin. HSV can be shed by asymptomatic individuals. HSV can be transmitted by health care workers.

b. **Herpetic whitlow** is HSV infection of the finger and can be caused by occupational exposure to HSV I or HSV II. Lesions are painful and inflamed and may be accompanied by fever and localized lymphadenopathy. Anesthetists may acquire herpetic whitlow (primarily HSV I) through contact with oral secretions of an infected source. Persons with active herpetic whitlow can transmit HSV and should avoid contact with patients during the period of transmissibility.

5. **Cytomegalovirus (CMV)** is a herpesvirus. Although usually asymptomatic, certain situations predispose to life-threatening CMV infection, including infections that occur *in utero* and in hosts that are severely ill or are immunocompromised.

Infection can result from reactivation of latent infection lying dormant in the host and from exposure to an external source such as a blood transfusion or organ transplantation.

a.   Transmission occurs via direct contact between the susceptible host and the infected source and through blood transfusion or transplantation of infected organs.

b.   Blood products commonly contain CMV. To reduce the chance of CMV transmission, CMV-negative immunosuppressed patients and CMV-negative parturients should receive blood from CMV-seronegative donors if transfusion is necessary.

6.   VZV causes chickenpox and herpes zoster (shingles).

a.   Transmission. VZV is highly contagious and is spread through direct contact or through airborne routes via respiratory secretions. Anesthetists may be exposed to VZV when caring for patients with primary infection or who have shingles. Infected health care workers can transmit VZV to other health care workers and to patients.

b.   Infection is extremely common in children who generally have an uncomplicated course. Severe infection can occur in adults and in immunocompromised persons. Infection during pregnancy can have disastrous effects on the fetus.

c.   Nonimmune health care workers that are likely to be in contact with high-risk patients should receive VZV vaccination. They should not have patient contact during the contagious stage of active infection and should not have direct patient contact between 10 and 21 days after significant exposure to active VZV.

7.   Influenza virus outbreaks occur annually. Influenza virus causes more severe manifestations than most other viral respiratory infections. Generally, infection is not life threatening, but there are roughly 20,000 deaths attributable to influenzae virus every year. Severe infections most often occur in elderly, debilitated, and chronically ill persons.

a.   Transmission. Influenza virus spreads through viral-containing droplets that are produced by coughing or sneezing. Anesthetist may acquire and then spread influenza virus because of their close involvement with respiratory secretions.

b.   Annual vaccination is recommended for health care workers caring for patients that are at risk of severe influenza-related complications.

8.   Prion diseases, such as **Creutzfeldt-Jakob disease** and **kuru**, are caused by an unusual group of protein-containing infectious particles. Prions can cause slowly progressive fatal neurodegenerative disorders. **Transmission** appears to result from direct inoculation of infected material into a host. There are numerous reports of transmission through transplantation of dura. The long incubation time has made epidemiologic evaluation of the occupational risk of these diseases difficult. Nevertheless, the **risk of transmission to health care workers is believed to be low**, and there have been no reports of transmission via transfused blood. In addition to the universal precautions that apply to all patients, reusable equipment (such as laryngoscopes) should be completely sterilized before reuse.

B. Bacteria
   1. MTB causes tuberculosis. MTB infection usually is localized to the lungs but can also disseminate and cause extrapulmonary disease. Tuberculosis infection frequently is asymptomatic
   and the bacteria become inactive. Nevertheless, the bacteria
   remain alive and can eventually become active and cause disease. Generally, active disease occurs in patients that are chronically ill, debilitated, or immunocompromised. The incidence of
   tuberculosis infection has increased recently, and antibiotic-resistant strains have become more problematic.
      a. Transmission is through inhalation of aerosolized MTB-
      containing droplets that are suspended in the air after an in-
      fected host coughs, sneezes, or talks. Health care workers
      that routinely deal with respiratory secretions are at signifi-
      cant risk for contracting MTB, particularly from patients in
      whom the diagnosis is not yet suspected.
      b. Preventing transmission
         (1) Respiratory precautions should be used in all cases
         of known or suspected tuberculosis until it is confirmed
         that the sputum does not contain acid-fast bacilli.
         **(2) Health care workers should be routinely
         screened for tuberculosis** using skin testing. Recent con-
         version can be treated with isoniazid.
         (3) Specialized face masks (respirators) should be
         worn. These are designed to filter out very small particles
         (see section II.C.3.a).
   2. Antibiotic-resistant bacteria have become a major problem in hospitalized patients and often severely limits the treatment options for serious bacterial infections. Frequent and prolonged use of antibiotics has contributed significantly to their
   emergence.
      a. Transmission can occur through physical contact with
      contaminated health care workers or equipment.
      b. MRSA and VRE require contact precautions that should
      be maintained throughout their time in the OR and PACU.
IV. Antibiotics in the OR
Tables 7-1 and 7-2 include guidelines for perioperative prophylaxis
against surgical wound infections and endocarditis.
   A. Indications for antibiotics in the OR
      1. Prophylaxis against surgical wound infections and endo-
      carditis.
      2. Continuation of treatment for active infection.
   B. Basic principals of antibiotic prophylaxis
      1. Guidelines for routine perioperative antibiotic prophylaxis
      are summarized in Table 7-1.
      2. Indications for antibiotic prophylaxis include surgical pro-
      cedures with a high risk of postoperative infection, procedures
      involving implantation of foreign materials, and if the conse-
      quences of postoperative infection would be disastrous. Prophy-
      lactic antibiotics are not necessary for all surgical procedures
      in all patients.
      **3. Timing and duration of perioperative antibiotics are
      extremely important.**
         a. Preoperative intravenous antibiotics should be given

Table 7-1. Partners Healthcare System Infection Control Unit guidelines for routine perioperative antibiotic prophylaxis for procedures involving incision of skin or mucosa

Procedure or Site	Preoperative Antibiotic	For Allergy[a]	Postoperative Antibiotic
Appendix or esophagus	Cefazolin 1 g and metronidazole 500 mg	#1	Same q8h × 2
Colon or rectum	2 d and 1 d before surgery: oral neomycin 500 mg and erythromycin base 250 mg at 7 a.m., 12 noon, 6 p.m., and bedtime and Preop: cefazolin 1 g and metronidazole 500 mg	#1	Cefazolin 1 g and metronidazole 500 mg q8h × 2
Biliary tract or other gastrointestinal	Cefazolin 1 g	#1	Cefazolin q8h × 2
Open gynecologic	Cefazolin 1 g	#1	Cefazolin q8h × 2
Thoracic or head and neck	Cefazolin 1 g when procedure involves the oropharynx or esophagus add metronidazole 500 mg	#3	None
Cardiac	Cefazolin 1 g[b]	#3	Cefazolin q8h × 3–5
Vascular	Cefazolin 1 g	#3	Cefazolin q8h × 3–5

Neurosurgery	Cefazolin 1 g	#2	Cefazolin q8h × 2
Orthopedic (includes joint replacement and other procedures)	Cefazolin 1 g	#3	Cefazolin q8h × 2
Plastic	Cefazolin 1 g	#3	None
Breast	Cefazolin 1 g	#3	None
Pacemaker/AICD insertion	Cefazolin 1 g	#3	None
Other clean surgery	Cefazolin 1 g at surgeon's direction	#3	None
Genitourinary			
TURP, sterile urine	None		
Open surgery, sterile urine	Cefazolin 1 g	#2	Cefazolin q8h × 2

AICD, automatic implantable cardioverter/defibrillator; TURP, transurethral resection of prostate.

Prophylaxis should be given shortly before the start of surgery. The drug should be redosed if the elapsed time from the start of administration until incision is more than 90 minutes for cefazolin or 150 minutes for vancomycin. Intraoperative redosing: Cefazolin should be redosed every 4 h intraoperatively. Vancomycin should be redosed after 8 h intraoperatively. Patients with open wounds and those at risk for endocarditis may require additional antibiotic therapy. Patients undergoing genitourinary surgery who have nonsterile urine require additional therapy. Patients at extremes of weight and age and those with abnormal renal or hepatic function may require alterations of dose or frequency. All doses are intravenous, except where noted.

[a]For allergy to cephalosporins or history of immediate type hypersensitivity, exfoliation, or other life-threatening reaction to penicillin: 1, Clindamycin 600 mg q8h and gentamicin 5 mg/kg ×1; 2, Vancomycin 1,000 mg q12h and gentamicin 5 mg/kg ×1; 3, Vancomycin 1,000 mg preoperative dose; if postoperative dosing is indicated, then repeat q12h × 3–5 doses.

[b]For prosthetic valve surgery, vancomycin may be substituted for cefazolin. Use 1 g, repeat q12 h × 3–5 doses

Table 7-2.   Endocarditis prophylaxis regimens recommended by the American Heart Association for dental and surgical procedures

Surgical Site	Endocarditis Risk	Standard Regimen		Alternative for Penicillin Allergy[b]	
		Antibiotic (Route)	Dose[a] and Timing Relative to Surgery	Antibiotic (Route)	Dose[b] and Timing Relative to Surgery
Mouth; Pharynx; resp. tract; esophagus	High and moderate	Amoxicillin (PO)	Adults: 2 g Children: 50 mg/kg 1 h before	Clindamycin (PO)	Adults: 600 mg Children: 20 mg/kg 1 h before
				Cephalexin or cefadroxil (PO)	Adults: 2 g Children: 50 mg/kg 1 h before
				Azithromycin or clarithromycin (PO)	Adults: 500 mg Children: 15 mg/kg 1 h before
		Ampicillin[c] (IV or IM)	Adults: 2 g Children: 50 mg/kg Within 30 min before	Clindamycin (IV)	Adults: 600 mg Children: 20 mg/kg Within 30 min before
				Cefazolin (IV)	Adults: 1 g Children: 25 mg/kg Within 30 min before

Site	Risk	Agent	Regimen[a]	Alternative agent	Alternative regimen
GU tract, GI tract other than esophagus	High	Ampicillin (IV) and gentamicin (IV)	Adults: ampicillin 2 g, gentamicin 1.5 mg/kg (up to 120 mg) Children: ampicillin 50 mg/kg, gentamicin 1.5 mg/kg (up to 120 mg) Within 30 min before; second dose of ampicillin recommended 6 h after initial dose[d]	Vancomycin (IV) and gentamicin (IV or IM)	Adults: vancomycin 1 g, gentamicin 1.5 mg/kg (up to 120 mg) Children: vancomycin 20 mg/kg, gentamicin 1.5 mg/kg (up to 120 mg) Complete within 30 min before; administer vancomycin over 1–2 h
GU tract; GI tract (other than esophagus)	Moderate	Amoxicillin (PO)	Adults: 2 g Children: 50 mg/kg 1 h before	Vancomycin (IV)	Adults: 1 g Children: 20 mg/kg Complete within 30 min before; administer vancomycin over 1–2 h
		Ampicillin (IV)	Adults: 2 g Children: 50 mg/kg Within 30 min before		

GI, gastrointestinal; GU, genitourinary.
[a] Maximum dose for children = adult dose.
[b] Cephalosporins should not be used if there is a history of anaphylaxis, urticaria, or angioedema with penicillins.
[c] For patients unable to take PO prophylaxis.
[d] Second dose of amoxicillin (adults; 1 g; children, 25 mg/kg) or ampicillin (adults, 25 mg/kg) recommended 6 h after the initial dose.

within 30 to 60 minutes of incision to ensure adequate levels at the time of incision.

b.   Repeated intraoperative dosing should be considered for longer surgeries. For example, cefazolin often is administered every 4 hours in the OR, particularly when surgery is accompanied by large blood losses and volume requirements.

c.   Postoperatively, antibiotics usually are continued for 24 to 48 hours. Prolonged administration is not recommended because of lack of benefit and the risk of colonization and subsequent infection with antibiotic-resistant bacteria.

4.   Antibiotics may have adverse effects that impact on anesthetic care and postoperative course.

a.   Hypersensitivity reactions can occur with virtually any class of antibiotic and can vary in severity from rash to anaphylaxis.

b.   Hypotension may occur because of histamine release (e.g., vancomycin) or anaphylaxis.

c.   Neuromuscular blockade and potentiation of neuromuscular blocking drugs can occur with aminoglycosides, clindamycin, lincomycin, polymyxins, and tetracyclines. Rarely, profound and prolonged weakness of the respiratory muscles can occur.

d.   Hypernatremia can be produced from the large sodium load associated with administration of penicillin derivatives such as ticarcillin and piperacillin.

e.   Nephrotoxicity (e.g., aminoglycosides) and **ototoxicity** (e.g., aminoglycosides and vancomycin) can occur.

f.   Bleeding can occur because of platelet dysfunction (e.g., ticarcillin, piperacillin) or impaired production of vitamin K-dependent clotting factors (e.g., cefotetan).

5.   Rate of infusion. Some antibiotics can be rapidly administered without difficulty. Others, such as vancomycin and aminoglycosides, should be given more slowly to prevent adverse effects.

C.   Postoperative surgical infections. Many factors influence the development and severity of postoperative infections. Prophylactic measures are effective in preventing wound infections. Bacteria that cause wound infections reflect the site of origin of the infection and are altered by recent treatment with antibiotics, prolonged preoperative hospitalization, and coexisting diseases. Severe wound infections that occur in the first 48 hours after surgery can be caused by *Clostridium* or group A streptococcus (*Streptococcus pyogenes*), which can require emergent surgical debridement in addition to intensive antibiotic therapy.

1.   Surgical wound classifications may be helpful in guiding antibiotic therapy.

a.   Clean. No entry into internal organs that harbor bacteria. Clean surgical wound infections are most often caused by aerobic gram-positive bacteria that colonize the skin, such as *S. aureus*, coagulase-negative *Staphylococcus*, and *Streptococcus* spp.

b.   Contaminated. Bacteria causing contaminated wound infections reflect the origin of contamination (respiratory, gastrointestinal [GI], or genitourinary tract) and often include

enteric gram-negative bacteria and anaerobic bacteria such as *Bacteroides*.
(1) **Clean-contaminated**. Organs are entered in elective surgery without spillage of contents.
(2) **Contaminated**. Spillage of organ contents occurs without formation of pus.
(3) **Dirty**. Pus formation occurring with spillage of organ contents.
2. Pathogens. Infections after "clean" surgeries tend to be caused by gram-positive bacteria, such as *S. aureus* and streptococci. Infections after "contaminated surgeries" may be polymicrobial, involving aerobic and anaerobic gram-positive and gram-negative bacteria. Many factors influence the colonizing flora, including length of hospitalization, use of antacids and histamine-2 blockers, recent use of antibiotics, GI dysmotility or obstruction, and the immune status of the host.
D. Commonly used antibiotics
1. β-Lactams include **penicillins**, **cephalosporins**, carbapenems (such as imipenem/cilastatin), and monobactams (such as aztreonam).
a. Cefazolin is a first-generation cephalosporin that is widely used for prophylaxis because it is active against most gram-positive and many gram-negative bacteria that are likely to cause infections of clean wounds in the early postoperative period. Second-generation cephalosporins, such as **cefoxitin** and **cefotetan**, provide additional gram-negative and anaerobic coverage and are sometimes used for "contaminated" surgeries, particularly those involving the GI tract. Third-generation cephalosporins, such as **ceftriaxone** and **ceftazidime**, are used infrequently in the OR and are usually administered as continuation of treatment for a known or suspected gram-negative bacterial infection. **Penicillin** often is used as prophylaxis for dental surgery.
b. Adverse reactions
(1) **Hypersensitivity reactions** ranging from rash to anaphylaxis. Five percent to 10% of patients with a history of allergy to penicillin are allergic to cephalosporins.
(2) **Bleeding** (see section IV.B.4.f).
(3) **Volume overload or hypernatremia** (see section IV.B.4.d).
(4) **Interstitial nephritis** (especially nafcillin).
(5) **Central nervous system toxicity**.
2. Vancomycin is used as an alternative to β-lactams in allergic patients or in those colonized with antibiotic-resistant gram-positive bacteria such as MRSA. Additional antibiotics are required if coverage of gram-negative organisms is needed.
a. Adverse reactions
(1) **Red man syndrome** is characterized by flushing of the face, neck, and trunk and variable degrees of hypotension. It results from histamine release and is not allergic in nature. Red man syndrome can be minimized by delivering the drug in a large volume and slowing the rate of infusion.
(2) **Hypersensitivity reactions** ranging from rash to anaphylaxis.
(3) **Ototoxicity** can be permanent and occurs more fre-

quently in patients receiving vancomycin and an aminoglycoside. High peak plasma drug levels have been implicated in the occurrence of ototoxicity.

(4) Nephrotoxicity used to be a major concern with vancomycin but does not appear to be significant with current preparations.

b. **Vancomycin-resistant gram-positive bacteria** (such as VRE) have become a problematic consequence of vancomycin therapy. Although *Enterococcus* spp. generally are not pathogenic, they have emerged as nosocomial pathogens that can cause significant infection in debilitated critically ill patients. Of great concern is the possibility that vancomycin resistance will emerge in more virulent gram-positive bacteria. Such concerns are validated by multiple recent reports of MRSA with decreased susceptibility to vancomycin (vancomycin-intermediate *S. aureus*).

3. **Aminoglycosides**. In the OR aminoglycosides are sometimes used in combination with other agents, such as a β-lactam and an antianaerobic agent, particularly when there has been spillage of bowel contents due to perforation. Aminoglycosides are active against gram-negative bacteria and are sometimes used in conjunction with vancomycin or a β-lactam for synergistic coverage of serious gram-positive infection such as endocarditis due to *S. aureus* or *Enterococcus*.

a. **Adverse reactions**

(1) Nephrotoxicity is the most common adverse effect and is generally mild, nonoliguric, and reversible. Risk factors include advanced age, debilitation, baseline renal insufficiency, hypotension, hypovolemia, and concomitant administration of other nephrotoxins such as intravenous contrast agents.

(2) Ototoxicity, with damage to inner ear components and the eighth cranial nerve, can produce vertigo and deafness. High peak plasma drug levels appear to increase the risk for ototoxicity. Slow rates of administration have been suggested to potentially decrease the risk.

(3) Weakness and potentiation of neuromuscular blockade (see section IV.B.4.c).

4. **Clindamycin** sometimes is used for prophylaxis in head and neck surgery or as an alternative to β-lactams in patients that are allergic. Clindamycin is active against most anaerobes and gram-positive aerobes. **Adverse reactions** include GI upset, rash, and elevated liver enzymes. Clindamycin is notorious as a cause of *Clostridium difficile* colitis.

5. **Metronidazole** sometimes is used in combination with other agents, such as a β-lactam and an aminoglycoside, particularly when there has been spillage of bowel contents. Metronidazole is only active against anaerobic bacteria. **Adverse reactions** are uncommon and include GI symptoms (metallic taste, anorexia, nausea) and neurologic dysfunction (peripheral neuropathy, seizures, ataxia, vertigo).

V. **Miscellaneous considerations**

A. **Aspiration pneumonia**

1. **Infectious and noninfectious complications** can result from aspiration during induction and intubation or at other

times in the perioperative period. Distinguishing noninfectious from infectious complications is important in determining the treatment plan and deciding whether to administer antibiotics.

   a. **Aspiration pneumonitis** (Mendelson syndrome) is a **noninfectious** chemical pneumonitis caused by aspiration of sterile gastric contents.

   b. **Aspiration pneumonia** is an infectious process resulting from aspiration of oropharyngeal or nonsterile gastric secretions that contain pathogenic bacteria. The chest radiograph often shows an infiltrate in dependent portions of the lung (often the right lower lobe).

2. **Microbiology.** Aspiration pneumonia is caused by gram-positive bacteria such as *S. aureus*, gram-negative bacteria such as *Pseudomonas aeruginosa, Escherichia coli, Klebsiella pneumoniae*, and sometimes anaerobes.

3. **Risk factors for development of aspiration pneumonia** include large volume aspiration, impaired immunity, colonization of oropharyngeal secretions with pathogenic bacteria, and poor dentition (lower likelihood in edentulous individuals).

4. **Antibiotics and aspiration.** Unnecessary use of antibiotics should be avoided to decrease the chance of colonization with antibiotic-resistant bacteria.

   a. Antibiotics should not be included routinely in the initial management of **witnessed aspiration of gastric contents**. Exceptions include situations that predispose to colonization of the usually sterile stomach, such as intestinal obstruction and antacid or histamine-2 receptor blocker use. Antibiotics should be considered if pneumonitis fails to improve after 48 hours.

   b. **Antibiotics are indicated for aspiration pneumonia**. The choice of antibiotics depends on multiple factors, including the presence of periodontal disease, antibiotic allergies, and recent antibiotic therapy. Initial therapy targets gram-negative and gram-positive bacteria and possibly anaerobic bacteria. Subsequent antibiotic choice should be guided by Gram stain and culture of lower respiratory tract secretions.

B. **Endocarditis.** Patients with congenital and acquired cardiac abnormalities are at risk for developing infective endocarditis after certain surgical and dental procedures and may require perioperative antibiotic endocarditis prophylaxis.

1. **Risk of postoperative endocarditis.** Endocarditis is an uncommon disease and very few cases of bacterial endocarditis are caused by surgery.

2. **Endocarditis prophylaxis.** The American Heart Association has published guidelines for endocarditis prophylaxis that include risk stratification based on the underlying cardiac abnormality and the surgical or dental procedure being performed (Table 7-2).

3. **The risk of endocarditis** depends on the cardiac abnormality.

   a. **High risk (prophylaxis recommended)** conditions include prosthetic valve, complex congenital heart disease, surgically placed systemic pulmonary shunts and conduits, and prior endocarditis.

b.   Moderate risk (prophylaxis recommended) conditions include less complex congenital heart disease (e.g., coarctation of the aorta), bicuspid aortic valve, acquired valvular disease, hypertrophic cardiomyopathy, and mitral valve prolapse with regurgitation.

c.   Negligible risk (not greater than the general population, routine prophylaxis not recommended) conditions include less complex congenital heart disease such as isolated secundum atrial septal defect, mitral valve prolapse without regurgitation, cardiac pacemakers and defibrillators, and innocent heart murmurs.

4.   Bacterial pathogens in postoperative endocarditis include *Streptoccocus*, *Staphylococcus*, and *Enterococcus*.

5.   Endocarditis prophylaxis is recommended for procedures that cause bacteremia. Provided that the skin has been appropriately cleaned before incision, surgeries that do not invade viscera or cross mucosal barriers do not produce significant bacteremia. Bacteremia occurs with many procedures that cross mucosal barriers or enter an internal viscus such as the GI tract. Antibiotic prophylaxis is recommended for dental and intraoral procedures that may result in significant bleeding such as dental extractions, periodontal surgery, root canal work, and placement of dental implants.

C.   Immunocompromised patients are at increased risk of community-acquired, nosocomial, and opportunistic infections. **Causes of immunocompromise** include immunosuppressive therapy such as for solid organ and bone marrow transplants, burns, malignancy, HIV infection, chemotherapy, corticosteroids, and severe malnutrition.

1.   Elective surgery should be delayed, if possible, in patients that are severely immunocompromised (such as total neutrophil count < 500 cells/mm^3).

2.   Personnel with respiratory infections should not be involved in the care of severely immunocompromised patients. If this is not possible, then the provider should wear a surgical mask during contact with the patient.

3.   Careful adherence to sterile technique is extremely important in preventing line-related and other infections.

4.   Antibiotic prophylaxis is used in organ transplant recipients for short-term prophylaxis against postoperative wound infection and for long-term prevention of opportunistic infections. Some antibiotics have significant interactions with immunosuppressive agents. In particular, cyclosporine metabolism may be altered (with fluoroquinolones, erythromycin, fluconazole, rifampin, isoniazid) and toxicity increased (with aminoglycosides, amphotericin B, vancomycin, pentamidine, high-dose trimethoprim/sulfamethoxazole) by concomitant administration of various antibiotics. Cyclosporine levels should be monitored in patients receiving these agents.

5.   It may be appropriate for severely immunocompromised patients to wear masks during transport.

SUGGESTED READING

Cardo DM, Culver DH, Ciesielski CA, et al. A case-control study of HIV seroconversion in health care workers after percutaneous exposure. *N Engl J Med* 1997;337:1485–1490.

Centers for Disease Control. Guidelines for preventing the transmission of *Mycobacterium tuberculosis* in health-care facilities, 1994. *MMWR Morb Mortal Wkly Rep* 1994;43:1–132.

Centers for Disease Control and Prevention. Immunization of health-care workers. *MMWR Morb Mortal Wkly Rep* 1997;46:1–42.

Centers for Disease Control and Prevention. Recommendations for prevention and control of hepatitis C virus (HCV) infection and HCV-related chronic disease. *MMWR Morb Mortal Wkly Rep* 1998;47:1–15.

Centers for Disease Control and Prevention. Updated US Public Health Service guidelines for the management of occupational exposures to HBV, HCV, and HIV and recommendations for postexposure prophylaxis. *MMWR Morb Mortal Wkly Rep* 2001;50(RR11):1–42.

Cheng EY, Numphius N, Hennen CR. Antibiotic therapy and the anesthesiologist. *J Clin Anesth* 1995;7:425–439.

Dajani AS, Taubert KA, Wilson W, et al. Prevention of bacterial endocarditis: recommendations by the American Heart Association. *JAMA* 1997; 277:1794–1801.

Ludwig KA, Carlson MA, Condon RE. Prophylactic antibiotics in surgery. *Annu Rev Med* 1993;44:385–393.

Marik PE. Aspiration pneumonitis and aspiration pneumonia. *N Engl J Med* 2001;344:665–671.

Moran GJ. Emergency department management of blood and body fluid exposures. *Ann Emerg Med* 2000;35:47–62.

Osmon DR. Antimicrobial prophylaxis in adults. *Mayo Clin Proc* 2000; 75:98–109.

II

Administration of Anesthesia

8

Safety in Anesthesia

Jeffrey B. Cooper

I. The risk of anesthesia

A. There is no accurate measure of the overall risk of anesthesia nor can the risk to an individual patient be predicted.

1. In the 1950s it was estimated that anesthesia care contributed to three deaths in 10,000 surgical procedures. More recent data suggest that the figure may be on the order of one per 10,000, but these estimates are speculative because control of the conditions is impossible.

2. Mortality rates for healthy patients (American Society of Anesthesiologists [ASA] classes 1 and 2) may be on the order of one in 100,000 from extrapolation of studies in the United Kingdom and Australia. Higher risk patients undergoing increasingly complex surgical interventions are more likely to be affected by adverse outcomes.

3. Additional patients suffer serious and costly nonfatal injuries such as permanent neurologic damage.

4. Although anesthesiology is recognized as a leading specialty in patient safety and adverse outcomes have been markedly reduced, the risks of anesthesia remain substantial. Past successful efforts to promote safety and reduce preventable deaths and injuries must be maintained and strengthened.

B. Seventy percent of accidents during anesthesia can be attributed to some level of human error compounded by a systems failure.

1. At least half of these events could have been prevented and may have resulted from deviations from accepted anesthesia practices.

2. There is rarely one cause leading to accidents. Most evolve from one or more trigger events, complicated by a systems failure, that is, a breakdown in the system of checks and balances required for the smooth operation of the system. The accepted approach to accident prevention now focuses on flaws in the system rather than on flaws in the operator.

3. The number of near mishaps is at least several times more prevalent than the number of events that result in injury. These "near-miss" events are an indicator of the overall safety of the system.

4. Adverse outcomes are not reported uniformly but are usually attributed to hypovolemia, hypoxia, hypotension, hypoventilation, airway obstruction, drug overdose, aspiration, or inadequate preparation, supervision, or crisis management.

C. Vigilance and attention to detail are essential for a safely conducted anesthetic. Coordinating different cognitive levels (thinking vs. doing) and managing many problems simultaneously are essential parts of dynamic decision making and distinguish the competent from the expert clinician.

D. Serious mishaps typically are the result of a combination of lapses in vigilance and judgment errors, which may be triggered by the interactions of the patient, the equipment, the anesthetist, the surgeon, and the environment (Fig. 8-1). These factors can combine to obscure the prompt detection or the appropriate correction of a problem. Disorderly personal routines, disorganized workspace ergonomics, and faulty or intermittent charting can contribute to accidents.

II. General safety strategies

A. Prepare a preoperative plan. Construct a sound anesthesia plan (including prioritization of goals, planned interruption points, and contingencies for crisis); become familiar with the procedure, equipment, and anesthetic technique; prepare the patient; prepare the workspace (including ergonomic considerations of maneuverability, unobstructed visual field, and access to patient and machine); check backup equipment; and label all medications (double-checking labels and concentrations). Know the location of emergency supplies and equipment.

B. Develop situational awareness. Arrange equipment and appropriate monitors in a way that facilitates scanning of monitors, the surgical field, and the operating room (drains, suctions, towel count, blood products, etc.). Constantly assess the "big picture," follow and construct "mental maps" of the different possible outcomes.

C. Enhance teamwork; communicate. Teamwork enhances safety and may be critical for prevention of or recovery from a critical situation. A healthy team has mutual collegial respect; the members share tasks, goals, and key information to enable all to do their jobs well. To enhance teamwork and communicate effectively, address surgeons and nurses early in the case by knowing names and establishing eye contact. Make requests and delegate tasks clearly and specifically by name; request verbal confirmation (e.g., "Jack, give 1 mg of epinephrine." "Got it—1 mg epinephrine coming" or "1 mg epinephrine given"). Delegate tasks to those who can best perform them. Never assume without confirmation that crucial interventions or medications have been given as planned.

D. Compensate for stressors. Recognize conditions that decrease performance: production pressure, noise, low ambient temperature, low light levels, long hours, fatigue, boredom, illness, hunger, and interpersonal tension (e.g., uncooperative colleagues, nurses, or staff). When possible, change the temperature in the room, ask for the noise to be reduced, get needed illumination, and ask for relief when needed. If you feel tired, you are probably more tired than you think. To compensate, ask for relief breaks more often during the case, particularly when you are ill. If you are unable to finish the case, ask to be relieved.

E. Verify observations. Repeat observations, cross-check with redundant systems (e.g., check heart rate with both the electrocardiogram and with pulse or pulse oximeter), check covarying variables (e.g., expect a concomitant change in heart rate with an increase in blood pressue), and review the situation with a second person.

F. Implement compensatory responses. React to a developing problem by implementing time-buying measures until a more

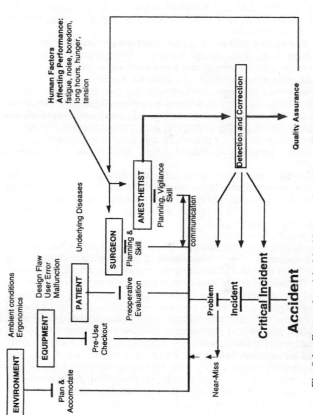

Fig. 8-1. Factors in critical incidents and accidents. (Modified from Gaba DM. Human error in anesthetic mishaps. *Int Anesth Clin* 1989; 27(3):137–147, with permission.)

definitive solution of the problem is found (e.g., increase the fraction of inspired oxygen when oxygen saturation falls; administer intravenous fluids when hypotension occurs).

G. Prepare for crisis. Be prepared for critical events. Be proactive, plan for contingencies, and be prepared to revise the plan. **Calling for help is an appropriate response when confronted with potentially overwhelming circumstances.** Learn to call for help early, because it may not be available immediately. Review, practice, and use accepted protocols for emergencies and resuscitation (e.g., Advanced Cardiac Life Support, malignant hyperthermia protocols).

H. Recognize and address production pressures, time constraints (e.g., preventing adequate preoperative evaluation, preparation, monitoring), and **economic constraints** (e.g., mitigating against cancellation of a case for medical reasons). If you feel uncertain about proceeding with the case or that it is unsafe to anesthetize the patient, address your concerns to anesthesia and surgical colleagues. Pressure to put efficiency and output ahead of safety has caused catastrophic accidents in various industries. Despite overt or covert pressures and incentives on personnel to emphasize production, patient safety must remain the highest priority.

I. Learn from close calls. An event that nearly results in an adverse outcome should be used to improve future performance under similar circumstances. Every mistake is an opportunity to learn and improve. Report such events via your department's quality assurance mechanism.

III. Quality assurance

Quality assurance programs take many different forms but must include a spectrum of activities aimed at maintaining and improving the quality of care and minimizing the risk of injury from anesthesia.

A. Documentation. An incident report is completed for any unusual occurrence or unforeseen outcome, especially if follow-up action may be required to prevent recurrence. The report should include the relevant facts and document unanticipated outcomes, avoiding judgmental statements. Incidents are reviewed by the departmental quality assurance committee, which receives additional information from those involved in the event and may suggest remedial steps as systematic factors are identified. Cases with special educational value should be presented at departmental case conferences. There should be an ongoing analysis and feedback of adverse events (actual and near-miss events) to identify and assess system problems and developing patterns.

B. The postoperative visit by the anesthesiologist is a key component of quality care and is required by the Joint Commission on Accreditation of Healthcare Organizations. The discussion should address the overall well-being of the patient and focus on the efficacy of pain and anxiety management, symptoms of postoperative nausea, and possible intraoperative awareness. The visit should be documented in the chart.

C. Standards and guidelines. Departments should develop safety policies appropriate to local practices; policies should be readily available. These should include, but not be limited to, those for monitoring, postanesthesia care units, response to an adverse event, relief protocol, and resuscitation protocols. Developing preoperative testing consensus guidelines and criteria for safe and timely surgical intervention could reduce production pressures. The website of the American Society of Anesthesiologists contains many such standards and guidelines (www.asahq.org).

D. Safety training. Training in safety of various forms is necessary to teach and maintain basic skills and for developing and nurturing a culture of safety. Such training should include the following:

1. **Basic environmental safety.** Fire and evacuation, electrical safety (see Chapter 18), and prevention and avoidance of cross-infection (see Chapter 7).

2. **Crisis management skills.** Including but not limited to the following: Advanced Cardiac Life Support, Advanced Trauma Life Support, Pediatric Advanced Life Support, Anesthesia Crisis Resource Management.

3. **Simulators.** Realistic simulation environments are used to train and educate operating room personnel in basic skills management of critical events and other topics.

E. Anesthesia Crisis Resource Management is used to train in generic skills of managing critical events. It stresses role clarity (e.g., leadership, followership), communication (clarity of directions, closing the loop of instructions), resource management (e.g., allocating personnel, time, and equipment), appropriate use of support (e.g., task delegation, assignment of responsibilities, priority assessment, monitoring and cross-checking of information), and global assessment (e.g., avoiding fixation errors, maintaining situational awareness).

F. Safety is a function of an institution's work culture; it should be an integral part of the evaluation of an organization's quality and outcomes. Prevention of most errors lies outside the direct control of a system's managers. The chain of responsibility to prevent incidents may be long and complex, so the entire system needs to be addressed. **A constant commitment to safety, including the presence of redundant systems, continuous training, and a dedication to learning from mistakes, is needed in an organization's culture.**

IV. Standards and protocols

A. American Society of Anesthesiologists' standards for basic anesthetic monitoring (approved by House of Delegates on October 21, 1986 and last amended on October 21, 1998; effective July 1, 1999). These standards apply to all anesthesia care, although in emergency circumstances appropriate life support measures take precedence. These standards may be exceeded at any time based on the judgment of the responsible anesthesiologist. They are intended to encourage quality patient care, but observing them cannot guarantee any specific patient outcome. They are subject to revision from time to time, as warranted by the evolution of technology and practice. They apply to all general anesthetics, regional anesthetics, and monitored anesthesia care. This set of standards addresses only the issue of basic anesthetic monitoring, which is one component of anesthesia care. In certain rare or unusual circumstances, some of these methods of monitoring may be clinically impractical and appropriate use of the described monitoring methods may fail to detect untoward clinical developments. Brief interruptions of continual monitoring may be unavoidable. Note that "continual" is defined as "repeated regularly and frequently in steady rapid succession," whereas "continuous" means "prolonged without any interruption at any time." Under extenuating circumstances, the responsible anesthesiologist may waive the requirements marked with an asterisk (*) below; it is recommended that when this is done, it should be so stated (including the reasons) in a note in the patient's medical record. These standards are not intended for application to the care of the obstetrical patient in labor or in the conduct of pain management.

1.   Qualified anesthesia personnel shall be present in the room throughout the conduct of all general anesthetics, regional anesthetics, and monitored anesthesia care.

a.   Objective. Because of the rapid changes in patient status during anesthesia, qualified anesthesia personnel shall be continuously present to monitor the patient and provide anesthesia care. In the event there is a direct known hazard (e.g., radiation) to the anesthesia personnel, which might require intermittent remote observation of the patient, some provision for monitoring the patient must be made. In the event that an emergency requires the temporary absence of the person primarily responsible for the anesthetic, the best judgment of the anesthesiologist will be exercised in comparing the emergency with the anesthetized patient's condition and in the selection of the person left responsible for the anesthetic during the temporary absence.

2.   During all anesthetics, the patient's oxygenation, ventilation, circulation, and temperature shall be continually evaluated.

a.   Oxygenation

(1)   Objective: To ensure adequate oxygen concentration in the inspired gas and the blood during all anesthetics.

(2)   Methods

(a)   Inspired gas. During every administration of general anesthesia using an anesthesia machine, the concentration of oxygen in the patient breathing system shall be measured by an oxygen analyzer with a low oxygen concentration limit alarm in use.*

(b)   Blood oxygenation. During all anesthetics, a quantitative method of assessing oxygenation such as pulse oximetry shall be used.* Adequate illumination and exposure of the patient are necessary to assess color.*

b.   Ventilation

(1)   Objective: To ensure adequate ventilation of the patient during all anesthetics.

(2)   Methods

(a) Every patient receiving general anesthesia shall have the adequacy of ventilation continually evaluated. Qualitative clinical signs such as chest excursion, observation of the reservoir breathing bag, and auscultation of breath sounds are useful. Continual monitoring for the presence of expired carbon dioxide shall be performed unless invalidated by the nature of the patient, procedure, or equipment. Quantitative monitoring of the volume of expired gas is strongly encouraged.*

(b) When an endotracheal tube or laryngeal mask is

inserted, its correct positioning must be verified by clinical assessment and by identification of carbon dioxide in the expired gas. Continual end-tidal carbon dioxide analysis, in use from the time of endotracheal tube/laryngeal mask placement until extubation/removal or initiating transfer to a postoperative care location, shall be performed using a quantitative method such as capnography, capnometry, or mass spectroscopy.*

(c) When ventilation is controlled by a mechanical ventilator, there shall be in continuous use a device that is capable of detecting disconnection of components of the breathing system. The device must give an audible signal when its alarm threshold is exceeded.

(d) During regional anesthesia and monitored anesthesia care, the adequacy of ventilation shall be evaluated, at least, by continual observation of qualitative clinical signs.

c. Circulation

(1) Objective: To ensure the adequacy of the patient's circulatory function during all anesthetics.

(2) Methods

(a) Every patient receiving anesthesia shall have the electrocardiogram continuously displayed from the beginning of anesthesia until preparing to leave the anesthetizing location.*

(b) Every patient receiving anesthesia shall have arterial blood pressure and heart rate determined and evaluated at least every 5 minutes.*

(c) Every patient receiving general anesthesia shall have, in addition to the above, circulatory function continually evaluated by at least one of the following: palpation of a pulse, auscultation of heart sounds, monitoring of a tracing of intraarterial pressure, ultrasound peripheral pulse monitoring, or pulse plethysmography or oximetry.

d. Body temperature

(1) Objective: To aid in the maintenance of appropriate body temperature during all anesthetics.

(2) Methods. Every patient receiving anesthesia shall have temperature monitored when clinically significant changes in body temperature are intended, anticipated, or suspected.

B. Relief protocol guideline

1. It is the policy at the Massachusetts General Hospital to provide periodic breaks for the primary individuals providing anesthesia. **The decision should be based on the individual's needs, the general caseload, and the timing of the procedure** (weekdays, weeknights, weekends). However, current practice is to afford a 15- to 20-minute break approximately every 2 to 3 hours.

2. Relief should be avoided in short cases and should be used with caution in cases characterized by complexity, that is, where the primary anesthesiologist's intuitive sense of anesthetic management cannot be satisfactorily transferred to another person.

3. When an anesthesiologist is relieved, the record should indicate the time of the change.

4. During a relief changeover, the following information should be relayed before the original anesthesiologist leaves the room:

  a. The clinical situation

    (1) Presentation of the patient's diagnosis, operation, past medical history, allergies, abnormal laboratory values, chest x-ray, and electrocardiogram.

    (2) Description of the anesthetic technique and the reasoning behind it.

  b. Surgical course

    (1) Determination of anesthetic course and the status of the surgical procedure.

    (2) Assessment of blood loss and adequacy of fluid replacement.

    (3) Inspection of intravenous catheters and monitoring lines.

    (4) Present level of anesthesia (lightening or deepening); time at which the patient will need additional medications.

    (5) Inspection of drug administration syringes and containers for drug names and concentrations.

    (6) Determination of current settings of gas flows and anesthetic concentration, readings on the oxygen analyzer, and the cylinder and pipeline supply pressures.

    (7) Measurement of current clinical vital signs.

  c. Anticipated course

    (1) The availability of blood products.

    (2) The anesthetic plan, including fluid and drug therapies.

    (3) Disposition plan for postoperative respiratory and drug support.

C. Guidelines for action following an adverse anesthesia event (abbreviated from Cooper et al. 1993; see Suggested Reading). The following guidelines for action should be used when a patient has died or has been injured from causes suspected to be related to the anesthesia management:

1. The objectives are to limit patient injury from a specific adverse event associated with anesthesia and to ensure that the causes of the event are identified so that a recurrence can be prevented. The activities aim at ensuring care of the patient, preventing loss or alteration of equipment or supplies related to the event, documenting information, informing appropriate personnel, and providing necessary guidance and support to caregivers.

2. The guidelines dictate the responsibilities for the primary anesthesiologist, the incident supervisor (preferably someone other than the primary anesthesiologist[s] involved in the event), the equipment manager, and the follow-up supervisor.

3. The anesthesiologist involved in an adverse event should:

  a. Provide for continuing care of the patient.

  b. Notify the anesthesia operating room administrator (or, if a resident or certified registered nurse anesthetist, the attending staff) as soon as possible.

  c. Not discard supplies or tamper with equipment.

d. Document events in the patient record (including the serial number of the anesthesia machine).
e. Not alter the record.
f. Stay involved with the follow-up care.
g. Contact consultants as needed.
h. Submit a follow-up report.
i. Document continuing care in the patient's record.

SUGGESTED READING

American Society of Anesthesiologists (www.asahq.org), accessed October 22, 2001.

Anesthesia Patient Safety Foundation (www.apsf.org) accessed October 22, 2001.

Beckmann U, Runciman WB. The role of incident reporting in continuous quality improvement in the intensive care setting. *Anaesth Intensive Care* 1996;24:311–313.

Berwick DM. A primer on leading the improvement of systems. *BMJ* 1996;312:619–622.

Bognar SM. *Human error in medicine.* Hillsdale, NJ: Lawrence Erlbaum, 1994.

Cheney FW, Posner K, Caplan RA, et al. Standard of care and anesthesia liability. *JAMA* 1989;261:1599–1603.

Cooper JB, Cullen DJ, Eichhorn JH, et al. Administrative guidelines for response to an adverse anesthesia event. *J Clin Anesth* 1993;5:79–84.

Cooper JB, Gaba DM. A strategy for preventing anesthesia accidents. *Int Anesthesiol Clin* 1989;27:148–152.

Derrington MC, Smith G. A review of studies of anaesthetic risk, morbidity and mortality. *Br J Anaesth* 1987;59:815–833.

Forrest JB, Rehder K, Cahalan MK, et al. Multicenter study of general anesthesia. III. Predictors of severe perioperative adverse outcomes. *Anesthesiology* 1992;76:3–15.

Gaba DM, Fish K, Howard S. *Anesthesia crisis management.* New York: Churchill Livingstone, 1994.

Howard SK, Gaba DM, Fish KJ, et al. Anesthesia crisis resource management training: teaching anesthesiologists to handle critical incidents. *Aviat Space Environ Med* 1992;63:763–770.

Institute for Safe Medication Practice (www.ISMP.org), accessed October 22, 2001.

Keats AS. Anesthesia mortality in perspective. *Anesth Analg* 1990;71:113–119.

Kohn LT, Corrigan JM, Donaldson MS, eds. *To err is human: building a safer healthcare system.* Washington, DC: National Academy Press, 1999.

Leape LL. Error in medicine. *JAMA* 1994;272:1851–1857.

Morrell RC, Eichhorn JH. *Patient safety in anesthetic practice.* New York: Churchill Livingstone, 1997.

National Patient Safety Foundation (www.npsf.org), accessed October 22, 2001.

The Anesthesia Machine

Jane C. Ballantyne

I.   Overview. The function of the anesthesia machine is to prepare a gas mixture of precisely known but variable composition. The
machine provides a controlled flow of oxygen, nitrous oxide, air,
and anesthetic vapors. These are delivered to a breathing system,
which provides a means to deliver positive pressure ventilation and
to control alveolar carbon dioxide by minimizing rebreathing and/or
by absorbing carbon dioxide. A mechanical ventilator is connected to
the breathing system, freeing up the anesthetist's hands for other
tasks. Several types of monitors are used to observe the function of
the system, to detect equipment failures, and to provide information
about the patient.

II.   The gas delivery system (Fig. 9-1)

A.   Gas supplies

1.   Piped gases. Wall outlets supply oxygen nitrous oxide and
air at a pressure of 50 to 55 pounds/in^2 (psi). These outlets and
the supply hoses to the machine are diameter indexed and color-
coded.

2.   Cylinders

a.   A full cylinder (size E) of oxygen has a pressure of
2,000 to 2,200 psi and contains the equivalent of 660 L of gas
at atmospheric pressure and room temperature. The oxygen
cylinder pressure decreases in direct proportion to the
amount of oxygen in the cylinder.

b.   A full cylinder (size E) of nitrous oxide has a pressure
of 745 psi and contains the equivalent of 1,500 L of gas at
atmospheric pressure and room temperature. The nitrous
oxide in the cylinder is a liquid; the cylinder pressure does
not decrease until the liquid content is exhausted, at which
time one-fourth of the total volume of gas remains.

c.   Air cylinders are present on some machines. A full cylinder (size E) has a pressure of 1,800 psi and contains the equivalent of 630 L at atmospheric pressure and room temperature.

d.   Pressure regulators reduce the high pressure from the
cylinders to about 45 psi (just below pipeline pressure) so
that when using cylinder gases adjustments at the rotameter
are not needed to compensate for the changing pressure that
occurs as the cylinders empty. If both cylinders and pipelines
are connected and open, gas flows preferentially from the
pipeline because its pressure is slightly higher than the regulated cylinder pressure. The regulators divide the machine
into high-pressure (proximal to the regulator) and low-pressure (distal to the regulator) systems.

⟶

**Fig. 9-1.   A schematic diagram of an anesthesia machine. There are many
variations in design depending on the vintage and manufacturer.**

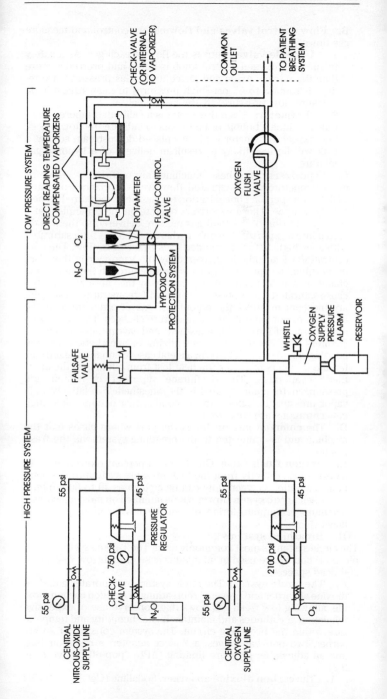

B. Flow control valves and flowmeters control and measure gas flows.

   1. A needle valve controls the flow of each gas. As a safety feature, the oxygen control knob is fluted and protrudes more than the nitrous oxide and air controls. Gas pressures are reduced from 45 to 55 psi (high pressure) to near atmospheric pressure (low pressure) by the needle valves.

   2. Flowmeters. Each flowmeter is a calibrated tapered glass tube in which a bobbin or ball floats to indicate the flow of gas. The oxygen flowmeter is always placed downstream so that a leak will be less likely to result in delivery of a hypoxic gas mixture.

C. Vaporizers. Anesthesia machines are outfitted with one or more temperature-compensated flow-over vaporizers calibrated to deliver a specific concentration of anesthetic measured as percent by volume. These vaporizers operate on the principle that a small proportion of the total gas mixture delivered to them is diverted into a vaporizing chamber where it becomes fully saturated with anesthetic before it is added back to the main flow. The concentration of anesthetic delivered by the vaporizer is therefore proportional to the amount of gas passing through the vaporizing chamber, which is controlled primarily by the vaporizer dial. Because saturated vapor pressure varies with temperature, a secondary mechanism alters the amount of gas diverted through the chamber to compensate for temperature changes. The vaporizers are calibrated for a specific anesthetic and have pin-indexed filling adapters to prevent inadvertent mixing of anesthetics. The vaporizing chamber is enclosed in a metal case to enhance heat transfer and to compensate for the heat lost from cooling as the anesthetic evaporates. The desflurane vaporizer is heated and pressurized to compensate for the anesthetic's relatively high vapor pressure and the extreme cooling that occurs when high concentrations are vaporized.

D. The **common gas outlet** is the port where gases exit the machine and is connected to the breathing system via the fresh gas hose.

E. Oxygen flush valve. One hundred percent oxygen at 45 to 55 psi comes directly from the high pressure system to the common gas outlet. Oxygen flow can be as high as 40 to 60 L/min.

F. A separate **oxygen flowmeter** is mounted on most anesthesia machines for administering oxygen by nasal cannulas or face mask.

III. Breathing systems

The circle system is most commonly used. The T-piece systems (Mapleson D and F) are used in infants because of their low resistance and dead space.

   A. The circle system. The circle system incorporates a carbon dioxide absorber and prevents rebreathing of exhaled carbon dioxide, allowing low fresh gas flows that conserve use of expensive inhalation anesthetics and maintain higher humidity and temperature within the breathing circuit. The system consists of an absorber, two one-way valves, a Y-piece adapter, a reservoir bag, and an adjustable pressure limiting (APL) "pop-off" valve (Fig. 9-2).

     1. The **carbon dioxide absorber**. Sodalime ($CaOH_2$ + NaOH

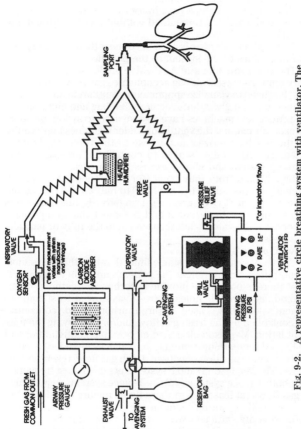

Fig. 9-2. A representative circle breathing system with ventilator. The airway pressure gauge may sense on the patient side of the inspiratory valve. The positive end-expiratory pressure (PEEP) valve may be integral to the ventilator. Other variations are possible depending on the manufacturer.

+ KOH + silica) or Baralyme (Ba[OH]$_2$ + Ca[OH]$_2$) contained in the absorber combines with carbon dioxide, forming CaCO$_2$ and liberating heat and moisture (H$_2$O). A pH-sensitive dye changes to a blue-violet color, indicating exhaustion of the absorbing capacity. The canister should be changed when 25% to 50% of the contents has changed color, although it should continue to absorb satisfactorily until at least the contents of the top canister have changed color.

2.   Two **one-way valves** (inspiratory and expiratory) ensure that exhaled gas is not rebreathed without passing through the carbon dioxide absorber.

3.   The **Y-piece adapter** is used to connect the inspiratory and expiratory sides of the system to the patient.

4.   The **reservoir bag and APL valve** are located on the expiratory limb. The reservoir bag accumulates gas between inspirations. It is used to visualize spontaneous ventilation and to assist ventilation manually. Adults require a 3-L bag and children a 2-L bag. Most new machines have a valve used to switch between the reservoir bag and the ventilator. Older machines may require that the bag be removed and a hose to the ventilator be connected. The APL valve is used to control the pressure in the breathing system and allows excess gas to escape. The valve can be adjusted from fully open (for spontaneous ventilation, minimal peak pressure 1 to 3 cm H$_2$O) to fully closed (maximum pressure 75 cm H$_2$O or greater). Dangerously high pressures that can produce barotrauma and hemodynamic compromise may occur if the valve is left unattended in the fully or partially closed position.

B.   The T-piece systems

The T-piece systems are single-limbed rebreathing systems. Fresh gas enters the system at the patient end, thus forming a T. Because there is no carbon dioxide absorber, rebreathing of carbon dioxide is inevitable unless a fresh gas flow at least equal to the patient's peak flow is used. Inspired carbon dioxide concentration is controlled by the fresh gas flow and/or by varying the minute ventilation. Mapleson classified all possible configurations of single-limbed rebreathing systems (the T-pieces included) according to the relative position of patient, fresh gas flow, reservoir bag, and valve. The Mapleson D and F systems are used most frequently and are both T-piece systems. All the T-piece systems require high fresh gas flows (at least two to three times minute ventilation) to prevent rebreathing during spontaneous ventilation. Capnography is useful to verify sufficient washout of carbon dioxide.

1.   The **Mapleson D** circuit is a semiclosed system with a reservoir bag and APL valve at the machine end with fresh gas entering at the patient end (Fig. 9-3).

2.   The **Bain** circuit is a coaxial version of the Mapleson D. The fresh gas delivery tube is a small-diameter uncorrugated tube that runs inside the corrugated wide diameter expiratory limb. Inspired gases are warmed and the system appears simpler, but there is a risk of hypoxia if leaks develop, so the circuit should always be carefully checked for leaks before use.

3.   The **Mapleson F** circuit (Jackson-Rees modification of the Ayres T-piece or Mapleson E) is particularly useful in neonates and small infants. It consists simply of an open-ended reservoir

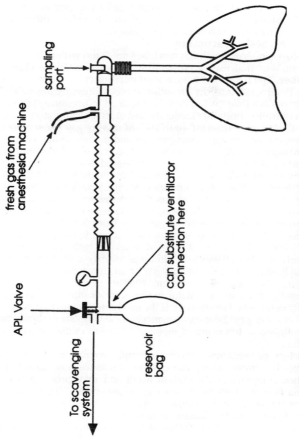

Fig. 9-3. Schematic diagram of a Mapleson D breathing system. In the Bain modification, the fresh gas flows through a tube that runs through the corrugated tubing.

bag and a defined length of corrugated breathing tube, with fresh gas entering the system at the patient end. Manual ventilation of small patients is accomplished well with this system because the anesthetist can adjust the filling of the open-ended reservoir bag with his or her hand, making the bag a sensitive indicator of lung compliance. The system also allows the anesthetist to be close to the infant while manually ventilating. The advantages of this system have been reduced by the introduction of scavenging systems that increase its weight and by improvements in alternative systems (e.g., low compliance breathing tubes and improvements in mechanical ventilators).

IV. Anesthesia ventilators

A. Most modern anesthesia machines are fitted with a mechanical ventilator that uses a **collapsible bellows within a closed chamber**. The bellows is compressed intermittently when oxygen or air is directed into the chamber, thereby pressurizing it. The ventilators are time cycled flow (as opposed to pressure) generators, controlled both mechanically and electronically, and pneumatically driven (requiring 10 to 20 L of driving gas per minute). Ventilator controls vary among makes and models. Some ventilators require setting of minute ventilation, rate, and inspiratory-expiratory (I:E) ratio to produce the desired tidal volume; other ventilators allow direct adjustment of tidal volume, with I:E ratio being dependent on the inspiratory flow rate, which is set independently. A portion of the fresh gas flow delivered by the machine adds to the set tidal volume during the inhalation phase. For example, an increase in total fresh gas flow from 3 to 6 L/min will increase delivered minute ventilation by an additional 1 L/min at an I:E ratio of 1:2 or by 1.5 L/min at an I:E ratio of 1:1 (more inspiratory time in the latter). Although gas-driven ventilators can be safely driven with either oxygen or air, most often oxygen is chosen and is supplied by pipeline. Whether or not cylinder gases are used to drive the ventilator in the event of pipeline failure is usually determined by the user. If the machine is set up to drive the ventilator using cylinder oxygen, mechanical ventilation should be discontinued in the event of pipeline failure to conserve oxygen supplies.

B. **Flow generators** deliver a set tidal volume regardless of changes in patients' compliance (unlike pressure generators) but will not compensate for system leaks and may produce barotrauma because high pressures can be generated. They reliably deliver the preset tidal volume (even in the presence of a small leak). The risk of barotrauma is minimal because most patients presenting to the operating room have healthy normally compliant lungs.

C. For infants and patients with diseased lungs, the maintenance of preset tidal volumes may produce unacceptably high airway pressures and increased risk of barotrauma. **Pressure generators** are more appropriate in these situations, because airway pressure is controlled and barotrauma risk minimized.

D. The lack of flexibility of most current anesthesia machine ventilators severely limits their use in setting of abnormal lung mechanics. In these situations sometimes the use of manual ventilation or a critical care ventilator is necessary. New "next generation" anesthesia machines have versatile microprocessor-controlled ventilators that can safely and effectively ventilate patients with lung disease. These ventilators have sophisticated interfaces and controls, additional monitoring of airway pressures and flow rates, and are capable of many ventilation modes.

V. Safety features

A. An **audible oxygen alarm** is fitted in the oxygen supply line of the high pressure system. It consists of a pressure regulator and a reed or whistle that will sound when the pressure in the supply line is greater than 0 and less than about 25 psi.

B. A pressure-operated **"fail-safe" valve** in the high pressure system of the nitrous oxide supply line opens only when oxygen pressure in the high pressure system is above 25 psi. If the oxygen pressure falls below that, nitrous oxide will cease to flow. Because both the audible oxygen alarm and the fail-safe valve respond specifically to low pressure in the oxygen supply line of the high pressure system, neither protects against the delivery of an hypoxic mixture downstream in the low pressure system (e.g., if the oxygen flow control valve is accidentally shut off).

C. **Oxygen ratio control**. All new anesthetic machines are fitted with a device to control the proportion of oxygen delivered. This may take the form of a mechanical link between the oxygen and nitrous oxide flow control knobs that will not allow a fraction of inspired oxygen (F_{IO_2}) of less than 25% to be set. Alternatively, some machines incorporate an oxygen ratio monitor that sounds an alarm if a low F_{IO_2} is set. Older machines may lack any mechanism to control oxygen ratio.

D. **Pressure alarms** are incorporated into all anesthesia machines, but different manufacturers use different pressure alarm systems.

1. A **low pressure alarm** is triggered by a period of no pressure in the system or by a sustained pressure drop below atmospheric pressure. Low pressure may be caused by a disconnection or large leak in the system. Negative pressure usually indicates a scavenging system malfunction or that the patient is inhaling against an obstruction.

2. A **high pressure alarm** may have a variable or a preset (e.g., 65 cm H_2O) limit. A high-pressure alarm may indicate obstruction in the tubing or endotracheal tube or a change in pulmonary compliance (e.g., bronchospasm or pneumothorax).

3. A **continuing pressure alarm** alerts the user in the event of high pressure being sustained for more than a few seconds. A blocked or closed pop-off valve, a malfunctioning ventilator pressure relief valve, or an obstruction in the scavenging system could create this condition.

VI. Scavenging. A scavenging system channels waste gases away from the operating room to a location outside the hospital building or a location where the gases can be discharged safely (e.g., to a nonrecirculating exhaust ventilating system). The ambient concentration of anesthetic gases in the operating room should not exceed 25 ppm for nitrous oxide and 2 ppm for halogenated agents. Specific anesthetic gas-scavenging systems should be used routinely. These systems consist of a collecting system, a transfer system, a receiving system, and a disposal system.

A. The **collecting system** delivers waste gases to the transfer system and operates from the APL valve and from the expiratory valve of the ventilator. In addition, waste gases may be collected from the gas analyzers.

B.   The **transfer system** consists of tubing that connects the collecting and receiving systems.

C.   The **receiving system** ensures that neither positive nor negative pressure builds at the patient end of the system. The system may be open or closed. An open system consists of a reservoir canister opened to atmosphere at one end. Suction usually is applied to the canister, exhausting the waste gas. A closed system consists of a reservoir bag with positive and negative pressure relief valves to maintain the pressure in the bag within an acceptable range.

D.   The **disposal system** may be passive or active, although passive systems are inadequate for modern hospitals. A passive system consists of wide-bore tubing that carries gases directly to the exterior or into the exhaust ventilation ducts. Active systems can be powered by vacuum systems, fans, pumps, or Venturi systems.

VII.   Gas analysis. Several methods are used to monitor concentrations of oxygen, carbon dioxide, and anesthetic gases in the breathing system. The oxygen analyzer is the single most important monitor for detection of a hypoxic gas mixture. Capnometry, the measurement of carbon dioxide, has many uses, including monitoring the adequacy of ventilation and detection of breathing system faults. Breath-to-breath monitoring of anesthetic concentrations provides tracking of anesthetic uptake and distribution. Most gas analyzers incorporate alarms. Among the techniques for measurement are the following:

A.   Mass spectrometry can provide rapid response measurement of the concentration of any gas, but the spectrometer itself is very large and must be housed in a central location where it can serve a number of operating rooms. A sample of gas is withdrawn through a side port in the breathing system near the Y piece and carried through a nylon catheter to the central mass spectrometer. The sample is ionized in an electron beam. The resulting fragments are accelerated through a high voltage field and then subjected to a deflecting magnetic field. The specific fragments are detected on collectors, and the relative concentration of each agent is determined. Calibration is performed automatically at the central system. By a switching system, the mass spectrometer can sample from as many as 32 locations. The time between measurements in each room may be one or several minutes depending on the number of rooms "on line." A "stat" sample may be requested.

B.   Infrared analysis uses spectrophotometry and Beer's law to provide continuous measurement of the concentration of gas or anesthetic in a gas mixture. Gases that have two or more different atoms in the molecule absorb infrared radiation; thus, infrared analysis can be used to measure concentrations of carbon dioxide, nitrous oxide, and halogenated anesthetics but not oxygen. Typically, some gas is withdrawn from the breathing system at a steady rate (50 to 300 mL/min) and passed into a small measurement chamber in the instrument. Pulses of infrared energy at a wavelength that is absorbed only by the gas of interest are beamed through the gas and the difference of energy absorbed is used to determine the gas concentration. In some capnographs, a miniaturized measurement chamber and sensor are placed in the breathing system. In most infrared instruments only one preselected volatile anesthetic can be measured at a time.

C. Oxygen analyzers. Continuous measurements of oxygen concentrations in a mixture of gases can be provided by mass spectrometry, polarographic, galvanic or fuel cell analysis, or paramagnetic analysis.

1. **Polarographic oxygen analyzers**. The analyzer sensor is placed in the inspiratory limb of the circuit. The sensor consists of an anode and a cathode in an electrolyte solution with a polarizing voltage. Oxygen diffuses through a semipermeable membrane into the electrolyte solution, after which a current flows dependent on the uptake of oxygen at the cathode and thus on the partial pressure of oxygen. Sensors have a limited lifespan; replacement cells are needed periodically. The sensor should be placed in the upright position to avoid accumulation of moisture and may require occasional removal and drying. The response time of these analyzers (30 seconds) is not rapid enough to provide breath-to-breath analysis. When first switched on, the analyzers require a warm-up time.

2. **Galvanic or fuel cell analyzers** are similar to polarographic cell analyzers except that different anode, cathode, and electrolyte materials are used and no polarizing voltage is applied. This cell is similar to a battery that consumes oxygen.

3. **Paramagnetic analyzers**. These analyzers are based on the principle that oxygen is paramagnetic and therefore attracted into a magnetic field, whereas most other gases are weakly diamagnetic and therefore repelled from a magnetic field. Modern miniaturized paramagnetic analyzers incorporate a rapidly oscillating magnetic chamber and are capable of breath-to-breath analysis. They are often combined with another gas analysis technique in an anesthetic agent monitor.

VIII. **Accessories**

A. A **backup means of positive-pressure ventilation** (self-inflating bag, e.g., Ambu) should be available for any anesthetic procedure.

B. A **humidifier** may be used and is indicated especially for infants and small children and during high flow anesthesia. Two types generally are used during anesthesia: water bath and condenser humidifiers. Water bath humidifiers are associated with a risk of overheating with consequent injury to the patient and with risk of infection. Condenser humidifiers increase the resistance of the breathing system but are simpler to use than water bath humidifiers. High resistance makes them unsuitable for use with small children.

C. A **positive end-expiratory pressure (PEEP) valve** can be connected to the expiratory limb of the breathing system. Many new machines have built-in PEEP capability.

D. A **flashlight** should be available in case of power failure.

IX. **New generation anesthesia machines**

The present day anesthesia machine works well and meets almost all needs. Current machines are at the end of their evolutionary cycle, however, and production of this generation of machines will end soon. New generation anesthesia machines are likely to present many challenges to anesthetists in terms of their increased complexity, changed layout and function, and integration of new technologies.

X.   **Anesthesia machine checkout recommendations**
This checkout, or a reasonable equivalent, should be conducted before administration of anesthesia. These recommendations are only valid for an anesthesia system that conforms to current and relevant standards and includes an ascending bellows ventilator and at least the following monitors: capnograph, pulse oximeter, oxygen analyzer, respiratory volume monitor (spirometer), and breathing system pressure monitor with high and low pressure alarms. This is a guideline that users are encouraged to modify to accommodate differences in equipment design and variations in local clinical practice. Such local modifications should have appropriate peer review. Users should refer to the operator's manual for manufacturer's specific procedures and precautions, especially the manufacturer's low-pressure leak test (see section X.C.2).
Note: If an anesthesia provider uses the same machine in successive cases, the steps denoted by an asterisk (*) below do not need to be repeated or may be abbreviated after the initial checkout.

A.   **Emergency ventilation equipment. Verify backup ventilation equipment is available and functioning.***

B.   **High pressure system**
   1.   **Check oxygen cylinder supply.***
      a.   Open oxygen cylinder and verify that it is at least half full (about 1,000 psi).
      b.   Close cylinder.
   2.   **Check central pipeline supplies.*** Check that hoses are connected properly and pipeline gauges read about 50 psi.

C.   **Low pressure system**
   1.   **Check initial status of low pressure system.***
      a.   Close flow control valves and turn vaporizers off.
      b.   Check fill level and tighten vaporizers' filler caps.
   2.   **Perform leak check of machine low pressure system.***
      a.   Verify that the machine master switch and flow control valves are "OFF."
      b.   Attach suction bulb to common (fresh) gas outlet.
      c.   Squeeze bulb repeatedly until it is fully collapsed.
      d.   Verify bulb stays fully collapsed for at least 10 seconds.
      e.   Open one vaporizer at a time and repeat "c" and "d" as above.
      f.   Remove suction bulb, and reconnect fresh gas hose.
   3.   **Turn on machine master switch and all other necessary electrical equipment.***
   4.   **Test flowmeters.***
      a.   Adjust flow of all gases through their full range, checking for smooth operation of floats and undamaged flow tubes.
      b.   Attempt to create a hypoxic O_2/N_2O mixture and verify correct changes in flow and/or alarm.

D.   **Scavenging system. Adjust and check scavenging system.***
   1.   Ensure proper connections between the scavenging system and both APL (pop-off) valve and ventilator relief valve.
   2.   Adjust waste gas vacuum (if necessary).
   3.   Fully open APL valve and occlude Y-piece.
   4.   With minimum O_2 flow, allow scavenger reservoir bag to

collapse completely and verify that absorber pressure gauge reads about 0.

5. With the O_2 flush activated, allow the scavenger reservoir bag to distend fully and then verify that absorber pressure gauge reads less than 10 cm H_2O.

E. Breathing system

1. Calibrate O_2 monitor.*

   a. Expose sensor to room air and verify monitor reads 21%.

   b. Verify low O_2 alarm is enabled and functioning.

   c. Reinstall sensor in circuit and flush breathing system with O_2.

   d. Verify that monitor now reads greater than 90%.

2. Check initial status of breathing system.

   a. Set selector switch to "bag" mode.

   b. Check that breathing circuit is complete, undamaged, and unobstructed.

   c. Verify that CO_2 absorbent is adequate.

   d. Install breathing circuit accessory equipment (e.g., humidifier, PEEP valve) to be used during the case.

3. Perform leak check of the breathing system.

   a. Set all gas flows to 0 (or minimum).

   b. Close APL (pop-off) valve and occlude Y-piece.

   c. Pressurize breathing system to 30 cm H_2O with O_2 flush.

   d. Ensure that pressure remains fixed for at least 10 seconds.

   e. Open APL (pop-off) valve and ensure that pressure decreases.

F. Manual and automatic ventilation systems. Test ventilation systems and unidirectional valves.

1. Place a second breathing bag on the Y-piece.

2. Set appropriate ventilator parameters for next patient.

3. Switch to automatic ventilation (Ventilator) mode.

4. Fill bellows and breathing bag with O_2 flush and then turn ventilator "ON."

5. Set O_2 flow to minimum and other gas flows to 0.

6. Verify that during inspiration bellows delivers appropriate tidal volume and that during expiration bellows fills completely.

7. Set fresh gas flow to about 5 L/min.

8. Verify that the ventilator bellows and simulated lungs fill and empty appropriately without sustained pressure at end expiration.

9. Check for proper action of unidirectional valves.

10. Test breathing circuit accessories to ensure proper function.

11. Turn ventilator "OFF" and switch to manual ventilation mode.

12. Ventilate manually and assure inflation and deflation of artificial lungs and appropriate feel of system resistance and compliance.

13. Remove second breathing bag from Y-piece.

G. Monitors. Check, calibrate, and/or set alarm limits of all monitors.

H. Final position. Check final status of the machine.

1. Vaporizers off.

2. APL valve open.

3. Selector switch to "Bag."
4. All flowmeters to 0.
5. Patient suction level adequate.
6. Breathing system ready to use.

SUGGESTED READING

Dorsch JA, Dorsch SE, eds. *Understanding anesthesia equipment*, 4th ed. Philadelphia: Lippincott, Williams & Wilkins, 1999.

Ehrenwerth J, Eisencraft JB. *Anesthesia equipment*, 2nd ed. St. Louis: Mosby Year Book, 2001.

10

Monitoring

John L. Walsh and Barry M. Stowe

I. Standard monitoring. Monitoring helps the anesthetist support and control vital organ functions during anesthesia, surgery, and critical illness. Standards of care for monitoring in anesthesiology have evolved:

A. Standard monitoring for general anesthesia includes electrocardiogram (ECG), blood pressure, respiratory rate, oxygen saturation by pulse oximetry (Sao_2), end-tidal carbon dioxide, and inspired oxygen concentration.

B. Standard monitoring for regional anesthesia includes ECG, blood pressure, respiratory rate, and oxygen saturation.

II. Cardiovascular monitoring. The goal of monitoring of cardiovascular hemodynamics is to maintain adequate organ perfusion and hemodynamic stability.

A. Signs and symptoms of individual organ dysfunction may result from inadequate end-organ flow:

1. Central nervous system. Decreased mental status, focal neurologic deficit.

2. Cardiac. Chest pain, ischemia on ECG, wall motion abnormalities on echocardiography.

3. Renal. Decreased urine output, increased blood urea nitrogen to creatinine ratio, decreased fractional excretion of sodium.

4. Gastrointestinal. Abdominal pain, decreased bowel sounds, hematochezia.

5. Periphery. Cool limbs, poor capillary refill, weak pulses.

B. End-organ blood flow is determined by that organ's perfusion pressure divided by its resistance to flow. In most cases, the perfusion pressure is the difference between the arterial pressure and venous pressure; in cases of increased intracerebral pressure, the cerebral perfusion pressure is the difference between the arterial pressure and the increased intracerebral pressure. Because the arterial pressure is time varying, **mean arterial pressure** is generally chosen as a static substitute for defining an average perfusion pressure.

III. ECG. The ECG is used for the determination of heart rate, detection and diagnosis of arrhythmias, pacemaker function, and myocardial ischemia. The presence of an ECG signal does not guarantee cardiac contraction or output. The ECG also may suggest electrolyte abnormalities.

A. Mechanism of measurement

1. Electrode application. Because the ECG is a small electrical signal (about 1 mV), its measurement is very susceptible to electrical interference from improper application of electrodes. Electrodes should have adequate contact and be applied to a clean dry skin area.

2. Electrode location. For the ECG to be interpreted properly, the electrodes must be placed in consistent locations. The limb leads must be located on or near their appropriate limbs, and the precordial lead typically over V_5 (fifth intercostal space, anterior axillary line).

3.   Mode. Frequently, monitors have a diagnostic and monitor mode. The **monitor mode** filters out more noise because of a narrower frequency bandpass (0.5 to 40 Hz); it consequently creates a more stable tracing for simple rhythm monitoring. The **diagnostic mode**, with a wider bandpass (0.05 to 100 Hz), should be used whenever evaluating ST segment changes for ischemia. Newer monitors permit continuous analysis and trending of ST segment changes.

B.   Rhythm detection. Lead II is monitored most commonly because the P wave is easily seen, allowing detection of arrhythmias. Inferior ischemia may also be detected.

C.   Ischemia detection. Typically, a five-lead system is used (with simultaneous monitoring of leads II and V_5) in patients with significant cardiac disease. Lead II is monitored for right coronary artery ischemia because the inferior wall is supplied by the right coronary in 90% of patients. Lead V_5 is monitored for the detection of left anterior descending artery ischemia, because the bulk of the left ventricular myocardium lies beneath it. For patients in whom the left circumflex artery is at risk, lead I may be monitored.

IV.   Monitoring arterial blood pressure. In the normal state, most organs are able to maintain relatively constant blood flow over a wide range of perfusion pressures (i.e., autoregulation). Blood pressure is monitored to ensure that an adequate perfusion pressure exists. In some pathologic states, however, a low perfusion pressure may be enough to provide adequate flow; conversely, a high perfusion pressure may be inadequate if an organ's resistance to flow is high.

A.   Noninvasive blood pressure measurement involves occluding an artery by a pressurized cuff and then measuring the oscillations in cuff pressure or the pressure at which flow resumes through the artery as the cuff is deflated. Multiple techniques exist for determining blood pressure by this method:

1.   Automated techniques are the most common methods for noninvasive blood pressure measurement in the operating room. Typically, the cuff is inflated about 40 mm Hg above the previous systolic pressure (or about 170 mm Hg initially) and then incrementally deflated while sensing pressure oscillations in the cuff. The mean arterial blood pressure correlates well with the lowest pressure at which maximum oscillations occur. The systolic and diastolic pressures are determined by algorithm but generally correlate with the initial rise and final fall of oscillations about the maximum.

  a.   Limitations

    (1)   Cuff size. The cuff should cover about two-thirds of the upper arm or thigh; that is, the width of the cuff should be 20% greater than the diameter of the limb. A cuff that is too narrow may produce falsely high measurements; a cuff that is too wide may produce falsely low values.

    (2)   Arrhythmias, such as atrial fibrillation, may make a measured value difficult to interpret.

(3) **Motion artifact** is rejected by some instruments but still increases the cycle time.

(4) **Rapid pressure changes**. Venous congestion may occur if the instrument is set to cycle too frequently; cycle times less than 2 minutes apart should be avoided for routine monitoring.

(5) **Very low or high blood pressures** may not correlate with intraarterial measurements. The exact difference is generally not clinically relevant, however.

2. **Auscultation of Korotkoff's sounds**. An occlusive cuff is inflated above the systolic blood pressure. As the cuff is slowly (3 to 5 mm Hg/sec) deflated, a pressure will be reached at which blood begins to flow turbulently through the artery. The pressure at which the sound of this turbulent flow is heard through a stethoscope is the systolic blood pressure. As the pressure in the cuff decreases below the diastolic blood pressure, the sounds muffle or disappear.

a. **Limitations**

(1) Requires a human operator.

(2) Vasoconstriction may decrease flow, making the sounds difficult to hear.

(3) Prone to observer error.

(4) Rapid deflation may produce an erroneously low pressure reading.

3. **Palpation or Doppler detection of flow**. As the cuff is deflated, the distal pulse is palpated or detected by Doppler ultrasound. The pressure in the cuff at which the pulse is first detected correlates with the systolic blood pressure. This technique only measures systolic blood pressure.

B. **Invasive blood pressure monitoring** most commonly measures pressure directly by means of an indwelling arterial catheter coupled through fluid filled tubing to an external pressure transducer. The transducer converts the pressure into an electrical signal, which is subsequently filtered and displayed on a screen.

1. The clinical indications for invasive arterial monitoring include:

a. Necessity for rigorous **control of blood pressure** (e.g., arterial aneurysms).

b. Hemodynamically unstable patient.

c. Necessity for frequent arterial blood sampling.

2. **A disposable transducer** is connected to a pressurized bag of saline or heparinized saline. The line is continuously flushed at 3 mL/hr to prevent clot formation at the tip of the cannula.

3. **Tubing** should be rigid and as short as possible to properly transmit the pressure wave. Air bubbles should be purged from the system.

4. **The signal** from the transducer setup should have a relatively flat frequency response below 20 Hz and consequently provide an accurate representation of the pressure for all physiologic heart rates.

5. The system should be electronically **zeroed** when the transducer is open to air. This may be done with the transducer at any height. When measuring pressures, the transducer should remain at a stable height with respect to the patient. This is

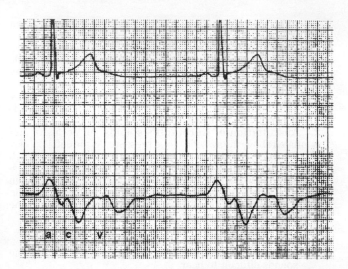

Fig. 10-1.   A normal central venous pressure tracing is shown in the bottom half of the figure with its corresponding electrocardiogram in the top half. Waves a, c, and v on the venous pressure tracing are labeled. The *x* descent occurs between waves c and v; the *y* descent occurs after the v wave. (From Kaplan JA. *Cardiac anesthesia*, 2nd ed. Philadelphia: WB Saunders, 1987:186, with permission.)

generally chosen as the height of the coronary sinus. In practice, the fourth intercostal space, mid-axillary line is a reasonable approximation.

C.   Interpretation of the blood pressure depends on the clinical question being asked.

   1.   The systolic blood pressure may be of interest when monitoring patients with aneurysms in whom a sudden high pressure might induce a rupture.

   2.   The mean arterial pressure is the most accurately measured and may be the most useful for assessing perfusion pressure of vital organs.

V.   Monitoring central pressures and cardiac output

A.   Central venous pressure (CVP)

   1.   **The measurement of CVP** is achieved by coupling the intravascular space through a fluid-filled tube to an external pressure transducer. The intravascular space is typically monitored at the junction of the superior vena cava and the right atrium. The transducer is set up in the same way as the arterial line; special care is taken to ensure that the transducer is maintained at the same level with respect to the patient during sequential measurements (e.g., at the level of the coronary sinus).

   2.   **Waveform**. A CVP trace contains three positive deflections, the **a**, **c**, and **v** waves (Fig. 10-1). These correspond roughly with atrial contraction, change in the shape of the heart in systole including tricuspid bulging, and right atrial filling.

   3.   **Value**. The CVP is often read after the a wave and before the c wave to reflect presystolic right ventricular pressure. To reflect transmural-filling pressure, the CVP, like all central vascular pressures, is read at end-expiration. **The CVP is normally approximately 2 to 6 mm Hg**.

    a. If the waveform does not contain pathologic a or v waves, the difference between the **mean value** (at end-expiration) and the value between the a and c waves is usually small and clinically unimportant.

4. Physiologic interpretation (Fig. 10-2). By itself, the CVP does not indicate the volume status of the patient; some assumption, or assessment, of the cardiac function needs to be included.

    a. A decrease in CVP (Fig. 10-2B) indicates either an increase in cardiac performance, increased impedance to venous return, or a decrease in mean systemic pressure (volume). With a concomitant increase in blood pressure, the reason for a decrease in CVP is most likely an increase in cardiac performance; if the blood pressure falls, the drop in CVP is likely due to a decrease in volume or increased resistance to venous return. This analysis assumes that the systemic vascular resistance has not changed.

    b. An increase in CVP (Fig. 10-2C) indicates either a decrease in cardiac performance, a decrease in impedance to venous return, or an increase in mean systemic pressure (volume). With a concomitant decrease in blood pressure, the reason for an increase in CVP is likely decreased cardiac performance, whereas with a concurrent increase in blood pressure, the reason for an increase in CVP is probably increased volume or decreased resistance to venous return.

5. Effects of pathology on interpretation

    a. Cannon a waves occur when the atrium contracts against a closed tricuspid valve. It occurs with atrioventricular dissociation.

    b. Abnormally large v waves occur with tricuspid regurgitation.

6. Effect of positive airway pressure on interpretation. The addition of positive airway pressure affects both the cardiac output and venous return relationships (Fig. 10-3). The Starling curve is based on transmural pressure, which is the difference between the atrial pressure and the transmitted extracardiac pressure. Because of this, positive end-expiratory pressure shifts the curve to the right by an amount equal to the transmitted pressure. At high levels of positive end-expiratory pressure, the curve can be depressed, reflecting increased right ventricular afterload. The net result is that CVP increases, whereas venous return and cardiac output decreases.

7. Indications for central venous cannulation

    a. Measurement of right heart filling pressures as a guide to intravascular volume, impedance to venous return, and right heart function.

    b. Injection of indicator for cardiac output determination (see below).

    c. Access into the central circulation for administration of drugs or parenteral nutrition.

    d. Intravenous access for patients with poor peripheral venous access.

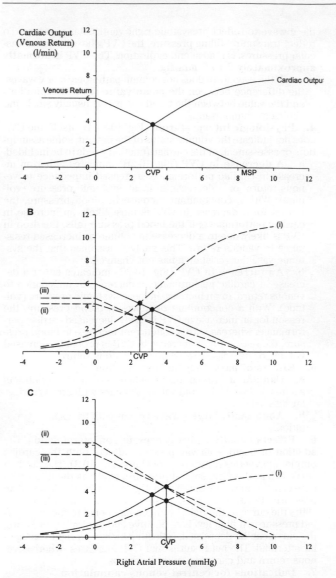

Fig. 10-2. **Venous return (VR)/cardiac output (CO) curves. A: In steady state, VR = CO. Thus, the measured central venous pressure (CVP) will occur at the point on the independent axis where the VR and CO curves cross. B: A fall in CVP could be caused by an increase in cardiac performance (*i*), an increased impedance to venous return (*ii*), a decrease in the mean systemic pressure (MSP) (*iii*), or a combination of these. C: An increase in CVP could be caused by a decrease in cardiac performance (*i*), a decreased impedance to VR (*ii*), an increase in MSP (*iii*), or a combination of these.**

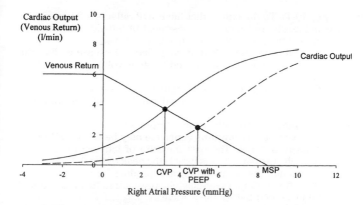

Fig. 10-3. Effect of positive end-expiratory pressure (PEEP) on the venous return/cardiac output curves. PEEP has the effect of shifting the Starling curve to the right by a degree equal to the transmitted extracardiac pressure. At high levels of PEEP (>15 cm H_2O), the curve can be depressed secondary to increased right ventricular afterload. The central venous pressure measured is consequently higher. *MSP*, mean systemic pressure.

B. Pulmonary artery catheter (PAC). The PAC is a catheter that passes sequentially through the vena cava, right atrium, right ventricle, and into the pulmonary artery. The PAC provides useful information including the CVP, pulmonary artery pressure (PAP), pulmonary artery occlusion pressure (PAOP), mixed-venous blood chemistries, and cardiac output.

    1. Measuring PAP and PAOP. As with the CVP, the PAP and PAOP are determined by coupling the intravascular space through a fluid-filled tube to an external pressure transducer. For an accurate measure of PAOP, the tip of the catheter should reside in a lung zone where pulmonary venous pressure is greater than alveolar pressure (West zone III), which, because the design of the catheter, is the usual case.

        a. Waveform. The morphology of the PAP waveform is similar to that of the systemic arterial waveform but is smaller and precedes it slightly. When the balloon at the tip of the catheter is inflated, the catheter occludes flow in the artery and the morphology of the waveform changes to more closely approximate that of the CVP. A and **v** waves are present; the **c** wave, however, often is not apparent.

        b. Value. The PAP is normally 15 to 25 mm Hg systolic and 5 to 12 mm Hg diastolic. The **PAOP** provides an estimate of the left atrial pressure. Because of the interposed lung, this estimate is delayed and dampened. The a and c waves typically are not very large. Consequently, the mean pressure at end-expiration reflects the left atrial pressure. **The PAOP is normally 5 to 12 mmHg.**

    2. Physiologic interpretation. The performance of the left heart can be described by two curves: the end-systolic pressure-volume curve and the diastolic pressure-volume relationship

(Fig. 10-4). To the extent that the PAOP reflects left ventricular end-diastolic pressure, an assessment of left-sided heart function may be made by the change in PAOP value.

  a.   An increase in PAOP can reflect a decrease in diastolic compliance, an increase in end-diastolic volume, or both (Fig. 10-4).

  b.   A decrease in PAOP reflects an increase in diastolic compliance, a decrease in end-diastolic volume, or both (Fig. 10-4).

  3.   Effects of pathology on interpretation.

  a.   A poorly compliant ventricle may be responsible for a large a wave. The best measure of left ventricular end-diastolic pressure in this case is the peak of the a wave. Atrioventricular dissociation may also produce large a waves, but the left ventricular end-diastolic pressure in this case should be measured before the a wave.

  b.   Mitral regurgitation may result in abnormally large v waves.

  c.   Ventricular interdependence. When the right ventricle dilates (e.g., in response to acute pulmonary hypertension or pulmonary embolus), the interventricular septum stiffens and shifts toward the left ventricular cavity. The altered septal behavior decreases left ventricular diastolic compliance. Left ventricular end-diastolic pressure for a given end-diastolic volume will be increased as a result.

  4.   Indications. The use of PACs continues to be controversial. PACs should be used only if the potential benefit in terms of diagnosis or guidance of treatment outweighs the risk of insertion and complications associated with their use (see below). Common indications include acute myocardial infarction with shock, unexplained hypotension, multiorgan dysfunction, pulmonary artery hypertension, access for cardiac pacing, and surgical procedures associated with profound physiologic changes (e.g., lung transplantation or thoracoabdominal aneurysm repair).

  5.   Types of PACs include

  a.   Venous infusion port (VIP, VIP+) catheters that provide additional infusion ports.

  b.   Paceport that provide specially positioned ports to pass temporary pacing wires or infuse drugs.

  c.   Oximetric catheters that provide monitoring of mixed venous oxygen saturation.

  d.   Continuous cardiac output catheters that use a special algorithm to perform frequent automated determinations of thermodilution cardiac output.

  e.   Right ventricular ejection fraction catheters that use a rapid response thermistor to calculate right ventricular ejection fraction in addition to cardiac output.

C. Cardiac output

  1.   Thermodilution cardiac outputs are determined by injecting a fixed volume of cold (room temperature or less) solution into the CVP port of the PAC. The cold tracer mixes with the blood as it passes through the right heart, and the temperature of the mixture is measured as it passes a thermistor near the tip of the PAC. The computation of the cardiac output uses a

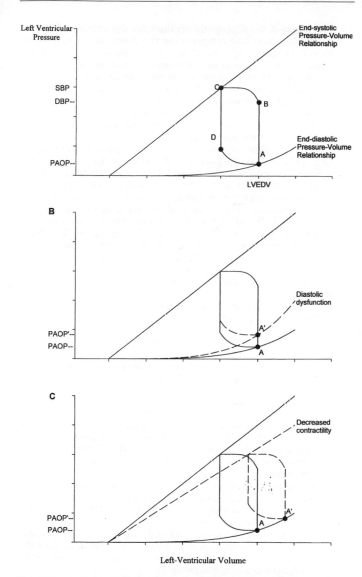

Fig. 10-4. **Left ventricular pressure–volume relationships. The cardiac cycle (A-B-C-D-A) is limited by the end-systolic pressure–volume relationship (describing the contractility) and the end-diastolic pressure–volume relationship. The pulmonary artery occlusion pressure (PAOP) approximates the left ventricular end-diastolic pressure. An increase in PAOP may be ascribed to decreased diastolic compliance (B), an increase in left ventricular end-diastolic volume (LVEDV) (C), or a combination of both. An increase in LVEDV often results from decreased contractility in the setting of a properly performing right ventricle (C).** *SBP,* **systolic blood pressure;** *DBP,* **diastolic blood pressure.**

formula that must properly account for the volume of the injectate; the injectate temperature; the thermodynamic properties of the blood, injectate solution, and the particular catheter used; and the integral of the temperature–time curve. Consequently, the proper volume of an appropriate solution must be injected to satisfy these assumptions. Typically, 10 mL of cold saline or 5% dextrose in water is injected within 4 seconds. The simultaneous rapid infusion of cold intravenous fluid into the central venous circulation may interfere with thermodilution cardiac output measurements.

2.   Dye dilution may be used as an alternative to thermodilution. This requires the injection of a nontoxic dye (usually indocyanine green) into the central venous circulation. Arterial blood is withdrawn at a known rate using a syringe pump. The arterial concentration of dye is continuously measured as the blood is withdrawn and a curve of dye concentration versus time constructed. The algorithm used to calculate cardiac output is analogous to that used for a thermodilution output. This technique requires that a central venous and an arterial line be present but does not require a PAC. A properly calibrated sensor is required to measure the arterial dye concentration. Alternative tracers, including radioisotopes, are sometimes used for research purposes.

3.   Interpretation of cardiac output usually is done in the setting of hypotension. Determining the cardiac output allows diagnosis of a low tone state (low systemic vascular resistance), a low cardiac output, or both. If the cardiac output is low, a concurrent measurement of heart rate will help determine whether the reason is related to the heart rate or ventricular performance (i.e., **stroke volume = cardiac output/heart rate**).

4.   Physiologic interpretation

   a.   Respiration. During spontaneous breathing, negative intrathoracic pressure enhances venous return and increases left ventricular afterload. During positive pressure breathing, inspiration reduces venous return and left ventricular afterload. Cardiac output can vary over the respiratory cycle, depending on the mode of ventilation and baseline levels of venous return and cardiac performance. Accordingly, the timing of injection affects the interpretation of a thermodilution cardiac output measurement. If a consistent trend is desired, **it is probably best to inject at a constant point in the respiratory cycle, usually at end-expiration**. If an average over the respiratory cycle is desired, it is usual to take the mean of three measurements obtained at random times throughout the respiratory cycle.

   b.   Tricuspid regurgitation may produce both erroneously high and low readings. Rarely do they vary more than 20% from the actual value.

   c.   Intracardiac shunts can also produce erroneous measurements.

VI.   Echocardiography

A.   Mechanism. Echocardiography (echo) uses high frequency (2.5 to 10 MHz) ultrasonic waves to generate images of the heart and surrounding structures. The two common approaches used in the perioperative period are **transthoracic** and **transesophageal**.

B.   Advantages of transesophageal echo over transthoracic echo are

1.   Better resolution of left-sided heart structures.
2.   Separation from the surgical field (infraclavicular), thereby allowing continuous monitoring.

C.   Echo can provide many of the parameters that a PAC can provide (estimates of cardiac ejection and blood flow).

D.   Echo can also provide much information that a PAC cannot, such as valvular function, assessment of ventricular contractility, diastolic relaxation, and assessment of the pericardium. Intracardiac structures such as vegetations, tumor, or thrombus can be visualized. Consequently, echo can be invaluable for intermittent assessment of cardiac function and diagnosis of cardiac and pericardial pathology.

E.   Indications include assessment of:

1.   Low blood pressure when the cardiac output is unknown.
2.   Low cardiac output accompanied by unexplained high filling pressures.
3.   Valvular lesions and suspected vegetations.
4.   Intracardiac shunts.
5.   Intracardiac thrombi.
6.   Intracardiac air.
7.   Pericardial disease.
8.   Thoracic aortic aneurysms or dissections.

VII.   Procedures

A.   Arterial cannulation

1.   **Location**. The radial artery is most commonly used. Other sites include the ulnar, brachial, axillary, femoral, and dorsalis pedis arteries. With increasing distance from the heart, systolic blood pressure increases, mean arterial blood pressure generally decreases, and the pressure waveform displayed on the monitor narrows.

2.   **Radial artery catheter insertion technique**

a.   Immobilize the forearm and hand with the wrist slightly hyperextended over a padded arm board (Fig. 10-5). The thumb may be extended to place the volar surface of the wrist exactly parallel to the floor. Palpate the radial artery medial to the head of the radius.

b.   After preparing the skin, a 25-gauge needle is used to raise a skin wheal with 1% lidocaine. A 15-gauge needle skin puncture may facilitate catheter passage.

c.   Select the appropriate-sized catheter (22 to 24 gauge for infants, 20 to 22 gauge for larger children, and 18 or 20 gauge for adults).

d.   **Transfixion method**. The catheter is advanced slowly and completely through the artery. Blood will often show in the hub of the needle but may not with the 22- or 24-gauge needle. The needle is removed from the cannula (keeping it sterile for possible reuse), and the catheter is firmly connected to a T-connector stopcock and flush syringe. The system should allow blood to flow back into the syringe. The catheter is lowered almost parallel to the skin of the wrist and slowly withdrawn until blood pulsates freely in the sys-

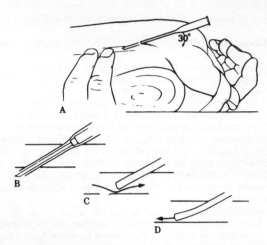

Fig. 10-5.   Percutaneous radial artery cannulation. A: Direct threading method. B–D: Transfixing method. The positioning of the hand and forearm is the same for both methods.

tem. The catheter is then advanced into the vessel. The catheter should be flushed free of blood and the stopcock turned off until connected to the transducer. A sterile arterial guide wire can be used if catheter insertion is difficult.

e.   Direct threading technique. The needle is advanced slowly until the artery is entered and free flow of blood is observed. The catheter is advanced over the needle while rigidly fixing the needle. Proximal pressure is applied to occlude the artery while the needle is removed and the flush system attached.

f.   The catheter and T-connector are securely attached to the skin and the T-connector is joined to the transducer system.

g.   At least 2 mL of blood should be removed to clear the volume in the catheter and T-connector before taking each blood sample.

h.   Do not flush the line with more than 3 mL of solution, because retrograde flow has been demonstrated into the cerebral circulation.

3.   Specific considerations for arterial cannulation.

a.   The **Allen test** has been advocated to assess the relative contribution of the radial and ulnar arteries to blood flow to the hand. However, it does not accurately predict complications and is not performed routinely.

b.   Arterial pulsation distal to old arterial cannulation sites may represent collateral flow. Proximal pulsation should be assessed prior to insertion to confirm that thrombosis has not occurred.

c.   Whenever there is a left- versus right-sided disparity in measured blood pressure, in general pressure should be measured on the side with the higher pressure.

d. For femoral and axillary arterial pressure measurement, a 6-inch 18-gauge catheter is inserted by Seldinger technique after cannulation by a 2-inch 18- or 20-gauge catheter.

e. Damped waveforms may be caused by proximal pressure on the artery, transducer malfunction, and mechanical problems such as air and clot within the system. The catheter should aspirate and flush easily. It may require repositioning, rewiring, or replacing with a larger gauge or longer cannula. The blood pressure should be measured by another technique in the interim.

4. Complications are rare but include thrombosis, distal ischemia, infection, and fistula or aneurysm formation. If the hand or digit appears ischemic, the cannula should be removed as soon as possible. In this case, if the radial artery had been cannulated, do not choose the ipsilateral ulnar artery as the alternative site.

B. Insertion of central venous catheters

1. Sites. The internal jugular vein, subclavian vein, external jugular vein, cephalic vein, axillary vein, and femoral vein all provide access to the central circulation. **Portable two-dimensional ultrasound imaging** (e.g., Siterite, Dymax Corporation, Pittsburgh, PA) can be used to define the anatomy of central vessels and determine their patency. Subsequently, cannulation can be performed under ultrasonic guidance or visualization.

2. Cannulation of the right internal jugular vein (Seldinger technique) (Fig. 10-6).

a. An oxygen mask is applied, and the patient's head is turned toward the left and slightly extended. The neck is cleaned with an antiseptic solution.

b. Under aseptic conditions (mask, hat, sterile gloves and gown), the chosen site is draped with sterile towels to expose the suprasternal notch, clavicle, lateral border of the sternocleidomastoid (SCM) muscle and the lower border of the mandible.

c. The midpoint between the mastoid process and the sternal attachment of the SCM is located.

d. The internal jugular vein can be entered medial to the SCM at this point (anterior approach) or more laterally, at the apex of the two heads of the SCM (central approach). The external jugular vein should be identified to avoid puncture.

e. The patient is placed in Trendelenburg position, unless contraindicated by conditions such as intracranial hypertension or congestive heart failure.

f. The carotid artery is gently palpated, and the skin and deep tissues are infiltrated with 1% lidocaine just lateral to the carotid artery. A finder needle (22 or 25 gauge) is advanced lateral to the artery at a 30-degree angle to the skin, pointing approximately toward the ipsilateral axilla (anterior approach) or nipple (central approach) until venous blood is aspirated.

g. A Valsalva maneuver may increase vein size during difficult cannulations.

h. Once the vein is localized, the finder needle is removed, and an 18-gauge thin wall needle (or intravenous catheter) is

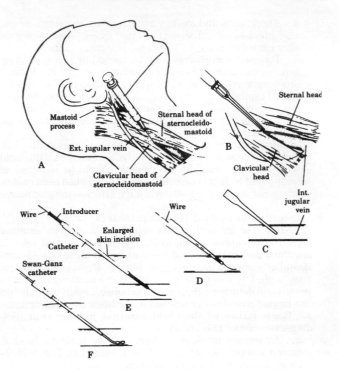

Fig. 10-6.   Cannulation of the right internal jugular vein (Seldinger technique). See text for details.

inserted at the same angle and depth. Blood should be easily aspirated when the vein is entered.

i. The syringe is removed from the needle and a guidewire is passed through the needle or catheter while the ECG is observed. The wire should pass easily. The thin-walled needle (or catheter) is removed over the guidewire. The insertion site may be superficially enlarged with a no. 11 scalpel blade inserted parallel to skin and pointed laterally (to avoid the carotid artery). With countertraction on the skin, a dilator is advanced over the wire; gentle twisting of the dilator may aid insertion. While maintaining proximal control of the guidewire at all times, the dilator is withdrawn, the central catheter passed, and the wire removed. Infusion ports are flushed after residual air is aspirated. The catheter is secured to the skin, and an occlusive dressing is applied.

j. A **chest radiograph** should be obtained to check the position of the radiopaque catheter and to exclude a pneumothorax. Correct tip position is at the junction of the SVC and the right atrium. Make certain that the tip of a catheter placed via the left jugular vein does not abut the wall of the SVC at a right angle.

3. The **external jugular vein** runs superficially from the edge of the mid-SCM toward the clavicle laterally. An external jugular catheter can be inserted in a manner similar to that described above in section VII.B.2. Occlusion of the vein at the clavicle will make it larger and less mobile. The external jugular vein bends to join the subclavian vein. Consequently, threading the catheter centrally may be more difficult. A "J"-shaped guidewire should be used.

4. The **subclavian vein** crosses under the clavicle just medial to the mid-clavicular line. The needle is inserted inferior to the outer third of the clavicle. The periosteum of the clavicle is identified with the needle and the tip "walked" posteriorly under the clavicle and directed toward the sternal notch. It should remain close to the posterior edge of the clavicle to avoid a pneumothorax. The catheter is inserted into the vein as described in section VII.B.2.

5. The **basilic vein** can be used as well. Long catheters threaded through an introducer needle are made for this purpose. If the catheter is difficult to thread, the arm can be abducted and the head turned toward the side of the insertion to decrease the incidence of catheter passage up into the jugular vein. A 140-cm guidewire may also be used.

6. Percutaneously inserted central catheters can be inserted via peripheral arm veins. Single- and double-lumen catheters are available. These provide long-term intravenous access for infusion of drugs and total parenteral nutrition and have low rates of complications and infection.

7. Cannulation of the femoral vein can be accomplished by entering the vein just medial to the femoral artery (inferior to the inguinal ligament) and proceeding as described in section VII.B.2. The leg should be slightly abducted before insertion.

8. Complications of CVP catheter insertion and use include the following:

    a. Arrhythmias, both atrial and ventricular, which generally are short-lived and corrected by withdrawing the catheter from the heart.

    b. Carotid or subclavian artery puncture. If unnoticed, a large intravenous catheter can be threaded into the artery and cause damage that requires surgical repair. Attention must be paid throughout the cannulation to the color and pulsations of the blood. The color or oxygen saturation of a venous sample drawn through the finder or thin-walled needle can be compared with a simultaneously drawn arterial sample. With the patient breathing an enriched oxygen concentration, a different in saturation usually is apparent. Additionally, the pressure in the finder needle or cannula can be measured by connecting it to a pressure transducer or to a free-flowing intravenous fluid bag. Whenever the suspicion of arterial cannulation remains, a fresh puncture site should be sought. Subclavian cannulation may be relatively contraindicated in anticoagulated patients because of difficulty in compressing the subclavian artery if it is punctured.

    c. Pneumothorax, pericardial tamponade, hemothorax, hydrothorax, chylothorax, infection, and air embolism.

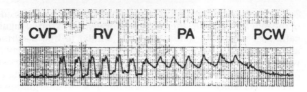

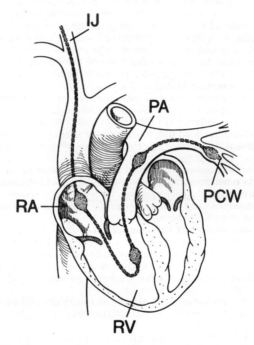

Fig. 10-7.   Characteristic pressure waves seen during insertion of a pulmonary artery catheter. *CVP*, central venous pressure; *IJ*, internal jugular; *RA*, right atrium; *RV*, right ventricle; *PA*, pulmonary artery; *PCW*, pulmonary capillary wedge.

C.   PAC insertion (Fig. 10-7). The right internal jugular vein is used most commonly because of easy access from the head of the patient and the lower incidence of pneumothorax, but all the access sites previously mentioned can be used.

1.   Oxygen is supplied by face mask, and the ECG is monitored. The Seldinger technique is used as described in section VII.B.2. The dilator/introducer assembly is placed over the wire, with care not to burr the end of the introducer as it is manipulated through skin and soft tissue.

2.   The wire and dilator are removed from the introducer, and the side port of the introducer is aspirated for blood and then flushed. The patient may now be taken out of Trendelenburg position.

3. A **protective sheath** is placed over the PAC so that the distal 70 cm will remain sterile. The PAC is then checked for symmetric balloon inflation with 1.5 mL of air. The PAC and CVP lumens are flushed with saline and attached to calibrated pressure transducers through three-way stopcocks. Raising and lowering the PAC distal end while observing the resulting change in the pressure tracing can serve as a quick test of the calibration and sensitivity of the system prior to insertion.

4. The PAC can be held over the patient to observe its natural curve, which is designed to facilitate flotation through the heart. **The PAC is inserted to a depth of 20 cm**; the monitor should confirm a **CVP waveform**. The balloon is inflated with 1.0 to 1.5 mL of air, and the PAC is advanced until a **right ventricular pressure waveform** is seen. This should occur **at a depth of about 30 to 35 cm**.

5. The PAC is then advanced until **a pulmonary artery tracing is obtained (at about 40 to 45 cm)**. Transient premature ventricular contractions often are encountered.

6. The PAC is inserted until **a pulmonary artery occlusion pressure tracing is obtained (at a depth of about 50 to 55 cm)**. The pulmonary artery tracing should reappear with deflation of the balloon. If it does not, withdraw the catheter slightly until the pulmonary artery tracing reappears.

7. The sterile sheath is connected to the introducer, and an occlusive tape is applied at the sheath's proximal end, allowing the position of the PAC to be adjusted about 10 cm. The introducer is secured to the skin, a sterile occlusive dressing applied, and the PAC secured to the patient.

8. During PAC insertion, difficulty in passing the catheter into the right ventricle and pulmonary artery may be encountered because of balloon malfunction, valvular lesions, a low flow state, or a dilated right ventricle. The monitoring equipment should be rechecked for calibration and scale. Inflating the balloon with a full 1.5 mL of air, slow PAC advancement, and large inspirations by the patient to augment blood flow may be helpful. The PAC may have to be withdrawn to a depth of 20 to 30 cm, rotated slightly, and readvanced.

9. The PAC is placed with **fluoroscopic visualization** when a permanent pacemaker has been placed within the past 6 weeks, when selective pulmonary artery placement is necessary (e.g., a patient undergoing a right pneumonectomy) or if a PAC is required in the presence of significant structural abnormalities (e.g., Eisenmenger complex).

10.   Complications are as follows:

   a.   A transient right bundle branch block. In the patient with first-degree block and left bundle branch block, insertion of the PAC may result in complete heart block. Appropriate medications (e.g., atropine, isoproterenol) and pacing capability (e.g., external transcutaneous, transvenous pacer, or Paceport PAC) should be available.

   b.   Pulmonary artery rupture or infarction. Balloon inflation should be slow, stopped immediately when a PAOP tracing is obtained, and never kept inflated for an extended period because of the possibility of pulmonary artery rupture or infarction. PAPs always should be monitored when a PAC is in place. Occurrence of a persistent "wedge" waveform indicates that the catheter should be pulled back immediately.

   c.   PACs may rarely knot. Fluoroscopic guidance may be needed to untangle and remove the catheter.

   d.   Balloon rupture. At no time should the balloon be filled with more than 1.5 mL of air.

   e.   Other complications as previously described for CVP catheters (see section VII.B.8.).

VIII.   Respiratory monitoring. Mandatory respiratory monitors during general anesthesia include pulse oximetry, capnography, a fraction of inspired oxygen analyzer, and a disconnect alarm.

   A.   Precordial and esophageal stethoscopes allow continuous evaluation of heart and breath sounds.

     1.   Precordial stethoscopes may be placed over the suprasternal notch to listen to the quality of airflow through the trachea. Alternatively, they may be placed over the heart to monitor the quality of heart sounds. Precordial stethoscopes often are used during breathe-down inductions in children and during mask anesthetics.

     2.   Esophageal stethoscopes are placed after tracheal intubation and offer the ability to monitor respirations, heart sounds, and often temperature.

   B.   Pulse oximetry uses spectrophotometry to measure changes in light absorption by hemoglobin. Two separate light sources (light-emitting diodes) alternately transmit light through a vascular bed (usually the finger). One light is in the infrared frequency range (e.g., 940 nm) and the other in the visible-red frequency range (e.g., 660 nm). At each frequency, oxyhemoglobin and deoxyhemoglobin absorb light differently and a change in either causes a change in the amount of each wavelength absorbed relative to the other. A photodetector on the opposite side of the vascular bed measures the transmitted light. By analyzing only the pulsatile component of absorption, the pulse oximeter reading (Sp_{O_2}) provides a measure of Sa_{O_2}.

     1.   A **high Sp_{O_2}** generally indicates that oxygen is getting to the lungs, crossing the alveolar membrane, and being transported to the site of monitoring. It does not by itself indicate the amount of oxygen being delivered.

     2.   A **low Sp_{O_2}** may reflect a problem with the patient (a low Sa_{O_2}, see Chapter 35), or a problem with the monitor (measurement artifact).

     3.   Measurement artifacts for Sp_{O_2} may produce values that are:

       a.   Falsely low in the presence of methylene blue, indocyanine green, indigo carmine, or isosulfan blue.

       b.   Falsely high in the presence of carboxyhemoglobin.

       c.   Tending toward 85% in the presence of large amounts of methemoglobin.

       d.   Erratic or unreliable in the presence of surgical cautery, motion, ambient light interference, or poor perfusion.

   C.   Capnometry. Capnometers are used in all anesthetizing locations (see Chapter 9 for principles).

     1.   Clinical uses include confirmation of proper endotracheal

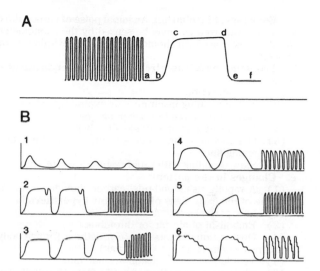

Fig. 10-8.   A: Normal capnograph. *a*, inspiration; *b*, beginning of
exhalation; *c*, beginning of plateau phase of expiration.; *d*, end-
expiration; *e*, ending of steep downstroke with normal inspiration; *f*,
return to zero baseline at end of inspiration. B: Capnographs that may be
seen in practice. *1*, rapidly extinguishing uncharacteristic waveform,
compatible with esophageal intubation; *2*, regular dips in end-expiratory
plateau, seen in underventilated lungs or in patients recovering from
neuromuscular blockade; *3*, upward shift in baseline and topline, seen
with rebreathing of carbon dioxide, miscalibration, and so forth; *4*,
restrictive pulmonary disease; *5*, obstructive pulmonary disease; *6*,
cardiogenic oscillations.

intubation, assessment of adequate ventilation, and detection of
pathologic conditions (e.g., malignant hyperthermia, pulmonary
thromboembolism, air embolism). The end-tidal carbon dioxide
value is typically several mm Hg below $Paco_2$ and follows
changes fairly well under most conditions. Nevertheless, with
changes in matching of ventilation to perfusion, dead space,
and pulmonary blood flow, end-tidal values may not accurately
reflect the change in $Paco_2$. The end-tidal value itself may be
misleading, because a plateau in CO_2 concentration at the end
of expiration is necessary to represent alveolar gas accurately.
Display of the waveform is strongly recommended. In some
cases, $Paco_2$ should be measured directly from an arterial blood
sample.

2.   Normal end-tidal carbon dioxide waveform ($Petco_2$)
(Fig. 10-8).

   a.   Carbon dioxide increases during exhalation as the distal
airways empty.

   b.   A plateau phase at end expiration approximates end-tidal
carbon dioxide values.

   c.   A rapid decline to zero should be seen with inspiration.

3.   Abnormal end-tidal carbon dioxide waveforms occur
during many important clinical conditions:

    a.   Esophageal intubation. An initial pulse of carbon dioxide from swallowed gas may be sensed by the capnometer. However, the waveform should return to zero within several breaths.

    b.   Problems with the circle system or endotracheal tube.

      (1)   Disconnection.

      (2)   Malfunctioning inspiratory or expiratory valves.

      (3)   Leak in the circuit or sampling system.

      (4)   Exhausted carbon dioxide absorber.

      (5)   Obstruction in breathing system, endotracheal tube, or sampling line.

      (6)   Slow sampling with rapid respiratory rate.

    c.   Changes in the patient:

      (1)   A rapidly rising end-tidal carbon dioxide waveform is one of the early signs of **malignant hyperthermia**.

      (2)   Low perfusion/shock states.

      (3)   Embolism of air, fat, or thrombus.

      (4)   Obstruction to expiration (e.g., asthma, foreign body, extrinsic compression of the airway).

      (5)   Ventilation and perfusion mismatching.

      (6)   Absorption of carbon dioxide from the peritoneal cavity during laparoscopic procedures.

      (7)   Reperfusion after release of long-standing tourniquet or arterial clamp.

      (8)   Early sign of return of neuromuscular function after pharmacologic blockade.

  4.   The capnograph can also be used during monitored anesthesia care to assess the presence or absence of ventilation. This can be accomplished by attaching the capnograph sampling line to a simple face mask by way of an intravenous cannula. This method provides a qualitative reflection of ventilation, but is not an accurate estimate of end-tidal CO_2.

IX.   Temperature monitoring

  A.   Indications

    1.   Malignant hyperthermia is an ever-present danger, and temperature monitoring must always be available.

    2.   Infants and small children with a high ratio of body surface area to mass have poor thermal stability and tolerate hypothermia poorly.

    3.   Adults subjected to low ambient temperatures and large evaporative losses (from burns, exposed peritoneum, transfusion of cold fluids, or extensive irrigation) may become hypothermic.

    4.   Cardiopulmonary bypass with induced hypothermia.

    5.   The febrile patient.

    6.   The patient with **autonomic dysfunction**.

  B.   Several sites may be used for temperature monitoring, including the skin, axilla, rectum, esophagus, nasopharynx, tympanic membranes, bladder, and blood.

    1.   Changes in skin temperature may not reflect changes in core temperature (skin temperature on the forehead is on average 3 to 4°C below core temperature).

    2.   The axilla can be used for temperature determination if the probe is secured over the axillary artery and the arm fully

adducted to the patient's side. The measured temperature will usually be 1°C lower than core temperature after equilibration.
3. **Rectal temperatures** changes lag behind early changes in core body temperature during anesthesia. Because of this hysteresis, in combination with nasopharyngeal monitoring, it is useful during rewarming from cardiopulmonary bypass to indicate slower "shell" warming. Rectal perforation is a rare complication.
4. **Esophageal temperature** should be measured in the lower third of the esophagus. Esophageal temperature is an accurate reflection of core and blood temperature.
5. **Nasopharyngeal temperature** accurately reflects brain temperature. The probe can be placed correctly by measuring the distance between the external meatus of the ear and the external nares and inserting the probe to that distance. Care should be taken to make sure the probe does not continuously press against the margin of the nostril during long procedures, because skin necrosis could occur. Nasopharyngeal probes can cause significant bleeding, especially in pregnant patients (engorged nasal mucosa) and those with coagulopathies or receiving anticoagulants or thrombolytic therapy. They are relatively contraindicated in patients with head trauma and cerebrospinal fluid rhinorrhea.
6. **Tympanic membrane temperature** measures core temperature by the placement of a special probe near the eardrum. It is rapid and reasonably accurate if the ear canal is free of cerumen.
7. **Blood temperature** can be measured directly by the thermistor of an indwelling PAC.
X. **Neuromuscular blockade monitoring** (see Chapter 12)
XI. **Central nervous system monitoring** (see Chapter 24)

SUGGESTED READING

Jacobsohn E, Chorn R, O'Connor M. The role of the vasculature in regulating venous return and cardiac output: historical and graphical approach. *Can J Anaesth* 1997;44:849–867.

Lake CL. *Clinical monitoring: practical applications for anesthesia & critical care*, 1st ed. Philadelphia: WB Saunders, 2001.

Mark JB. *Atlas of cardiovascular monitoring*. New York: Churchill Livingstone, 1998.

Pagel PS, Grossman W, Haering JM, et al. Left ventricular diastolic function in the normal and diseased heart (pt 1). *Anesthesiology* 1993;79: 836–854.

Pagel PS, Grossman W, Haering JM, et al. Left ventricular diastolic function in the normal and diseased heart (pt 2). *Anesthesiology* 1993;79: 1104–1120.

Perret C, Tagan D, Feihl F, et al. *The pulmonary artery catheter in critical care*. Oxford: Blackwell Science, 1996.

Sagawa K, Maughan L, Suga H, et al. *Cardiac contraction and the pressure-volume relationship*. Oxford: Oxford University Press, 1988.

Intravenous and Inhalation Anesthetics

Mark Dershwitz

I. Pharmacology of intravenous (IV) anesthetics

A. Propofol (2,6-diisopropylphenol) is used for induction or maintenance of general anesthesia. It is prepared as a 1% isotonic oil-in-water emulsion, which contains egg lecithin, glycerol, and soybean oil. Bacterial growth is inhibited by either ethylenediaminetetraacetic acid or sulfite, depending on the manufacturer.

1. Mode of action. Increases activity at inhibitory γ-aminobutyric acid (GABA) synapses.

2. Pharmacokinetics

a. Elimination occurs primarily through hepatic metabolism to inactive metabolites.

b. The **context sensitive half-time** (CSHT) of propofol is shown in Fig. 11-1. CSHT is defined as the time for a 50% decrease in the central compartment drug concentration after an infusion of specified duration. For example, the CSHT of propofol is 15 minutes after a 2-hour infusion.

c. Induction doses rapidly produce unconsciousness (approximately 30 to 45 seconds), followed by rapid reawakening due to redistribution.

3. Pharmacodynamics

a. Central nervous system (CNS)

(1) Induction doses produce unconsciousness, whereas low doses produce conscious sedation.

(2) No analgesic properties.

b. Cardiovascular system

(1) A cardiovascular depressant.

(2) Produces dose-dependent decreases in arterial blood pressure and cardiac output.

(3) Heart rate is minimally affected, and barostatic reflex is blunted.

c. Respiratory system

(1) Produces a dose-dependent decrease in respiratory rate and tidal volume.

(2) Ventilatory response to hypercarbia is diminished.

4. Dosage and administration

a. Induction: 2.0 to 2.5 mg/kg IV.

b. Sedation: 25 to 75 μg/kg/min by IV infusion is often sufficient (titrate to effect).

c. Maintenance of general anesthesia: 100 to 150 μg/kg/min IV (titrate to effect).

d. Reduce dosages in elderly or hemodynamically compromised patients or if administered with other anesthetics.

e. May be diluted, if necessary, only in 5% dextrose in water to a minimum concentration of 0.2%.

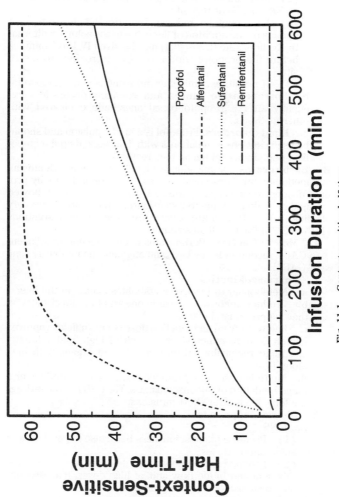

Fig. 11-1. Context-sensitive half-time.

f. Propofol emulsion supports bacterial growth; prepare drug under sterile conditions and discard unused opened propofol after six hours to prevent inadvertent bacterial contamination.

5. **Other effects**
   a. **Venous irritation**
      (1) May cause pain during IV administration in as many as 50% to 75% of patients.
      (2) Pain may be reduced by prior administration of opioids or the addition of lidocaine to the solution; alternatively, lidocaine (0.5 mg/kg) may be given IV 1 to 2 minutes before the propofol with a tourniquet proximal to the IV site.
      (3) If possible, administer intravenously in a large vein.
   b. **Postoperative nausea and vomiting** occurs less frequently after a propofol-based anesthetic compared with other methods.
   c. **Lipid disorders.** Propofol is a lipid emulsion and should be used cautiously in patients with disorders of lipid metabolism (e.g., hyperlipidemia, pancreatitis).

B. **Barbiturates** for anesthesia include thiopental, thiamylal, and methohexital. These medications, like propofol, rapidly produce unconsciousness (approximately 30 to 45 seconds), followed by rapid reawakening due to redistribution. Barbiturates are very alkaline (pH > 10) and are usually prepared as dilute solutions (1.0% to 2.5%) for IV administration.

1. **Mode of action.** Barbiturates occupy receptors adjacent to GABA receptors in the CNS and augment the inhibitory tone of GABA.

2. **Pharmacokinetics**
   a. Metabolism to inactive metabolites occurs in the liver.
   b. Produce unconsciousness in one arm-to-brain circulation time (approximately 30 seconds).
   c. Recovery from an induction dose occurs quickly (approximately 5 to 10 minutes) as a result of high lipid solubility and rapid redistribution into muscle and organs with high blood flow.
   d. Multiple doses or a prolonged infusion may produce prolonged sedation or unconsciousness. The CSHT of these drugs are long, even after short infusions.

3. **Pharmacodynamics**
   a. **CNS**
      (1) Produce unconsciousness but cause hyperalgesia in subhypnotic doses.
      (2) Produce a dose-dependent decrease in cerebral metabolism and blood flow and, at high doses, may produce an isoelectric electroencephalogram.
   b. **Cardiovascular system**
      (1) Decrease arterial blood pressure and cardiac output in a dose-dependent manner.
      (2) May increase heart rate via baroreceptor reflexes.
   c. **Respiratory system.** Produce a dose-dependent decrease in respiratory rate and tidal volume. Apnea may result for 30 to 90 seconds after a sleep dose.

4. Dosage and administration. Induction doses are as follows:

   a. Thiopental and thiamylal: 3 to 5 mg/kg IV.

   b. Methohexital: 1 to 2 mg/kg IV or 25 to 30 mg/kg per rectum (see Chapter 28).

   c. Reduce doses in sick, elderly, or hypovolemic patients.

5. Adverse effects

   a. Allergy. Do not administer to patients with a history of allergy to any barbiturate. Anaphylactic and anaphylactoid reactions occur rarely.

   b. Porphyria

   (1) **Absolutely contraindicated** in patients with acute intermittent porphyria, variegate porphyria, and hereditary coproporphyria.

   (2) Barbiturates induce the enzyme δ-aminolevulinic acid synthetase, the rate-limiting step in porphyrin synthesis, and may precipitate an acute attack.

   c. Venous irritation and tissue damage

   (1) May cause pain at the site of administration because of venous irritation.

   (2) Infiltration or intraarterial administration of a barbiturate may cause severe pain, tissue damage, and necrosis due to its high alkalinity. If intraarterial administration occurs, heparinization and regional sympathetic blockade may be helpful in treatment.

   d. Myoclonus and hiccoughing are often associated with the administration of methohexital.

C. Benzodiazepines include midazolam, diazepam, and lorazepam. They are often used for sedation and amnesia or as adjuncts to general anesthesia.

1. Mode of action: Bind at specific receptors in the CNS and enhance the inhibitory tone of GABA receptors.

2. Pharmacokinetics

   a. Metabolized in the liver.

   b. Peak CNS effects occur 4 to 8 minutes after an IV dose of diazepam, and its terminal half-life is approximately 20 hours. Repeated doses result in accumulation and a prolonged effect. Active metabolites of diazepam are longer lasting than the parent drug.

   c. Both midazolam and diazepam redistribute rapidly and similarly after bolus injections.

   d. Metabolism may be significantly slower in elderly patients or those with hepatic disease.

3. Pharmacodynamics

   a. CNS

   (1) Produce amnestic, anticonvulsant, hypnotic, muscle-relaxant, and sedative effects in a dose-dependent manner.

   (2) Do not produce significant analgesia.

   (3) Reduce cerebral blood flow and metabolic rate.

   b. Cardiovascular system

   (1) Produce a mild systemic vasodilation and reduction in cardiac output. Heart rate is usually unchanged.

   (2) Hemodynamic changes may be pronounced in hypovolemic patients or in those with little cardiovascular reserve, if rapidly administered in a large dose, or if administered with an opioid.

  c. Respiratory system
  (1) Produce a mild dose-dependent decrease in respiratory rate and tidal volume.
  (2) Respiratory depression may be pronounced if administered with an opioid, in patients with pulmonary disease, or in debilitated patients.
  4. **Dosage and administration**
    a. **Sedation**(incremental doses)
    (1) **Midazolam:** 0.5 to 1.0 mg IV or 0.07-0.1 mg/kg intramuscularly (IM). Midazolam is the only benzodiazepine that can be given reliably by the intramuscular route.
    (2) **Diazepam:** 2.5 to 5.0 mg IV or orally.
    (3) **Lorazepam:** 0.5 to 2.0 mg IV or orally.
    (4) Preoperative benzodiazepine administration may lead to prolonged sedation postoperatively.
  5. **Adverse effects**
    a. **Drug interactions.** Administration of a benzodiazepine to a patient receiving the anticonvulsant valproate may precipitate a psychotic episode.
    b. **Pregnancy and labor**
    (1) May be associated with birth defects (cleft lip and palate) when administered during the first trimester.
    (2) Cross the placenta and may lead to a depressed neonate.
  6. **Flumazenil** is a competitive antagonist for benzodiazepine receptors in the CNS.
    a. Reversal of benzodiazepine-induced sedative effects occurs within 2 minutes; peak effects occur at approximately 10 minutes.
    b. Flumazenil is shorter acting than the benzodiazepines it is used to antagonize. Repeated administration may be necessary due to its short duration of action.
    c. Metabolized to inactive metabolites in the liver.
    d. **Dose:** 0.3 mg IV every 30 to 60 seconds (to a maximum dose of 5 mg).
    e. Flumazenil is **contraindicated** in patients with tricyclic antidepressant overdose and patients receiving benzodiazepines for control of seizures or elevated intracranial pressure. Use cautiously in patients who have had long-term treatment with benzodiazepines because acute withdrawal may be precipitated.
D. **Ketamine.** An arylcyclohexylamine and a congener of phencyclidine (PCP), ketamine is usually employed as an induction agent.
  1. **Mode of action:** Not well defined but may include antagonism at the N-methyl-D-aspartate receptor
  2. **Pharmacokinetics**
    a. Metabolized in the liver to multiple metabolites, some of which are active.
    b. Produces unconsciousness in 30 to 60 seconds after an IV induction dose; unconsciousness may last 15 to 20 minutes. After IM administration, the onset of CNS effects is delayed for approximately 5 minutes, with peak effect at approximately 15 minutes.

    c. Repeated bolus doses or an infusion results in accumulation.

3. Pharmacodynamics

    a. CNS

      (1) Produces a "dissociative" state accompanied by amnesia and profound analgesia.

      (2) Increases cerebral blood flow, metabolic rate, and intracranial pressure.

    b. Cardiovascular system

      (1) Increases heart rate and systemic and pulmonary artery blood pressure by causing release of endogenous catecholamines.

      (2) Often used for induction of general anesthesia in hemodynamically compromised patients.

      (3) May act as a myocardial depressant if administered in the presence of hypovolemia, autonomic nervous system blockade, or maximal sympathetic nervous system stimulation.

    c. Respiratory system

      (1) Mildly depresses respiratory rate and tidal volume.

      (2) Minimal effect on responsiveness to hypercarbia.

      (3) Laryngeal protective reflexes tend to be maintained longer than with other intravenous anesthetics.

      (4) Alleviates bronchospasm by a sympathomimetic effect.

4. Dosage and administration

    a. It may be especially useful for IM induction in patients in whom IV access is not available (e.g., children). Ketamine is water soluble and may be administered either IV or IM.

    b. Induction dosages are 1 to 2 mg/kg IV or 5 to 10 mg/kg IM (a concentrated 10% solution is available for IM use only).

    c. IV sedative doses may be significantly lower (e.g., 0.2 mg/kg) and should be titrated to the desired effect.

5. Adverse effects

    a. Oral secretions are markedly stimulated by ketamine. Coadministration of an antisialagogue (e.g., glycopyrrolate) may be helpful.

    b. Emotional disturbance: Administration of ketamine may occasionally result in restlessness and agitation during emergence; hallucinations and unpleasant dreams may occur postoperatively. Patient characteristics associated with adverse effects include increased age, female gender, and dosages greater than 2 mg/kg. The incidence (up to 30%) of these untoward sequelae may be greatly reduced with coadministration of a benzodiazepine (e.g., midazolam) or propofol. Children seem to be less troubled by the hallucinations than adults. Alternatives to ketamine should be considered in patients with psychiatric disorders.

    c. Muscle tone. May lead to random myoclonic movements, especially in response to stimulation. Muscle tone is often increased.

    d. Increases intracranial pressure and is relatively contraindicated in patients with head trauma or intracranial hypertension.

    e. Eye movements. May lead to nystagmus, diplopia, blepharospasm, and increased intraocular pressure; alternatives should be considered during ophthalmologic surgery.

f.   Anesthetic depth may be difficult to assess. Common signs of anesthetic depth (e.g., respiratory rate, blood pressure, heart rate, eye signs) are less reliable when ketamine is used.

D.   Etomidate is an imidazole-containing hypnotic unrelated to other anesthetics; it is most commonly used as an IV induction agent for general anesthesia.

1.   Mode of action: Augments the inhibitory tone of GABA in the CNS.

2.   Pharmacokinetics

a.   Metabolized in the liver and by circulating esterases to inactive metabolites.

b.   Times to loss of consciousness and awakening after a sleep dose are similar to those of propofol.

3.   Pharmacodynamics

a.   CNS

(1)   Does not possess analgesic properties.

(2)   Cerebral blood flow and metabolism decrease in a dose-dependent manner.

b.   Cardiovascular system. Produces minimal changes in heart rate, blood pressure, and cardiac output; accordingly, etomidate may be a preferred agent for induction of general anesthesia in a hemodynamically compromised patient.

c.   Respiratory system. Produces a dose-dependent decrease in respiratory rate and tidal volume; transient apnea may occur. The respiratory depressant effects of etomidate appear to be less than those of propofol or the barbiturates.

4.   Dosage and administration: Available as a solution in propylene glycol. An IV induction dose is 0.3 mg/kg.

5.   Adverse effects

a.   Myoclonus may occur after administration, particularly in response to stimulation.

b.   Nausea and vomiting occur more frequently in the postoperative period than with other anesthetic agents.

c.   Venous irritation may be minimized by administration into a free-flowing IV carrier infusion.

d.   Adrenal suppression. Suppresses adrenal steroid synthesis for up to 24 hours (probably an effect of little clinical significance). Repeated doses or infusions are not recommended because of the risk of significant adrenal suppression.

F.   Opioids. Morphine, meperidine, fentanyl, sufentanil, alfentanil, and remifentanil are the major opioids commonly used in general anesthesia. Their primary effect is analgesia, and therefore they are used to supplement other agents during induction or maintenance of general anesthesia. In high doses, opioids are occasionally used as the sole anesthetic (e.g., cardiac surgery). The opioids differ in their potency, pharmacokinetics, and side effects.

1.   Mode of action: Opioids bind at specific receptors in the brain and spinal cord.

2.   Pharmacokinetics

Table 11-1. Dose, time to peak effect, and duration of analgesia for intravenous opioid agonists and agonist-antagonists[a]

Opioid	Dose (mg)[b]	Peak (min)	Duration (h)[c]
Morphine	10	30–60	3–4
Meperidine	80	5–7	2–3
Hydromorphone	1.5	15–30	2–3
Oxymorphone	1.0	15–30	3–4
Methadone	10	15–30	3–4
Fentanyl	0.1	3–5	0.5–1
Sufentanil	0.01	3–5	0.5–1
Alfentanil	0.75	1.5–2	0.2–0.3
Remifentanil	0.1	1.5–2	0.1–0.2
Pentazocine	60	15–30	2–3
Butorphanol	2	15–30	2–3
Nalbuphine	10	15–30	3–4
Buprenorphine	0.3	<30	5–6
Dezocine	10	15–30	3–4

[a]Data for fentanyl derivatives are derived from intraoperative studies; the remainder from postoperative pain studies.
[b]Approximately equianalgetic doses (see text).
[c]Average duration of first single dose.

    a. Pharmacokinetic data are presented in Table 11-1, and the CSHTs for alfentanil, sufentanil, and remifentanil are shown in Fig. 11-1.
    b. Elimination is primarily by the liver and is dependent on hepatic blood flow. Most opioids have inactive metabolites that are excreted in the urine. Remifentanil is metabolized by circulating and skeletal muscle esterases.
    c. After IV administration of opioids, onset of action is within minutes; those opioids with greater lipid solubility have a more rapid clinical onset.
  3. Pharmacodynamics
    a. CNS
      (1) Produce sedation and analgesia in a dose-dependent manner; euphoria is common.
      (2) In large doses may (but not reliably) produce amnesia and loss of consciousness.
      (3) Reduce the minimum alveolar concentration (MAC) of volatile and gaseous anesthetic agents.
      (4) Decrease cerebral blood flow and metabolic rate. Meperidine, in large doses, may produce CNS excitation and seizures, possibly secondary to the effects of normeperidine, a metabolite.
    b. Cardiovascular system
      (1) Produce minimal changes in cardiac contractility

(with the exception of meperidine, which is a direct myocardial depressant).

(2)   Systemic vascular resistance usually is moderately reduced because of reduced medullary sympathetic outflow.

(3)   Systemic resistance may be greatly reduced with the administration of meperidine or morphine because of histamine release.

(4)   May markedly enhance the myocardial depressant effects of other agents.

(5)   Produce bradycardia in a dose-dependent manner by a centrally mediated mechanism.

(6)   Meperidine may produce an increase in heart rate, possibly because of its atropine-like structure.

(7)   The relative hemodynamic stability offered by opioids often leads to their use as the primary anesthetic in hemodynamically compromised or critically ill patients.

c.   Respiratory system

(1)   Produce respiratory depression in a dose-dependent manner. Initially, respiratory rate decreases; with larger doses tidal volume decreases. Effect may be accentuated in the presence of other respiratory depressants or preexisting pulmonary disease.

(2)   Decrease ventilatory response to Pa_{CO_2}.

(3)   May produce apnea from respiratory depression or muscle rigidity.

(4)   Opioids produce a decrease in the cough reflex in a dose-dependent manner.

d.   Pupil size. Decrease in pupil size (miosis) by stimulation of the Edinger-Westphal nucleus.

e.   Muscle rigidity may occur after opioid administration, especially in the chest, abdomen, and upper airway, resulting in the inability to ventilate the patient; the incidence increases with drug potency, dose, rate of administration, and presence of nitrous oxide. This rigidity may be overcome by administration of neuromuscular relaxants or opioid antagonists. The incidence may be decreased by pretreatment with a small dose of a nondepolarizing muscle relaxant or a sedative dose of a benzodiazepine or propofol.

f.   Gastrointestinal system.

(1)   Produce an increase in the tone and secretions of the gastrointestinal tract and a decrease in motility.

(2)   May produce biliary colic; the incidence may be lower with the agonist-antagonist agents.

g.   Nausea and vomiting can occur because of direct stimulation of the chemoreceptor trigger zone.

h.   Urinary retention may occur because of stimulation of the vesical sphincter and a decrease in awareness of the need to urinate.

i.   Allergy is rare.

j.   Drug interactions. Administration of meperidine to a patient who has received a monoamine oxidase inhibitor may result in delirium, hyperthermia, and may be fatal.

4.   Dosage and administration. Opioids are usually administered IV, either by bolus or infusion. Appropriate dosages are presented in Table 11-1. Clinical dosing must be individualized and based on the patient's underlying condition and clinical response. Larger doses may be required in patients chronically receiving opioids.

5. Naloxone is a pure opioid antagonist used to reverse unanticipated or undesired opioid-induced effects such as respiratory or CNS depression.

   a. Mode of action. Naloxone is a competitive antagonist at opioid receptors in the brain and spinal cord.

   b. Pharmacokinetics
      (1) Peak effects are seen within 1 to 2 minutes; a significant decrease in its clinical effects occurs after 30 minutes.
      (2) Metabolized in the liver.

   c. Pharmacodynamics
      (1) Reverses the pharmacologic effects of opioids such as CNS and respiratory depression.
      (2) Crosses the placenta; administration to the mother before delivery will decrease the degree of respiratory depression in the neonate secondary to opioids.

   d. Dosage and administration: Titrated every 2 to 3 minutes in IV boluses of 0.04 mg until the desired effect is attained.

   e. Adverse effects
      (1) Pain. May lead to the abrupt onset of pain as opioid analgesia is reversed. This may be accompanied by abrupt hemodynamic changes (e.g., hypertension, tachycardia).
      (2) Cardiac arrest. Naloxone administration has, in rare cases, precipitated pulmonary edema and cardiac arrest.
      (3) Repeated administration may be needed due to its short duration of action.

II. Pharmacology of inhalation anesthetics

Inhalation anesthetics are usually administered for maintenance of general anesthesia but also can be used for induction, especially in pediatric patients. General properties of inhalation anesthetics are presented in Table 11-2. Dosages of inhalation anesthetics are ex-

Table 11-2. Properties of inhalation anesthetics

| Anesthetic | Vapor Pressure (mm Hg, 20°C) | Partition coefficients | | MAC (% with O$_2$ only) |
		Blood Gas[a] (37°C)	Brain-blood (37°C)	
Halothane	243	2.3	2.0	0.74
Enflurane	175	1.8	1.4	1.68
Isoflurane	239	1.4	1.6	1.15
Desflurane	664	0.42	1.3	6.0
Sevoflurane	157	0.69	1.7	2.05
Nitrous oxide	39,000	0.47	1.1	104

MAC, minimum alveolar concentration that inhibits movement in response to a skin incision in 50% of patients.

[a]The blood-gas partition coefficient is inversely related to the rate of induction.

pressed as **MAC**, the **minimum alveolar concentration** at one atmosphere at which 50% of patients do not move in response to a surgical stimulus.

A.   **Nitrous oxide** is a clear, colorless, and odorless gas.

1.   **Mode of action.** Produces general anesthesia through interaction with the cellular membranes of the CNS; exact mechanisms are not clear.

2.   **Pharmacokinetics**

a.   Uptake and elimination of nitrous oxide are relatively rapid compared with other inhaled anesthetics, primarily as a result of its low blood-gas partition coefficient (0.47).

b.   Elimination of nitrous oxide is via exhalation.

c.   Significant biotransformation has not been demonstrated.

3.   **Pharmacodynamics**

a.   **CNS**

(1)   Produces analgesia.

(2)   Concentrations greater than 60% may produce amnesia, although not reliably.

(3)   Because of its high MAC (104%), it is usually combined with other anesthetics to attain surgical anesthesia.

b.   **Cardiovascular system**

(1)   Mild myocardial depressant and a mild sympathetic nervous system stimulant.

(2)   Heart rate and blood pressure are usually unchanged.

(3)   May increase pulmonary vascular resistance in adults.

c.   **Respiratory system.** Nitrous oxide is a mild respiratory depressant, although less than the volatile anesthetics.

4.   **Adverse effects**

a.   **Expansion of closed gas spaces.** The predominant constituent in closed gas-containing spaces in the body is nitrogen. Because nitrous oxide is 31 times more soluble in blood than nitrogen, closed air spaces will expand as more nitrous oxide diffuses into these spaces than nitrogen diffuses out. Spaces such as a pneumothorax, occluded middle ear, the bowel lumen, an air bubble, or pneumocephalus will markedly enlarge if nitrous oxide is administered. Nitrous oxide will diffuse into the cuff of an endotracheal tube and may markedly increase pressure within the cuff; this pressure should be intermittently assessed and, if necessary, adjusted.

b.   **Diffusion hypoxia.** After discontinuation of nitrous oxide, its rapid diffusion from the blood into the lung may lead to a partial pressure of oxygen in the alveoli dramatically lower than the inspired Po_2, resulting in hypoxia and hypoxemia if supplemental oxygen is not administered.

c.   **Inhibition of tetrahydrofolate synthesis.** Inactivates methionine synthetase, a vitamin B_{12}-dependent enzyme necessary for the synthesis of DNA. Nitrous oxide should be used with caution in pregnant patients and those deficient in vitamin B_{12}.

B.   Volatile agents are liquids whose potent evaporative vapors (in a carrier gas) are used in inhalation anesthesia. Those currently in use include halothane, enflurane, isoflurane, desflurane, and sevoflurane.

1. **Mode of action:** Produce general anesthesia through interaction with the cellular membranes of the CNS; exact mechanisms are not clear.

2. **Pharmacokinetics**

   a. **Determinants of speed of onset and offset.** The alveolar anesthetic concentration (F_A) may differ significantly from the inspired anesthetic concentration (F_I). The rate of rise of the ratio of these two concentrations (F_A/F_I) determines the speed of induction of general anesthesia (Fig. 11-2). Two opposing processes, anesthetic delivery to and uptake from alveoli, determine the F_A/F_I at a given time. Determinants of uptake include the following:

      (1) **Blood-gas partition coefficient.** A lower solubility will lead to more rapid absorption and excretion (nitrous oxide > desflurane > sevoflurane > isoflurane > enflurane > halothane). Decreasing anesthetic solubility in blood decreases uptake, thereby increasing the rate of rise of F_A/F_I. The solubility of halogenated volatile anesthetics in blood is increased somewhat with hypothermia and hyperlipidemia.

      (2) **Inspired anesthetic concentration**, which is influenced by circuit size, fresh gas inflow rate, and solubility of volatile anesthetic in circuit components.

      (3) **Alveolar ventilation.** Increased ventilation, without alteration of other processes that affect anesthetic delivery or uptake, increases F_A/F_I. This effect is more pronounced with the more blood-soluble agents.

      (4) **Concentration effect.** For a given uptake (e.g., 50%), the resulting decrease in alveolar anesthetic concentration is proportionately less at higher inspired concentrations (a decrease to 0.5% for a 1% inspired concentration, compared with a decrease to 67% for an 80% inspired concentration). In addition, as anesthetic is removed from the alveoli by blood uptake, additional fresh gas is drawn into the alveoli, augmenting the inspired tidal volume. This effect is also more significant at higher alveolar concentrations. The net effect of these two processes is an increase in the rate of rise of an anesthetic's alveolar concentration as its inspired concentration is increased.

      (5) **The second gas effect.** When two inhalation anesthetics are administered together, uptake by blood of large volumes of a "first" gas (e.g., nitrous oxide) increases both the alveolar concentration of a "second" gas (e.g., isoflurane) and the input of additional second gas into alveoli via augmentation of inspired volume.

      (6) **Cardiac output.** An increase in cardiac output (and pulmonary blood flow) will increase anesthetic uptake and decrease the rate of rise in alveolar concentration (and speed of induction). Conversely, a decrease in cardiac output will have the opposite effect. This effect of cardiac output is pronounced with nonrebreathing circuits or highly soluble anesthetics. It is also accentuated early in the course of anesthetic administration.

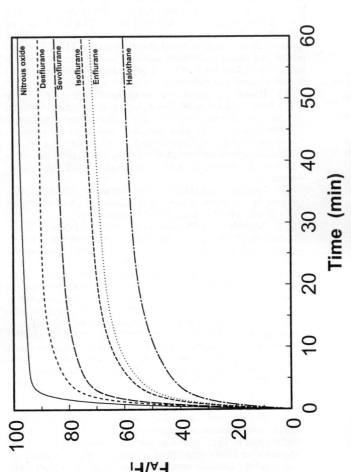

Fig. 11-2.   The ratio of alveolar to inspired gas concentration (F_A/F_I) as

(7) Gradient between alveolar and venous blood.
The uptake of anesthetic by blood perfusing the lung will increase (and the rate of rise of F_A/F_I will decrease) as the gradient between the partial pressure of anesthetic between the alveoli and blood increases. This gradient will be particularly large early in the course of anesthetic administration.

b. Distribution in tissues. The partial pressure of an inhalation anesthetic in arterial blood usually approximates its alveolar pressure. The arterial partial pressure may be significantly less, however, when marked ventilation-perfusion abnormalities (e.g., shunt) are present, especially with less-soluble anesthetics (e.g., nitrous oxide). The rate of equilibration of anesthetic partial pressure between blood and a particular organ system is dependent on the following factors:

(1) Tissue blood flow. Equilibration occurs more rapidly in tissues receiving increased perfusion. The most highly perfused organ systems receive approximately 75% of cardiac output; these include the brain, kidney, heart, liver, and endocrine glands and are referred to as the vessel-rich group. The remainder of the cardiac output perfuses predominantly muscle and fat.

(2) Tissue solubility. For a given arterial anesthetic partial pressure, anesthetic agents with a high tissue solubility are slower to equilibrate. Solubilities of anesthetic agents differ among tissues. Blood–brain partition coefficients of inhalation agents are shown in Table 11-2.

(3) Gradient between arterial blood and tissue. Until equilibration is reached between the anesthetic partial pressure in the blood and a particular tissue, a gradient exists that leads to uptake of anesthetic by the tissue. The rate of uptake will decrease as the gradient decreases.

c. Elimination

(1) Exhalation. This is the predominant route of elimination. After discontinuation, an anesthetic's tissue and alveolar partial pressures decrease by reversal of the processes that occurred when the anesthetic was introduced.

(2) Metabolism. Inhalation anesthetics may eventually undergo varying degrees of hepatic metabolism (halothane, 15%; enflurane, 2% to 5%; sevoflurane, 1.5%; isoflurane, <0.2%; desflurane, <0.2%). When anesthetizing concentrations of an agent are present (e.g., induction, maintenance), metabolism probably has little effect on the alveolar concentration because of saturation of hepatic enzymes. After discontinuation of the anesthetic, metabolism may contribute to the decrease in the alveolar concentration; however, the effect is not clinically significant.

(3) Anesthetic loss. Inhalation anesthetics can be lost from the body both percutaneously and through visceral membranes; these losses are probably negligible.

3. Pharmacodynamics

a. CNS

(1) Produce unconsciousness and amnesia at relatively low inspired concentrations (25% MAC).

(**2**)   Produce a dose-dependent generalized CNS depression and depression of electroencephalographic activity up to and including burst suppression.

(**3**)   **Enflurane** can produce electroencephalographic epileptiform activity at high inspired concentrations (>2%).

(**4**)   Produce decreased amplitude and increased latency of somatosensory evoked potentials.

(**5**)   Increase cerebral blood flow (halothane > enflurane > isoflurane, desflurane, or sevoflurane)

(**6**)   Decrease cerebral metabolic rate (isoflurane, desflurane, or sevoflurane > enflurane > halothane).

(**7**)   Uncouple autoregulation of cerebral blood flow; decreased cerebral metabolic rate does not lead to decreased cerebral blood flow.

b.   **Cardiovascular system**

(**1**)   Produce dose-dependent myocardial depression (halothane > enflurane > isoflurane $\geq$ desflurane or sevoflurane) and systemic vasodilation (isoflurane > desflurane or sevoflurane > enflurane > halothane).

(**2**)   Heart rate tends to be unchanged, although desflurane has been associated with sympathetic stimulation, tachycardia, and hypertension at induction or when the inspired concentration is abruptly increased. Isoflurane administration may lead to similar effects, but to a lesser degree than desflurane.

(**3**)   Sensitize the myocardium to the arrhythmogenic effects of catecholamines (halothane > enflurane > isoflurane or desflurane > sevoflurane), which is of particular concern during infiltration of epinephrine-containing solutions or the administration of sympathomimetic agents. With halothane, subcutaneous infiltration with epinephrine should not exceed 2 μg/kg/20 min. In a subgroup of patients with coronary artery disease, isoflurane may contribute to myocardial ischemia; the clinical significance of this is not clear (see Chapter 23).

c.   **Respiratory system**

(**1**)   Produce dose-dependent respiratory depression with a decrease in tidal volume, an increase in respiratory rate, and an increase in $Paco_2$.

(**2**)   Produce airway irritation (desflurane > isoflurane > enflurane > halothane > sevoflurane) and, during light levels of anesthesia, may precipitate coughing, laryngospasm, or bronchospasm, particularly in patients who smoke or have asthma. The lesser pungency of sevoflurane and halothane may make them more amenable as inhalation induction agents.

(**3**)   Equipotent doses of volatile agents possess similar bronchodilator effects with the exception of desflurane, which has mild bronchoconstricting activity.

d.   **Muscular system**

(**1**)   Produce a dose-dependent decrease in muscle tone, often enhancing surgical conditions.

(**2**)   May precipitate malignant hyperthermia in a susceptible patient (see Chapter 18).

e.   **Liver.** May cause a decrease in hepatic perfusion (halo-

thane > enflurane > isoflurane, desflurane, or sevoflurane).
Rarely, a patient may develop hepatitis secondary to exposure
to a volatile agent, most notably halothane ("halothane hepatitis") (see Chapter 5).
   f.   Renal system. Decrease renal blood flow through either
   a decrease in mean arterial blood pressure or an increase in
   renal vascular resistance.
4.   Reaction with carbon dioxide absorbent
   a.   Desflurane can be degraded in carbon dioxide absorbents (especially Baralyme when new or dry from the passage
   of large volumes of dry gas) to carbon monoxide; a few cases
   of clinically significant carbon monoxide poisoning have been
   reported.
   b.   Sevoflurane can be degraded in carbon dioxide absorbents (especially Baralyme) to fluoromethyl-2,2,-difluoro-1-
   vinyl ether (Compound A), which has been shown to produce
   renal toxicity in animal models. Compound A concentrations
   increase at low fresh gas rates. So far, there has been no
   evidence of consistent renal toxicity with sevoflurane usage
   in humans.

SUGGESTED READING

Ebert TJ, Frink EJ Jr, Kharasch ED. Absence of biochemical evidence for
   renal and hepatic dysfunction after 8 hours of 1.25 minimum alveolar
   concentration sevoflurane anesthesia in volunteers. *Anesthesiology*
   1998;88:601–610.

Eger EI. *Anesthetic uptake and action.* Baltimore: Williams & Wilkins,
   1974.

Eger EI. Uptake and distribution. In: Miller RD, ed. *Anesthesia*, 5th ed.
   New York: Churchill Livingstone, 2000:74–95.

Philbin DM, Rosow CE, Schneider RC, et al. Fentanyl and sufentanil
   anesthesia revisited: how much is enough? *Anesthesiology* 1990;73:
   5–11

Rosow CE, Dershwitz M. Pharmacology of opioid analgetic agents. In:
   Longnecker D, Tinker JH, Morgan GE Jr, eds. *Principles and practice
   of anesthesiology*, 2nd ed. Philadelphia: Mosby-Year Book, 1997.

Shafer SL, Varvel JR. Pharmacokinetics, pharmacodynamics, and rational opioid selection. *Anesthesiology* 1991;74:53–63.

12

Neuromuscular Blockade

Jason A. Campagna and Peter F. Dunn

The principal pharmacologic effect of neuromuscular blocking drugs (NMBDs) is to interrupt transmission of synaptic signaling at the neuromuscular junction (NMJ) by antagonism of the nicotinic acetylcholine receptor (AChR).

I. Anatomy and physiology of the NMJ

A. **The NMJ** comprises portions of three cell types: motor neuron, muscle fiber, and Schwann cell. It is a chemical synapse located in the peripheral nervous system that is composed of **the neuronal presynaptic terminal**, where **acetylcholine** (ACh) is stored and released, and the postsynaptic muscle cell (**motor endplate**), where high densities of the AChR reside. In the nerve terminal, ACh is stored for eventual release in specialized organelles known as **synaptic vesicles**. These vesicles are found in high concentrations in the regions of the nerve terminal that lie in direct apposition to areas of muscle membrane with high concentrations of AChRs. On the folds of the postsynaptic muscle membrane, AChRs are found in densities as high as $10,000/\mu m^2$ at the synapse and fall to concentrations as low as 10 to $100/\mu m^2$ at extrajunctional regions of the muscle cell.

B. In response to an action potential in the nerve, **voltage dependent N-type calcium channels**, which are also highly concentrated at the nerve terminal in close proximity to synaptic vesicles, open and cause a rapid influx of calcium into the nerve terminal. These calcium transients, lasting approximately 0.5 ms, elevate calcium concentrations intracellularly to approximately 100 μM and induce fusion of synaptic vesicles with the plasma membrane and release of the stored ACh. The ACh then diffuses across the synaptic cleft where two molecules of ACh bind simultaneously to a single AChR.

C. **Junctional AChRs** are composed of five subunits (α, α, β, δ, ϵ). Of these, the α subunits constitute the binding sites for ACh. When two molecules of ACh are bound, the AChR undergoes a conformational change, "activation," that allows influx of Na^+ and Ca^{2+} into the muscle cell, depolarizes the membrane, and causes contraction. As the membrane becomes depolarized, Na^+ and Ca^{2+} cease to enter and K^+ begins to move out, beginning the process of repolarization. At this point, the AChR is "inactivated." The amount of ACh released and the number of postsynaptic AChRs is much greater than that actually needed to induce contraction. This is termed the "safety factor" for neuromuscular transmission and plays a crucial role in neuromuscular transmission under certain pathologic conditions.

D. After triggering depolarization, the ACh diffuses into the synaptic cleft where it is broken down by **acetylcholinesterase** into choline and acetyl-CoA. These molecules are then recycled to synthesize new ACh for use in synaptic vesicles and synaptic transmission. Inactivated AChRs are now returned to their "resting" state, able to be activated once more.

II. General pharmacology of the NMJ

The precise apposition of a motor nerve terminal and the muscle membrane make the NMJ a very efficient specialized structure. AChR and acetylcholinesterase are the primary targets of most NMBDs used in clinical anesthesia.

A. Cholinergic receptors are categorized as **nicotinic** or **muscarinic** by their responses to the alkaloids nicotine and muscarine, respectively. There are two broad classes of nicotinic cholinergic receptors, muscular (N_M) and neuronal (N_N). N_M receptors are found at the NMJ, whereas N_N are in autonomic ganglia and the central nervous system (CNS). The various classes of muscarinic receptor are found in autonomic ganglia, at end-organ sites of parasympathetic innervation, and in the CNS. All these cholinergic receptors have different subunit composition and are affected differently by various agonists and antagonists. Nonspecific cholinergic agonists (e.g., reversal agents) can affect all of them, however.

B. There are well-described **signaling systems** that regulate the distribution and density of AChR at the NMJ. Conditions that affect AChR distribution are quite common clinically. For example, with burns, trauma, or disuse, the density of postsynaptic junctional AChRs decreases, whereas extrajunctional densities increase.

C. All NMBDs are antagonists of the AChR. Each is designated **depolarizing** or **nondepolarizing** based on whether it induces a depolarization of the muscle membrane after binding to the receptor. The agents differ substantially in their onset, duration of blockade, metabolism, side effects, and interactions with other drugs.

D. Succinylcholine (SCh) is currently the only available depolarizing NMBD. Nondepolarizing NMBDs are often divided by chemical class: **aminosteroid derivatives** (e.g., pancuronium, vecuronium, and rocuronium) and **benzylisoquinolines** (e.g., *d*-tubocurarine, cisatracurium, and mivacurium). The NMBDs also are commonly classified by duration of effect: ultrashort (SCh), short (mivacurium), intermediate (vecuronium, rocuronium, cisatracurium), and long (pancuronium, *d*-tubocurarine).

III. Neuromuscular Blockade

A. Depolarizing blockade occurs when a drug mimics the action of the neurotransmitter ACh. SCh, like ACh, binds and activates the AChR, which leads to depolarization of the endplate and adjacent muscle membrane. Because SCh is not degraded as quickly as ACh, persistent endplate depolarization inhibits the inward flow of sodium ions, and there is accommodation or inexcitability of the perijunctional muscle membrane. Inactivation of sodium channels explains how muscle relaxation can occur in the presence of an endplate potential sufficient to trigger an action potential.

1. Depolarizing blockade (Fig. 12-1) is characterized by:

a. Muscle fasciculation followed by relaxation.

b. Absence of fade after tetanic or train-of-four (TOF) stimulation (see Section IV.)

c. Absence of posttetanic potentiation (PTP).

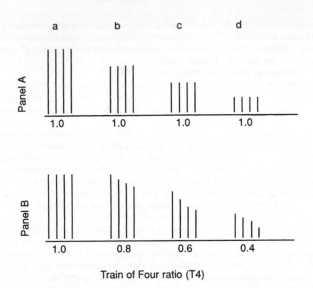

Fig. 12-1. A schematic representation of train-of-four responses to a depolarizing (A) and a nondepolarizing (B) relaxant, showing the control response before the relaxant (*a*) and afterward (*b, c, d*). Note no fade with the depolarizing relaxant and progressive fade with the nondepolarizing relaxant.

    d. Potentiation of the block by anticholinesterases.

    e. Antagonism of the block by nondepolarizing relaxants.

2. Depolarizing blockade from SCh ends when the molecule diffuses away from the receptor and is broken down to choline and succinic acid in the plasma. First, SCh is hydrolyzed by plasma cholinesterase to choline and succinylmonocholine (a depolarizing agent with 1/20 the potency of the dicholine). Second, and much more slowly, succinylmonocholine is converted to choline and succinic acid by both plasma cholinesterase and a nonspecific liver factor.

3. Side effects of SCh are related to its transient agonist effects at both the nicotinic and muscarinic AChRs.

    a. Myalgias are common postoperatively. They occur more frequently in women and in ambulatory patients after minor surgical procedures. The incidence of myalgias may be reduced by administering a small dose of a nondepolarizing relaxant (e.g., *d*-tubocurarine 3 mg intravenously [IV] or rocuronium 3 mg IV) 3 minutes before SCh. When pretreating for a rapid sequence induction, the subsequent dose of SCh is increased to 1.5 mg/kg IV. Awake patients pretreated with a nondepolarizing relaxant may experience diplopia, weakness, or dyspnea. Pretreatment with lidocaine, propofol, benzodiazepines, Mg^{2+}, vitamin C, and combinations have been tried but remain unproved. No technique can completely eliminate myalgias.

    b. Arrhythmias. Ganglionic stimulation may increase

heart rate and blood pressure in adults. **SCh** may produce sinus bradycardia, junctional rhythm, and sinus arrest in children after the first dose and in adults receiving a second dose within a short dose interval (i.e., 5 minutes). Pretreatment with atropine (0.4 mg IV) immediately before SCh may block this bradycardia.

c. SCh normally causes serum K^+ to increase 0.5 to 1.0 mEq/L but may produce dangerous **hyperkalemia** and cardiovascular collapse in patients with burns, upper and lower motor neuron disease, trauma, prolonged bed rest, muscle diseases, and closed head injuries. This effect is due to up-regulation of extrajunctional ACh receptors. In burned patients, the time of greatest risk is from 2 weeks to 6 months after the burn has been sustained; however, it is advisable to avoid SCh in burned patients after the first 24 hours and for 2 years from the injury. Patients with renal failure may safely receive SCh if they are not already hyperkalemic or acidemic.

d. **A transient increase in intraocular pressure** occurs after an intubating dose of SCh due to contraction of the extraocular muscles. The use of SCh in open eye injuries is controversial (see Chapter 25, section I.C.1.a for a full discussion).

e. **Increased intragastric pressure** results from fasciculation of abdominal muscles. The pressure increase averages 15 to 20 mm Hg in an adult but does not occur to a significant extent in infants and children.

f. SCh produces a mild brief **increase in cerebral blood flow and intracranial pressure** (see Chapter 24, section II.C).

g. A history of **malignant hyperthermia** is an absolute contraindication to the use of SCh. Malignant hyperthermia may be triggered in susceptible patients. Failure of the masseter muscle to relax or generalized myotonia after SCh should alert one to this possibility (see Chapter 18, section XVII).

h. **Pretreatment with nondepolarizing NMBDs** can block visible fasciculations but is not uniformly effective in attenuating the above-mentioned side effects.

i. **The occurrence of phase II block** is most likely after repeated or continuous administration of SCh. Phase II block may occur with dosages of 2 to 5 mg/kg IV in conjunction with inhalation anesthetics and 8 to 12 mg/kg with nitrous oxide-opioid anesthesia. Phase II blockade is characterized by

(1) Fade after tetanic or TOF stimulation.

(2) Tachyphylaxis (increasing dose requirement).

(3) Partial or complete reversal with anticholinesterases.

j. **Prolonged blockade** may be caused by low levels of plasma cholinesterase, drug-induced inhibition of cholinesterase activity, or a genetically atypical enzyme.

(1) **Decreased plasma cholinesterase levels** are seen in the last trimester of pregnancy, liver disease, starvation, carcinomas, hypothyroidism, burn patients, shock, uremia, cardiac failure, and after therapeutic radiation.

(2) **Inhibition of plasma cholinesterase** occurs with the use of organophosphate compounds (e.g., insecticides, echothiophate eye drops), drugs that inhibit acetylcholinesterase (e.g., neostigmine, pyridostigmine), and certain other drugs (e.g., the monoamine oxidase inhibitor, phenelzine). Plasma cholinesterase levels are not usually altered after hemodialysis.

(3)   Heterozygous atypical plasma cholinesterase occurs in 4% of the general population, whereas the incidence of **homozygous atypical cholinesterase** enzyme is about 0.04% (1 of 2,800 patients). Homozygous atypical patients have prolonged neuromuscular blockade and respiratory insufficiency for 2 to 3 hours after SCh administration. The **dibucaine number** is a laboratory assay to characterize plasma cholinesterase abnormality. Normal plasma cholinesterase is 80% inhibited *in vitro* by the local anesthetic, dibucaine (dibucaine number 80), whereas the homozygous atypical plasma cholinesterase is only 20% inhibited (dibucaine number 20). A range of dibucaine numbers from 30 to 65 occurs in heterozygotes. Less commonly, individuals sensitive to SCh may have a fluoride-resistant enzyme (with a normal dibucaine number but low fluoride number) or a silent gene with complete absence of plasma cholinesterase (dibucaine number 0) and no esterase activity.

B.   Nondepolarizing blockade is reversible competitive antagonism of ACh at the α subunits of the AChR.

1.   Other mechanisms can be involved under certain circumstances:

a.   Physical block of the ion channel can occur during rapid stimulation (open channel or "use-dependent blockade").

b.   Noncompetitive blockade around the extracellular entrance of the channel may be produced by some antibiotics, quinidine, tricyclic antidepressants, and naloxone.

c.   Binding of the NMBD to another "allosteric" site on the receptor may render it unresponsive to ACh.

d.   Desensitization can be produced by long duration of exposure of the AChR to an agonist resulting in a conformational change in the receptor.

e.   Interference with presynaptic ACh mobilization or Ca^{2+} influx. The commonly used nondepolarizing relaxants probably mediate these prejunctional effects by binding to cholinergic receptors on the presynaptic terminal.

2.   Nondepolarizing blockade (Figs. 12-1 and 12-2) is characterized by:

a.   Absence of fasciculations.

b.   Fade during tetanic and TOF stimulation.

c.   PTP.

d.   Antagonism of block by depolarizing agents and anticholinesterases.

e.   Potentiation of block by other nondepolarizing agents.

3.   Synergistic blockade may result when steroidal NMBDs (e.g., vecuronium or rocuronium) are combined with benzylisoquinolines (e.g., atracurium or cisatracurium). The combined effects of agents with similar chemical structure, such as *d*-tubocurarine and atracurium, are additive.

4.   The clinical pharmacology of the commonly used nondepolarizing NMBDs is outlined in Table 12-1.

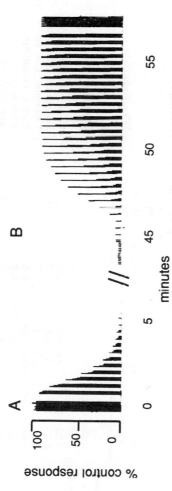

Fig. 12-2. A: The electromyographic response to repeated train-of-four (TOF) stimulation after the injection of a nondepolarizing agent. Fade of TOF response eventually leaves only one twitch (approximately 90% block). B: Reversal of the blockade by neostigmine and atropine given 45 minutes later shows a progressive recovery of the TOF response and reduction in fade with a TOF ratio of 0.9.

Table 12-1.   Comparative clinical pharmacology of relaxants[a,b]

	$ED_{95}{}^{c}$ (mg/kg IV)	Intubating Dose (mg/kg IV)[d]	Time to Intubation (min)[e]	Time to 25% Recovery (min)[f]	Elimination
Depolarizing drug					
Succinylcholine	0.25	1	1	5–20	Hydrolysis by plasma cholinesterase.
Nondepolarizing drug					
Atracurium	0.25	0.4–0.5	2–3	25–30	Ester hydrolysis and Hoffman elimination
Cisatracurium	0.05	0.15–0.2	2–2.5	50–60	Hoffman elimination
d-tubocurarine	0.51	0.5–0.6	3–5	80–100	70% renal, 15%–20% biliary secretion
Doxacurium	0.03	0.05–0.08	4–5	100–160	Excreted unchanged in urine and bile
Gallamine	3.0	3.0–4.0	3–5	80–120	100% renal
Metocurine	0.28	0.3–0.4	3–5	80–100	80%–100% renal
Mivacurium	0.09	0.15–0.25	1.5–2.0	16–20	Hydrolysis by plasma cholinesterase
Pancuronium	0.07	0.08–1.0	3–5	80–100	70%–80% renal, 15%–20% biliary excretion and hepatic

Pipecuronium	0.05–0.06	0.07–0.085	5	47–124	Excreted in urine and to lesser extent bile
Rocuronium	0.3	0.6–1.2	1–1.5	40–150	Primarily excreted by liver
Vecuronium	0.06	0.1–0.12	2–3	25–30	10%–20% renal, 80% biliary excretion and hepatic
Synergistic combinations					
Pancuronium and d-tubocurarine		0.02 + 0.15	3–5	40–60	
Pancuronium and metocurine		0.02 + 0.07	3–5	40–60	

[a]All doses were determined under balanced (nitrous oxide–opioid) technique.

[b]There is a large variability in the response to all relaxants, especially at the extremes of age and with profound illness. Therefore, all patients should be monitored as described in the text.

[c]An ED$_{95}$ dose of a relaxant gives adequate surgical relaxation with nitrous oxide–opioid anesthesia.

[d]These are customary intubating doses and not all equipotent. All relaxants are potentiated by potent inhalational anesthetics, including newer agents such as desflurane and sevoflurane.

[e]These times reflect the use of customary intubating doses and may be altered by very substantially by very light or very deep anesthesia. For rapid sequence induction with nondepolarizing agents, onset time can be reduced by using a "priming dose" 3–5 min before the full dose. No nondepolarizing relaxant has as rapid an onset as succinylcholine.

[f]Maintenance doses to be given when the twitch height reaches 25% of control are generally 20%–25% of the initial dose.

5.   Cisatracurium is one of 10 stereoisomers that constitute atracurium. It is two to three times as potent as atracurium. Unlike atracurium, it does not produce histamine release or hemodynamic effects after rapid injection of doses as high as eight times its 95% effective dose (ED_{95}). In usual doses, intubating conditions are achieved in 3 to 5 minutes. The drug is cleared primarily by nonenzymatic Hoffman degradation, so its duration of action is largely independent of renal or hepatic function.

6.   Rocuronium is an analogue of vecuronium that has lower potency. Low potency (large intubating dose) results in a fast onset time. At a dose of 0.6 mg/kg, good to excellent intubating conditions occur by 60 seconds. Increasing the dose to 1.2 mg/kg (4 times the ED_{95}) shortens the time even more but significantly prolongs the duration of action.

7.   Mivacurium is a short-acting nondepolarizing NMBD that is rapidly hydrolyzed by plasma cholinesterase. It should be used with caution in patients with known atypical plasma cholinesterase activity. Histamine release can occur with higher doses.

8.   The **cardiovascular side effects** of nondepolarizing NMBDs are summarized in Table 12-2. Hypotension caused by histamine release (e.g., with curare, atracurium, or mivacurium) can be reduced or prevented if the drug is administered over 30 seconds or by prior administration of histamine (H_1 and H_2) receptor blockers.

C.   **Clinical choice of NMBD**

1.   Many factors must be considered simultaneously when selecting an NMBD: the urgency of the need for tracheal intuba-

Table 12-2.   **Cardiovascular side effects of relaxants**

Drugs	Histamine Release[a]	Ganglionic Effects	Vagolytic Activity	Sympathetic Stimulation
Atracurium	+	0	0	0
Cisatracurium	0	0	0	0
Doxacurium	0	0	0	0
d-Tubocurarine	+++	−	0	0
Gallamine	0	0	+++	+
Metocurine	+	0	0	0
Mivacurium	+	0	0	0
Pancuronium	0	0	++	++
Pipecuronium	0	0	±	0
Rocuronium	0	0	0	0
Succinylcholine	±	+	0	0
Vecuronium	0	0	0	0

[a]Histamine release is dose and rate dependent, and, therefore, less pronounced if drugs are given slowly.

tion, the duration of the procedure, other coexisting medical conditions that effect the NMJ, and side effects and metabolism of the drug. For example, SCh is a good choice for rapid intubation of the trachea, but mivacurium may be a better choice in the burned patient. Pancuronium can produce a tachycardia that is undesirable in patients with severe ischemic heart disease but appropriate in pediatric patients.

2. Cost effectiveness is also a consideration in the choice of drug, and some have suggested that the additional expense of newer short-acting NMBDs is not justified in longer cases. A large Danish study (Berg et al., 1997) compared pancuronium with vecuronium and atracurium. Despite the use of intraoperative neuromuscular monitoring, pancuronium-treated patients had a significantly higher incidence of postoperative residual blockade and pulmonary complications. The cost of any drug-induced morbidity should be a part of assessing cost effectiveness.

IV. Monitoring neuromuscular function

A. There are several reasons to monitor neuromuscular function under anesthesia:

1. To facilitate timing of intubation.

2. To provide an objective measurement of relaxation during surgery and degree of recovery before extubation.

3. To titrate dosage according to patient response.

4. To monitor for the development of phase II block.

5. To permit early recognition of patients with abnormal plasma cholinesterase.

B. Peripheral nerve stimulators use various patterns of stimulation: single-twitch, tetanus, TOF, and double-burst stimulation, as well as the "posttetanic count." The **adductor pollicis response to ulnar nerve stimulation** at the wrist is most often used, because it is easily accessible and results are not complicated by direct muscle activation. Cutaneous electrodes are placed at the wrist over the ulnar nerve and attached to a battery-driven pulse generator, which delivers a graded impulse of electrical current at a specified frequency. For maximal twitch response, the negative pole (active) should be placed over the ulnar nerve at the wrist. Evoked muscle tension can be estimated by feeling for thumb adduction or measured by using a force transducer attached to the thumb. The response to nerve stimulation may also be quantified by analyzing the integrated electromyogram of the muscle. After the administration of a muscle relaxant, the developed tension and twitch height decrease with the onset of neuromuscular blockade. If the ulnar nerve is unavailable, other sites may be used (e.g., facial, posterior tibial, peroneal, or lateral popliteal nerves).

C. The twitch response to various patterns of stimulation has been correlated with clinical endpoints, and these data are summarized in Table 12-3.

1. Single twitch is a supramaximal stimulus, typically lasting 0.2 ms at a frequency of 0.1 Hz. The height of the muscle twitch (its amplitude for a given load and peak tension) is determined as a percent of control. A supramaximal stimulus ensures recruitment of all muscle fibers, and a short duration prevents repetitive nerve firing. The stimulus frequency is important be-

Table 12-3. Clinical assessment of blockade

Twitch Response	Clinical Correlate
95% suppression of single twitch at 0.15–0.1 Hz	Adequate intubating conditions
90% suppression of single twitch; train-of-four count of one twitch	Surgical relaxation with nitrous oxide-opioid anesthesia
75% suppression of single twitch; train-of-four count of three twitches	Adequate relaxation with inhalation agents
25% suppression of single twitch	Decreased vital capacity
Train-of-four ratio > 0.75; sustained tetanus at 50 Hz for 5 s	Head lift for 5 s; vital capacity = 15–20 mL/kg; inspiratory force = −25 cm H_2O; effective cough
Train-of-four ratio > 0.9	Sit up unassisted; intact carotid body response to hypoxemia; normal pharyngeal function
Train-of-four ratio = 1.0	Normal expiratory flow rate, vital capacity, and inspiratory force. Diplopia resolves

cause it affects twitch height and degree of fade. Single twitch is not a sensitive measure of onset or recovery from blockade, because 75% of receptors must be blocked before twitch height begins to decrease and 75% may still be blocked when it returns to control height.

2. Tetanic stimulus frequencies vary from 50 to 200 Hz. All NMBDs reduce twitch height, but with nondepolarizing block and phase II block, tetanic fade is also demonstrated. This occurs when NMBDs bind to presynaptic receptors and decrease mobilization of ACh during high frequency stimulation. A tetanic stimulus at 50 Hz for 5 seconds is clinically useful, because a sustained tension at this frequency corresponds to that achieved with maximum voluntary effort. However, tetanic stimuli are painful and can speed recovery in the stimulated muscle, thus misleading the observer with respect to the degree of recovery in important respiratory and upper airway muscles.

3. Posttetanic single twitch is measured by single-twitch stimulation 6 to 10 seconds after a tetanic stimulus. An increase in this twitch is called **PTP**. This transient reversal is due to partial increased mobilization and synthesis of ACh during and after tetanic stimulation. Both nondepolarizing and phase II blockade will cause PTP, but depolarizing blockade will not. Repeated tetanic stimuli can change contractile function and may occasionally cause an artifactual PTP.

4. **The TOF** is four supramaximal stimuli at a frequency of 2 Hz, repeated at intervals of at least 10 seconds. Responses at this frequency show fade during partial curarization. During nondepolarizing neuromuscular blockade, elimination of the fourth response corresponds to 75% depression of single twitch. Disappearance of the third, second, and first responses correspond to 80%, 90%, and 100% depression of single twitch, respectively. The ratio of the height of the fourth to the first twitch (TOF ratio) correlates with the degree of clinical recovery. A TOF ratio of 0.75 correlates with some indices of clinical recovery (Table 12-3). Recent studies have demonstrated that functional impairment of the muscles of the upper airway may exist up to TOF ratios as high as 0.9, with the potential for greater risk of regurgitation and aspiration. In addition, NMBDs may impair the carotid body hypoxic response, even at a TOF ratio of 0.7. Nevertheless, TOF is a very useful method for clinical monitoring, because it does not require a control measurement, it is not as painful as tetanic stimulation, and it does not induce changes in subsequent recovery. It is a good measure in the range of blockade required for surgical relaxation (75% to 90%) and is useful in assessing recovery from blockade. It is not helpful in quantifying the degree of depolarizing blockade because no fade will be evident. However, TOF monitoring may be used to detect fade, signifying the onset of phase II blockade during continuous or repeated administration of SCh.

5. **Posttetanic count** is used to quantify deep levels of nondepolarizing block. A 50-Hz tetanic stimulus is given for 5 seconds, followed 3 seconds later by repeated single stimuli at 1.0 Hz. The number of responses detectable predicts the time for spontaneous recovery.

6. **Double-burst stimulation** uses a burst of two to three tetanic stimuli at 50 Hz followed 750 ms later by a second burst. A decrease in the second response indicates residual curarization. It has been suggested that fade in response to double-burst stimulation is more easily detected than fade in response to TOF stimulation.

V. Reversal of neuromuscular blockade

A. **Recovery from SCh-induced depolarizing blockade** usually occurs in 10 to 15 minutes. Patients with atypical or inhibited plasma cholinesterase will have a greatly prolonged duration of blockade. Reversal of phase II blockade occurs spontaneously within 10 to 15 minutes in approximately 50% of patients. The remaining patients have prolonged responses. It is advisable to allow these patients to recover spontaneously for 20 to 25 minutes, and then reversal with an anticholinesterase may be attempted if there is no further improvement in twitch height. Earlier reversal could worsen the block.

B. **Nondepolarizing block** spontaneously recovers when the drugs diffuse from their sites of action. Reversal can be accelerated by administering agents that inhibit acetylcholinesterase (anticholinesterases), thereby increasing the ACh available to compete for binding sites.

C. **Anticholinesterases**. The three principal drugs are **edro-**

phonium, **neostigmine**, and **pyridostigmine**. Table 12-4 summarizes the clinical pharmacology of these three relaxant antagonists. Because they work by increasing ACh, the three reversal drugs have muscarinic and nicotinic effects. Salivation, bradycardia, tearing, miosis, and bronchoconstriction can be minimized by administration of an antimuscarinic drug (e.g., atropine or glycopyrrolate) before the anticholinesterase.

D.   Time to adequate reversal is related to the degree of spontaneous recovery, so it will take longer to reverse a deeper block. Reversal may be more difficult with the use of long-acting NMBDs, high total doses, and large amounts of inhalation anesthetics. Other factors that may prolong the blockade include hypothermia, antibiotics (particularly aminoglycosides, clindamycin, uridopenicillins), electrolyte disturbances (hypokalemia, hypocalcemia, hypermagnesemia), and acid-base disturbances (alkalosis prolongs blockade, acidosis impairs reversal). If residual weakness is present after attempted reversal, the endotracheal tube should be left in place to provide adequate ventilation and airway protection. Reversal should not be attempted unless at least one response to TOF stimulation is present. Attempts to reverse a deep or resistant block with excessive doses of neostigmine may increase the degree of residual weakness.

E.   Evidence of neuromuscular recovery should include a TOF ratio more than 0.75, adequate ventilation and oxygenation, sustained grip strength, the ability to sustain head lift or movement of an extremity without fade, and the absence of discoordinated muscle activity. These may be sufficient for a patient emerging from major surgery or remaining in the hospital overnight. However, an outpatient may not tolerate residual diplopia, inability to sit up unassisted, fatigue, or malaise. For these patients, more stringent criteria (TOF ratio > 0.9, ability to clench down on an oral airway and prevent its withdrawal) may be more appropriate.

VI.   Disorders that influence the response to NMBDs
Certain illnesses, both those confined to the NMJ and those affecting more general systems, dramatically affect the use and safety of NMBDs. Generally, transmission at the NMJ is abnormal in these disorders and there are ultrastructural and biochemical changes in motor nerves, muscle, or both.

A.   Burns and immobilization

1.   Thermal injury affects fluid and electrolyte regulation, cardiovascular and pulmonary function, drug metabolism, and musculoskeletal structure and function.

2.   Burn patients and many immobilized patients (such as those found in intensive care unit [ICU] settings) have a greatly exaggerated response to depolarizing agents and a decreased responsiveness to nondepolarizing agents. Burn patients exhibit ultrastructural and biochemical alterations in both muscle cells and neuromuscular contacts. Administration of SCh can cause dramatic, and sometimes fatal, hyperkalemia. These effects can be seen for greater than 1 year after the initial thermal insult.

B.   Critical illness

1.   The prevalence of neuromuscular dysfunction in critical illness is exceedingly high. The frequency of diagnosis

Table 12-4. Clinical pharmacology of reversal drugs

Drugs	Dosage	Time to peak Antagonism (min)	Duration of Antagonism (min)	Excretion Pattern[a]	Dosage of Atropine Required[b] (μg/kg)
Edrophonium	0.05–1.0 mg/kg	1	40–65	70% renal 30% hepatic	7–10
Neostigmine	0.03–0.06 mg/kg up to 5 mg	7	55–75	50% renal 50% hepatic	15–30
Pyridostigmine	0.25 mg/kg	10–13	80–130	75% renal 25% hepatic	15–20

[a]The increased duration during renal failure exceeds the increased durations of pancuronium and curare and so there is no "recurarization."
[b]Dosage of glycopyrrolate = $\frac{1}{2}$ dosage of atropine. The onset time of atropine is much faster than that of glycopyrrolate, and it peaks in a little over a minute compared with 4–5 min for glycopyrrolate. Therefore, glycopyrrolate is a good choice with pyridostigmine, which has a longer time to peak antagonism. However, glycopyrrolate should be given at least 3 min before edrophonium. There appears to be less tachycardia, fewer arrhythmias, and a greater secretory drying effect with glycopyrrolate.

ranges from 30% to 70%, and the incidence approaches 76% with more sensitive electrophysiologic tests.

2.   Myopathy of critical illness is the name given the collective group of disorders that can cause weakness in ICU patients. The underlying pathology is quite heterogeneous, ranging from pure neuropathies and myopathies to mixed neuromuscular–transmission disorders. Sepsis and multiorgan systems failure are commonly associated with myopathy of critical illness.

3.   Weakness is the common manifestation of all these disorders. In critically ill patients, such weakness can cause ventilator dependence and increased morbidity and mortality. Other signs and symptoms that may be present include altered deep tendon reflexes, increased creatine kinase (CK) levels, and electrophysiologic alterations in nerve, muscle, or both.

4.   Corticosteroids, NMBDs, and certain antibiotics can contribute to or precipitate weakness in ICU patients. One subtype of myopathy of critical illness, acute necrotizing myopathy, has been linked to the repeated administration of NMBDs, often in conjunction with high doses of corticosteroids. These patients exhibit profound weakness, elevated serum CK levels, and sparing of sensory-nerve action potentials. Limitation of steroid and NMBD use in critically ill patients is advisable.

C.   Myasthenia gravis (MG)

1.   MG is an autoimmune disease with a prevalence of 1 in 20,000 in the general population. It is most common in young adult women.

2.   The loss of AChR at motor endplates in MG is induced by anti-receptor antibodies that increase the degradation of junctional and extrajunctional receptors. The antibodies are detectable in the serum of 90% of MG patients, but antibody titers correlate poorly with clinical signs.

3.   MG often presents with the gradual onset of **pharyngeal or ocular weakness**. All muscle groups may be affected. The hallmark of MG is weakness that becomes worse with exercise.

4.   The diagnosis is supported by the clinical history and confirmed by transiently improved muscle strength after 10 mg of intravenous edrophonium (the **Tensilon test**), by characteristic electromyographic findings, and most specifically by the presence of anti-AChR antibodies in the patient's serum.

5.   Treatment includes anticholinesterases (e.g., pyridostigmine), corticosteroids, immunosuppressive drugs such as azathioprine or cyclophosphamide, plasmapheresis, and thymectomy. Remission of the disease is common after thymectomy.

6.   Special attention needs to be given to MG patients receiving either regional or general anesthetics.

    a.   The use of neuraxial regional anesthesia is associated with skeletal muscle relaxation and some degree of diaphragmatic weakness. This normal effect of regional anesthesia often unmasks underlying weakness that may have been only partially treated by cholinesterase inhibitors. These patients therefore may suffer from profound respiratory weakness even when not challenged with neuromuscular blocking agents. They need careful respiratory monitoring throughout anesthesia and recovery.

b. Anticholinesterase therapy should not be discontinued before surgery.

c. These patients are often resistant to depolarizing agents although clearance of SCh is inhibited by pyridostigmine. They are also extremely sensitive to nondepolarizing agents. Both longer acting agents such as pancuronium and shorter acting agents such as cisatracurium have been associated with prolonged blockade, refractoriness to reversal agents, and profound postoperative weakness. NMBDs are probably best avoided, if possible.

d. Monitoring of the degree of neuromuscular blockade is strongly advised, although complete recovery of the TOF does not ensure recovery of either the muscles of the upper airway or of ventilation.

e. Surgery and anesthesia may exacerbate the underlying illness. Postoperative ventilation may be required for these patients, even after minor surgical procedures.

D. Muscular dystrophies are a heterogeneous group of inherited muscle disorders that are characterized by a progressive loss of skeletal muscle function. **Duchenne muscular dystrophy** is the most common and the most severe of the disorders. The gene responsible encodes a membrane-associated protein known as dystrophin that is critical for the stability of the muscular membrane. The disorder is X-linked recessive and clinically evident in boys. The clinical course is characterized by painless degeneration and atrophy of skeletal muscle, which manifests as weakness by the age of 5 years. By the preteen years, the patient often is confined to a wheelchair, and death usually occurs by the mid-twenties secondary to congestive heart failure.

1. Serum CK levels are elevated and track the progression of muscular degeneration. By the late stages of the disease, CK levels are near normal due to significant loss of muscle mass.

2. Cardiac (progressive systolic dysfunction and ventricular thinning) and smooth muscle (gastrointestinal hypomotility with delayed gastric emptying) are affected to variable degrees.

3. Although the diaphragm is spared, accessory muscle weakness produces a restrictive pattern on pulmonary function testing. Because coughing is impaired, pneumonia is a frequent complication.

4. SCh can cause massive rhabdomyolysis, hyperkalemia, and death. **Volatile inhalational agents**, particularly halothane, can have exaggerated myocardial depressant effects. **Malignant hyperthermia** occurs with increased frequency, but there are no good predictive tests for which patients are at risk. The delayed gastric emptying and ineffective cough places these patients at greater risk for regurgitation and aspiration. Because the intensity and duration of drug effect is hard to predict, short-acting agents may be preferable. Postoperatively, these patients require aggressive pulmonary physiotherapy to ensure adequate secretion clearance. Opioids, which may further depress deep breathing and cough, should be used cautiously.

E. The myotonic syndromes are a group of disorders characterized by a defect in skeletal muscle relaxation and persistent contraction of skeletal muscles after stimulation. The persistent contraction is a consequence of ineffectual calcium removal from the cytoplasm to the sarcoplasmic reticulum. **Myotonic dystrophy** (Steinert disease) is the most common syndrome in this group of disorders.

1.   Myotonic dystrophy patients have progressive involvement and deterioration of skeletal, cardiac, and smooth muscle throughout the body, with weakened respiratory effort, a restrictive pattern on pulmonary function testing, and diminished gastrointestinal motility. Other symptoms include cataracts, cardiac conduction abnormalities, baldness, and mental retardation.

2.   Regional anesthesia, neuromuscular blocking agents, and increasing depth of general anesthesia do not relieve myotonic muscle rigidity. Pregnancy exacerbates this condition, and cesarean section is often indicated because of uterine muscle dysfunction. These patients are exquisitely sensitive to the respiratory depressant effects of opioids, benzodiazepines, and inhalational agents. Neuraxial opiates that have minimal effect on respiratory function in normal persons can have a substantial effect in these patients. Like patients with Duchenne muscular dystrophy, these patients have frequent cardiac arrhythmias and are at increased risk for cardiac arrest during general anesthesia.

SUGGESTED READING

Ali HH, Savarese JJ. Monitoring of neuromuscular function. *Anesthesiology* 1976;45:216–249.

Baraka A. Onset of neuromuscular block in myasthenic patients. *Br J Anaesth* 1992;69:227–228.

Baraka A, Taha S, Yazbeck V, et al. Vecuronium block in the myasthenic patient. Influence of anticholinesterase therapy. *Anaesthesia* 1993;48:588–590.

Belmont MR, Lien CA, Quessy S, et al. The clinical neuromuscular pharmacology of 51W89 in patients receiving nitrous oxide/opioid/barbiturate anesthesia. *Anesthesiology* 1995;82:1139–1145.

Berg H, Roed J, Viby-Mogensen J, et al. Residual neuromuscular block is a risk factor for postoperative pulmonary complications. A prospective, randomised, and blinded study of postoperative pulmonary complications after atracurium, vecuronium and pancuronium. *Acta Anaesthesiol Scand* 1997;41:1095–1103.

Chiu JW, White PF. The pharmacoeconomics of neuromuscular blocking drugs. *Anesth Analg* 2000;90:S19–S23.

De Jonghe B, Cook D, Sharshar T, et al. Acquired neuromuscular disorders in critically ill patients: a systematic review. Groupe de Reflexion et d'Etude sur les Neuromyopathies En Reanimation. *Intensive Care Med* 1999;24:1242–1250.

Eriksson LI. The effects of residual neuromuscular blockade and volatile anesthetics on the control of ventilation. *Anesth Analg* 1999;89:243–251.

Eriksson LI, Sundman E, Olsson R, et al. Functional assessment of the pharynx at rest and during swallowing in partially paralyzed humans. *Anesthesiology* 1997;87:1035–1043.

Ibebunjo C, Martyn JA. Fiber atrophy, but not changes in acetylcholine receptor expression, contributes to the muscle dysfunction after immobilization. *Crit Care Med* 1999;27:275–285.

Kim C, Fuke N, Martyn JA. Burn injury to rat increases nicotinic acetyl-choline receptors in the diaphragm. *Anesthesiology* 1988;68:401–406.

Kopman AF, Yee SY, Neuman GG. Relationship of the train-of-four fade ratio to clinical signs and symptoms of residual paralysis in awake volunteers. *Anesthesiology* 1997;86:765–771.

Lin RC, Scheller RH. Mechanisms of synaptic vesicle exocytosis. *Annu Rev Cell Dev Biol* 2000;16:19–49.

Lubarsky DA, Glass PS, Ginsberg B, et al. The successful implementation of pharmaceutical practice guidelines. Analysis of associated outcomes and costs savings. *Anesthesiology* 1997;86:1145–1160.

Martyn JA, Matteo RS, Szyfelbein SK, et al. Unprecedented resistance to neuromuscular blocking effects of metocurine with persistence after complete recovery in a burned patient. *Anesth Analg* 1982;61:614–617.

Martyn JA, Szyfelbein SK, Ali HH, et al. Increased d-tubocurarine requirement following major thermal injury. *Anesthesiology* 1980;52:352–355.

Martyn JA, Vincent A. A new twist to myopathy of critical illness. *Anesthesiology* 1999;91:337–339.

Pino RM, Basta SJ. Pharmacology of neuromuscular blocking drugs. In: Rogers MC, Tinker JH, Covino BG, et al., eds. *Principles and practice of anesthesiology.* St. Louis, MO: Mosby, 1998:765–790.

Sanes JR, Lichtman JW. Development of the vertebrate neuromuscular junction. *Annu Rev Neurosci* 1999;22:389–442.

Airway Evaluation and Management

Harish Lecamwasam and Peter F. Dunn

I. Applied Anatomy

A. The pharynx is divided into the nasopharynx, the oropharynx, and the laryngopharynx.

1. The **nasopharynx** consists of the nasal passages, including the septum, turbinates, and adenoids.

2. The **oropharynx** consists of the oral cavity, including the dentition and tongue.

3. The **epiglottis** separates the **laryngopharynx** into the larynx (leading to the trachea) and the **hypopharynx** (leading to the esophagus).

B. The larynx

1. The **larynx**, located at the level of the fourth to the sixth cervical vertebrae, originates at the laryngeal inlet and ends at the inferior border of the cricoid cartilage. It consists of nine cartilages, three unpaired (thyroid, cricoid, and epiglottis) and three paired (corniculates, cuneiforms, arytenoids); ligaments; and muscles.

2. The **cricoid cartilage** (C5-6), located just inferior to the **thyroid cartilage**, is the only complete cartilaginous ring in the respiratory tree.

3. The **cricothyroid membrane** connects the thyroid and cricoid cartilages and measures 0.9×3.0 cm in the adult. The membrane is superficial, thin, and devoid of major vessels in the midline, making it an important site for emergent surgical airway access (see cricothyroidotomy below).

4. The **laryngeal muscles** can be divided into two groups: muscles that open and close the glottis (lateral cricoarytenoid [adduction], posterior cricoarytenoid [abduction], transverse arytenoid) and muscles that control the tension of the vocal ligaments (cricothyroid, vocalis, and thyroarytenoid).

5. Innervation

a. Sensory. The **glossopharyngeal nerve** (cranial nerve IX) provides sensory innervation to the posterior one-third of the tongue, the oropharynx from its junction with the nasopharynx, including the pharyngeal surfaces of the soft palate, epiglottis, and the fauces, to the junction of the pharynx and esophagus. The **internal branch of the superior laryngeal nerve**, a branch of the vagus nerve (cranial nerve X), provides sensory innervation to the mucosa from the epiglottis to and including the vocal cords. The sensory fibers of the **inferior laryngeal nerve**, a branch of the recurrent laryngeal nerve (also a branch of the vagus nerve), provides sensory innervation to the mucosa of the subglottic larynx and trachea.

b. **Motor**. The external branch of the **superior laryngeal nerve** provides motor innervation to the cricothyroid muscle. Activation of this muscle results in tensing of the vocal cords. The motor fibers of the **inferior laryngeal nerve** provide motor innervation to all other intrinsic muscles of the larynx. **Bilateral injury to the inferior laryngeal nerves** (e.g., via injury to the recurrent laryngeal nerves) can produce unopposed activation of the cricothyroideus, leading to tensing of the vocal cords and airway closure.

C. The **glottis** is comprised of the vocal folds (true and "false" cords) and the rima glottidis.

    1. The **rima glottidis** describes the aperture between the true vocal cords.

    2. The **glottis** represents the narrowest point in the adult airway (more than 8 years of age), whereas the cricoid cartilage represents the narrowest point in the infant airway (birth to 1 year of age).

D. **The lower airway** extends from the subglottic larynx to the bronchi.

    1. The subglottic larynx extends from the vocal folds to the inferior border of the cricoid cartilage (C-6).

    2. The **trachea** is a fibromuscular tube that is approximately 10 to 12 cm long with a diameter of approximately 20 mm in the adult. It extends from the cricoid cartilage to the carina. The trachea is supported by approximately 16 to 20 U-shaped cartilages, with the open end facing posteriorly. Noting the posterior absence of cartilaginous rings provides anterior–posterior orientation during fiberoptic exam of the tracheobronchial tree.

    3. The trachea bifurcates into the right and left main stem bronchi at the carina. The right main stem bronchus is approximately 2.5 cm long with a take-off angle of approximately 25 degrees. The left main stem bronchus is approximately 5 cm long with a take-off angle of approximately 45 degrees.

II. **Evaluation**

A. **History**. A history of difficult airway management in the past may be the best predictor of a challenging airway. If old medical records are available, prior anesthetic records should be reviewed for the ease of intubation and ventilation (number of intubation attempts, ability to mask ventilate, type of laryngoscope blade used, use of stylet, or any other modifications of technique). Particular importance should also be placed on diseases that may affect the airway. Specific symptoms related to airway compromise should be sought, including hoarseness, stridor, wheezing, dysphagia, dyspnea, and positional airway obstruction.

    1. **Arthritis or cervical disk disease** may decrease neck mobility. Cervical spine instability and limitation of mandibular motion are common in rheumatoid arthritis; the temporomandibular and cricoarytenoid joints may also be involved. Aggressive neck manipulation in these patients may lead to atlantoaxial subluxation and spinal cord injury. The risk of atlantoaxial subluxation is highest in patients with severe hand deformities and skin nodules.

    2. **Infections** of the floor of the mouth, salivary glands, tonsils, or pharynx may cause pain, edema, and trismus with limited mouth opening.

3. **Tumors** may obstruct the airway or cause extrinsic compression and tracheal deviation.

4. **Morbidly obese** individuals may have a history of obstructive sleep apnea from hypertrophied tonsils and adenoids, as well as a short neck or increased soft tissue at the neck and upper airway.

5. **Trauma** may be associated with airway injuries, cervical spine injury, basilar skull fracture, or intracranial injury.

6. **Previous surgery, radiation, or burns** may produce scarring, contractures, and limited tissue mobility (also see Chapter 32).

7. **Acromegaly** may cause mandibular hypertrophy and overgrowth and enlargement of the tongue and epiglottis. The glottic opening may be narrowed because of enlargement of the vocal cords.

8. **Scleroderma** may produce skin tightness and decrease mandibular motion and narrow the oral aperture.

9. **Trisomy 21 patients** may have atlantoaxial instability and macroglossia.

10. **Dwarfism** may be associated with atlantoaxial instability and potentially difficult airway management because of mandibular hypoplasia (micrognathia).

11. **Other congenital anomalies** may complicate airway management, particularly patients with craniofacial abnormalities such as Pierre-Robin syndrome, Treacher-Collins syndrome, or Goldenhar syndrome.

B. **Physical examination**

1. **Specific findings** that may indicate a difficult airway include:

   a. Inability to open the mouth.

   b. Poor cervical spine mobility.

   c. Receding chin (micrognathia).

   d. Large tongue (macroglossia).

   e. Prominent incisors.

   f. Short muscular neck.

   g. Morbid obesity.

2. **Injuries** to the face, neck, or chest must be evaluated to assess their contribution to airway compromise.

3. **Head and neck examination**

   a. **Nose.** The patency of the nares or the presence of a deviated septum should be determined by occluding one nostril at a time and assessing ease of ventilation through the other nostril. This is especially important should nasotracheal intubation be required.

   b. **Mouth.** Identify macroglossia and conditions that reduce mouth opening (e.g., facial scars or contractures, temporomandibular joint disease). **Poor dentition** may increase the risk of tooth injury or loss during airway manipulation. Loose teeth should be identified preoperatively and protected or removed before initiation of airway management.

   c. **Neck**

   (1) If the **thyromental distance** (the distance from the lower border of the mandible to the thyroid notch with the neck fully extended) is less than 6 cm (three to four finger breadths), there may be difficulty visualizing the glottis.

The mobility of laryngeal structures should be assessed, and the trachea should be palpable in the midline above the sternal notch. Look for scars from previous neck surgery, an enlarged thyroid, and other paratracheal masses.

(2) Cervical spine mobility. Patients should be able to touch their chin to their chest and extend their neck posteriorly. Lateral rotation should not produce pain or paresthesia.

(3) The presence of a healed or patent tracheostomy stoma may be a clue to subglottic stenosis or prior complications with airway management. Smaller diameter endotracheal tubes (ETTs) should be available for these patients.

4. The **Mallampati classification** is based on the finding that visualization of the glottis is impaired when the base of the tongue is disproportionately large. Assessment is made with the patient sitting upright, with the head in the neutral position, the mouth open as wide as possible, and the tongue protruded maximally. The modified classification includes four categories (Fig. 13-1):

   a. **Class I**. Faucial pillars, soft palate, and uvula are visible.

   b. **Class II**. Faucial pillars and soft palate may be seen, but uvula is masked by the base of the tongue.

   c. **Class III**. Only soft palate is visible. Intubation is predicted to be difficult.

   d. **Class IV**. Soft palate not visible. Intubation predicted to be difficult.

C. **Special studies**. In most patients, a careful history and physical examination will be all that is needed to evaluate an airway. Useful adjuncts may include the following:

   1. **Laryngoscopy** (direct, indirect, or fiberoptic) will provide information regarding the hypopharynx, laryngeal inlet, and vocal cord function. It can be performed in a conscious patient using topical anesthesia or nerve blocks.

   2. **Chest or cervical radiographs** may reveal tracheal devia-

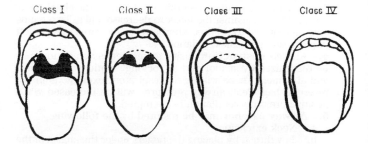

Fig. 13-1. **Mallampati classification of the oropharyngeal structures as modified by Samsoon and Young, as defined in a patient sitting upright with mouth maximally opened and tongue protruded without phonation. (From Samsoon GLT, Young JRB. Difficult tracheal intubation, a retrospective study.** *Anesthesia* **1987;42:487–490, with permission.)**

tion or narrowing and bony deformities in the neck. Cervical spine films are particularly important in trauma cases and should be performed whenever there is an injury above the clavicle or serious multiple traumatic injuries. Lateral cervical spine films may be useful in the rheumatoid patient to assess for atlantoaxial subluxation.

3.   Tracheal tomograms or computed tomography can delineate masses obstructing the airway.

4.   Pulmonary function tests and flow volume loops can help determine the degree and site of airway obstruction (see Chapter 3).

5.   Baseline arterial blood gas tensions can indicate the functional consequences of airway abnormalities and alert the clinician to patients who are chronically hypoxemic or hypercarbic.

III.   Mask airway

A.   Indications

1.   To provide inhalation anesthesia for short procedures in patients not at risk for regurgitation of gastric contents.

2.   To preoxygenate (denitrogenate) a patient before endotracheal intubation.

3.   To assist or control ventilation as part of initial resuscitation.

B.   Technique involves the placement of a face mask and maintenance of a patent airway.

1.   The mask should fit snugly around the bridge of the nose, cheeks, and mouth. Clear plastic masks allow for observation of the lips (for color) and mouth (for secretions or vomitus).

2.   Mask placement. The mask is held in the left hand so that the little finger is at the angle of the mandible, the third and fourth fingers are along the mandible, and the index finger and thumb are placed on the mask. The right hand is available to control the reservoir bag. Two hands may be required to maintain a good mask fit, necessitating an assistant to control the bag. Head straps may be used to assist mask fit.

3.   Edentulous patients may present a problem when attempting to achieve an adequate seal with the face mask because of decreased distance between the mandible and the maxilla. An oral airway should correct this problem, and the cheeks may be compressed against the mask to decrease leaks. Two hands may be required to do this. Alternatively, dentures may be left in place during mask ventilation.

4.   Airway obstruction during spontaneous ventilation may be recognized by stridor and a "rocking" motion of the chest and abdomen. There will be no respiratory excursions in the reservoir bag. Peak airway pressures will be increased when positive pressure ventilation is attempted.

5.   Airway patency may be restored by the following:

    a.   Neck extension.

    b.   Jaw thrust, by placing the fingers under the angles of the mandible and lifting forward.

    c.   Head rotation.

    d.   Insertion of an oral airway. An airway may not be well tolerated if the gag reflex is intact. Complications from use of oral airways include vomiting, laryngospasm, and dental trauma. The wrong size oral airway may worsen obstruction. If the oral airway is too short, it may compress the tongue; if it is too long, it may lie against the epiglottis.

e. A nasal airway helps maintain upper airway patency in a patient with minimal to moderate obstruction and is reasonably tolerated by awake or sedated patients. Nasal airways can cause epistaxis and should be avoided in patients who are anticoagulated.

C. Difficult mask ventilation may be anticipated in a patient with a beard, body mass index greater than 26 kg/m², lack of teeth, age older than 55 years, or a history of snoring. Appropriate oral and nasal airways and laryngeal mask airways (LMA) should be available.

D. Complications. The mask may cause pressure injuries to soft tissues around the mouth, mandible, eyes, or nose. Loss of the airway may produce laryngospasm or vomiting. Mask ventilation does not protect the airway from aspiration of gastric contents. **Laryngospasm,** a tonic contraction of the laryngeal and pharyngeal muscles, causes airway obstruction that may be relieved by jaw thrust and the application of constant positive airway pressure. If this fails, a small dose of succinylcholine (20 mg intravenously or intramuscularly in the adult) may be required.

IV. Laryngeal mask airway

A. The LMA is a reusable airway management device that can be used as an alternate to both mask ventilation and endotracheal intubation in appropriate patients. The LMA also plays an important role in the management of the difficult airway. When inserted appropriately, the LMA lies with its tip resting over the upper esophageal sphincter, cuff sides lying over the pyriform fossae, and cuff upper border resting against the base of the tongue. Such positioning allows for effective ventilation with minimal inflation of the stomach.

B. Indications

1. As an alternate to mask ventilation or endotracheal intubation for airway management. The LMA is not a replacement for endotracheal intubation when endotracheal intubation is indicated.

2. In the management of a known or unexpected difficult airway.

3. In airway management during the resuscitation of an unconscious patient.

C. Contraindications

1. Patients at risk of aspiration of gastric contents.

2. Patients with decreased respiratory system compliance, because the low pressure seal of the LMA cuff will leak at the high inspiratory pressures and gastric insufflation may occur. Peak inspiratory pressures should be maintained at less than 20 cm H_2O to minimize cuff leaks and gastric insufflation.

3. Patients in whom long-term mechanical ventilatory support is anticipated or required.

4. Patients with intact upper airway reflexes, because insertion can precipitate laryngospasm.

D. Use

1. LMAs are available in a variety of pediatric and adult sizes

Table 13-1.   Laryngeal mask airway (LMA) sizes

Patient Age/Size	LMA Size	Cuff Volume	ETT Size (ID)
Neonates/infants to 5 kg	1	Up to 4 mL	3.5 mm
Infants, 5–10 kg	1.5	Up to 7 mL	4.0 mm
Infants/children, 10–20 kg	2.0	Up to 10 mL	4.5 mm
Children, 20–30 kg	2.5	Up to 14 mL	5.0 mm
Children, 30 kg to small adults	3.0	Up to 20 mL	6.0 cuffed
Average adults	4.0	Up to 30 mL	6.0 cuffed
Large adults	5.0	Up to 40 mL	7.0 cuffed

ETT, endotracheal tube; ID, inner diameter.

(Table 13-1). Using the proper size maximizes the probability of appropriate cuff fit. Maneuvers for the appropriate insertion of the LMA are shown in Fig. 13-2.

2.   Ensure correct cuff deflation and lubrication. Lubrication of the LMA inner surface should be avoided because any lubricant dripping into the larynx can precipitate laryngospasm.

3.   Follow usual preoxygenation and monitoring requirements.

4.   Ensure an adequate level of anesthesia and suppression of upper airway reflexes.

5.   Position the patient's head appropriately. The "sniffing" position (slight flexion of the lower cervical spine with extension of C1-2) used to optimize endotracheal intubation also typically provides the best positioning for LMA insertion.

6.   Insert the LMA (Fig. 13-2). A soft bite block can be used to protect against a patient biting down on the LMA tube.

7.   Inflate cuff (Table 13-1). Typically, one sees a smooth ovoid expansion of the tissues above the thyroid cartilage with adequate inflation of the appropriately positioned LMA.

8.   Ensure adequate ventilation.

9.   Connect to anesthetic circuit. The LMA can be secured with tape, if necessary.

10.   **LMA removal.** The LMA generally is well tolerated by a patient emerging from general anesthesia as long as the cuff is not overinflated (cuff pressure less than 60 cm H_2O). The LMA can be removed by deflating the cuff once the patient has emerged from general anesthesia and has return of upper airway reflexes.

11.   The LMA is a suitable airway for some patients having procedures in the prone position. If this technique is chosen, patients can position themselves on the operating table before induction. After induction of anesthesia, the LMA can be inserted with the patient's head turned to the side and resting on either a pillow or blankets.

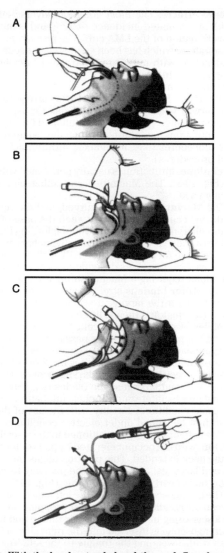

Fig. 13-2. A: With the head extended and the neck flexed, carefully flatten the laryngeal mask airway (LMA) tip against the hard palate. B: With the index finger, push the LMA in a cranial direction following the contours of the hard and soft palate. C: Maintaining pressure with the finger on the tube in the cranial direction, advance the mask until definite resistance is felt at the base of the hypopharynx. D: Inflation without holding the tube allows the mask to seat itself optimally. (From Brain AIJ, Denman WY, Goudsouzian NG. *Laryngeal mask airway instructional manual.* Berkshire, UK: Brain Medical Ltd., 1996:21–25.)

E.   Adverse effects. The most common adverse effect is sore throat, with an estimated incidence of 10%, and is most often related to overinflation of the LMA cuff. The primary major adverse effect is aspiration, which has been estimated to occur at a comparable incidence as with mask or endotracheal anesthesia.

V.   Endotracheal intubation

A.   Orotracheal intubation

    1.   Indications. Endotracheal intubation is required to provide a patent airway when patients are at risk for aspiration, when airway maintenance by mask is difficult, and for prolonged controlled ventilation. Intubation also may be required for specific surgical procedures (e.g., head/neck, intrathoracic, or intraabdominal procedures).

    2.   Technique. Intubation is usually performed with a laryngoscope (Fig. 13-3). The Macintosh and Miller blades are most commonly used.

        a.   The **Macintosh blade** is curved, and the tip is inserted into the vallecula (the space between the base of the tongue and the pharyngeal surface of the epiglottis) (Fig. 13-3D). It provides a good view of the oro- and hypopharynx, thus allowing more room for passage of the ETT with decreased epiglottic trauma. Size ranges as designated as no. 1 through 4, with most adults requiring a Macintosh no. 3 blade.

        b.   The **Miller blade** is straight, and it is passed so that the tip lies beneath the laryngeal surface of the epiglottis (Fig. 13-3C). The epiglottis then is lifted to expose the vocal cords. The Miller blade provides excellent exposure of the glottic opening but provides a smaller passageway through the oro- and hypopharynx. Sizes are designated as no. 0 through 4, with most adults requiring a Miller no. 2 or 3 blade.

        c.   Many specially modified laryngoscopes (e.g., Bullard, Upsher, Wu) and laryngoscope blades (e.g., Siker) are available that may facilitate endotracheal intubation under difficult or unusual conditions. Facility with the use of these devices should first be gained under elective conditions.

        d.   The patient should be positioned in the so-called **sniffing position**, with the occiput elevated by pads or folded blankets and the neck extended. This position aligns the oral, pharyngeal, and laryngeal axes so that the pathway from the lips to the glottis is nearly in a straight line (Fig. 13-3, A and B).

        e.   The laryngoscope is held in the left hand near the junction between the handle and blade. After propping the mouth open with a scissoring motion of the right thumb and index finger, the laryngoscope is inserted into the right side of the patient's mouth while sweeping the tongue to the left. The lips should not be pinched by the blade and the teeth should be avoided. The blade is then advanced toward the midline until the epiglottis comes into view. The tongue and pharyngeal soft tissues are then lifted to expose the glottic opening. The laryngoscope should be used to lift (Fig. 13-3C) rather than act as a lever (Fig. 13-3D) to prevent damage to the maxillary incisors or gingiva.

        f.   An appropriate ETT size depends on the patient's age, body habitus, and type of surgery. A 7.0-mm ETT is used for most women and an 8.0-mm ETT for most men. The ETT is

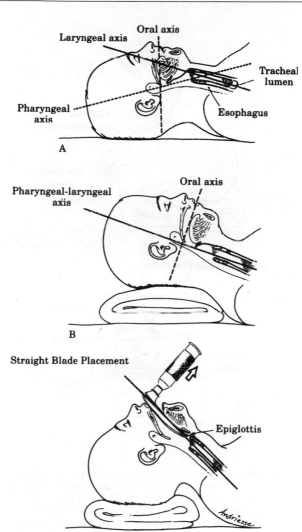

Fig. 13-3. Anatomic relations for laryngoscopy and endotracheal intubation. *(figure continues)*

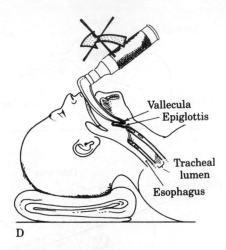

Vallecula
Epiglottis

Tracheal
lumen

Esophagus

D

Curved Blade Placement

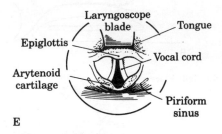

Laryngoscope
blade

Tongue

Epiglottis

Vocal cord

Arytenoid
cartilage

Piriform
sinus

E

Fig. 13-3.   *Continued.*

held in the right hand as one would hold a pencil and advanced through the oral cavity from the right corner of the mouth and then through the vocal cords. The anatomic view for visualization with a Macintosh laryngoscope is seen in Fig. 13-3E. If visualization of the glottic opening is incomplete, it may be necessary to use the epiglottis as a landmark, passing the ETT immediately beneath it and into the trachea. External pressure on the cricoid and/or thyroid cartilage may aid in visualization. The proximal end of the ETT cuff is placed just below the vocal cords, and the markings on the tube are noted in relation to the patient's incisors (or lips). The cuff is inflated just to the point of obtaining a seal in the presence of 20 to 30 cm H_2O positive airway pressure.

g.   Proper placement of the ETT can be verified by the detection of carbon dioxide in end-tidal or mixed expiratory gas and inspection and auscultation of the stomach and both lung fields chest during positive pressure ventilation. If breath sounds are heard on one side of the thorax only, a mainstem intubation should be suspected and the ETT should be withdrawn until breath sounds are heard bilaterally. Listening for breath sounds high in each axilla may decrease the chances of being misled by transmitted breath sounds from the opposite lung. No single verification technique is fool-proof, and the consequences of misdiagnosis may be disastrous. Additional confirmatory techniques, such as use of an esophageal bulb detector, bronchoscopy, and radiography, may be necessary. A high index of suspicion of an esophageal intubation should be maintained until adequate oxygenation and ventilation are ensured.

   h. The ETT should be fastened securely with tape, preferably to taut skin overlying bony structures.

3. Complications of orotracheal intubation include injury of the lips or tongue, teeth, pharynx, or tracheal mucosa. There may rarely be avulsion of arytenoid cartilages or damage to vocal cords or trachea.

B. Nasotracheal intubation

   1. Indications. Nasotracheal intubation may be required in patients undergoing an intraoral procedure. Compared with oral ETTs, the maximal diameter that can be accommodated is usually smaller, and, accordingly, resistance to breathing may be higher. The nasotracheal route is now rarely used for long-term intubation because of increased airway resistance and the increased risk of sinusitis.

   2. Contraindications. Basilar skull fractures, especially of the ethmoid bone, nasal fractures, epistaxis, nasal polyps, coagulopathy, and planned systemic anticoagulation and/or thrombolysis (i.e., the patient with acute myocardial infarction), are relative contraindications to nasal intubation.

   3. Technique. The nasal mucosa is anesthetized and vasoconstricted, usually using cotton-tipped pledgets to apply a phenylephrine–lidocaine mixture. If both nares are patent, the right naris is preferred because the bevel of most ETTs, when introduced through the right naris, will face the flat nasal septum, reducing damage to the turbinates. The inferior turbinates can interfere with passage and limit the size of the ETT. Usually, a 6.0- to 6.5-mm ETT is used for women and a 7.0- to 7.5-mm ETT for men. After passage through the naris into the pharynx, the tube is advanced through the glottic opening. Intubation may be performed blindly, under direct vision using a laryngoscope or fiberoptic bronchoscope, and assisted by Magill forceps.

   4. Complications are similar to those described for orotracheal intubation (see section V.A.3). Additionally, epistaxis, submucosal dissection, and dislodgement of enlarged tonsils and adenoids may occur. Compared with orotracheal intubation, the nasotracheal route has been associated with an increased incidence of sinusitis and bacteremia.

C. Fiberoptic intubation. The flexible fiberoptic laryngoscope consists of glass fibers that are bound together to provide a flexible unit for the transmission of light and images. The fiberoptic bundle is fragile, and excessive bending can damage the fibers. Working channels are usually present that can be used to administer topical anesthetics and provide suction. The visual field often becomes limited as the fiberoptic bronchoscope nears the glottic opening.

Secretions, blood, or fogging of the lens may obscure the view. Immersion of the tip of the fiberoptic scope in warm water helps to prevent fogging.

1. Standard equipment for oral or nasal fiberoptic intubation includes an oral bite block or Ovassapian airway, topical anesthetics and vasoconstrictors, suction, and a sterile fiberoptic scope with light source.

2. Indications

   a. The flexible fiberoptic laryngoscope or bronchoscope can be used in both awake and anesthetized patients to evaluate and intubate their airways. It can be used for both nasal and oral endotracheal intubation and should be used as a first option in an anticipated difficult airway rather than as a "last resort."

   b. Initial fiberoptic intubation is recommended for patients with known or suspected cervical spine pathology, head and neck tumors, morbid obesity, or a history of difficult ventilation or intubation.

3. Technique. An ETT is placed over a lubricated fiberoptic scope, suction tubing is attached to the suction port, and the control lever is grasped with one hand while the scope is advanced or maneuvered with the other hand. An oral Ovassapian airway is helpful and well tolerated for oral laryngoscopy. It is important to keep the fiberoptic scope in the midline to prevent entering the piriform fossa. The tip of the scope is positioned anteriorly when in the hypopharynx and advanced toward the epiglottis. If mucosa or secretions impair the view, the scope should be retracted or removed to clean the tip and then reinserted in the midline. As the scope slides beneath the epiglottis, the vocal cords will be seen. The scope is advanced with the tip in a neutral position until tracheal rings are noted. If topical anesthesia is adequate, the patient will tolerate this without coughing. The scope is stabilized within the trachea, and the ETT is advanced over it and into the trachea. If there is resistance to passage, the ETT may need to be turned 90 degrees in the counterclockwise direction to avoid the anterior commissure and permit passage through the vocal cords.

D. The **light wand** consists of a malleable lighted stylet over which an oral ETT can be passed blindly into the trachea. To insert, the operating room lights are dimmed, and the light wand and ETT are advanced following the curve of the tongue. A glow noted in the lateral neck indicates that the tip of the ETT lies in the piriform fossa. If the tip enters the esophagus, there is a marked diminution in the light's brightness. When the tip is correctly positioned in the trachea, a glow is noted in the anterior neck. At this point, the ETT is slid off the stylet and into the trachea.

E. Retrograde tracheal intubation can be performed when previously described techniques have been unsuccessful. It is performed in a conscious patient who is ventilating with a stable airway. For this technique, the cricothyroid membrane is identified and punctured in the midline with an 18-gauge intravenous (IV) catheter. An 80-cm, 0.025-inch guidewire is introduced and directed cephalad. A laryngoscope is used to visualize and retrieve the wire. An ETT is passed over the wire, which serves as a guide through the vocal cords.

VI. The difficult airway and emergency airway techniques
A. Difficult Airway. The most recent American Society of Anesthesiologists (ASA) algorithm for the management of the difficult airway is shown in Fig. 13-4. Familiarity with this algorithm is crucial for the anesthesiologist given that 30% of anesthesia-related deaths and a disproportionately large number of closed malpractice claims against anesthesiologists are related to airway management issues.

    1. The difficult airway can be divided into the recognized difficult airway and the unrecognized difficult airway, with the latter presenting the greater challenge for the anesthesiologist.

    2. The ASA defines **a difficult airway** as failure to intubate with conventional laryngoscopy after three attempts and/or failure to intubate with conventional laryngoscopy for more than 10 minutes. Others have suggested that a more appropriate definition of a difficult airway would be that of failure to intubate with conventional laryngoscopy after an optimal/best attempt. This optimal/best attempt is defined as an attempt with a reasonably experienced laryngoscopist, no significant resistive muscle tone, use of optimal sniffing position, use of external laryngeal manipulation, change of laryngoscope blade type a single time, and change of laryngoscope blade length a single time.

    3. The role of **regional anesthesia** in the airway algorithm deserves special mention. Although the algorithm advocates the consideration of regional anesthesia in the management arm of a difficult airway, it should be kept in mind that the use of a regional anesthetic does not solve the issue of a difficult airway. The choice of a regional anesthetic may not preclude the need for general anesthesia. It is generally not recommended to elect a regional anesthetic for a patient with a known difficult airway if the surgery is not amenable to rapid termination (if the patient cannot tolerate the regional anesthetic) or access to the patient's airway is compromised.

    4. The **LMA** (basic and intubating) appears in five places in the 1996 ASA difficult airway algorithm: as a choice for awake intubation, as an airway option for patients with an unrecognized airway who can be mask ventilated but cannot be intubated (nonemergency limb), as a conduit for intubation in patients who can be mask ventilated but cannot be intubated with conventional laryngoscopy (nonemergency limb), as an emergency airway option in patients who cannot be intubated and cannot be ventilated (emergency limb; the Combitube and transtracheal jet ventilation are other options here), and as a conduit for intubation in patients who cannot be intubated and cannot be ventilated (when a supraglottic airway is insufficient and intubation *per se* is needed).

    5. The **intubating LMA** (Fastrach) includes a curved stainless steel tube (13 mm inner diameter [ID]) covered with silicone, a 15-mm end connector, a handle, cuff, and an epiglottic lifting bar (Fig. 13-5). The tube is of sufficient diameter to accept a cuffed 8 mm ID ETT and is long enough to ensure that the ETT cuff will rest beyond the vocal cords. The primary differences between the intubating LMA and the basic LMA are the steel tube, handle, and epiglottic lifting bar.

    a. The intubating LMA is inserted similarly to the basic LMA.

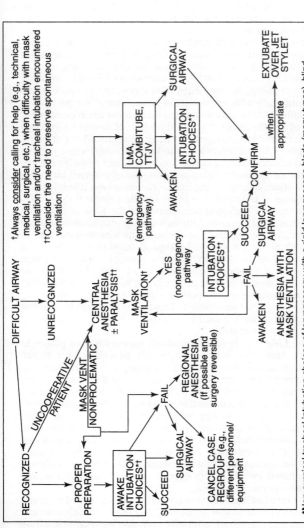

Fig. 13-4. American Society of Anesthesiologists difficult airway

*Non-surgical tracheal intubation choices of laryngoscopy with a rigid laryngoscope blade (many types), blind orotracheal or nasotracheal technique, fiberoptic technique, retrograde technique, illuminating stylet, rigid bronchoscope, percutaneous dilational tracheal entry.

†Always consider calling for help (e.g., technical, medical, surgical, etc.) when difficulty with mask ventilation and/or tracheal intubation encountered
††Consider the need to preserve spontaneous ventilation

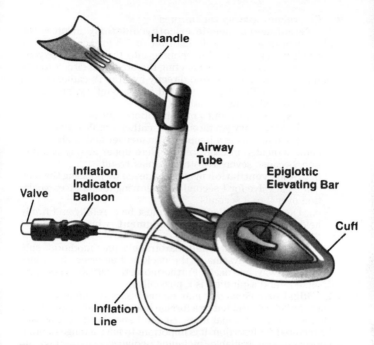

Fig. 13-5. Features of the laryngeal mask airway Fastrach. (From Brain AIJ, Verghese C. *LMA-Fastrach instruction manual.* San Diego: LMA North America, Inc., 1998.)

Once inserted, it can be used with the cuff inflated as the sole airway device. It can also be used as a conduit for either fiberoptic or blind intubation.

b. For intubation, a special ETT with a blunt bullnose tip (the Euromedical ILM ETT) can be used to minimize soft tissue damage. If attempting blind intubation, the tube should be lubricated and gently inserted into the LMA tube. At 15 cm, the ETT tip will lie at the epiglottic lifting bar. The ETT should be gently pushed into the trachea while grasping the LMA handle for support. Using the Fastrach handle as a lever while intubating is not recommended. Once the intubation is deemed successful, the tube position should be verified, and the cuff inflated and ETT secured (see section V).

c. **After intubation**, the intubating LMA can either be left in place or removed leaving the ETT in place. If the intubating LMA is left in place, the LMA cuff should be deflated. If the intubating LMA is removed, the LMA cuff should be deflated and the LMA gently removed by manipulating the handle while using an ETT stabilizer to keep the ETT in place. The ETT stabilizer can be removed once the LMA has cleared the patient's mouth and the ETT stabilized with the operator's other hand or by an assistant.

B. Emergency airway techniques

1. Percutaneous needle cricothyroidotomy involves the placement of a 14-gauge IV catheter or 7.5 French introducer through the cricothyroid membrane into the trachea. Oxygen can be administered by connecting the breathing circuit to a 3-mm ID ETT adapter inserted directly into the IV catheter or to a 7.5-mm ID ETT adapter inserted into a 3-mL syringe barrel and connected to the IV catheter.

    a. Oxygenation, but not ventilation, can be achieved by administering oxygen through the catheter at flow rates of 10 to 12 L/min. This is a temporary maneuver and is absolutely contraindicated in cases of complete upper airway obstruction, because severe barotrauma may result.

    b. Some ventilation may be achieved by pressing the oxygen flush valve for 1 second and allowing for passive exhalation over 2 to 3 seconds.

    c. Once in place, the catheter must be carefully and firmly held in position to **avoid dislodgment**, which can be life threatening.

    d. Complications include barotrauma, pneumothorax, subcutaneous emphysema of the neck and anterior chest, loss of the airway, and death. Furthermore, the airway is not "protected," and aspiration is a possibility.

2. Rigid bronchoscopy may be necessary to support an airway partially obstructed by a foreign body, traumatic disruption, stenosis, or mediastinal mass. General anesthesia will usually be required for insertion. It is important to have a range of bronchoscope sizes available (including pediatric sizes). An inhalation induction with spontaneous ventilation is most commonly used (see Chapter 21).

3. Cricothyroidotomy is a rapid effective method for relieving severe upper airway obstruction. With the neck extended, a small incision is made in the cricothyroid membrane in the midline. The handle of a scalpel or a Kelley forceps is used to separate the tissues while a tracheostomy tube or ETT is inserted percutaneously.

4. Tracheostomy may be performed under local anesthesia before the induction of general anesthesia for a patient with a particularly difficult airway.

    a. Technique. After careful dissection of vessels, nerves, and the thyroid isthmus, a tracheal incision is made, usually between the third or fourth cartilaginous rings. Percutaneous dilational tracheostomy, using commercially available techniques and a modified Seldinger technique, may also be performed.

    b. Complications include hemorrhage, false passage, and pneumothorax.

VII. Special considerations

A. Rapid sequence induction

1. Indications. Patients at risk for aspiration include those who have recently eaten (full stomach), pregnant patients, those with bowel obstruction, morbid obesity, or symptomatic reflux.

2. Technique

    a. Equipment necessary for a rapid sequence induction should include the following:

(1) Functioning tonsil-tip (Yankauer) suction.

(2) Several different laryngoscope blades (Macintosh and Miller).

(3) Several styletted ETT's, including one that is a size smaller than normal.

(4) An assistant who can apply cricoid pressure effectively.

b. The patient is **preoxygenated** using high flow rates of 100% oxygen for 3 to 5 minutes (denitrogenation). Four vital capacity breaths of 100% oxygen achieve nearly the same results when time is of the essence.

c. **The neck is extended** so the trachea is directly anterior to the esophagus. After the IV administration of an induction agent (e.g., thiopental, propofol, or ketamine), followed immediately by succinylcholine (1 to 1.5 mg/kg intravenously), an assistant places firm downward digital pressure on the cricoid cartilage, effectively compressing and occluding the esophagus (**Sellick maneuver**). This maneuver reduces the risk of passive regurgitation of gastric contents into the pharynx and may bring the vocal cords into better view by displacing them posteriorly. It will not prevent active vomiting.

d. There should be no attempt to ventilate the patient by mask. Intubation can usually be performed within 30 to 60 seconds. Cricoid pressure is maintained until successful endotracheal intubation is verified.

e. If intubation attempts are unsuccessful, cricoid pressure should be maintained continuously during subsequent intubation maneuvers and while mask ventilation is in progress.

B. Awake intubation

1. Indications. Awake oral or nasal intubation should be considered when there is:

a. A difficult intubation anticipated in a patient at risk for aspiration.

b. Uncertainty about the ability to ventilate or intubate after induction of general anesthesia (e.g., morbidly obese patients).

c. A need to assess neurologic function after intubation or positioning for surgery.

2. Technique

a. To perform an awake intubation, a 4% lidocaine gargle, followed by a lidocaine spray or nebulizer, is used to decrease upper airway sensation.

(1) **Superior laryngeal nerve block** may be used to anesthetize supraglottic structures. A 25-gauge needle is directed anterior to the greater cornu of the hyoid bone and walked off in a caudal direction until inserted in the thyrohyoid membrane. After negative aspiration, 2 mL of 2% lidocaine is injected on each side.

(2) **Translaryngeal injection of local anesthetic** can anesthetize the glottis and upper trachea. A 25-gauge needle is inserted through the cricothyroid membrane in the midline. After aspiration of air to confirm placement within the tracheal lumen, 2 mL of 2% lidocaine is injected, and the

needle is withdrawn. The patient will cough when local anesthetic is injected, aiding in anesthetic spread. This block is usually not performed in the patient with a full stomach because of the risk for aspiration.

b. Awake oral laryngoscopy often allows one to assess the airway. Sedatives such as midazolam, propofol, and fentanyl may be used in addition to the nerve blocks described above.

c. Awake nasal intubation may be performed after adequate topical anesthesia and regional airway blocks.

(1) Incremental doses of sedatives are useful adjuncts.

(2) A well-lubricated ETT is passed into the nasopharynx with gentle pressure.

(3) Deep resonant breath sounds may be noted as the tube is advanced toward the glottis. An exaggerated sniffing position may be useful. The ETT is usually passed into the trachea during inspiration.

(4) Successful intubation is noted when the patient is unable to phonate, breath sounds and humidification within the ETT are noted with ventilation, and carbon dioxide is noted on the capnograph.

3. Complications are as previously described in section V.B.4.

C. ETT changes. Occasionally, ETT cuff leaks or partial obstruction of the ETT necessitates changing an ETT in a patient with a difficult airway.

1. The oropharynx is suctioned and the patient is ventilated with 100% oxygen.

2. A **tracheal tube changer** is a specialized stylet that is placed through the ETT and into the distal trachea. The old ETT is slid off the changer, and a new ETT is passed over the changer into the trachea.

3. A **fiberoptic bronchoscope** can also be used for reintubation. An ETT is placed over the bronchoscope, the tip of which is passed into the trachea alongside the existing tube. The cuff of the existing ETT is deflated, the bronchoscope is advanced, and tracheal rings are noted to confirm position. The existing ETT is removed (a tracheal tube changer may be left in its place) and the new one advanced as described in section V.C.

SUGGESTED READING

Benumof JL. The LMA and the ASA difficult airway algorithm. *Anesthesiology* 1996;84:686–689.

Cormack RS, Lehane J. Difficult tracheal intubation in obstetrics. *Anaesthesia* 1984;39:1105–1111.

Crosby ET, Cooper RM, Douglas MI, et al. The unanticipated difficult airway with recommendations for management. *Can J Anaesth* 1998; 45:757–776.

Domino KB, Posner KL, Capan RA, et al. Airway during anesthesia: a closed claim analysis. *Anesthesiology* 1999;91:1703–1711.

Hurford WE. Nasotracheal intubation. *Respir Care* 1999;44:643–649.

Langeron O, Masso E, Huraux C, et al. Prediction of difficult mask ventilation. *Anesthesiology* 2000;92:1229–1236.

Samsoon GLT, Young JRB. Difficult tracheal intubation: a retrospective study. *Anaesthesia* 1987;42:490–497.

Scmitt H, Buchfelder M, Radespil-Troger M, et al. Difficult intubation in acromegalic patients. *Anesthesiology* 2000;93:110–114.

Sellick B. Cricoid pressure to control regurgitation of stomach contents during induction of anesthesia. *Lancet* 1961;2:404–406.

Administration of General Anesthesia

Stuart A. Forman

The **primary goals** of general anesthesia are to maintain the health and safety of the patient while providing amnesia, analgesia, and optimal surgical conditions. **Secondary goals** may vary, depending on the patient's medical condition, the surgical procedure, and the surgical setting (e.g., outpatient surgical unit vs. inpatient operating room [OR]; see Chapters 30 and 31). Perioperative planning involves the integration of pre-, intra-, and postoperative care. Flexibility is an essential component in this planning; multiple approaches to induction, maintenance, and emergence should be considered. Furthermore, intraoperative changes in the surgical procedure or the patient's condition may occur, requiring modification of anesthetic goals and plans.

I. Preoperative preparation. The anesthetist assumes responsibility for the patient when the preoperative medication is administered. An anesthetist should accompany an unstable patient during transport to the OR.

A. Preoperative evaluations may be performed minutes to weeks before the administration of the anesthetic and sometimes not by the anesthetist of record. The administering anesthetist performs an airway examination and checks for interim changes in the patient's condition, medications, laboratory data, and consultant notes. Time of last oral intake is confirmed, the anesthetic plan is reviewed with the patient, and proper informed consent for the administration of anesthesia is obtained.

B. Intravascular volume. Patients may arrive in the OR with intravascular or total body hypovolemia due to prolonged lack of oral intake, severe inflammatory illness, hemorrhage, fever, vomiting, or diuretic use. Currently available isotonic bowel preparations do not directly induce water loss but can decrease absorption of fluids ingested before surgery. The patient's volume status is evaluated either clinically or with appropriate monitors. If a **fluid deficit** is present, the patient should be adequately hydrated before the induction of anesthesia. The fluid deficit for fasting adults is estimated at 60 mL/h plus 1 mL/kg/h for each kilogram greater than 20 kg (maintenance fluids). In general, at least half of this deficit is corrected before induction; the remainder may be corrected intraoperatively.

C. Intravenous (IV) access. The size and number of IV catheters placed varies with the procedure, anticipated blood loss, and the need for continuous drug infusions. At least one 14- or 16-gauge catheter should be placed when rapid fluid or blood infusion is anticipated. When continuous drug infusions are to be delivered concurrently with rapid fluid infusion, an additional IV catheter often is dedicated for this purpose. Some medications used for cardiovascular support (e.g., norepinephrine) are best delivered via a central venous catheter.

D. Preoperative medications

  1. Anxiety. The preoperative period is one of high anxiety, especially for patients who have not had a prior interview with an anesthetist. Anxiety may be managed effectively with calm reassurance and expression of interest in the patient's well-being. When deemed appropriate, a benzodiazepine (e.g., diazepam, midazolam) with or without a small dose of an opioid (e.g., fentanyl, morphine) may be administered. Oral diazepam or lorazepam may be given with a small amount of water 30 to 60 minutes before the procedure. Patients complaining of pain on arrival in the OR may be given opioids in incremental amounts to alleviate symptoms. Dosages are based on the patient's age, medical condition, and anticipated time of discharge (see Chapters 1 and 11). Appropriate monitoring should be used and resuscitative equipment available.

  2. Drugs to neutralize gastric acid and decrease gastric volume are used when the patient is at increased risk of aspiration of gastric contents (i.e., recent meal, trauma, morbid obesity, bowel obstruction, pregnancy, history of gastric surgery, or history of active reflux; see Chapter 1).

E. Monitoring. Standard monitoring (see Chapter 10) is established before the induction of anesthesia. Invasive monitors (e.g., arterial catheter, central venous line, pulmonary artery catheter) should be placed before induction of anesthesia when indicated by the patient's medical condition (e.g., an arterial line for a patient at risk for cerebral ischemia). Invasive monitors may be placed after induction of anesthesia when indicated primarily by the surgical procedure (e.g., a central line for a patient undergoing elective aortic surgery).

F. Trauma and cardiac, thoracic, aortic, neurologic, and carotid surgery pose significant risks to the patient that prolong the need for close monitoring and highly skilled care (see Chapters 21, 22, 23, and 32). If necessary, intensive care unit (ICU) bed availability must be confirmed before elective cases and planned for during emergency surgery.

II. Induction of anesthesia produces an unconscious patient with depressed reflexes who is entirely dependent on the anesthetist for maintenance of homeostatic mechanisms and safety.

  A. The environment in the OR should be warm, with minimal noise, and all attention focused on the patient.

  B. The patient's position for induction is usually supine, with extremities resting comfortably on padded surfaces in a neutral anatomic position. The head should rest comfortably on a firm support, which is raised in a "sniff" position (see Chapter 13). Routine preinduction administration of oxygen minimizes the risk of hypoxia developing during induction of anesthesia. High flow (8 to 10 L/min) oxygen should be delivered via a face mask placed gently on the patient's face. The patient can be instructed to take deep breaths and exhale fully to speed the exchange of oxygen.

  C. Induction techniques. The choice of induction technique is guided by the patient's medical condition, anticipated airway management (i.e., risk of aspiration, difficult intubation, or compromised airway), and patient preference.

1.   IV induction begins with administration of a potent short-acting hypnotic drug (specific agents and doses are given in Chapter 11). After loss of consciousness, inhalation or additional IV agents are administered to maintain anesthesia. The patient may continue to breathe spontaneously or with assistance.

2.   An induction using only inhalational anesthetics may be used to maintain spontaneous ventilation when there is a compromised airway or to defer the placement of an IV catheter (e.g., in pediatric patients). The classic stages of anesthesia should be anticipated (Table 14-1). After preoxygenation, inhalational anesthetics are added at low concentration (0.5 times minimum alveolar concentration [MAC]) and then increased in in-

Table 14-1.   Stages of general anesthesia

Stage I: Amnesia	This period begins with induction of anesthesia and continues to loss of consciousness. The threshold of pain perception is not lowered during stage I.
Stage II: Delirium	This period characterized by uninhibited excitation and potentially injurious responses to noxious stimuli, including vomiting, laryngospasm, hypertension, tachycardia, and uncontrolled movement. The pupils are often dilated, gaze may be divergent, respiration is frequently irregular, and breath holding is common. Desirable induction drugs accelerate transition through this stage.
Stage III: Surgical anesthesia	In this target depth for anesthesia, the gaze is central, pupils are constricted, and respirations are regular. Anesthesia considered sufficient when painful stimulation does not elicit somatic reflexes or deleterious autonomic responses (e.g., hypertension, tachycardia).
Stage IV: Overdosage	Commonly described as "too deep," this stage is marked by shallow or absent respirations, dilated and nonreactive pupils, and hypotension that may progress to circulatory failure. Anesthesia should be lightened immediately.

The "stages" or planes of anesthesia were defined by Guedel after careful observation of patient responses during induction with diethyl ether. Induction with modern anesthetic agents is sufficiently rapid that these descriptions of individual stages are often not applicable or appreciated. However, modification of these categories still provides useful terminology to describe progression from the awake to the anesthetized state.

crements of 0.3 to 0.5 MAC every three to four breaths until the depth of anesthesia is adequate for IV placement or airway manipulation. Alternatively, a "single vital capacity breath" inhalation induction can be achieved using a high concentration of a less pungent agent like halothane or sevoflurane.

3. Intramuscular injection of ketamine, rectal methohexital, oral transmucosal fentanyl, and oral midazolam are induction techniques more commonly used in uncooperative patients or young children (see Chapters 11 and 28).

D. **Airway management** (see Chapter 13). The patency of the patient's airway is critically important during induction of anesthesia. Patients with difficult or unstable airways may be endotracheally intubated most safely before the induction of anesthesia. The anesthetized patient's airway may be managed using a face mask, oral or nasopharyngeal airway, cuffed oropharyngeal airway, laryngeal mask airway (LMA), or endotracheal tube (ETT). If tracheal intubation is planned, a muscle relaxant may be given to facilitate laryngoscopy and intubation, but the ability to ventilate the patient via face mask should be assessed before muscle relaxant administration. An exception to this rule is the "rapid sequence induction" for patients at risk for pulmonary aspiration (see Chapter 13).

E. **Laryngoscopy** and **intubation** may cause profound sympathetic responses such as hypertension and tachycardia; these can be attenuated by the prior administration of additional hypnotics, volatile anesthetics, opioids, or β-adrenergic blockers.

F. **Positioning for surgery** usually occurs after the induction of general anesthesia. Patients at risk for neurologic injury during positioning may undergo awake intubation and then be assisted into their surgical position before induction of anesthesia. Movement of a supine anesthetized patient into a different position may cause hypotension because of the lack of intact compensatory hemodynamic reflexes. Positioning should occur at a controlled pace with frequent assessments of the patient's cardiovascular status and with close attention to the patient's airway and ventilation. The anesthetist should ensure that the patient's head and limbs are protected and sufficiently padded to prevent compressive ischemia or neurologic damage. Hyperextension or over-rotation of the patient's neck and joints must be avoided.

III. **Maintenance** begins when the patient is sufficiently anesthetized to provide analgesia, unconsciousness, and muscle relaxation for surgery. Vigilance on the part of the anesthetist is required to maintain homeostasis (vital signs, acid-base balance, temperature, coagulation, and volume status) and regulate anesthetic depth.

A. **Ensuring lack of awareness and amnesia** are implicit goals of a general anesthetic. **Intraoperative awareness** with recall is estimated to occur in 0.1% to 0.2% of general anesthetics and is more frequent in certain high risk populations (e.g., trauma, cardiac surgery, obstetrics). Factors that increase the risk of awareness include the use of muscle relaxants and nitrous oxide-narcotic or low concentrations of volatile anesthetics (i.e., "light" anesthesia). **Depth of anesthesia** should be continuously assessed from induction through emergence. Changes in the intensity of surgical stimulation may cause rapid changes in anesthetic depth, which should be anticipated. Responses suggesting inadequate anesthetic depth are relatively nonspecific. These may be somatic (movement, coughing, changes of respiratory pattern) or autonomic (tachycardia, hypertension, mydriasis, sweating, or tearing). Purposeful movements in response to surgical stimulation or voice command are evidence of "perceptive awareness" but can occur without recall. These should be attenuated by first ensuring adequate hypnosis and analgesia and then, if indicated, by the administration of muscle relaxants. Changes in physiologic signs (Table 14-1) may indicate inadequate anesthesia in paralyzed patients, but awareness has been reported to occur without any autonomic signs. **Sympathetic activation** may be caused by stimuli other than awareness or pain (e.g., hypoxia, hypercarbia, hypovolemia, caval compression, adrenal manipulation) and can be controlled with increased concentrations of volatile anesthetics, IV analgesics, regional anesthesia, and adrenergic antagonists. The coherence of the cortical encephalogram (bispectral electroencephalographic analysis) and the mid-latency auditory evoked potential has been shown to correlate with the hypnotic state under many types of general anesthesia and may supplement monitoring of anesthetic depth.

B. Methods

    1. The use of volatile agents with minimal opioid use usually permits spontaneous ventilation. The concentration of the volatile anesthetic is titrated to patient movement (if muscle relaxants are not used), blood pressure (which decreases with increasing depth), and ventilation. Nitrous oxide, if used, is adjusted to ensure adequate oxygenation. High concentrations of nitrous oxide may be contraindicated in patients with closed air-filled compartments (e.g., pneumothorax, pneumocephalus, bowel obstruction, intravitreal bubbles in eye surgery).

    2. In a nitrous oxide–opioid relaxant technique, an inspired gas mixture of 65% to 70% nitrous oxide is combined with IV opioids, which are titrated to the patient's heart rate and blood pressure in response to surgical stimulation. Ventilation is controlled during the procedure to prevent hypoventilation because of the combination of muscle relaxants and opioids. An estimate of the total opioid requirement should be calculated and large doses avoided near the end of surgery to prevent delayed emergence and hypoventilation. Depending on the nitrous oxide concentration, patient's age, and physical status, awareness during surgery may be a concern requiring additional amnestic agents.

    3. IV anesthesia uses the continuous infusion or repeated boluses of a short-acting hypnotic drug (e.g., propofol) with or without opioids (e.g., remifentanil) and a muscle relaxant. This technique is particularly useful in situations where ventilation is frequently interrupted (e.g., bronchoscopy, laser airway surgery) and allows for a rapid emergence.

    4. Combinations of the above methods are often used. A low concentration of a volatile anesthetic (0.3 to 0.5 × MAC) may be added to a nitrous oxide–opioid relaxant technique to decrease the possibility of awareness. Nitrous oxide is frequently used in conjunction with IV anesthetics. Multiple anesthetics reduce the need for and the potential toxicity of large doses of single anesthetic agents. However, adverse medication reactions and interactions increase with the number of anesthetics administered.

5. General anesthesia can be combined with a regional anesthetic technique (i.e., peripheral or neuraxial nerve block). The required depth of general anesthesia is significantly reduced with blockade of painful surgical stimulation but still needs to be sufficient to ensure lack of awareness.

C. Ventilation of the patient during general anesthesia may be spontaneous, assisted, or controlled.

1. Spontaneous or assisted ventilation allows for the ability to assess the depth of anesthesia by observing the respiratory rate and pattern. A patient may breathe spontaneously with or without assistance, via a mask, LMA, or ETT. Intraoperatively, respiratory function may be significantly compromised because of the patient's medical condition, positioning, external pressure on the thorax and abdomen, surgical maneuvers (e.g., peritoneal insufflation, open chest, surgical packing), and medications (e.g., opioids). Most inhaled and IV anesthetic agents depress respiration in a dose-dependent manner, with a moderate rise in arterial partial pressure of carbon dioxide (Pa_{CO_2}).

2. Controlled ventilation. Although a mask or LMA may be used, an ETT and mechanical ventilator are generally used if ventilation is to be controlled for a significant period of time. Initial ventilator settings in healthy patients usually consist of a tidal volume of 10 to 12 mL/kg and a respiratory rate of 8 to 10 breaths/min. Lower tidal volumes (6 mL/kg) and the addition of positive end-expiratory pressure (PEEP) reduce the likelihood of barotrauma in patients with pulmonary pathology (see Chapter 35). Peak inspiratory pressure (PIP) should be noted. High airway pressure (greater than 25 to 30 cm H_2O) or changes of PIP must be immediately investigated and may signal a breathing circuit leak, ETT obstruction or movement, altered lung compliance or resistance, change in muscle relaxation, or surgical compression.

3. Assessment of ventilation. Adequate ventilation is confirmed by continual observation of the patient, auscultation of breath sounds, inspection of the anesthesia machine (e.g., reservoir breathing bag, ventilator bellows, airway pressures and flows), and patient monitors (e.g., capnograph, pulse oximeter). Arterial blood gas analysis and adjustments in the patient's ventilation may be required intraoperatively. If gas exchange is inadequate, manual controlled ventilation, increased inspired oxygen concentrations, PEEP, or special ventilator modes (sometimes requiring a stand-alone ventilator) may be used (see Chapter 35) while the source of the problem is sought and treated.

D. IV fluids

1. Intraoperative IV fluid requirements

  a. Maintenance fluid requirements as described in section I.B. should be continued intraoperatively. In some instances (e.g., extremity surgery with tourniquet use) this may be the major component of the fluid requirement.

  b. "**Third space losses**" are due to tissue edema from surgical trauma, whereas "**insensible losses**" are due to evaporation from the airways and surgical wounds. These losses are difficult to assess and may be substantial (up to 20 mL/kg/ h) depending on the site and extent of surgery. The rate of evaporative loss is increased in febrile patients.

   c.   Blood losses may be difficult to estimate. The amount present in the suction canisters should be monitored, taking into consideration the presence of other fluids (e.g., irrigation, ascites). Used surgical sponges should be checked and may be weighed to improve estimates of blood loss. Blood lost on the surgical field (e.g., surgical drapes) and on the floor should be estimated. If blood loss is substantial, serial monitoring of hematocrits is warranted.

   2.   IV fluids are administered to correct preoperative deficits and intraoperative losses.

   a.   Crystalloid solutions are used to replace maintenance fluid requirements, evaporative losses, and third space losses. The IV solution should be an isotonic balanced salt solution (e.g., lactated Ringer's). Other IV solutions may be indicated for patients with specific metabolic conditions (e.g., added glucose for diabetic patients receiving insulin, reduced sodium in diabetes insipidus, or increased sodium in syndrome of inappropriate secretion of antidiuretic hormone). Blood loss also may be replaced with balanced salt solution, administered in a 3:1 ratio of volume to estimated blood loss. With continued blood loss, this ratio will increase.

   b.   Colloid solutions (e.g., 5% albumin, 6% hydroxyethyl starch) may be used to replace blood loss or restore intravascular volume. To replace blood loss, colloid solutions should be administered in an approximately 1:1 ratio of volume to estimated blood loss (see Chapter 33).

   c.   Blood transfusion is discussed in Chapter 33.

   3.   Assessment. Trends in heart rate, blood pressure, and urine output may serve as guides to intravascular volume status and adequacy of replacement therapy. Measurement of central venous pressure, pulmonary artery occlusion pressure, right and left end-diastolic volumes (using transesophageal echocardiography), and cardiac output provide additional data to guide fluid administration when intraoperative losses are large or when cardiopulmonary disease mandates strict control of the patient's central pressures. Hematocrit, platelet count, fibrinogen concentration, prothrombin time, and partial thromboplastin time are used to assess adequacy of blood product therapy.

IV.   Emergence from general anesthesia. During this period, the patient makes the transition from an unconscious state to an awake state with intact protective reflexes.

   A.   Goals. Patients should be awake and responsive, with full muscle strength. This minimizes the risk of airway obstruction or pulmonary aspiration upon extubation and facilitates immediate neurologic assessment. In patients with cardiovascular disease, hemodynamics should be controlled.

   B.   Technique. Surgical stimulation diminishes as the procedure nears completion and anesthetic depth is reduced, enabling rapid emergence. Residual muscle relaxation is reversed, and the patient may start to breathe spontaneously. Analgesic requirements should be estimated and addressed before awakening.

C. Environment. The OR should be warmed, blankets placed on the patient, and noise and conversation minimized.

D. Positioning. The patient is usually returned to the supine position before extubation. The patient may be extubated in a lateral or prone position if the anesthetist is confident that the airway can be maintained and protected. A method for quickly returning the patient to the supine position must be available.

E. Mask ventilation. A patient who has received mask ventilation should continue to breathe 100% oxygen by mask during emergence. A period of light anesthesia (stage II; Table 14-1) often occurs before regaining consciousness. Stimulation (especially of the airway) during this period may precipitate laryngospasm and is best avoided. The patient can be moved when fully awake, following verbal commands, breathing spontaneously, and oxygenating adequately.

F. Extubation. Removal of the ETT from the trachea of an intubated patient is a critical moment. Patients with respiratory failure, hypothermia, impaired sensorium, marked hemodynamic instability, or whose airway may be significantly jeopardized (e.g., extensive oral surgery or possible glottic edema after prolonged headdown positioning) may remain intubated postoperatively until these conditions have improved.

   1. Awake extubation. Extubation of the airway usually occurs after the patient fully regains protective reflexes. Awake extubation is indicated in patients at risk of aspiration of gastric contents, patients who have difficult airways, and patients who have just undergone tracheal or maxillofacial surgery.

   a. Criteria. Before extubation, the patient should be awake and hemodynamically stable. The patient should have regained full muscle strength (see Chapter 12), follow simple verbal commands (e.g., lift head), and breathe spontaneously with acceptable oxygenation and ventilation.

   b. Technique. The presence of an ETT may be irritating to patients emerging from anesthesia. Lidocaine (0.5 to 1.0 mg/kg IV) can be given to suppress coughing but may prolong emergence. The patient breathes 100% oxygen, and the oropharynx is suctioned. Mild positive airway pressure (20 cm H_2O) is applied via the ETT, the ETT cuff is deflated, and the tube is removed. Oxygen (100%) administration is continued by face mask. The anesthetist's attention should remain focused on the patient until the patient's ability to ventilate, oxygenate, and protect the airway is confirmed. The extubated patient may become unconscious again and lose protective airway reflexes when stimulation decreases.

   c. Removal of the ETT over a flexible stylette (e.g., ETT exchanger, jet stylette, fiberoptic bronchoscope) can be performed when the patency of the patient's airway is uncertain or reintubation may be difficult. The airway is first anesthetized with 0.3 to 0.5 mg/kg lidocaine administered via the ETT and the patient is allowed to breathe spontaneously. A lubricated ETT exchanger is passed into the trachea through the ETT, the ETT cuff is deflated, and the ETT removed, leaving the exchange device in place until the anesthetist is certain that the patient's airway is stable. If airway obstruction develops, oxygen can be insufflated via the hollow exchange device or an ETT can be inserted over the device, which acts as a guide.

2.   Deep extubation. Stimulation of airway reflexes by the ETT during emergence can be avoided by extubating the trachea while the patient is still deeply anesthetized (stage III). This reduces the risk of laryngospasm and bronchospasm, making it a useful technique for severely asthmatic patients. It also avoids coughing and straining that may be undesirable after middle-ear surgery, open-eye procedures, and abdominal or inguinal herniorrhaphy.

    a.   Criteria. Contraindications to deep extubation are noted above (section IV.F.1.). Anesthetic depth must be sufficient to avoid responses to airway stimulation. Anesthesia may be deepened with a short-acting IV anesthetic or brief inhalation of a high concentration of a volatile agent.

    b.   Technique. All necessary airway equipment and medications should be readily available for replacement of the ETT. Surgical positioning must allow unrestricted access to the head for airway management. The oropharynx should be suctioned, the ETT cuff deflated, and, if there is no response to cuff deflation, the ETT is removed. Inhalation anesthesia is continued by mask and emergence is managed as described above (section IV.F.).

G.   Agitation. Severe agitation is occasionally seen on emergence from general anesthesia, especially in adolescents. Physiologic causes (e.g., hypoxia, hypercarbia, airway obstruction, or a full bladder) must be excluded. Pain, a common reason for agitation, may be treated with cautious titration of opioids (e.g., fentanyl, 0.025 mg IV, or meperidine, 25-mg IV increments).

H.   Delayed awakening. On occasion, a patient will not awaken promptly after the administration of general anesthesia. Ventilatory support and airway protection should be continued, and specific etiologies should be investigated (see Chapter 34).

V.   Transport. The anesthetist should accompany the patient from the OR to the postanesthesia care unit (PACU) or ICU. Monitoring of blood pressure, hemoglobin saturation, and electrocardiogram is continued during transport to an ICU but generally are not needed for transport of stable patients to the PACU. Supplemental oxygen should be available, and the patient's airway, ventilation, and overall condition should be continually observed. Placing the patient in the lateral position may help to prevent aspiration and upper airway obstruction. Medications and airway equipment should be available during transport if the patient is unstable or if transport is over a significant distance. Upon transfer of responsibility for patient care in the PACU or ICU, the anesthetist should provide a concise but thorough summary of the patient's past medical history, intraoperative course, postoperative condition, and current therapy.

VI.   Postoperative visit. A postoperative evaluation of the patient should be performed by the anesthetist within 24 to 48 hours of surgery and documented in the patient's medical record. The visit should include a review of the medical record, examination of the patient, and discussion of the patient's perioperative experience. Specific complications such as nausea, sore throat, dental injury, nerve injury, ocular injury, pneumonia, or change in mental status should be sought. Complications that require further therapy or consultations should be addressed.

SUGGESTED READING

Stanski DR. Monitoring depth of anesthesia. In: Miller RD, ed. *Anesthesia*, 5th ed. Philadelphia: Churchill Livingstone, 2000:1087–1116.

Willenkin RL, Polk SL. Management of general anesthesia. In: Miller RD, ed. *Anesthesia*, 4th ed. New York: Churchill Livingstone, 1994: 1045–1056.

15

Local Anesthetics

Tania Haddad and Jeannie Min

I. General principles

A. Chemistry. Local anesthetics are weak bases whose structure consists of an aromatic moiety connected to a substituted amine through an ester or amide linkage. The pK_a values of local anesthetics are near physiologic pH; thus, *in vivo*, both charged and uncharged forms are present to a significant degree. The degree of ionization is important because the uncharged form is most lipid soluble and able to gain access to the axon. The clinical differences between the ester and amide local anesthetics involve their potential for producing adverse effects and the mechanisms by which they are metabolized.

1. Esters. Procaine, cocaine, chloroprocaine, and tetracaine. The ester linkage is cleaved by plasma cholinesterase. The half-life of esters in the circulation is very short (about 1 minute). The degradation product of ester metabolism is para-aminobenzoic acid.

2. Amides. Lidocaine, mepivacaine, bupivacaine, etidocaine, and ropivacaine. The amide linkage is cleaved through initial *N*-dealkylation followed by hydrolysis, which occurs primarily in the liver. Patients with severe hepatic disease may be more susceptible to adverse reactions from amide local anesthetics. The elimination half-life for amide local anesthetics is approximately 2 to 3 hours.

B. Mechanism of action

1. Local anesthetics block nerve conduction by impairing propagation of the action potential in axons. They have no effect on the resting or threshold potentials but decrease the rate of rise of the action potential such that the threshold potential is not reached.

2. Local anesthetics interact directly with specific receptors on the Na^+ channel, inhibiting Na^+ ion influx. The anesthetic molecule must traverse the cell membrane through passive nonionic diffusion in the uncharged state and then bind to the sodium channel in the charged state.

3. Physiochemical properties of the local anesthetics affect neural blockade.

    a. High lipid solubility increases the potency, because lipophilic local anesthetics more easily cross nerve membranes.

    b. Agents with a high degree of **protein binding** will have a prolonged duration of effect.

    c. pK_a determines speed of onset of neural blockade. pK_a is the pH at which 50% of the local anesthetic is in the charged form and 50% uncharged. Agents with a lower pK_a value will have a faster onset because a greater fraction of the molecules

Table 15-1. Classification of nerve fibers

Fiber Type	Myelin	Diameter (μm)	Function
A-α	++	6–22	Motor efferent, proprioception afferent
A-β	++	6–22	Motor efferent, proprioception afferent
A-γ	++	3–6	Muscle spindle efferent
A-δ	++	1–4	Pain, temperature, touch afferent
B	+	<3	Preganglionic autonomic
C	–	0.3–1.3	Pain, temperature, touch afferent, postganglionic autonomic

will exist in the uncharged form and thus will more easily diffuse across nerve membranes.

   d. Lower pH of the drug solution, by decreasing the proportion of molecules in the uncharged form, results in a slower onset time of anesthesia.

4. Differential blockade of nerve fibers

   a. Peripheral nerves are classified according to size and function (Table 15-1). Traditionally, thin nerve fibers were believed to be more easily blocked than thick ones; however, the opposite susceptibility has been found. Myelinated fibers are more readily blocked than unmyelinated ones because of the need to produce blockade only at the nodes of Ranvier.

   b. By careful selection of an appropriate agent and concentration, it is often possible to block pain and temperature sensation (A-δ and C fibers) in the absence of significant motor blockade (A-α fibers). Nevertheless, the concentration of local anesthetic required to block a particular sensory modality is not a reliable guide to the nerve fibers involved.

   c. Differential blockade is a reflection of the arrangement of the fibers within the peripheral nerve; the outermost layer is blocked first with a concentration gradient toward the center.

5. Sequence of clinical anesthesia. Neural blockade of peripheral nerves usually progresses in the following order:

   a. Sympathetic block with peripheral vasodilation and skin temperature elevation.

   b. Loss of pain and temperature sensation.

   c. Loss of proprioception.

   d. Loss of touch and pressure sensation.

   e. Motor paralysis.

6. Pathophysiologic factors

   a. A decrease in cardiac output reduces the volume of distribution and plasma clearance of local anesthetics, increasing plasma concentration and the potential for toxicity.

b. Severe hepatic disease may prolong the duration of action of amino amides.

c. Renal disease has minimal effect.

d. Patients with **reduced cholinesterase activity** (newborns and pregnant patients) and patients with **atypical cholinesterase** may have an increased potential for toxicity.

e. Fetal acidosis may result in greater transplacental transfer and trapping of local anesthetics from mother to her fetus and thus may have an increased potential for fetal toxicity.

C.   **Commercial preparations**

1.   Commercially available solutions of local anesthetics are supplied as **hydrochloride salts** to increase solubility in water. These solutions are usually acidic to enhance the formation of the water-soluble ionized form. Plain solutions usually are adjusted to a pH of 6. Those containing a vasoconstrictor are adjusted to a pH of 4 because of the lability of catecholamine molecules at alkaline pH.

2.   **Antimicrobial preservatives** (paraben derivatives) are added to multidose vials. Only preservative-free solutions should be used in spinal, epidural, or caudal anesthesia to prevent potentially neurotoxic effects.

3.   **Antioxidants** (sodium metabisulfite, sodium ethylenediamine tetraacetic acid [EDTA]) may be added to slow breakdown of local anesthetics.

II.   **Clinical uses of local anesthetics.** The choice of local anesthetic must take into consideration the duration of surgery, regional technique used, surgical requirements, the potential for local or systemic toxicity, and any metabolic constraints (Tables 15-2 and 15-3).

A.   **Combinations of local anesthetics**

1.   Chloroprocaine–bupivacaine, lidocaine–bupivacaine, and mepivacaine–tetracaine mixtures are reported to have a rapid onset and long duration. The systemic toxicity of combinations appears to be additive. The potential benefit of combinations of drugs is unclear.

2.   **Eutectic mixture of local anesthetics (EMLA)** cream is a mixture of 2.5% lidocaine and 2.5% prilocaine for use as a topical skin anesthetic.

B.   **Epinephrine**

1.   **Epinephrine** may be added to local anesthetics as follows:

   a. To prolong the duration of anesthesia. This varies with the type of regional block and concentration of local anesthetic.

   b. To decrease systemic toxicity by decreasing the rate of absorption of anesthetic into the circulation, thus minimizing peak blood levels of local anesthetics.

   c. To increase intensity of the block by direct α agonist effect on antinociceptive receptors in the spinal cord.

   d. To provide local vasoconstriction and decrease surgical bleeding.

   e. To assist in the evaluation of a test dose.

2.   **Adding epinephrine** (1:200,000 solution) to plain solutions of local anesthetics just before administration permits the use of a solution with high pH, which speeds onset of the block. A 1:200,000 dilution is achieved by adding 0.1 mL of 1:1,000

epinephrine (with a tuberculin syringe) to 20 mL of local anesthetic solution.

3. The **maximum dose of epinephrine** should probably not exceed 10 μg/kg in pediatric patients and 200 to 250 μg in adults.

4. Epinephrine should not be used in peripheral nerve blocks in areas with poor collateral blood flow (e.g., digits, penis, toes) or in intravenous regional techniques. Caution is advised in patients with severe coronary artery disease, arrhythmias, uncontrolled hypertension, hyperthyroidism, and uteroplacental insufficiency.

C. **Phenylephrine** has been used like epinephrine, but no particular advantages have been demonstrated. Five milligrams of phenylephrine can be added to solutions of local anesthetics to prolong spinal anesthesia.

D. **Sodium bicarbonate** added to local anesthetic solutions raises the pH and increases the concentration of non-ionized free base. The increased percentage of uncharged drug will increase the rate of diffusion and speed the onset of neural blockade. Typically, 1 mEq of sodium bicarbonate is added to each 10 mL of lidocaine or mepivacaine; only 0.1 mEq of sodium bicarbonate may be added to each 10 mL of bupivacaine to avoid precipitation. Carbonated local anesthetics (e.g., lidocaine carbonate) are thought to augment neural block by lowering intraneural pH and promoting the formation of the active (charged) species.

E. **Local anesthetic substitutes.** Meperidine and other phenylpiperidine derivatives have local anesthetic properties. Meperidine has been used as the sole anesthetic agent in spinals for cesarean section but there seems little advantage to using the drug this way.

III. **Toxicity** (Table 15-4)

A. **Allergic reactions.** True allergic reactions to local anesthetics are rare. It is important to differentiate these from common nonallergic responses such as vasovagal episodes and responses to intravascular injection of local anesthetic and/or epinephrine.

1. **Ester-type local anesthetics** may cause allergic reactions from the metabolite *p*-aminobenzoic acid. These anesthetics also may produce allergic reactions in persons sensitive to sulfa drugs (e.g., sulfonamides or thiazide diuretics.)

2. **Amide-type local anesthetics** are essentially devoid of allergic potential. Multidose vials of anesthetic solutions containing **methylparaben** as the preservative may produce an allergic reaction in patients sensitive to *p*-aminobenzoic acid.

3. **Local hypersensitivity reactions** may produce local erythema, urticaria, edema, or dermatitis.

4. **Systemic hypersensitivity reactions** are rare and can present with generalized erythema, urticaria, edema, bronchoconstriction, hypotension, and cardiovascular collapse.

5. **Treatment** is symptomatic and supportive (see Chapter 18).

B. **Local toxicity**

1. **Tissue toxicity** is rare.

2. **Transient radicular irritation (TRI) or transient neurologic symptoms (TNS)** can occur secondary to unintentional subarachnoid injection of large volumes or high concentrations of local anesthetics or chemical contamination of a

Table 15-2. Clinical uses of local anesthetics

Anesthetic	Onset	Duration	Potency	Toxicity	Remarks
Esters					
Procaine (Novocain)	Fast	Short	Low	Low	Local infiltration Spinal anesthesia (very short duration)
Chloroprocaine (Nescaine)	Very rapid	Short	Low	Very low	Local blocks Epidural anesthesia Rapid hydrolysis Previous bisulfite preservative removed
Tetracaine (Pontocaine)	Slow	Very long	High	Moderate	Spinal anesthesia Nerve blocks Produces motor and sensory blockade of similar duration and intensity

Amides					
Lidocaine (Xylocaine)	Rapid	Moderate	Moderate	Moderate	Most frequently used local anesthetic
Mepivacaine (Carbocaine)	Moderate	Moderate	Moderate	Moderate	Local infiltration Nerve blocks Epidural anesthesia
Bupivacaine (Marcaine, Sensorcaine)	Slow	Very long	High	High	All types of local and regional anesthesia requiring long duration
Levobupivacaine	Slow	Very long	High	Moderate	Epidural anesthesia Nerve blocks
Etidocaine (Duranest)	Rapid	Very long	High	Moderate	Epidural anesthesia Motor greater than sensory blockade
Ropivacaine	Slow	Long	High	Moderate	Sensory greater than motor blockade Less cardiotoxic than bupivacaine

Table 15-3.   Local anesthetic agents

Anesthetic Technique	Anesthetic	Concentration (%)	Duration (h)	Duration with epinephrine (h)	Dose Range (mL;70-kg patient)
Peripheral nerve block	Lidocaine	1–2	1.5–3.0	2–4	40–50
	Mepivacaine	1–2	3–5	3–5	40–50
	Bupivacaine	0.25–0.5	6–12	6–12	40–50
	Levobupivacaine	0.25–0.5	14–17	6–12	30
	Etidocaine	1.0–1.5	6–12	6–12	40–50
	Ropivacaine	0.5	5–8	5–8	35–50
Epidural and caudal	Chloroprocaine	2–3	0.25–0.5	0.5–1.0	20–30
	Lidocaine	1–2	0.5–1.0	0.75–1.5	20–30
	Mepivacaine	1–2	0.75–1.0	1–2	20–30
	Bupivacaine	0.25–0.75	1.5–3.0	2–4	20–30
	Levobupivacaine	0.5–0.75	3–9	2–4	20–30
	Etidocaine	0.5–1.5	1.5–3.0	2–4	20–30
	Ropivacaine	0.5–1.0	2–5	2–5	15–30

Table 15.? Recommended doses of local anesthetics

Local infiltration					
Procaine	0.5–1.0		0.25–0.5	0.5–1.5	1–60
Lidocaine	0.5–1.0	0.5–2.0	1–3	1–50	
Mepivicaine	0.5–1.0	0.25–2.0	1–3	1–50	
Bupivicaine	0.25–0.5	2–4	4–8	1–45	
Levobupivicaine	0.25–0.5	3–9	4–8	1–60	
Ropivicaine	0.5	2–6		1–40	
Spinal					
Lidocaine (hyperbaric)	5	0.75–1.5	0.75–1.5	60 mg	
Lidocaine (isobaric)	2	1–2	1–2	60 mg	
Bupivicaine (hyperbaric)	0.75	2–4	2–4	9 mg	
Bupivicaine (isobaric)	0.5	2–4	2–4	15 mg	
Levobupivicaine	0.5	4–7	2–4	15 mg	
Tetracaine (hyperbaric)	0.5	2–3	3–5	12 mg	
Tetracaine (isobaric)	0.5	3–5	5–8	15 mg	
Tetracaine (hypobaric)	0.1	3–5	5–8	10 mg	
Ropivicaine	0.5	2–4		15–22.5 mg	

Table 15-4.   Relative toxicity of local anesthetics

Agent	Approximate Potency Ratios		Maximum Recommended Dose	
	Anesthetic Potency	CNS Toxicity	Plain Solution	Epinephrine Containing (mg)
Procaine	1	1	400	600
Chloroprocaine	1	1	800	1,000
Lidocaine	2	3	300	500
Mepivicaine		2	300	500
Etidocaine		6	300	400
Bupivicaine	14	12	175	225
Tetracaine	10	8	100	200
Ropivicaine		9	300	
Levobupivicaine	14	ND	150	

ND, no data.

Potency ratios and equivalent doses depend on the method of anesthesia used. Maximum dose as recommended by the manufacturer in the United States for peripheral nerve blocks in 70-kg individuals. Tetracaine is used only for spinal anesthesia, primarily because of its toxic potential. When used at the recommended doses for spinal anesthesia, central nervous system (CNS) and cardiovascular toxicity are unlikely.

solution. An increased incidence of neurotoxicity associated with the subarachnoid administration of 5% lidocaine has been reported. It appears prudent to avoid the use of 5% lidocaine for spinal anesthesia; some practitioners suggest that the incidence of TRI may be increased with lower concentrations of lidocaine as well. The risk of TNS/TRI appears to be lower with bupivacaine. If lidocaine is to be used, commercially available 1.5% lidocaine with dextrose or preservative-free 2% lidocaine is recommended. Lithotomy position and outpatient status are additional factors found to contribute to TNS/TRI.

    3. Reports of sensory and motor deficits after intrathecal chloroprocaine solutions containing the antioxidant sodium bisulfite resulted in a change in its formulation. EDTA has replaced bisulfite. Nevertheless, intense back pain has been reported after administration of large volumes of solution. The back pain is thought to caused by spasms of the paraspinal muscles caused by the calcium binding properties of EDTA.

C.   Systemic toxicity usually results from either intravascular injection or overdose.

    1.   Intravascular injection most commonly occurs during nerve blockade in areas with large blood vessels (e.g., axillary or vertebral artery and epidural vein). This can be minimized by

        a.   Aspiration before injection.

        b.   Use of epinephrine-containing solutions for test doses.

c. Use of small incremental volumes in establishing the block.

d. Use of proper technique during intravenous regional anesthesia (see Chapter 17).

2. Central nervous system (CNS) toxicity

a. **Clinical features** of CNS toxicity include metallic taste, light-headedness, tinnitus, visual disturbances, and numbness of the tongue and lips. These may progress to muscle twitching, loss of consciousness, grand mal seizures, and coma.

b. **CNS toxicity is exacerbated** by hypercarbia, hypoxia, and acidosis.

c. **Treatment.** At the first sign of toxicity, injection of local anesthetic should be discontinued and oxygen administered. If seizure activity interferes with ventilation or is prolonged, anticonvulsant treatment is indicated with either benzodiazepines (e.g., midazolam, 1 to 2 mg) or barbiturates (e.g., thiopental, 50 to 200 mg in the adult). Succinylcholine can be given to facilitate intubation.

3. Cardiovascular toxicity. The cardiovascular system is more resistant than the CNS to toxic effects, but cardiovascular toxicity may be severe and difficult to treat.

a. **Clinical features.** Cardiovascular toxicity produces decreased ventricular contractility, refractory cardiac arrhythmias, and loss of peripheral vasomotor tone, which may lead to cardiovascular collapse. Cocaine is the only local anesthetic that causes vasoconstriction at all doses.

b. The **intravascular injection of bupivacaine or etidocaine** may produce cardiovascular collapse, which is often refractory to therapy because of the high degree of tissue binding displayed by these agents. Hypercarbia , acidosis, and hypoxia enhance the negative inotropic and chronotropic effects of these drugs.

  (1) **Ropivacaine**, similar to bupivacaine in potency and duration of action, lacks significant cardiac toxicity because it dissociates more rapidly from sodium channels.

  (2) **Levobupivacaine**, a single levorotary isomer of bupivacaine, has less cardiotoxic effects when compared with its racemate (bupivacaine).

c. **Treatment**

  (1) **Oxygen** must be administered and the circulation supported with volume replacement and vasopressors, including inotropes as necessary. Advanced cardiac life support should be performed if indicated (see Chapter 36).

  (2) **Ventricular tachycardia** should be treated by electrical cardioversion. Local anesthetic-induced cardiac arrhythmias are difficult to treat but usually subside over time if the patient can be maintained hemodynamically.

  (3) **Amiodarone** may be more effective than lidocaine for ventricular arrhythmias associated with intravascular injections of bupivacaine, and very large doses of epinephrine may be necessary for successful resuscitation.

  (4) **Prolonged cardiopulmonary resuscitation** may be required until the cardiotoxic effects subside with drug redistribution.

D. **Other adverse effects** include **Horner syndrome**, which can result from blockade of B fibers in the T1-4 nerve roots, and methemoglobinemia, which can follow administration of benzocaine, prilocaine, and EMLA cream. Methylene blue can be administered intravenously to convert methemoglobin to reduced hemoglobin.

SUGGESTED READING

Berde CB, Strichartz GR. Local anesthetics. In: Miller RE, ed. *Anesthesia*, 5th ed. New York: Churchill Livingstone, 2000:491–522.

Cousins MJ, Bridenbaugh PO. *Neural blockade in clinical anesthesia and management of pain*, 3rd ed. Philadelphia: Lippincott-Raven, 1998.

Cox CR, Faccenda KA, Gilhooly C, et al. Extradural S(-)-bupivacaine: comparison with racemic RS-bupivacaine. *Br J Anaesth* 1998;80: 289–293.

Reiz S, Nath S. Cardiotoxicity of local anaesthetic agents. *Br J Anaesth* 1986;58:736–746.

Spinal, Epidural, and Caudal Anesthesia

Shobana Chandrasekhar and May C. M. Pian-Smith

I. General considerations

A. Preoperative assessment of the patient for regional anesthesia is similar to that for general anesthesia. The details of the procedure to be performed, including its anticipated length, patient position, and a complete review of any coexisting diseases, should be taken into account in determining the appropriateness of a regional technique.

B. The area where the block is to be administered should be examined for potential difficulties or pathology. Preexisting neurologic abnormalities should be well documented and presence of kyphoscoliosis determined.

C. A history of abnormal bleeding and a review of the patient's medications may indicate a need for additional coagulation studies.

D. Patients should be given a **detailed explanation** of the planned procedure, with risks and benefits. In addition, they should be reassured that additional sedation and anesthesia can be given during the operation and that general anesthesia is an option if the block fails or the operation becomes more prolonged or extensive than originally thought.

E. As with general anesthesia, patients should receive appropriate monitoring (see Chapter 10) and have an intravenous (IV) line in place. Oxygen, equipment for intubation and positive-pressure ventilation, and drugs to provide hemodynamic support should be available.

II. Segmental level required for surgery

A. A knowledge of the sensory, motor, and autonomic distribution of spinal nerves will help the anesthetist determine the correct segmental level required for a particular operation and help anticipate the potential physiologic effects of producing a block to that level. Figure 16-1 illustrates the dermatomal distribution of the spinal nerves.

B. Afferent autonomic nerves innervate visceral sensation and viscerosomatic reflexes at spinal segmental levels much higher than would be predicted from skin dermatomes.

C. Minimal suggested levels for common surgical procedures are listed in Table 16-1.

III. Contraindications to peridural anesthesia

A. Absolute

1. Patient refusal.
2. Localized infection at skin puncture site.
3. Generalized sepsis (e.g., septicemia, bacteremia).

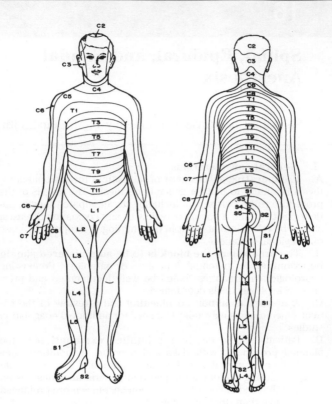

Fig. 16-1. Skin dermatomes corresponding to respective sensory innervation by spinal nerves.

Table 16-1.   Suggested minimum cutaneous levels for spinal anesthesia

Operative Site	Level
Lower extremities	T-12
Hip	T-10
Vagina, uterus	T-10
Bladder, prostate	T-10
Lower extremities with tourniquet	T-8
Testis, ovaries	T-8
Lower intraabdominal	T-6
Other intraabdominal	T-4

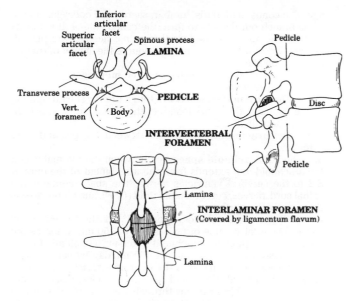

Fig. 16-2. Vertebral anatomy.

4. Coagulopathy.
5. Increased intracranial pressure.

B. Relative
1. Localized infection peripheral to regional technique site.
2. Hypovolemia.
3. Central nervous system disease.
4. Chronic back pain.

IV. Spinal anesthesia involves the administration of local anesthetic into the subarachnoid space.

A. Anatomy
1. The **spinal canal** extends from the foramen magnum to the sacral hiatus. The boundaries of the bony canal are the vertebral body anteriorly, the pedicles laterally, and the spinous processes and laminae posteriorly (Fig. 16-2).
2. Three **interlaminar ligaments** bind the vertebral processes together:
    a. Superficially, the **supraspinous ligament** connects the apices of the spinous processes.
    b. The **interspinous ligament** connects the spinous processes on their horizontal surface.
    c. The **ligamentum flavum** connects the caudal edge of the vertebrae above to the cephalad edge of the lamina below. This ligament is composed of elastic fibers and is usually recognized by its increased resistance to passage of a needle.
3. The **spinal cord** extends the length of the vertebral canal during fetal life, ends at about L-3 at birth, and moves progressively cephalad to reach the adult position near L-1 by 2 years of

age. The conus medullaris, lumbar, sacral, and coccygeal nerve roots branch out distally to form the cauda equina. It is in this area of the canal (below L-2) that spinal needles are placed, because the mobility of the nerves reduces the danger of trauma from the needle.

4.   The spinal cord is invested in three **meninges**:

   a.   The **pia mater**.

   b.   The **dura mater**, which is a tough fibrous sheath running longitudinally the entire length of the spinal cord and is tethered caudally at S-2.

   c.   The **arachnoid**, which lies between the pia and dura mater.

5.   The **subarachnoid space** lies between the pia mater and the arachnoid and extends from the attachment of the dura at S-2 to the cerebral ventricles above. The space contains the spinal cord, nerves, cerebrospinal fluid (CSF), and blood vessels that supply the cord.

6.   **CSF** is a clear colorless fluid that fills the subarachnoid space. The total volume of CSF is 100 to 150 mL, whereas the volume in the spinal subarachnoid space is 25 to 35 mL. CSF is continuously formed at a rate of 450 mL/day by secretion or ultrafiltration of plasma from the choroid arterial plexuses located in the lateral, third, and fourth ventricles. CSF is reabsorbed into the bloodstream through the arachnoid villi and granulations that protrude through dura to lie in contact with the endothelium of the cerebral venous sinuses.

B.   **Physiology**

1.   **Neural blockade**. Smaller C fibers conveying autonomic impulses are more easily blocked than the larger sensory and motor fibers. As a result, the level of autonomic blockade extends above the level of the sensory blockade by two to three segments. This is termed differential blockade. Similarly, fibers conveying sensation are more easily blocked than the larger motor fibers so that sensory blockade will extend above the level of motor blockade.

2.   **Cardiovascular**. Hypotension is directly proportional to the degree of **sympathetic blockade** produced. Sympathetic blockade results in dilatation of arteries and venous capacitance vessels, leading to decreased systemic vascular resistance and decreased venous return. If the block is below T-4, increased baroreceptor activity produces an increase in activity to the cardiac sympathetic fibers and vasoconstriction of the upper extremities. Blockade above T-4 interrupts cardiac sympathetic fibers, leading to bradycardia, decreased cardiac output, and a further decrease in blood pressure. These changes are more marked in patients who are hypovolemic, elderly, or have obstruction to venous return (e.g., pregnancy). These effects can be minimized with prehydration, vasopressors, and anticholinergics.

3.   **Respiratory**. Low spinal anesthesia has no effect on ventilation. With ascending height of the block into the thoracic area, there is a progressive ascending intercostal muscle paralysis. This has little effect on ventilation in the supine surgical patient who still has diaphragmatic function mediated by the phrenic nerve. Ventilation in patients with poor respiratory reserve, such

as the morbidly obese, however, may be profoundly impaired. Both intercostal and abdominal muscle paralysis decrease the efficiency of coughing, which may be important in patients with chronic obstructive pulmonary disease. Epidural analgesia with opioids and low dose local anesthetics, which produces minimal motor blockade, is helpful in the postoperative care of thoracic surgical patients.

4. Visceral effects

    a. Bladder. Sacral blockade (S2-S4) results in an atonic bladder that is able to retain large volumes of urine. Blockade of sympathetic efferents (T5-L1) results in an increase in sphincter tone, producing retention. A urinary catheter should be placed if anesthesia or analgesia is maintained for a prolonged period.

    b. Intestine. Sympathetic blockade (T5-L1) produced by spinal anesthesia has a promotility effect on the gut because of predominance of parasympathetic tone.

5. Renal blood flow is maintained, because of autoregulation by local tissue factors, except with severe hypotension. Urine production is usually unaffected.

6. Neuroendocrine. Peridural block to T-5 inhibits part of the neural component of the stress response, through its blockade of sympathetic afferents to the adrenal medulla and blockade of sympathetic and somatic pathways mediating pain. Other components of the stress response and central release of humoral factors are unaffected. Vagal afferent fibers from upper abdominal viscera are not blocked and can stimulate release of hypothalamic and pituitary hormones, such as antidiuretic hormone and adrenocorticotropic hormone. Glucose tolerance and insulin release are normal.

7. Thermoregulation. Vasodilation of the lower limbs can produce hypothermia.

C. Technique

1. Spinal needle. Newer needles such as the **Sprotte** and **Whitacre** feature a pencil-point design with a lateral opening. These needles may reduce the incidence of postdural puncture headache (to ≤1%) compared with traditional "cutting tip" needles by splitting rather than cutting dural fibers during insertion. Needles that are 24 and 25 gauge are easily bent and are often inserted through a 19-gauge introducer needle. The 22-gauge **Quincke** needle is more rigid and is more easily directed and inserted. It can be useful in older patients in whom access may be more difficult and the incidence of postdural puncture headache is low.

2. Patient position. The lateral decubitus, prone, and sitting positions can be used for administration of spinal anesthesia.

    a. In the **lateral position**, the patient is placed with the affected side up if a hypobaric or isobaric technique is to be used and with the affected side down if a hyperbaric technique is to be used. The spine is horizontal and parallel to the edge of the table. The knees are drawn up toward the chest and the chin flexed downward onto the chest to obtain maximal flexion of the spine.

    b. The **sitting position** is useful for low spinal blocks required in certain gynecologic and urologic procedures and is commonly used in obese patients to assist in identification of the midline. It is used in conjunction with hyperbaric anesthetics. The head and shoulders are flexed downward onto the trunk with the arms resting on a Mayo stand. An assistant should be available to stabilize the patient, and the patient should not be oversedated.

c. The **prone position** is used in conjunction with hypobaric or isobaric anesthetics for procedures on the rectum, perineum, and anus. A prone jackknife position can be used for both administration of spinal anesthesia and the subsequent surgery.

3. Procedure

   a. The L2-3, L3-4, or L4-5 interspaces are commonly used for spinal anesthesia. The L3-4 interspace or the spinous process of L-4 are aligned with upper borders of the superior iliac crests.

   b. Disinfect a large area of skin with an appropriate antiseptic solution. Care must be taken to avoid contamination of the spinal kit with antiseptic solution, which is potentially neurotoxic.

   c. Check the stylet for correct fit within the needle.

   d. Raise a skin wheal with 1% lidocaine and a 25-gauge needle at the spinal puncture site.

   e. Approaches

   (1) Midline. Place the spinal needle (or introducer) through the skin wheal and into the interspinous ligament. The needle should be in the same plane as the spinous processes and angulated slightly cephalad toward the interlaminar space (Fig. 16-3).

   (2) Paramedian. This approach is useful in patients who cannot adequately flex their back because of pain or whose interspinous ligaments may be ossified. Place the spinal needle 1.5 cm lateral and slightly caudad (approximately 1 cm) to the center of the selected interspace. Aim the needle medially and slightly cephalad, passing lateral to the supraspinous ligament. If the lamina is contacted, redirect the needle and walk the tip off the lamina in a medial and cephalad direction.

   (3) Needle placement. Always keep the stylet in place when advancing the needle so that the needle's lumen does not become plugged with tissue. If paresthesias occur during placement, immediately withdraw the needle. Allow the paresthesia to pass and reposition the needle before proceeding again. Advance the needle until increased resistance is felt as it passes through the ligamentum flavum. As the needle is advanced beyond this ligament, a sudden loss of resistance will occur as the needle "pops" through the dura.

   (4) Remove the stylet and confirm correct placement by noting free flow of CSF into the hub of the needle. Rotate the needle in 90-degree increments to confirm good flow of CSF at each position.

   (5) Administration of anesthetic. Connect the syringe containing the predetermined dose of local anesthetic to the needle. Gently aspirate CSF into the syringe, which pro-

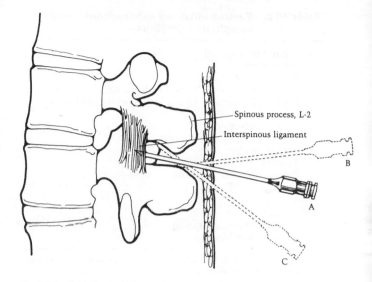

Fig. 16-3. Spinal needle insertion, lateral view. For the classic midline approach, the needle is introduced in the middle of the interspace and advanced with a slight cephalad angulation. If correctly angled (A), it will enter the interspinous ligament, ligamentum flavum, and epidural space. If bone is contacted, it may be the inferior spinous process (B), and cephalad redirection will identify the correct path. If angling cephalad causes contact with bone again at a shallower depth (C), it is probably the superior spinous process. If bone is encountered at the same depth after several attempts at redirection (not shown), the needle is most likely on the lamina lateral to the interspace, and the position of the true midline should be reassessed. (From Mulroy MF. *Regional anesthesia: an illustrated procedural guide*, 2nd ed. Boston: Little, Brown and Company, 1996:79, with permission.)

duces birefringence within dextrose-containing solutions and confirms free flow. Inject the drug slowly. Repeat aspiration of CSF at the end of the injection confirms that the needle point is still within the subarachnoid space. Remove the needle and place the patient gently into the desired position.

f. Closely monitor (every 60 to 90 seconds) blood pressure, pulse, and respiratory function for 10 to 15 minutes. Determine the ascending anesthetic level by noting the response to gentle pinprick or a cold alcohol swab. Stabilization of the local anesthetic level takes approximately 20 minutes.

g. Continuous spinal anesthesia allows small aliquots of drug to be injected repeatedly to produce the desired level of sensory blockade. With this technique, a high or rapid sympathetic block can be avoided (of particular concern in the compromised patient). The duration of anesthesia can be extended for longer surgical procedures by repeated administration of drug. Use a 17-gauge epidural needle and 20-gauge catheter for this technique. Place the epidural needle as de-

Table 16-2.   Factors affecting subarachnoid local anesthetic injections

Determinants of spread
  Major factors
    Baricity of solution
    Position of patients (except isobaric solution)
    Dose and volume of drug injected (except isobaric)
  Minor factors
    Level of injection
    Speed of injection/barbotage
    Size of needle
    Physical status of patients
    Intraabdominal pressure
Determinants of duration
  Drug used
  Dose injected
  Presence of vasoconstrictors
  Total spread of blockade

Adapted from Wildsmith JAW, Rocco AG. Current concepts in spinal anesthesia. *Reg Anesth* 1985;10:119, with permission.

scribed above, confirm free flow of CSF, and thread the catheter through the needle, advancing it 2 to 4 cm beyond the tip of the needle. Stimulation of nerve roots by the catheter tip is very painful, so avoid advancing the catheter further than 4 cm. **Neurotoxicity** from hyperbaric glucose-containing local anesthetic solutions injected through microbore spinal catheters (26 to 32 gauge) has been reported and may be due to the development of very high concentrations of local anesthetic around the nerves of the cauda equina. The use of such small-bore catheters is no longer recommended.

D. **Determinants of level of spinal blockade (Table 16-2)**
  1. **Drug dose**. The anesthetic level varies directly with the dose of agent used.
  2. **Drug volume**. The greater the volume of the injected drug, the further the drug will spread within the CSF. This is especially applicable to hyperbaric solutions.
  3. **Turbulence of CSF**. Turbulence created within the CSF during or after injection will increase spread of the drug and the level obtained. Turbulence is created by rapid injection, barbotage (the repeated aspiration and reinjection of small amounts of CSF mixed with drug), coughing, and excessive patient movement.
  4. **Baricity of local anesthetic solution**. Local anesthetic solutions can be described as hyperbaric, hypobaric, or isobaric in relation to the specific gravity of CSF.
      a. **Hyperbaric solutions** are typically prepared by mixing the drug with dextrose. They flow by gravity to the most dependent parts of the CSF column (Table 16-3).
      b. **Hypobaric solutions** are prepared by mixing the drug with

Table 16-3.   Drugs and dosages for hyperbaric spinal anesthesia

| Drug | Level (mg)[a] | | | Duration (min) |
	T-10	T-8	T-6	
Tetracaine	10	12	14	90–120
Bupivacaine	7.5	9.0	10.5	90–120
Lidocaine	50	60	70	30–90

[a]Doses are based on a 66-inch patient. An additional 2 mg of tetracaine, 10 mg of lidocaine, or 1.5 mg of bupivacaine should be added or subtracted for each 6 inches in height above or below 66 inches.

sterile water. They slowly rise to the highest part of the CSF column.

c.   **Isobaric solutions** may have the advantage of a predictable spread through the CSF that is less dependent on patient position. Increasing the dose of an isobaric anesthetic has more of an effect on the duration of anesthesia than on the dermatomal spread. Patient positioning can be altered to limit or increase the spread of these mixtures.

5.   **Increased intraabdominal pressure**. Pregnancy, obesity, ascites, and abdominal tumors increase pressure within the inferior vena cava. This increases blood volume within the epidural venous plexus, concomitantly reducing the volume of CSF within the vertebral column, which permits greater spread of injected local anesthetic. In obese patients, this effect is potentiated by increased fat within the epidural space.

6.   **Spinal curvatures**. Lumbar lordosis and thoracic kyphosis influence the spread of hyperbaric solutions. Drug injected above the L-3 level while the patient is in the lateral position will spread cephalad and will be limited by the thoracic curvature at T-4 (Fig. 16-4).

E.   **Determinants of duration of spinal blockade**

1.   **Drugs and dose**. The characteristic duration is specific for each drug (see Chapter 15). The addition of opioids to the injected solution can modify the character of the block (see Chapter 37, section III.E.7).

2.   **Vasoconstrictors**. The addition of epinephrine, 0.2 mg (0.2 mL of 1:1,000), or phenylephrine, 2 to 5 mg, can prolong the duration of spinal anesthesia by up to 50%.

F.   **Complications**

1.   **Hypotension** is a common complication of spinal anesthesia and may be profound in the hypovolemic patient. IV administration of 500 to 1,000 mL of Ringer lactate solution before performing the block decreases the incidence of hypotension. Patients with decreased cardiac function require care in administering large volumes of IV fluid, because translocation of fluid from the peripheral to central circulation during recession of the block and return of systemic vascular tone could produce volume overload and pulmonary edema. Oxygen should be avail-

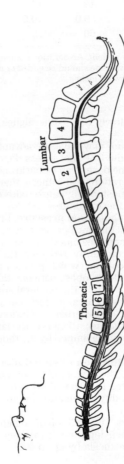

Fig. 16-4.   Spinal column curvatures that influence the spread of anesthetic solutions.

able. Ephedrine (5 to 10 mg IV bolus) or a phenylephrine infusion may be necessary.

2. Bradycardia can result from blockade of cardiac sympathetic fibers and may be treated with atropine, 0.4 to 0.8 mg IV, or, if severe and accompanied by hypotension, ephedrine or epinephrine.

3. Paresthesias. During placement of the spinal needle or injection of anesthetic, direct trauma to a spinal nerve or intraneural injection may occur.

4. Bloody tap. Puncture of an epidural vein during needle insertion may result in either blood or a mixture of blood and CSF emerging from the spinal needle. If the fluid does not rapidly clear, the needle should be withdrawn and reinserted.

5. Dyspnea is a common complaint with high spinal levels. It is caused by proprioceptive blockade of afferent fibers from abdominal and chest wall muscles. Reassurance of the patient may be all that is required, although adequate ventilation must be ensured.

6. Apnea can be caused by reduced medullary blood flow accompanying severe hypotension or from direct blockade of C-3 to C-5 ("total spinal"), inhibiting phrenic nerve output. Immediate ventilatory support is required.

7. Nausea and vomiting are usually caused by hypotension or unopposed vagal stimulation. Treatment involves restoration of blood pressure, administration of oxygen, and IV atropine. Care should be taken in giving the antiemetic droperidol, because it may augment the hypotension. Fentanyl, 10 μg, added to the spinal injectate may decrease nausea precipitated by peritoneal stimulation.

8. Postdural puncture headache characteristically is worsened by the patient sitting upright and improved by lying down. It is a severe occipital headache that radiates to the posterior cervical region. With increasing severity, the pain becomes circumferential and may be accompanied by tinnitus, blurred vision, and diplopia. Onset is usually 24 to 48 hours postoperatively. It is caused by a continued leak of CSF through the hole in the dura mater, which reduces CSF pressure and produces traction on meningeal vessels and nerves. The overall incidence of postdural puncture headache is approximately 1% to 5% but is increased in younger patients, with the use of larger gauge or cutting tip needles, and after multiple attempts. Initial treatment is conservative and includes bed rest, IV fluids, and analgesics. The use of caffeine (300 mg orally) or caffeine benzoate (500 mg in 500 mL of normal saline IV over 2 hours) has also been advocated. If the headache is severe or lasts longer than 24 hours, an **epidural blood patch** can be performed by sterilely withdrawing 10 to 15 mL of the patient's blood from an antecubital vein and injecting it into the epidural space. The success rate of the first treatment varies from 65% to 95%. Meningitis and arachnoiditis are rare but must be considered in the differential diagnosis of a postdural puncture headache.

9. Backache. Mild localized tenderness at the puncture site is common and usually self-limited. The incidence of generalized backache after spinal anesthesia is no different from that after general anesthesia. The suggested mechanism is flattening of the normal lumbar lordosis during muscle relaxation, with resultant stretching of joint capsules, ligaments, and muscles. Treatment is with analgesics and reassurance.

10.   Urinary retention. The mechanism of urinary retention is described in section IV.B.4.a. Urinary retention may outlast the sensory and motor blockade. This effect may be problematic, particularly if the patient has preexisting urinary obstructive symptoms or if large volumes of IV fluids have been administered during surgery.

11.   Neurologic impairment after spinal anesthesia is exceptionally rare, although it is often foremost in the patient's mind. Neurologic damage may be direct (e.g., needle trauma), toxic (e.g., introduction of chemicals, viruses, or bacteria), or ischemic (e.g., vascular compromise from compression by an extradural hematoma). Direct nerve trauma from surgical procedures or improper positioning of the patient may also occur. Neurologic impairment should be immediately evaluated by a neurologist because prompt diagnosis and treatment are essential to improving outcome. **Transient radicular irritation** or neurologic syndrome is a spontaneous severe radicular pain that is evident after resolution of the anesthetic and lasts 2 to 7 days after a spinal anesthetic. The incidence varies from 0% to 37% and seems to be higher with lidocaine administration (hyperbaric 5% or isobaric 2%) but has also been observed with other local anesthetics, including bupivacaine. The incidence is also greater in ambulatory surgical patients and with the lithotomy position.

12.   Infection after spinal anesthesia is exceedingly rare. Nevertheless, meningitis, arachnoiditis, and epidural abscess can occur. Possible etiologies include chemical contamination and viral or bacterial infection. Early consultation with a neurologist is essential for prompt diagnosis and treatment.

V.   Epidural anesthesia is achieved by introduction of anesthetics into the epidural space.

A.   Anatomy. The epidural space extends from the base of the skull to the sacrococcygeal membrane. Posteriorly, it is bounded by the ligamentum flavum, the anterior surfaces of the laminae, and the articular processes. Anteriorly, it is bounded by the posterior longitudinal ligament covering the vertebral bodies and intervertebral disks. Laterally, it is bounded by intervertebral foramina and the pedicles. It has direct communications with the paravertebral space. It contains fat and lymphatic tissue, as well as epidural veins, which are most prominent in the lateral part of the space. The veins have no valves and directly communicate with the intracranial veins. The veins also communicate with the thoracic and abdominal veins through the intervertebral foramina and with the pelvic veins through the sacral venous plexus. The space is widest in the midline and tapers off laterally. In the lumbar region, it is 5 to 6 mm wide in the midline; in the midthoracic region the space is 3 to 5 mm wide.

B.   Physiology

1.   Neural blockade. Local anesthetic placed in the epidural space acts directly on the spinal nerve roots located in the lateral part of the space. These nerve roots are covered by the dural sheath, and local anesthetic gains access to the CSF by uptake through the dura. The onset of the block is slower than with spinal anesthesia, and the intensity of the sensory and motor block is less. Anesthesia develops in a segmental manner, and selective blockade can be achieved.

2. Cardiovascular. Hypotension from sympathetic blockade is similar to that described for spinal anesthesia (see section IV.B.2). In addition, the large doses of local anesthetic used may be absorbed into the systemic circulation and may depress the myocardium. Epinephrine used with the local anesthetics may also be absorbed, producing systemic effects such as tachycardia and hypertension.

3. Other physiologic changes seen are similar to those described for spinal anesthesia (see section IV.B).

4. Epidural anesthesia has been reported to reduce venous thrombosis and subsequent pulmonary embolism after orthopedic surgery. This is probably because of increased lower limb perfusion. Decreased coagulability, decreased platelet aggregation, and improved fibrinolytic function during epidural anesthesia also has been reported.

C. Technique

1. Epidural needles. Most commonly, the 17-gauge **Tuohy** or **Weiss** needle is used for identification of the epidural space. These needles are styletted, have a blunt leading edge with a lateral opening, and have a thin wall to allow passage of a 20-gauge catheter.

2. Patient position. Patients can be positioned for epidural anesthesia in either the sitting or lateral positions. The same considerations apply as for spinal anesthesia (see section IV.C.2).

3. Approaches. Whether from a midline or paramedian approach, the needle should enter the epidural space in the midline, because the space is widest here and there is a decreased risk of puncturing epidural veins, spinal arteries, or spinal nerve roots, all of which lie predominantly in the lateral part of the epidural space. Palpation of landmarks, skin preparation, and draping are as described for spinal anesthesia (see section IV.C.3) (Fig. 16-5).

    a. Lumbar. Use a long 25-gauge needle for superficial and deep infiltration of local anesthetic into the supraspinous and interspinous ligaments. This needle also assists in defining the direction in which the epidural needle should be inserted. A skin puncture can be made with a 15-gauge needle to facilitate epidural needle passage. Advance the epidural needle through the supraspinous and interspinous ligaments in a slightly cephalad direction, until it comes to lie within the "rubbery" ligamentum flavum.

    (1) Loss of resistance techniques. Remove the stylet and attach a glass or plastic loss-of-resistance syringe containing approximately 3 mL of air or saline to the needle hub. Apply constant pressure to the plunger of the syringe while slowly advancing the needle. When the bevel enters the epidural space, there is a marked "loss of resistance" to plunger displacement. Alternatively, an "intermittent" technique can be used, where the change in resistance is tested repeatedly in between small careful advances of the epidural needle.

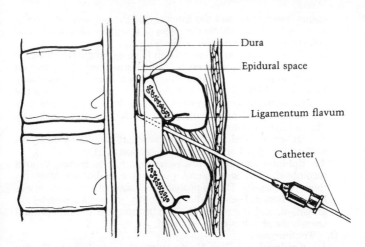

Fig. 16-5. Insertion of an epidural catheter. The needle is secured by resting one hand on the back and grasping the hub firmly (not shown) while the other hand inserts the catheter into the hub and gently advances it beyond the tip of the needle. The bevel is usually directed cephalad, which produces the most reliable insertion; caudad orientation may allow the catheter to exit one of the intervertebral foramina. Ideally, the catheter is advanced 3 to 4 cm beyond the needle tip; further placement increases the potential for lateral misdirection or foraminal exit. (From Mulroy MF. *Regional anesthesia: an illustrated procedural guide*. Boston: Little, Brown and Company, 1996:109, with permission.)

(2) The **hanging drop technique** relies on the principle that a drop of fluid placed on the hub of the epidural needle (once the ligamentum flavum has been entered) will retract into the needle as the tip of the needle is advanced into the epidural space. This negative pressure is provided by "tenting" of the dura by the needle tip but may be altered by transmitted changes in intraabdominal and intrathoracic pressure (e.g., pregnancy, obesity). Drop retraction only occurs about 80% of the time, so if a change in compliance is felt while advancing through the ligamentum flavum, it should be checked by "loss of resistance."

b. **Thoracic epidural anesthesia** provides upper abdominal and thoracic anesthesia with a smaller dose of local anesthetic. Postoperative analgesia can be produced without lower extremity blockade. Although the technique is the same as for lumbar placement, the thoracic vertebral spinous processes are much more sharply angulated downward such that the tip of the superior spinous process overlies the lamina of the vertebra below, and the epidural needle should be directed in a more cephalad direction. In addition, there is a risk of producing trauma to the underlying spinal cord if dural puncture occurs. Occasionally, a paramedian approach is necessary.

c. **Technique for catheter placement**. An epidural catheter permits repeated injections of local anesthetic for prolonged procedures and provides a route for postoperative analgesia.

(1)   Thread a 20-gauge radiopaque catheter with 1-cm graduations through the epidural needle. If the catheter contains a wire stylet, it should first be withdrawn 1 to 2 cm to decrease the incidence of paresthesia and dural or venous puncture. Polyvinyl chloride catheters are relatively stiff and resist kinking but can be associated with dural and venous puncture. Teflon catheters are very soft and flexible but may be more likely to kink and occlude. Newer catheters of nylon, polyamide, or polyvinyl offer compromises between flexibility and rigidity. When multipore catheters are used, the distance from the catheter tip to the most proximal lateral hole should be noted to ensure that all injected medication reaches the epidural space.

(2)   Advance the catheter 3 to 5 cm beyond the needle tip and into the epidural space. The patient may experience an abrupt paresthesia, which is usually transient. If it is sustained, the catheter must be repositioned. If the catheter must be withdrawn, the catheter and needle should be removed together to avoid shearing the catheter tip.

(3)   Measure the distance from the surface of the patient's back to a mark on the catheter.

(4)   Carefully withdraw the needle over the catheter and remeasure the distance from the patient's back to the mark on the catheter. If the catheter was advanced, withdraw it, leaving 4 to 5 cm within the epidural space.

d.   Administer a **test dose** of local anesthetic agent through the needle if a single-dose technique is used or through the catheter for continuous techniques. A test dose usually consists of 3 mL 2% lidocaine with 1:200,000 epinephrine. This should have little effect in the epidural space. If the solution has been injected into the CSF, a spinal block will occur rapidly. If the solution has been injected into an epidural vein, a 20% to 30% increase in heart rate may be seen. Other symptoms of an intravascular injection include perioral numbness, a metallic taste, tinnitus, and palpitations.

e.   Injection of anesthetic. Administer the anesthetic solution in 3- to 5-mL increments every 3 to 5 minutes until the total dose has been given. Aspirate the catheter or needle, checking for the appearance of blood or CSF, before each injection.

D.   Determinants of the level of epidural blockade

1.   Volume of local anesthetic. A maximum dose of 1.6 mL of local anesthetic per segment has been suggested for the induction of epidural blockade. This maximum can be exceeded if dilute mixtures of medications are used, as for postoperative or labor analgesia.

2.   Age. The volume of local anesthetic should be reduced by approximately 50% in the elderly and neonates. Stenosis of intervertebral foramina in the elderly reduces the lateral paravertebral spread of injected drug, allowing for more cephalad spread.

3.   Pregnancy. A 30% reduction in dose is expected in pregnant women. Hormonal effects during pregnancy render nerves more sensitive to the effects of local anesthetic, and inferior vena cava compression increases blood volume within the epidural venous plexus, reducing the potential volume of the epidural space.

4. Speed of injection. Rapid injection of drug into the epidural space may produce a less reliable block than a slow steady injection at approximately 0.5 mL/sec. Very rapid injection of large volumes of drug has the potentially hazardous effect of increasing pressure within the epidural space. Such a rise in pressure can produce headache, increased intracranial pressure, and possibly spinal cord ischemia by decreasing spinal cord blood flow.

5. Position. The position of the patient has a slight effect on the level of epidural blockade. Patients sitting upright have greater caudad spread of blockade; patients in the lateral position have a higher level of block on the dependent side.

6. Spread of epidural blockade. Onset of blockade occurs first and is most dense at the level of injection. Spread of the block usually occurs faster in a cephalad than a caudad direction. This is likely because of the relative difference in size between the large lower lumbar and sacral nerve roots compared with the smaller thoracic nerve roots. There is often anesthetic sparing of the L5-S1 nerve roots because of their large size.

E. Determinants of onset and duration of epidural blockade

  1. Selection of drug (see Chapter 15).

  2. Addition of epinephrine. Epinephrine, added in a concentration of 1:200,000, decreases the systemic uptake and plasma levels of local anesthetic and prolongs its duration of action (see Chapter 15).

3. Addition of opioid. For example, the addition of fentanyl, 50 to 100 µg, to the local anesthetic solution speeds the onset, increases the level, prolongs the duration, and improves the quality of the block. Fentanyl is thought to produce this effect by having a selective action at the substantia gelatinosa of the dorsal horn of the spinal cord to modulate pain transmission. This action appears to be synergistic with the actions of the local anesthetic drug.

4. pH adjustment of solution. The addition of sodium bicarbonate to the local anesthetic solution in a ratio of 1 mL of 8.4% sodium bicarbonate to each 10 mL of lidocaine (0.1 mL for each 10 mL of bupivacaine) decreases the onset time for blockade. It is thought that this effect is due to an increased amount of local anesthetic base, which increases the rate that drug crosses axonal membranes.

F. Complications

1. Unintentional dural puncture occurs in about 1% of epidural injections. If this occurs, several options are available. A conversion to spinal anesthesia can be made by injection of an appropriate amount of anesthetic into the CSF. Continuous spinal anesthesia can be performed by insertion of an epidural catheter into the subarachnoid space through the needle. If epidural anesthesia is required (e.g., for postoperative analgesia), the catheter can be repositioned at a different interspace than the one punctured so that the tip of the epidural catheter lies well away from the site of dural puncture. The possibility of spinal anesthesia occurring with injection of the epidural catheter should be considered.

2. **Catheter complications**

a. **Inability to thread the epidural catheter** is relatively common. This problem can occur if the epidural needle is inserted into the lateral part of the epidural space rather than the midline or the bevel of the needle is at too acute an angle to the epidural space for the catheter to emerge. It can also occur if the bevel of the needle is only partially through the ligamentum flavum when loss of resistance is found. In the latter case, slight (1 mm) advancement of the needle into the epidural space may facilitate catheter insertion.

b. **The catheter can be inserted into an epidural vein.** Blood can be aspirated from the catheter and tachycardia may be noted with the test dose. The catheter should be gently withdrawn until blood is no longer be aspirated, flushed with saline, and then retested. Withdrawal by more than 1 to 2 cm should prompt removal and reinsertion.

c. **Catheters can break off or become knotted** within the epidural space. In the absence of infection, a retained catheter is no more reactive than a surgical suture. The patient should be informed of the problem and reassured. The complications of surgical exploration and removal of the catheter are greater than conservative management.

d. **Cannulation of the subdural space.** The subdural space is a potential space between the dural and arachnoid membranes and may be entered with a needle or with a catheter. CSF is not aspirated but the effects of the local anesthetic are quite different from usual epidural anesthesia and often quite variable. In the absence of myelography, it is a diagnosis of exclusion. It can result in dissociation of blocked modalities (e.g., full sensory anesthesia without motor block or motor block with minimal sensory block). It should be suspected whenever an epidural dose produces a more extensive spread than expected.

3. **Unintentional subarachnoid injection.** The injection of a large volume of local anesthetic into the subarachnoid space can produce total spinal anesthesia. Treatment is similar to that described for spinal complications (see section IV.F).

4. **Intravascular injection of local anesthetic** into an epidural vein causes central nervous system and cardiovascular toxicity and may result in convulsions and cardiopulmonary arrest. Resistant ventricular fibrillation with IV bupivacaine 0.75% has been described (see Chapters 15 and 36).

5. **Local anesthetic overdose.** Systemic local anesthetic toxicity is possible because of the relatively large amounts of drug used.

6. **Direct spinal cord injury** is more likely if the epidural injection is above L-2. The onset of a unilateral paresthesia during needle insertion suggests lateral entry into the epidural space. Further injection or insertion of a catheter at this point may produce trauma to a nerve root. Small feeder arteries to the anterior spinal artery also run in this area as they pass through the intervertebral foramen. Trauma to these arteries

may result in anterior spinal cord ischemia or an epidural hematoma.

7. Bloody tap. Perforation of an epidural vein by the needle will result in blood return through the needle. The needle should be removed and repositioned. It is preferable to reposition the needle at a different interspace, because the presence of blood in the original space will make it difficult to determine correct needle placement.

8. Postdural puncture headache. If the dura is punctured with a 17-gauge epidural needle, there is a greater than 75% chance of a young patient developing a postdural puncture headache. Management is the same as that described under spinal anesthesia (see section IV.F.8).

9. Epidural abscess is an extremely rare complication of epidural anesthesia. The source of infection usually is from hematogenous spread to the epidural space from an infection in another area. Infection can also arise from contamination during insertion, contamination of an indwelling catheter used for postoperative pain relief, or a cutaneous infection at the insertion site. The patient presents with fever, severe back pain, and localized back tenderness. Progression to nerve root pain and paralysis occurs. Initial laboratory investigations reveal a leukocytosis and a lumbar puncture suggestive of a parameningeal infection. Definitive diagnosis is by magnetic resonance imaging (MRI). Treatment includes antibiotics and sometimes urgent decompression laminectomy. Rapid diagnosis and treatment is associated with good neurologic recovery.

10. Epidural hematoma is an extremely rare complication of epidural anesthesia. Trauma to epidural veins in the presence of a coagulopathy may result in a large epidural hematoma. The patient presents with severe back pain and persistent neurologic deficit after epidural anesthesia. Diagnosis is confirmed by MRI. Decompression laminectomy is required to preserve neurologic function.

VI. Combined spinal–epidural anesthesia

A. Spinal anesthesia offers the benefits of rapid onset. Placement of an epidural catheter at the same time offers the advantage of prolonged anesthesia and analgesia for procedures or postoperative pain management. This technique often is used in the labor and delivery setting (see Chapter 29).

B. Technique. Prepare the patient as for epidural placement (see section V.C). After placing the epidural needle in the epidural space, advance a long spinal needle (Sprotte 24-gauge × 120 mm or Whitacre 25 gauge) through the epidural needle until the characteristic pop of dural penetration occurs. At this point, withdraw the stylette from the spinal needle and confirm free flow of CSF. Inject medication into the subarachnoid space and withdraw the spinal needle. Thread an epidural catheter is through the epidural needle in the standard fashion.

VII. Caudal anesthesia

A. Anatomy. The caudal space is an extension of the epidural space. The sacral hiatus is formed by the failure of the laminae of S-5 to fuse. The hiatus is bound laterally by the sacral cornua, which are the inferior articulating processes of S-5. The **sacrococcygeal membrane** is a thin layer of fibrous tissue that covers the sacral hiatus. The caudal canal contains the sacral nerves, the sacral venous plexus, the filum terminale, and the dural sac, which usually ends at the lower border of S-2. In neonates the dural sac may extend to S-4.

B. Physiology. The physiology of caudal anesthesia is similar to that described for epidural anesthesia (see section V.B). It is indicated for surgical and obstetric procedures of the perineal and sacral areas.

C. Technique

1. Caudal epidural anesthesia is performed with the patient in the lateral, prone, or jackknife position.

2. Palpate the sacral cornua. If they are difficult to palpate directly, the location of the sacral hiatus can be estimated by measuring 5 cm from the tip of the coccyx in the midline.

3. Skin preparation and draping are as described for spinal anesthesia (see section IV.C.3).

4. Raise a skin wheal with 1% lidocaine between the sacral cornua.

5. Insert a 22-gauge spinal needle at an angle of 70 to 80 degrees to the skin. Advance the needle is advanced through the sacrococcygeal membrane, which is identified by a characteristic pop. Avoid attempting to thread the needle up the caudal canal, because this increases the likelihood of puncturing an epidural vein (Fig. 16-6).

6. Withdraw the stylet and inspect the hub of the needle for passive CSF or blood flow. The needle can be aspirated as a further check. Reposition the needle if either blood or CSF appears.

7. Administer a test dose of 3 mL of local anesthetic solution with epinephrine (1:200,000), similar to that for lumbar epidural anesthesia (see section V.C.3.d), observing the patient for signs of subarachnoid or IV injection. Because the caudal canal has a rich epidural venous plexus, IV injections are seen frequently and can occur even though blood cannot be aspirated from the needle.

8. A caudal catheter can be placed in a manner analogous to that for lumbar epidural anesthesia using a 17-gauge Tuohy needle (see section V.C.3.a). The catheter can be used for postoperative analgesia.

9. The level, onset, and duration for caudal anesthesia follow the same principles outlined for epidural anesthesia (see sections V.D and V.E). The extent of caudal block is less predictable than other epidural techniques because of the variability in content and volume of the caudal canal and the amount of local anesthetic solution that leaks out the sacral foramina. To obtain sacral anesthesia, a volume of 12 to 15 mL should be sufficient.

D. Complications. The complications of caudal anesthesia are similar to those of epidural anesthesia (see section V.F).

VIII. Anticoagulation and neuraxial blockade

Neuraxial blockade should be performed cautiously in the presence of prophylactic anticoagulation because of the increased risk of epidural hematoma formation.

A. Oral anticoagulants. In patients receiving low dose oral anticoagulants (warfarin), regional techniques may be performed if the thromboprophylaxis was initiated less than 24 hours previ-

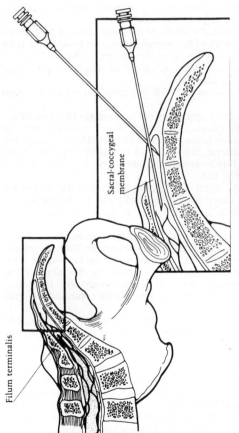

Fig. 16-6. Sacral anatomy, lateral view. A needle directed through the sacral-coccygeal membrane at a 45-degree angle will usually "pop" through the ligament and contact the anterior bone of the sacral canal. The needle needs to be rotated so that the bevel does not scrape the periosteum of this layer, and the angle of advancement changed to allow passage directly 2 to 3 cm up the canal without contacting the bone again. This space is generously endowed with blood vessels, and the terminal point of the dural sac extends a variable distance in the sacral canal but usually lies at the S-2 level. (From Mulroy MF. *Regional anesthesia: an illustrated procedural guide.* Boston: Little, Brown and Company, 1996:124, with permission.)

ously. Epidural catheters should be removed within 36 hours after starting warfarin. The prothrombin time and the international normalized ratio (INR) should be monitored daily and checked before removal of a catheter. An INR greater than 3 should be an indication to withhold or reduce the dose of warfarin if there is an indwelling neuraxial catheter. Neurologic testing and sensory and motor function should be checked routinely, and the analgesic solution should be tailored to minimize sensory and motor blockade.

B.   Unfractionated heparin. Subcutaneous (mini-dose) heparin prophylaxis is not necessarily a contraindication for the use of neuraxial techniques. Caution should be used in debilitated patients, in whom the action of the drug may be prolonged and in whom neurologic monitoring may be difficult. IV heparin should be stopped 6 hours before the initiation of neuraxial blockade and administration of further heparin should be delayed for at least 1 hour after placement. When patients with an indwelling catheter are receiving heparin anticoagulation, IV heparin should be stopped 2 to 4 hours before removal of the catheter and should not be restarted until 1 hour after removal.

C.   Low molecular weight heparin (LMWH). Patients receiving LMWH for thromboembolism prophylaxis have altered coagulation parameters. Spinal or epidural needle placement should occur at least 12 hours after the last dose. Patients receiving higher doses of LMWH (enoxaparin 1 mg/kg twice daily) will require longer delays (24 hours). In patients requiring continuing LMWH administration, spinal or epidural catheters should be removed before administration of LMWH. The subsequent administration of LMWH should be delayed for 2 hours after catheter removal.

D.   Antiplatelet drugs. Patients receiving aspirin or nonsteroidal anti-inflammatory drugs do not appear to be at higher risk for epidural hematoma formation. These drugs could contribute to an increased bleeding risk, however, if they are used concurrently with other anticoagulants. The risk of bleeding complications with medications affecting platelet glycoprotein IIb/IIIa receptors (e.g., ticlopidine and clopidogrel) is unknown. Neuraxial techniques should be undertaken with caution until additional data are available.

E.   Fibrinolytic and thrombolytic agents. Patients receiving heparin with fibrinolytic and thrombolytic drugs are at high risk of bleeding complications with neuraxial techniques. Patients receiving fibrinolytic and thrombolytics should be cautioned against receiving neuraxial techniques, but the length of time that neuraxial puncture should be avoided (or when indwelling catheters can be removed safely) after discontinuing these drugs is unclear.

SUGGESTED READING

American Society of Regional Anesthesia and Pain Medicine. Recommendations for neuraxial anesthesia and anticoagulation. www.asra.com/items_of_interest/consensus_statements (accessed October 22, 2001).

Caplan RA, Ward RJ, Posner K, et al. Unexpected cardiac arrest during spinal anesthesia: a closed claims analysis of predisposing factors. *Anesthesiology* 1988;68:5–11.

Cousins MJ, Bridenbaugh PO. *Neural blockade in clinical anesthesia and management of pain*. Philadelphia: Lippincott-Raven, 1998.

Fox J. Spinal and epidural anesthesia and anticoagulation. *Int Anesthesiol Clin* 2001;39:51–61

Horlocker TT, Wedel DJ, Offord KP. Does preoperative antiplatelet therapy increase the risk of hemorrhagic complications associated with regional anesthesia? *Anesth Analg* 1990;70:631–634.

Kane RE. Neurologic deficits following epidural or spinal anesthesia. *Anesth Analg* 1981;60:150–161.

Kehlet H. Surgical stress: the role of pain and analgesia. *Br J Anaesth* 1989;63:189–195.

Lambert DH. Complications of spinal anesthesia. *Int Anesthesiol Clin* 1989;27:51–55.

Mulroy MF. *Regional anesthesia: an illustrated procedural guide*, 2nd ed. Philadelphia: Lippincott Williams and Wilkins, 1996.

Pollock JE, Neal JM, Stephenson CA, et al. Prospective study of the incidence of transient radicular irritation in patients undergoing spinal anesthesia. *Anesthesiology* 1996;84:1361–1367.

Schneider M, Ettlin T, Kaufmann M, et al. Transient neurologic toxicity after hyperbaric subarachnoid anesthesia with 5% lidocaine. *Anesth Analg* 1993;76:1154–1157.

Scott NB, Kehlet H. Regional anaesthesia and surgical morbidity. *Br J Surg* 1988;75:299–304.

Vandermeulen EP, Van Aken H, Vermylen J. Anticoagulants and spinal-epidural anesthesia. *Anesth Analg* 1994;79:1165–1177.

Regional Anesthesia

James B. Mayfield and Margaret Gargarian

I. General considerations

A. Peripheral nerve blockade can be an excellent alternative to general anesthesia for many surgical procedures and does not significantly disrupt autonomic function. Regional blockade provides optimal surgical conditions while providing prolonged postoperative analgesia. Patient safety, satisfaction, and quicker initial recovery are among the benefits of regional anesthesia.

B. The preoperative assessment, preparation of the patient, and degree of monitoring are the same as for central neuraxial blockade. Patients should follow fasting (nothing by mouth) guidelines whenever possible, and regional anesthesia should not be chosen just to avoid complications of a full stomach or difficult airway. Any neurologic conditions should be documented fully before performance of any block.

C. Consent for regional anesthesia should include a through description of the risks, benefits, options, and common side effects. Need for supplemental local anesthesia or general anesthesia in case of block failure should also be discussed.

D. Preoperative medication may be prescribed as long as the patient remains cooperative and alert. Usually, short-acting agents such as fentanyl and midazolam are adequate.

E. All blocks should be performed with strict sterile technique (i.e., sterile equipment, preparation of the skin with an antiseptic solution). Before inserting any block needle, a skin wheal should be raised with local anesthetic.

II. Equipment

A. Needles used for nerve blockade

1. A block needle should be of the minimum diameter possible for patient comfort. However, regional block needles often are inserted into deep tissue and therefore need a more rigid shaft. For superficial blocks, such as an axillary block, a 23-gauge needle is suitable. For most peripheral regional blocks, a 22-gauge needle is preferable.

2. Short bevel needles are associated with less nerve trauma than the standard A-bevel needles and therefore have become standard for peripheral nerve blocks. Newer needles with a Sprotte or Whitacre tip may be less traumatic.

3. Upper and lower extremity blocks are best performed with a 50- to 150-mm needle. Brachial plexus blocks usually do not require more than a 100-mm needle and can frequently be accomplished, in the case of interscalene block, with a 25- to 50-mm needle.

B. Nerve stimulators (Fig. 17-1) designed for regional anesthesia deliver a current of 0.1 to 10.0 mA at a frequency of 1 to 2 pulse/sec. **Insulated needles** provide the best results.

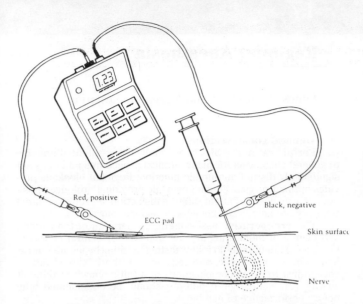

Fig. 17-1. Nerve stimulator attached to regional block needle. The negative (*black*) lead is attached to the exploring needle, whereas the positive (*red*) is connected to a reference electrocardiogram pad used as a "ground." The stimulator is set to deliver 1 to 2 mA of current to detect the nerve. The current is reduced further as the needle approaches the nerve. A current of 0.5 mA will produce motor stimulation when the needle is adjacent to the nerve. (From Mulroy MF. *Regional anesthesia: an illustrated procedural guide*, 2nd ed. Boston: Little, Brown and Company, 1996:65, with permission.)

C. Many blocks require depositing a large volume of local anesthetic in a single injection. Connecting a large-volume (20 mL) syringe to the block needle with sterile extension tubing will ensure stable needle position during aspiration and injection. For larger volumes of local anesthesia, multiple syringes can be attached with a stopcock.

D.   Continuous catheter techniques for nerve blockade are accomplished with commercially available kits.

III.   Nerve localization techniques

A.   Eliciting a paresthesia by contacting a nerve with a needle is a time-honored method of nerve localization. However, this may cause patient discomfort and possibly a higher incidence of post-anesthetic dysesthesia or neuropathy.

B.   Electrical stimulation of a mixed nerve produces a motor response without significant pain.

1. Ground the positive lead of the stimulator to the patient and attach the negative terminal of the stimulator to the needle.

2. Set the nerve stimulator to an initial current of 1 to 1.5 mA and move the needle toward the nerve until a motor response in the desired muscle group occurs. Twitches may also arise from local muscle stimulation. Regardless of its origin, if a twitch is uncomfortable the current should be reduced. The needle position and stimulator output should be adjusted to produce the maximum twitch at the lowest current (usually <0.5 mA, although many clinicians accept <0.3 mA as an end point for successful block). This suggests that the needle is close to the nerve and the local anesthetic may be injected.

3. The nerve stimulation technique may be used on patients who are unable to report paresthesias reliably. Patient discomfort and the incidence of postanesthetic neuropathies related to paresthesia may be reduced. However, performing blocks on heavily sedated patients or those under general anesthesia is contraindicated.

C. Infiltration without precise localization will block many nerves because of their consistent relationship to palpable anatomic landmarks. Blocks of the brachial plexus and sciatic nerve benefit from more precise localization to maintain a high success rate.

IV. General contraindications. Not all patients are suitable for regional anesthesia. Absolute contraindications to regional anesthesia include lack of patient consent or when nerve blockade would hinder the proposed surgery. Relative contraindications include coagulopathy, infection at the skin entry site, excessive anxiety, mental illness, anatomic distortion, and an unskilled anesthetist. Diseases such as multiple sclerosis, polio, neurologic trauma, or muscular dystrophy may be aggravated by peripheral nerve blockade.

V. Complications common to all nerve blocks

A. Complications of local anesthetics include intravascular injection (Fig. 17-2), overdose, and allergic responses. Test doses and intermittent aspiration during injection may help identify intravascular injection. Benzodiazepine premedication increases the seizure threshold and may decrease the central nervous system (CNS) toxicity of local anesthetics, as well as level of patient anxiety.

B. Nerve damage resulting from needle trauma or from painful intraneural injection is a rare complication. This pain can be confused with a paresthesia that is potentiated on injection. If the pain is severe or does not subside after a few milliliters of local anesthetic, the needle should be repositioned.

C. Hematomas may result from arterial puncture but usually resolve without residual problems.

VI. Cervical plexus block for regional anesthesia of the neck

A. Anatomy. The cervical plexus lies in the paravertebral region of the upper four cervical vertebrae (Fig. 17-3). It is formed from the ventral rami of the C-1 to C-4 spinal nerve roots. It is deep to the sternocleidomastoid muscle and anterior to the middle scalene muscle, in continuity with the nerve roots forming the brachial plexus (see section VII.A). The plexus has superficial and deep branches. The **superficial branches** pierce the cervical fascia anteriorly, just posterior to the sternocleidomastoid, and supply the skin of the back of the head, side of the neck, and anterior and lateral shoulder. The **deep branches** supply the muscles and deep structures of the neck and form the phrenic nerve.

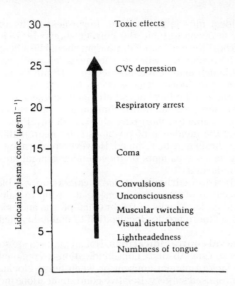

Fig. 17-2. **Progressive continuum of symptoms of lidocaine local anesthetic toxicity. These symptoms are seen in roughly the same progression and proportion with the other local anesthetics, except that cardiovascular system toxicity may be seen with of the more potent amino amides at blood levels closer to the convulsion threshold. (From Barash PG, Cullen BF, Stoelting RK, eds. *Clinical anesthesia*. Philadelphia: Lippincott, 1988:389, with permission.)**

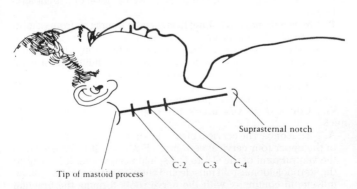

Fig. 17-3. **Superficial landmarks for cervical plexus block. A line is drawn from the mastoid process to the prominent tubercle of the sixth cervical vertebra. The transverse processes of the second, third, and fourth cervical vertebrae lie 0.5 cm posterior to this line and at 1.5 cm intervals below the mastoid. (From Mulroy MF. *Regional anesthesia: an illustrated procedural guide*, 2nd ed. Boston: Little, Brown and Company, 1996:235, with permission.)**

B. Indications. Superficial cervical plexus block produces only cutaneous anesthesia and is useful for superficial procedures on the neck and shoulder. **Deep cervical plexus block** is a paravertebral block of the C-1 to C-4 nerve roots that form the plexus, anesthetizing both the deep and superficial branches. Common indications for cervical plexus block are

1. Cervical lymph node biopsy/excision.
2. Carotid endarterectomy.
3. Thyroid operations.
4. Tracheostomy (when combined with topical airway anesthesia).

C. Techniques

1. **For a superficial block**, inject 10 mL of local anesthetic subcutaneously along the posterior border of the sternocleidomastoid.

2. **For a deep block**, position the patient supine with the neck slightly extended and the head turned toward the opposite side. Draw a line connecting the tip of the mastoid process and **Chassaignac tubercle** (the most prominent of the cervical transverse processes, located at C-6, the level of the cricoid cartilage). Draw a second line 1 cm posterior to the first line. The C-2 transverse process can be palpated 1 to 2 cm caudad to the mastoid process, with the C-3 and C-4 processes lying at 1.5-cm intervals along the second line. At each level, insert a 22-gauge 5-cm needle perpendicular to the skin with caudal angulation. Advance the needle 1.5 to 3.0 cm until it contacts the transverse process. After careful aspiration for cerebrospinal fluid or blood, inject 10 mL of local anesthetic solution at each transverse process.

D. Complications are possible with deep cervical plexus block because of the close proximity of the needle to neural and vascular structures.

1. **Phrenic nerve block** is the most common complication. This block should be used cautiously in patients with diminished pulmonary reserve. Bilateral deep cervical plexus block will produce bilateral phrenic and recurrent laryngeal nerve blockade and therefore should be avoided.

2. **Subarachnoid injection** resulting in total spinal anesthesia.

3. **Epidural injection** with resultant bilateral cervical epidural anesthesia.

4. **Vertebral artery injection** causing CNS toxicity with very small doses of local anesthetic.

5. **Recurrent laryngeal nerve block** causing hoarseness and vocal cord dysfunction.

6. **Cervical sympathetic nerve block** producing Horner syndrome.

VII. Regional anesthesia of the upper extremity

A. Anatomy

1. Except for the skin over the shoulder and axilla, the upper extremity is innervated by the brachial plexus. The skin over the shoulder is supplied by the branches of the cervical plexus (suprascapular nerve); the skin over the medial arm is served by the intercostobrachial nerve, a branch of the T-2 spinal nerve.

2. The **brachial plexus** is formed from the anterior roots of

the spinal nerves from C5-8 and T-1, with frequent contributions from C-4 and T-2. Each **root** exits posterior to the vertebral artery and travels laterally in the trough of its cervical transverse process, where it is directed toward the first rib and fuses with the other four roots to form the three trunks of the plexus. The roots are sandwiched between the anterior and middle scalene muscles. The fasciae form a sheath that envelops the plexus. This sheath encircles the plexus, providing a closed potential space for the injection of local anesthetics.

3. The **trunks** pass over the first rib through the space between the anterior and middle scalene muscles, in association with the subclavian artery, which shares the same fascial sheath. The roots and trunks have several branches, innervating the neck, shoulder girdle, and chest wall. Stimulating these nerves as they exit the plexus proximally is not reliable for plexus localization.

4. As the trunks pass over the first rib and under the clavicle, they reorganize to form the three **cords** of the plexus. The cords descend into the axilla, where each has one major branch, in addition to several minor branches, before becoming a major

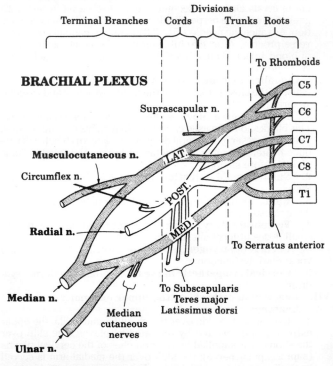

Fig. 17-4. Diagram of the brachial plexus and peripheral nerve formation.

terminal nerve of the upper extremity. Branches of the lateral and medial cords form the **median nerve**. The lateral cord gives off a branch that forms the **musculocutaneous nerve**, whereas the posterior cord becomes the **axillary and radial nerves**. The medial cord also forms the **ulnar nerve**, **medial antebrachial**, and **brachial cutaneous nerves**. In the axilla, the median nerve lies lateral to the axillary artery, the radial nerve posterior, and the ulnar nerve medial. The axillary and musculocutaneous nerves exit the sheath high up in the axilla, the musculocutaneous nerve traveling through the substance of the coracobrachialis muscle before becoming subcutaneous below the elbow. The median cutaneous nerves of the arm and forearm are minor branches of the medial cord (Fig. 17-4). The cutaneous peripheral nerve supply of the upper extremity is summarized in Fig. 17-5.

5. The **cutaneous and sclerotome distribution of the nerves** of the body is summarized in Fig. 17-6. Cutaneous innervation does not necessarily correlate with deep structures; therefore, knowledge of the sclerotomes can be very useful in predicting ultimate success of any regional technique.

6. The **major motor functions** of the five nerves are as follows:

    a. **Axillary (circumflex nerve):** shoulder abduction (deltoid contraction).

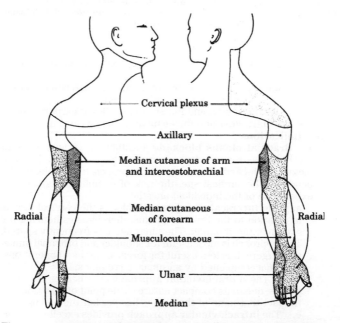

Fig. 17-5. **Cutaneous peripheral nerve supply of the upper extremity.**

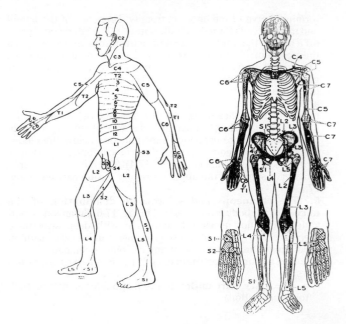

Fig. 17-6. A side view of the dermatomes (*left*) and an anterior view of the sclerotomes indicated by the different styles of shading (*right*). (From Haymaker W, Woodhall B. *Peripheral nerve injuries*. Philadelphia: WB Saunders, 1945:20, 41, with permission.)

    b. Musculocutaneous: elbow flexion (biceps contraction).
    c. Radial: elbow (triceps contraction), wrist, and finger extension (extensor carpi radialis longus).
    d. Median: wrist and finger flexion (flexor carpi radialis).
    e. Ulnar: wrist and finger flexion (flexor carpi ulnaris).
B. Indications
    1. Brachial plexus blockade anesthetizes various areas of the upper extremity, depending on which level the brachial plexus is blocked. The preferred approach to the plexus depends on the surgical site, the risk of complications, and the experience of the individual anesthetist.
    a. The **interscalene approach** blocks the cervical plexus in addition to the brachial plexus, thereby anesthetizing the skin over the shoulder. The ulnar nerve is frequently spared. This approach is most useful for shoulder and proximal humerus surgery. It is less useful for forearm and hand operations, unless accompanied by an ulnar nerve block.
    b. The **supraclavicular approach** anesthetizes the entire plexus, due to its compact nature at the point of injection and the fact that none of the nerves has yet left the plexus.
    c. The **infraclavicular approach** provides excellent coverage for surgery distal to mid-humerus.

d. The **axillary approach** is very common. However, because the musculocutaneous and medial cutaneous nerves of the arm exit the sheath more proximally, they are not blocked by this approach, making it unreliable for operations proximal to the elbow.

2. The **intercostobrachial nerve** must be blocked in addition to the plexus for procedures involving the medial arm or using a proximal humeral tourniquet.

3. **Blockade of an individual peripheral nerve** may be useful when limited anesthesia is required or a plexus block is incomplete. The musculocutaneous nerve may be blocked at the axilla or the elbow. Each of the other major terminal nerves may be blocked at either the elbow or the wrist.

C. Techniques

   1. Interscalene (Fig. 17-7)

     a. Position the patient supine with the head turned slightly away from the side to be blocked.

     b. Identify the lateral border of the sternocleidomastoid by having the patient lift his or her head off the bed. The anterior scalene muscle lies below the posterior edge of the sternocleidomastoid. By rolling your fingers posteriorly over the anterior scalene muscle, you will feel a groove between the ante-

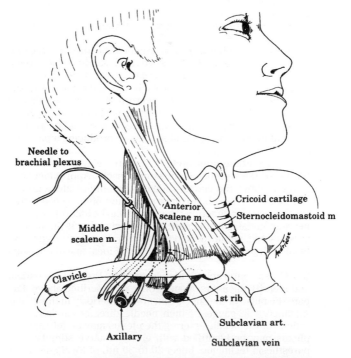

Fig. 17-7. Interscalene approach to brachial plexus block.

rior and middle scalenes. The intersection of this groove with a transverse plane at the level of the cricoid cartilage is the point at which the needle should enter the skin in a caudal direction. Because the scalenes are accessory muscles of respiration, asking the patient to take slow deep breaths while palpating for the groove may be helpful. The external jugular vein frequently crosses the groove at the level of the C-6 vertebra and may also be a useful landmark.

c. Advance a 25- to 50-mm needle into the groove in a 45-degree angle in the caudal direction. Stimulation of the plexus will result in a paresthesia or muscle twitch in either the deltoid, biceps, or pectoris major muscles. Paresthesia or twitches confined to the shoulder may result from suprascapular or cervical plexus stimulation and indicate that the needle is too posterior to the plexus. Paresthesia or twitches of the diaphragm (phrenic nerve) indicate that the needle is too anterior to the plexus. Despite being accurately placed in the groove, the needle will sometimes contact the cervical transverse process without stimulating the plexus. If this happens, withdrawing the needle and redirecting it slightly will likely elicit the correct response.

d. A volume of 30 to 40 mL of anesthetic solution should be injected.

e. If digital pressure is held distal to the injection site, cervical plexus block will accompany the brachial plexus block.

f. **Complications** are identical to those of the cervical plexus block (see section VI.D).

2. The **supraclavicular block** provides anesthesia of the brachial plexus at the level of the nerve trunks and produces reliable anesthesia of the elbow, forearm, and hand. Three approaches will be described; for each, place the patient in the supine position with his or her head turned to the contralateral side. With each of these techniques, it is generally safe to direct the needle laterally, but the medial direction should be avoided to prevent entering the pleural space and producing a pneumothorax.

a. **Parascalene approach**. Palpate the clavicle and lateral border of the sternocleidomastoid muscle. Approximately 1 to 2 cm above the clavicle, identify the interscalene groove as in section VII.C.1.b. Advance a 22-gauge 50-mm needle in an anteroposterior direction. The plexus can be identified using a nerve stimulator or the paresthesia technique. If the first rib is contacted, withdraw and redirect the needle in a stepwise fashion. Inject a total of 30 to 40 mL of local anesthetic solution.

b. **Classic supraclavicular approach**. Prepare the patient and identify the interscalene groove as described above. Palpate the pulse of the subclavian artery inferiorly in this space. Advance a 22-gauge 1.5-inch needle directly caudally. The "click" of the needle entering the plexus may be felt, and the plexus may be identified with either a nerve stimulator or paresthesia technique. Inject 20 to 30 mL of local anesthetic solution.

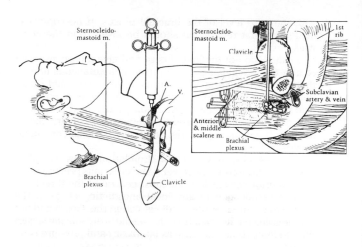

Fig. 17-8. The "plumb-bob" approach to the supraclavicular block. The needle is introduced directly posterior to the midpoint of the clavicle. If the nerves are not encountered at the first insertion, the needle is rotated in a caudad direction in very small steps and will encounter the neurovascular bundle before encountering the lung. (From Mulroy MF. *Regional anesthesia: an illustrated procedural guide*, 2nd ed. Boston: Little, Brown and Company, 1996:169, with permission.)

   c. Plumb-bob approach (Fig. 17-8). Identify the midpoint of the clavicle and advance a 22-gauge 1.5-inch needle in a caudal direction in a plane parallel to that of the head and neck until it contacts the first rib. If a paresthesia or motor response with a nerve stimulator is not elicited, walk the needle in an anterior and then posterior direction across the first rib. Once the plexus has been located, inject 25 to 40 mL of local anesthetic solution.
   d. Complications common to each of these approaches include pneumothorax and intravascular injection.
3. Infraclavicular approach to the brachial plexus is primarily used for anesthesia of the arm distal to the mid-humeral line. It is most useful for medium to long duration procedures where prolonged postoperative analgesia would be beneficial (e.g., bone and joint surgery). Soft tissue surgery may be most appropriately accomplished with a **Bier block (see section VII.C.10)**.
   a. Position the patient supine with the extremity slightly abducted and the palm upward.
   b. Landmarks to be palpated include the clavicle, coracoid process, and chest wall. After identifying the coracoid process, mark 2 cm inferior and 2 cm medial, making sure this needle insertion mark is superior to the chest wall (between coracoid process and chest wall).
   c. Using a 100-mm insulated needle with nerve stimulator starting between 1.0 and 1.5 mA, advance the needle in a plumb-bob direction until motor stimulation indicates contact

with the cord level of the brachial plexus. If no contact is made, the first redirection should be away from the chest wall.

d.   Stimulation of the lateral cord will give motor response of arm flexion and/or pronation (musculocutaneous nerve), flexor carpi radialis stimulation, and some wrist and finger flexion (median nerve). Stimulation of the posterior cord will give finger, hand, and arm extension (radial nerve). Stimulation of the medial cord produces flexor carpi ulnaris movement with flexion of the wrist and fingers (median and ulnar nerves).

e.   Success is seen with motor stimulation below 0.3 mA in any of the three cords, however some clinicians prefer to take the posterior cord as it is the most central of the three.

f.   Before injection of any local anesthetic, let go of the needle to ensure that the needle is within the sheath and not just pressing on the outside (if the needle is outside the sheath motor stimulation will cease as operator hand pressure is released).

g.   Inject 40 mL of local anesthetic after careful aspiration and in 3- to 5-mL aliquots. Use of a mixture of short onset and long duration local anesthetic will make the block most efficient and longer lasting.

h.   Complications include infection, hematoma, pneumothorax, nerve injury, and failed block.

4.   Axillary approach(Fig. 17-9)

a.   Position the patient supine with the arm abducted 90 degrees at the shoulder, externally rotated and flexed at the elbow.

b.   Palpate the axillary artery at its most proximal location in the axilla. If the artery is difficult to palpate, move the patient's hand laterally or reduce the degree of abduction at the shoulder.

c.   Advance a 23-gauge needle through the skin just superior to the palpating fingertip, directing the needle toward the apex of the axilla. Localization of one of the nerves of the plexus by either paresthesia or nerve stimulation confirms that the needle tip is within the plexus sheath; 40 to 50 mL of local anesthetic may be injected.

d.   If the axillary artery is penetrated (see section VII.C.5), advance the needle through the posterior wall of the artery.

e.   Frequently, a "pop" will be felt as the sheath is penetrated. If this occurs and the needle pulsates in synchrony with the pulse, the tip of the needle is located within the sheath and the anesthetic may be injected.

f.   While holding distal pressure on the upper arm, redirect the needle so that the tip of the needle is just superior to the artery and perpendicular to the skin in all planes. Advance the needle until the humerus is contacted and then, moving the tip through a 30-degree arc superiorly, 5 mL of local anesthetic solution can be injected in a fan-wise pattern. This will block the musculocutaneous nerve in the body of coracobrachialis muscle.

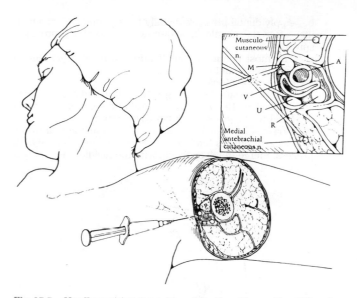

Fig. 17-9. Needle position for axillary injection. The median (*M*) and musculocutaneous nerves lie on the superior side of the artery (*A*). The latter usually lies within the body of the coracobrachialis muscle at this point. The ulnar (*U*) nerve lies inferior and the radial (*R*) nerve is inferior and posterior to the artery. These positions may vary with individual patients. The medial antebrachial cutaneous nerve usually lies in the subcutaneous tissues just inferior to the neurovascular bundle and is anesthetized by a subcutaneous wheal along that area, along with the intercostobrachial fibers. (From Mulroy MF. *Regional anesthesia: an illustrated procedural guide*, 2nd ed. Boston: Little, Brown and Company, 1996:172, with permission.)

    g.   Intercostobrachial nerve block requires subcutaneous injection of 5 mL of anesthetic, directly inferior to the axillary artery and extending to the inferior border of the axilla.

    h.   The most common complication specific to the axillary approach is injection of local anesthetic into the axillary artery.

    i.   After blocking the musculocutaneous and intercostobrachialis nerves, the needle should be withdrawn and the patient's arm replaced at their side while applying distal digital pressure.

    5. Axillary transarterial approach

    a.   Prepare the patient as previously described and palpate the axillary artery. Insert a 24-gauge medium bevel at an angle of 30 degrees to the skin and advance it cephalad toward the axillary artery. When blood is aspirated, advance the needle through the posterior wall of the artery. Inject 20 to 40 mL of local anesthetic solution posterior to the artery while aspirating for blood with every 5 mL of anesthetic injected.

      b. Apply digital pressure distally for a period of 3 to 5 minutes after the needle is withdrawn to maximize proximal spread.

      c. The most common complication with this approach is vascular spasm and hematoma.

6. Ulnar nerve block

      a.   Elbow. Locate the ulnar groove in the medial epicondyle and inject 5 to 10 mL of local anesthetic solution 3 to 5 cm proximal to the groove in a fan-wise pattern.

      b.   Wrist (Fig. 17-10). The ulnar nerve is just lateral to the flexor carpi ulnaris tendon at the level of the ulnar styloid process. Pierce the deep fascia with the needle oriented per-

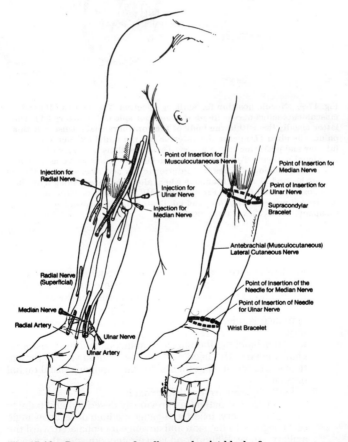

Fig. 17-10.   Deep anatomy for elbow and wrist block of musculocutaneous, radial, ulnar, and median nerves. (From Raj PP. *Clinical practice of regional anesthesia.* **New York: Churchill Livingstone, 1991.)**

pendicular to the skin, just lateral to the tendon, and inject 3 to 6 mL of solution.

7. **Median nerve block**

   a. **Elbow** (Fig. 17-10). The median nerve is just medial to the brachial artery. Palpate the artery 1 to 2 cm proximal to the elbow crease and inject 3 to 5 mL of anesthetic just medial to it in a fan-wise pattern.

   b. **Wrist** (Fig. 17-10). The median nerve lies between the palmaris longus tendon and the flexor carpi radialis tendon, 2 to 3 cm proximal to the wrist crease. Pierce the deep fascia with the needle oriented perpendicular to the skin close to the lateral border of the palmaris longus and inject 3 to 5 mL of anesthetic.

8. **Radial nerve block**

   a. **Elbow** (Fig. 17-10). The radial nerve lies lateral to the biceps tendon, medial to the brachioradialis muscle, at the level of the lateral epicondyle of the humerus. Insert the needle 1 to 2 cm lateral to the tendon and advance until it contacts the lateral epicondyle. Inject 3 to 5 mL of anesthetic solution.

   b. **Wrist**. The radial nerve divides into its terminal branches in the superficial fascia. Inject 5 to 10 mL of local anesthetic subcutaneously, extending from the radial artery anteriorly to the extensor carpi radialis posteriorly, beginning just proximal to the wrist.

9. **Musculocutaneous nerve block**. The musculocutaneous nerve may be blocked in the axilla, as described in section VII.C.4.f. Its terminal cutaneous component is blocked concomitantly with the radial nerve block at the elbow.

10. **Intravenous (IV) regional anesthesia (Bier block).** IV administration of local anesthetic distal to a tourniquet is a simple way to anesthetize an extremity.

    a. Place a 20- to 22-gauge IV catheter capped off with a heparin-lock device as distally as possible in the extremity. Apply a pneumatic double tourniquet proximally and exsanguinate the extremity by elevating it and wrapping it distally to proximally with an Esmarch bandage.

    b. Both tourniquet cuffs should be checked. Inflate the proximal cuff to 150 mm Hg greater than systolic pressure. Absence of pulses after inflation ensures arterial occlusion. Remove the Esmarch bandage and inject the anesthetic into the previously placed IV catheter. Average drug doses are 50 mL of 0.5% lidocaine for an arm and 100 mL of 0.25% lidocaine for a leg. No vasoconstrictors should be used.

    c. Anesthesia occurs within 5 minutes of local anesthetic injection. Tourniquet pain generally becomes unbearable after 1 hour and is the limiting factor for the success of this technique. When the patient complains of pain, the distal tourniquet that overlies anesthetized skin should be inflated and the proximal tourniquet released. Some advocate changing cuffs at 45 minutes, before the onset of pain.

    d. A **toxic reaction to the local anesthetic** is the major complication associated with IV regional anesthesia. It may occur during injection if the tourniquet fails or after tourniquet deflation, particularly with an inflation time of less than

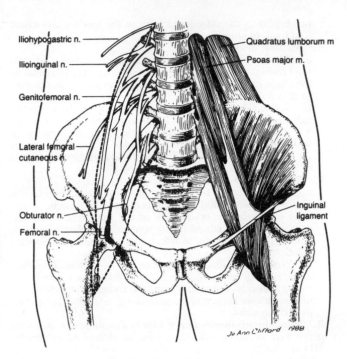

Fig. 17-11.   The lumbar plexus lies in the psoas compartment between to the psoas major and quadratus lumborum. (From Miller RD. *Anesthesia*, 3rd edition. New York: Churchill Livingstone, 1991.)

25 minutes. Careful attention to drug dosage and to the adequacy of vascular occlusion will minimize the risk of a local anesthetic reaction. If the tourniquet is deflated before 25 minutes, the patient should be observed closely for evidence of toxicity.

VIII.   **Regional anesthesia of the lower extremity**

  A.   **Anatomy.** There are two major plexuses that innervate the lower extremity: the lumbar plexus and the sacral plexus.

    1.   The **lumbar plexus** (Fig. 17-11) is formed within the psoas muscle from the anterior rami of the L-1 to L-4 spinal nerves, with a contribution from the twelfth thoracic nerve. The most cephalad nerves of the plexus are the **iliohypogastric, ilioinguinal, and genitofemoral nerves**. These nerves pierce the abdominal musculature anteriorly before supplying the skin of the hip and groin. The remainder of the lower abdomen is supplied by intercostal nerves. The three caudal nerves of the lumber plexus are the **lateral femoral cutaneous (LFC), femoral, and obturator nerves**.

      a.   The **LFC nerve** passes under the lateral end of the inguinal ligament, supplying sensory innervation to the lateral thigh and buttock.

b. The **femoral nerve** passes under the inguinal ligament just lateral to the femoral artery and supplies the muscles and skin of the anterior thigh, as well as the knee and hip joints. The **saphenous nerve** is the cutaneous termination of the femoral nerve, supplying the skin of the medial leg and foot. It is the only nerve of the lumbar plexus that innervates the leg below the knee.

c. The **obturator nerve** exits from the pelvis through the obturator canal of the ischium, innervating the adductor muscles of the thigh, the hip and knee joints, and a portion of the skin of the medial thigh.

2. The **sacral plexus** is formed from the anterior rami of the L4-5 lumbar nerves and the S1-3 sacral nerves. The two major nerves of the sacral plexus are the sciatic nerve and the posterior cutaneous nerve of the thigh.

a. The **posterior cutaneous nerve of the thigh** travels with the sciatic nerve in its proximal extent and supplies the skin of the posterior thigh. Techniques for blocking the sciatic nerve will also block the posterior cutaneous nerve of the thigh.

b. The **sciatic nerve** passes out of the pelvis through the greater sciatic foramen, becomes superficial at the lower border of the gluteus maximus, descends along the medial aspect of the femur supplying branches to the hamstrings, and becomes superficial again at the popliteal fossa. There it divides into the tibial nerve and the common peroneal nerve.

(1) The **tibial nerve** travels down the posterior calf and passes under the medial malleolus before dividing into its terminal branches. It supplies the skin of the medial and plantar foot and causes plantar flexion.

(2) The **common peroneal nerve** winds around the head of the fibula before dividing into the superficial and deep peroneal nerves.

(a) The **superficial peroneal nerve** is a sensory nerve that passes down the lateral calf, dividing into its terminal branches just medial to the lateral malleolus supplying the anterior foot.

(b) The **deep peroneal nerve** enters the foot just lateral to the anterior tibial artery, lying at the superior border of the malleolus, in between the anterior tibialis tendon and the extensor hallucis longus tendon. Although primarily a motor nerve causing dorsiflexion of the foot, it also sends a sensory branch to the web space between the first and second toes.

(3) The **sural nerve** is a sensory nerve formed from branches of the common peroneal and tibial nerves. It passes under the lateral malleolus, supplying the lateral foot.

B. Indications. Anesthetizing the entire lower extremity requires blocking components of both the lumbar and sacral plexuses. Because multiple injections may be required, lower extremity blocks are unpopular with many clinicians. However, they are useful when limited anesthesia is required (making a single injection feasible) or when a regional technique is preferable, but a central neuraxis block is contraindicated. Many of these blocks may be used as adjuncts to general anesthesia to provide postoperative analgesia.

1. Although **lower abdominal operations** can be performed with combined lumbar plexus block and intercostal nerve blocks, this is rarely done. However, an **ilioinguinal– iliohypogastric block** is a simple and very useful block, providing excellent analgesia for groin operations (e.g., hernia repair).

2. Hip operations require anesthesia of the entire lumbar plexus with the exception of the ilioinguinal and ilioinguinal nerves. This is most easily accomplished with a lumbar plexus block (psoas block).

3. Major thigh operations (e.g., placement of a femoral rod) require anesthesia of the LFC, femoral, obturator, and sciatic nerves. Obturator nerve block may be difficult to perform. Alternatively, these operations may be performed with a combined psoas–sciatic block.

4. Operations limited to the anterior thigh may be performed with a combined LFC–femoral block. The nerves may be blocked separately or together with a "3-in-1" block (see section VIII.C.2). Alone, an LFC block gives excellent analgesia for skin graft donor sites. An isolated femoral nerve block is particularly useful for providing postoperative analgesia for femoral shaft fractures or as the sole anesthetic for quadricepsplasty or repair of a patellar fracture.

5. For tourniquet pain, a combined LFC–femoral nerve block, in concert with a sciatic block, will usually provide adequate analgesia. This is because the area of skin that the obturator nerve supplies is generally small.

6. Open operations on the knee require anesthesia of the LFC, femoral, obturator, and sciatic nerves, which is most easily accomplished with a combined psoas–sciatic block. For knee arthroscopy, combined 3-in-1 and femoral–sciatic nerve blocks provide adequate anesthesia.

7. Operations distal to the knee require sciatic block and block of the saphenous component of the femoral nerve. The branches of the sciatic nerve can be blocked with multiple injections at the ankle or with a single injection in the popliteal fossa. The latter is particularly useful when cellulitis is present at the ankle. Ankle block will provide reliable anesthesia for transmetatarsal and toe amputations.

C. Techniques. Although paresthesias may be used for nerve localization in the lower extremity, in general, a nerve stimulator is more accurate.

1. Lumbar plexus block (psoas block)

a. Local anesthetic deposited into the substance of the psoas muscle will be confined by its fascia and will anesthetize the entire plexus.

b. Place the patient in the lateral position, hips flexed, with the surgical side uppermost. Insert a 22-gauge 3.5-inch spinal needle perpendicular to the skin at a point 3 cm cephalad to a line connecting the iliac crests and 4 to 5 cm lateral to the midline. If the transverse process of L-4 is contacted, redirect the needle. Localize the plexus by using a nerve stimulator, which will produce a quadriceps muscle twitch. Inject 30 to 40 mL of local anesthetic.

c. **Epidural blockade** is a complication of this approach, occurring with an incidence of approximately 10%.

2. **3-in-1 block**

a. The three branches of the lumbar plexus can be blocked with a single injection.

b. With the patient in the supine position, insert a 2.5- to 3-inch needle just caudad to the inguinal ligament and lateral to the femoral artery. Direct the needle cephalad at a 45-degree angle until a quadriceps twitch or paresthesia is elicited. While maintaining distal pressure, which may force the anesthetic more proximally onto lumbar nerve roots, inject 30 to 40 mL of local anesthetic.

c. An alternative approach is the **fascia iliaca compartment block**. It consists of injecting local anesthetic behind the fascia iliaca at the junction of the lateral and middle thirds of the inguinal ligament and forcing it upward by finger compression.

3. **Ilioinguinal–iliohypogastric nerve block**. Insert a 1.5-inch needle perpendicular to the skin and 3 cm medial to the anterior superior iliac spine (ASIS). Contact the ASIS and inject 10 to 15 mL of local anesthetic while withdrawing the needle to the skin.

4. **LFC nerve block** (Fig. 17-12). Insert a 1.5-inch needle 1.5 cm caudad and 1.5 cm medial to the ASIS. Direct the needle in a slightly lateral and cephalad direction, striking the iliac bone medially just below the ASIS, and inject 5 to 10 mL of local anesthetic.

5. **Femoral nerve block** (Fig. 17-12) is carried out identically to the 3-in-1 block (see section VIII.C.2), with the exception that the needle is directed perpendicular to the skin rather than at a 45-degree angle. A volume of 15 to 20 mL of local anesthetic suffices.

6. **Obturator nerve block** (Fig. 17-12). With the patient in the supine position, identify the pubic tubercle and insert a 3-inch needle 1.5 cm caudal and 1.5 cm lateral to the tubercle. After contacting the bone, withdraw the needle and redirect it slightly lateral and caudal while advancing 2 to 3 cm into the obturator foramen. After aspiration, inject 20 mL of local anesthetic while fanning lateral.

7. **Sciatic nerve block**

a. **Indications**

(1) **Surgery of the leg** when blocked proximally in combination with femoral nerve blockade.

(2) **Surgery of the knee** when combined with blockade of the femoral, LFC, and obturator nerves.

(3) **Foot and ankle surgery** when combined with saphenous nerve (femoral) blockade.

b. **Classic posterior approach**. Place the patient in the Sims position (the lateral decubitus position with the leg to be blocked uppermost and flexed at the hip and knee; Fig. 17-13). Identify the posterior superior iliac spine and greater trochanter and draw a straight line connecting the two structures. At its midpoint, draw a perpendicular line inferiorly for 3 to 4 cm. Insert a 3.5-inch 22-gauge needle perpendicularly to the skin, 3 cm below the midpoint, and connect the needle

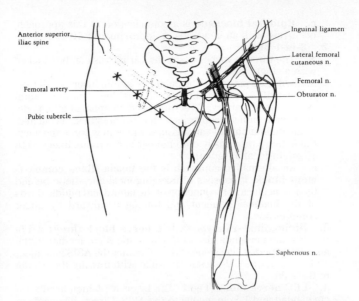

Fig. 17-12.   Block of the anterior lumbosacral branches in the groin. The lateral femoral cutaneous nerve emerges approximately 2.5 cm medial to the anterior superior iliac spine and is best blocked along that line 2.5 cm caudad to the anterior superior iliac spine. The femoral nerve emerges alongside and slightly posterior to the femoral artery and is again easily approached approximately 2.5 cm below the inguinal ligament. On that same line, the obturator nerve emerges from the obturator canal but is deeper and less reliably located. (From Mulroy MF. *Regional anesthesia: an illustrated procedural guide*, 2nd ed. Boston: Little, Brown and Company, 1996:204, with permission.)

to a nerve stimulator set at an initial current of 2.5 mA. Advance the needle to a depth of approximately 3 cm to elicit a motor response in the sciatic distribution (contraction of hamstring or gastrocnemius, foot dorsi- or plantar flexion) or paresthesia in the leg or foot. If buttock contraction is observed, the inferior or superior gluteal nerves are being stimulated, and the needle is simply redirected. When an appropriate motor response is noted, decrease the stimulus current in a stepwise fashion to determine the threshold for stimulation. Reposition the needle until the goal of a stimulus threshold less than 1.0 mA is reached. After a test dose, inject 20 to 30 mL of local anesthetic, aspirating the syringe after each 5 mL injected. A double injection technique identifies and injects the tibial and peroneal components of the sciatic nerve separately, through the same skin wheal.

c.   **Lithotomy approach**. With the patient supine, flex the lower extremity as far as possible at the hip and support it by stirrups or an assistant. Locate the midpoint of a line between the greater trochanter and the ischial tuberosity. Insert a 3.5-inch needle attached to a nerve stimulator perpendicular

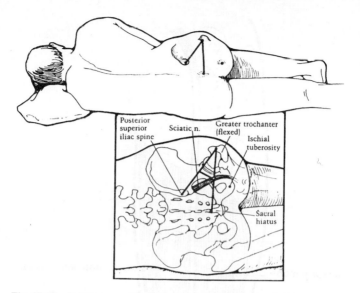

Fig. 17-13. Sciatic nerve block, classic posterior approach. With the patient in the lateral position and the hip and knee flexed, the muscles overlying the sciatic nerve are stretched to allow easier identification. The nerve lies beneath a point 5 cm caudad along the perpendicular line that bisects the line joining the posterior superior iliac spine and the greater trochanter of the femur. This is also usually the intersection of that perpendicular with another line joining the greater trochanter and the sacral hiatus. (From Mulroy MF. *Regional anesthesia: an illustrated procedural guide*, 2nd ed. Boston: Little, Brown and Company, 1996:202, with permission.)

to the skin at this point and advance the needle until a motor response is seen, indicating sciatic nerve stimulation. Inject 20 to 30 mL of local anesthetic, aspirating intermittently.

d. Sciatic block at the knee (Fig. 17-14). With the patient prone, flex the knee 30 degrees. This outlines the borders of the popliteal fossa, which is bounded by the knee crease inferiorly, the long head of the biceps femoris laterally, and the superimposed tendons of the semimembranosus and semitendinosus muscles medially. Draw a vertical line on the skin, dividing the fossa into two equilateral triangles. Insert a needle 6 cm superior to the knee crease and 1 cm lateral to the line bisecting the fossa. Use a nerve stimulator to localize the nerve and inject 30 to 40 mL of local anesthetic, aspirating intermittently.

8. Saphenous nerve block. The saphenous nerve (femoral) can be blocked at the ankle (see section VIII.C.9) or at the knee. At the knee, inject 10 mL of local anesthetic in the deep subcutaneous tissue, extending from the medial surface of the tibial condyle to the superimposed tendons of the semimembranosus and semitendinosus muscles.

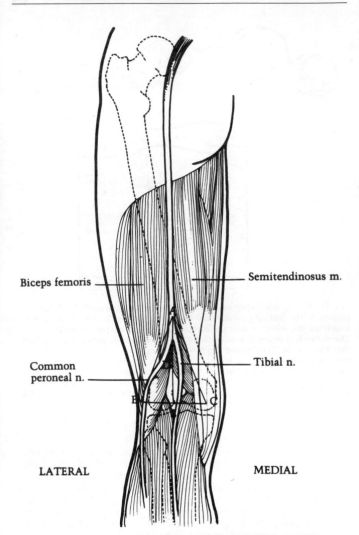

Fig. 17-14. Popliteal fossa block. The two major trunks of the sciatic
nerve bifurcate in the popliteal fossa 7 to 10 cm above the knee. A
triangle is drawn using the heads of the biceps femoris and the
semitendinous muscles and the skin crease of the knee; a long needle is
inserted 1 cm lateral to a point 6 cm cephalad on the line from the skin
crease that bisects this triangle. (From Mulroy MF. *Regional anesthesia.*
Boston: Little, Brown, 1989.)

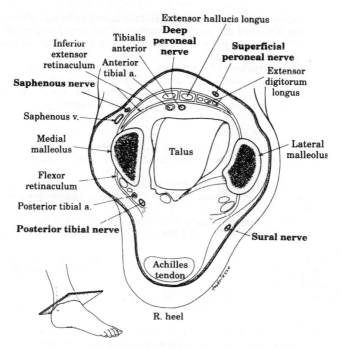

Fig. 17-15. Cross-section at the level of the ankle.

9. **Ankle block** (Fig. 17-15)

   a. The five nerves supplying the foot can be blocked at the ankle. Elevate the foot on a pillow to provide easy access to both sides of the ankle.

   b. At the superior border of the malleoli, the **deep peroneal nerve** is situated between the anterior tibialis tendon and the extensor hallucis longus tendon, which are easily palpable with dorsiflexion of the foot and extension of the great toe. Insert a 1.5-inch needle just lateral to the anterior tibial artery between the two tendons until contacting the tibia and then withdraw the needle while depositing 5 to 10 mL of local anesthetic.

   c. Then, inject a 10-mL volume of local anesthetic subcutaneously across the anterior surface of the tibia, from malleolus to malleolus. This will block the **superficial peroneal nerve** laterally and the **saphenous nerve** medially.

   d. To block the **posterior tibial nerve**, insert a needle posterior to the medial malleolus, directed toward the inferior border of the posterior tibial artery. A paresthesia may be noted in the sole of the foot. Withdraw the needle 1 cm from the point of bony contact and inject 5 to 10 mL of local anesthetic in a fan-shaped area.

   e. Block the **sural nerve** by inserting the needle midway between the Achilles tendon and the lateral malleolus, directing it toward the posterior surface of the lateral malleolus. After contacting bone, withdraw the needle and inject 5 mL of local anesthetic.

D. Complications of lower extremity blocks include epidural blockade with potential sympathectomy (psoas block), intravascular injection, inadvertent arterial puncture, and neural trauma (particularly if a paresthesia technique was performed).

SUGGESTED READING

Bailey SL, Parkinson SK, Little WL, et al. Sciatic nerve block. A comparison of single versus double injection technique. *Reg Anesth* 1994;19: 9–13.

Cousins MJ, Bridenbaugh PO. *Neural blockade in clinical anesthesia and management of pain*, 3rd ed. Philadelphia: Lippincott-Raven, 1998.

Dalens B, Vanneuville G, Tanguy A. Comparison of the fascia iliaca compartment block with the 3-in-1 block in children. *Anesth Analg* 1989; 69:705–713.

De Andres J, Sala-Blanch X. Peripheral nerve stimulation in the practice of brachial plexus anesthesia: a review. *Reg Anesth Pain Med* 2001; 26:478–483.

Franco CD, Vieira ZEG. 1,001 subclavian perivascular brachial plexus blocks: success with a nerve stimulator. *Reg Anesth Pain Med* 2000; 25:41–46.

Henderson CL, Warriner CB, McEwen JA, et al. A North American survey of intravenous regional anesthesia. *Anesth Analg* 1997;85:858–863.

Lanz E, Theiss D, Jankovic D. The extent of blockade following various techniques of brachial plexus block. *Anesth Analg* 1983;62:55–58.

Mulroy MF. *Regional anesthesia: an illustrated procedural guide*, 2nd ed. Philadelphia: Lippincott Williams & Wilkins, 1996.

Parkinson SK, Mueller JB, Little WL, et al. Extent of blockade with various approaches to the lumbar plexus. *Anesth Analg* 1989;68:243–248.

Pham-Dang C, Gunst J-P, Gouin F, et al. A novel supraclavicular approach to brachial plexus block. *Anesth Analg* 1997;85:111–116.

Raj PP. *Textbook of regional anesthesia*. New York: Churchill Livingstone, 2002.

Rorie DK, Byer DE, Nelson DO, et al. Assessment of block of the sciatic nerve in the popliteal fossa. *Anesth Analg* 1980;59:371–376.

Schroeder LE, Horlocker TT, Schroeder DR. The efficacy of axillary block for surgical procedures about the elbow. *Anesth Analg* 1996;83: 747–751.

Scott DB, Hakansson L, Buckhoj P. *Techniques of regional anesthesia*. New York: McGraw-Hill, 1996.

Stan TC, Krantz MA, Solomon DL, et al. The incidence of neurovascular complications following axillary brachial plexus block using a transarterial approach. A prospective study of 1,000 consecutive patients. *Reg Anesth* 1995;20:486–492.

Urban MK, Urquhart B. Evaluation of brachial plexus anesthesia for upper extremity surgery. *Reg Anesth* 1994;19:175–182.

Vloka JD, Hadzic A, April E, et al. The division of the sciatic nerve in the popliteal fossa: anatomical implications for popliteal nerve blockade. *Anesth Analg* 2001;92:215–217.

Vongvises P, Panijayanond T. A parascalene technique of brachial plexus anesthesia. *Anesth Analg* 1979;58:267–273.

Wedel DJ. Nerve blocks. In: Miller RD, ed. *Anesthesia*, 5th ed. New York: Churchill Livingstone, 2000:1520–1548.

Wildsmith JAW, Armitage EN. *Principles and practice of regional anesthesia*, 2nd ed. Edinburgh: Churchill Livingstone, 1993.

18

Intraanesthetic Problems

Keith Baker and Douglas E. Raines

I. **Hypotension** is a significant decrease of arterial blood pressure below the patient's normal range. It may be due to a decrease in cardiac function (contractility), systemic vascular resistance (SVR), venous return, or arrhythmias.

A. **Contractility**

   1. Most anesthetic agents, including inhalation agents, barbiturates, and benzodiazepines (see Chapter 11), cause dose-dependent direct myocardial depression. **Opiates** are not myocardial depressants in the usual clinical doses.

   2. **Cardiac medications**, such as beta-adrenergic antagonists, calcium channel blockers, and lidocaine, are myocardial depressants.

   3. **Cardiac dysfunction** may occur with myocardial ischemia or myocardial infarction (MI), hypocalcemia, severe acidosis or alkalosis, hypothermia less than 32°C, cor pulmonale, vagal reflexes, and systemic toxicity from local anesthetics (particularly bupivacaine).

B. **Decreased SVR**

   1. **Isoflurane** and, to a lesser extent, halothane and enflurane produce a decrease in SVR.

   2. **Opiates** produce loss of vascular tone by reducing sympathetic nervous system outflow. Morphine can release histamine with resultant vasodilation.

   3. **Benzodiazepines** may decrease SVR, particularly when administered at high doses with opiates.

   4. A decrease in SVR can be seen with many of the drugs used during anesthesia.

      a. **Direct vasodilators** (e.g., nitroprusside, nitroglycerin, hydralazine).

      b. **α-Adrenergic blockers** (e.g., droperidol, chlorpromazine, phentolamine, labetalol).

      c. **Histamine-releasing medications** (e.g., curare).

      d. **Ganglionic inhibitors** (e.g., trimethaphan).

      e. **Calcium channel blockers**.

      f. **Angiotensin-converting enzyme inhibitors**.

   5. **Sympathetic blockade** frequently occurs during spinal and epidural anesthesia.

   6. **Sepsis** causes release of vasoactive substances that mediate hypotension.

   7. **Vasoactive metabolites** (e.g., after bowel manipulation or tourniquet release) may cause hypotension.

   8. **Allergic reactions** (see section XVIII) may cause profound hypotension.

   9. **Profound hypoxia**.

C. Inadequate venous return
1. **Hypovolemia** may be caused by blood loss, insensible evaporative losses, preoperative deficits (e.g., nothing-by-mouth status, vomiting, diarrhea, nasogastric tube suction, enteric drains, and bowel preparations), polyuria (as a result of diuretics, diabetes mellitus, diabetes insipidus, or postobstructive diuresis), and adrenal insufficiency.
2. **Caval compression** may result from surgical maneuvers or a gravid uterus.
3. **Increased venous capacitance** may occur with sympathetic blockade from ganglionic blockers, regional anesthesia, vasodilators (e.g., nitroglycerin), histamine-releasing medications, and induction agents (e.g., barbiturates and propofol).
4. **Increased intrathoracic pressure** during mechanical ventilation with large tidal volumes, positive end-expiratory pressure (PEEP), or auto-PEEP (air trapping) will impair venous return.
5. **Other etiologies** include pneumothorax and cardiac tamponade.
D. Arrhythmias
1. **Tachyarrhythmias** often result in hypotension.
2. **Atrial fibrillation, atrial flutter, and junctional rhythms** cause hypotension from loss of the atrial contribution to diastolic filling. This is particularly pronounced in patients with valvular heart disease or diastolic dysfunction, in whom atrial contraction may augment end-diastolic volume more than 30%.
3. **Bradyarrhythmias** may cause hypotension if preload reserve is inadequate to maintain a compensatory increase in stroke volume.
4. **Treatment** should be directed toward correcting the underlying cause and may include:
   a. **Decreasing anesthetic depth**.
   b. **Volume expansion**.
   c. **Vasopressor support** to increase vascular resistance or decrease venous capacitance (e.g., phenylephrine) and increase stroke volume (e.g., dopamine).
   d. **Correction of mechanical causes**, such as placement of a chest tube for pneumothorax, reducing or eliminating PEEP, decreasing mean airway pressure, or relieving obstruction of the vena cava (e.g., left uterine displacement for a pregnant patient).
   e. **Antiarrhythmic (see section III) or antiischemic medical therapy**.
II. Hypertension
A. Etiologies
1. **Catecholamine excess**, which may be seen with inadequate anesthesia (especially during laryngoscopy, intubation, incision, and emergence), hypoxia, hypercarbia, patient anxiety, pain, and prolonged tourniquet use.
2. **Preexisting disease** (e.g., essential hypertension).
3. **Increased intracranial pressure**.
4. **Systemic absorption of vasoconstrictors** such as epinephrine and phenylephrine.
5. **Aortic cross-clamping**.

6. **Rebound hypertension** from discontinuation of clonidine or β-adrenergic blockers.

7. **Drug–drug interactions**. Tricyclic antidepressants or monoamine oxidase inhibitors given with ephedrine may cause an exaggerated hypertensive response.

8. **Bladder distention**.

9. **Administration of indigo carmine dye** (via an α-adrenergic effect).

B. **Treatment** is directed toward correcting the underlying cause and may include the following:

1. Improving oxygenation and ventilatory abnormalities.

2. Increasing depth of anesthesia.

3. Sedating an anxious patient or emptying a full bladder.

4. **Medications** (for further discussion, see Chapter 19).

a. **β-Adrenergic blocking agents** (e.g., labetalol, 5- to 10-mg increments intravenously [IV]; propranolol, 0.5- to 1.0-mg increments IV; or esmolol, 5- to 10-mg increments IV).

b. **Vasodilators** (e.g., hydralazine, 2.5- to 5-mg increments IV; nitroglycerin infusion starting at 30 to 50 μg/min IV and titrating to effect; nitroprusside infusion, 30 to 50 μg/min IV and titrating to effect).

III. **Arrhythmias**

A. **Sinus bradycardia** is a sinus node driven heart rate of less than 60 beats/min. Unless there is severe underlying heart disease, hemodynamic changes are minimal. With slow rates, atrial and ventricular ectopic escape beats or rhythms may occur.

1. **Etiologies**

a. **Hypoxia**.

b. **Intrinsic cardiac disease** such as sick sinus syndrome or acute MI (particularly inferior wall MI).

c. **Medications** such as succinylcholine (especially in young children), anticholinesterases, β-adrenergic blockers, calcium channel blockers, digoxin, and narcotics.

d. **Increased vagal tone** occurs with traction on the peritoneum or spermatic cord, the oculocardiac reflex, direct pressure on the vagus nerve or carotid sinus during neck or intrathoracic surgery, centrally mediated vagal response from anxiety or pain, and Valsalva maneuvers.

e. **Increased intracranial pressure**.

2. **Treatment**

a. **Verify adequate oxygenation and ventilation.**

b. Bradycardia due to increased vagal tone requires discontinuation of the provocative stimulus. **Atropine** (0.4 to 0.8 mg IV) may be needed.

c. In patients with intrinsic cardiac disease, treatment should proceed with atropine (0.4 to 0.8 mg IV), chronotropes (e.g., ephedrine, dopamine), and rarely, cardiac pacing.

B. **Sinus tachycardia** is a sinus node driven heart rate greater than 100 beats/min. The rate is regular and rarely exceeds 160 beats/min.

1. **Etiologies** include catecholamine excess, hypercarbia, hypoxia, hypotension, hypovolemia, medications (e.g., pancuronium, atropine, ephedrine), fever, MI, pulmonary embolism, malignant hyperthermia, pheochromocytoma, and thyrotoxicosis.

2. Treatment should be directed toward correcting the underlying cause and may include:
   a. Correcting oxygenation and ventilatory abnormalities.
   b. Increasing the depth of anesthesia.
   c. Correcting hypovolemia.
   d. Medications such as narcotics and β-adrenergic blockers. Patients with active coronary artery disease may benefit by treatment with β-adrenergic blockers to control heart rate while the cause is being determined.
C. Heart block
   1. First-degree atrioventricular (AV) block is prolongation of the PR interval for 0.2 seconds or longer. In first-degree block, every atrial pulse is transmitted to the ventricle.
   2. Second-degree AV block can be divided into two types: Mobitz 1 (Wenckebach) and Mobitz 2.
      a. Mobitz 1 usually occurs when a conduction defect is in the AV node and is manifested by a progressive PR prolongation culminating in a nonconducted P wave. It is generally benign.
      b. Mobitz 2 is a block in or distal to the AV node with a constant PR interval. It is more likely to progress to third-degree block.
   3. Third-degree heart block is usually due to lesions distal to the His bundle and is characterized by the complete absence of AV conduction. Usually, a slow ventricular rate is seen (<45/min). P waves occur regularly but are independent of QRS complexes (AV dissociation).
   4. Treatment
      a. First-degree heart block does not usually require specific treatment. First-degree heart block in combination with a bifascicular block may warrant temporary ventricular pacing.
      b. Second-degree heart block
         (1) Mobitz 1 requires treatment only if bradycardia, congestive heart failure, or bundle branch block occurs. Transcutaneous or transvenous pacing may be necessary, particularly during inferior MIs.
         (2) Mobitz 2 may progress to complete heart block thus necessitating the use of a pacemaker.
      c. Third-degree heart block may necessitate transcutaneous or transvenous pacing.
D. Supraventricular tachycardias originate at or above the bundle of His, and the resulting QRS complexes are narrow except during aberrant conduction.
   1. Atrial premature contractions (APCs) occur when ectopic foci in the atria fire before the next expected impulse from the sinus node. The P wave of an APC characteristically looks different from preceding P waves, and the PR interval may vary from normal. Early APCs may cause aberrant QRS complexes or be nonconducted to the ventricle, if the latter is still in a refractory period. APCs are common, benign, and usually require no treatment.
   2. Junctional or AV nodal rhythms are characterized by absent or abnormal P waves and normal QRS complexes. Although they may indicate ischemic cardiac disease, junctional rhythms are commonly seen in normal individuals receiving inhalation

anesthesia. In the patient whose cardiac output depends heavily on the contribution from atrial contraction, stroke volume and blood pressure may decline precipitously. Treatment should include the following:

   a. Reduction of anesthetic depth.

   b. Increasing intravascular volume.

   c. Atropine in increments of 0.2 mg IV may convert a slow junctional rhythm to sinus rhythm, particularly if secondary to a vagal mechanism.

   d. Paradoxically, propranolol may be used cautiously in increments of 0.25 mg IV.

   e. If the arrhythmia is associated with hypotension, increasing the blood pressure with vasopressors (e.g., ephedrine or norepinephrine) may be required.

   f. If necessary, atrial pacing may be instituted to restore atrial contraction.

3. **Atrial fibrillation** is an irregular rhythm with an atrial rate of 350 to 600 beats/min and a variable ventricular response. It may be seen with myocardial ischemia, mitral valvular disease, hyperthyroidism, excessive sympathetic stimulation, or digitalis toxicity; after thoracic surgery; or when the heart has been manipulated. Treatment is based on the hemodynamic status.

   a. **Rapid ventricular rate with stable hemodynamics** can be treated initially with β-adrenergic blockade, such as propranolol (0.5-mg increments IV), metoprolol (2.5- to 5-mg increments), esmolol (5- to 10-mg increments), or a calcium channel blocker such as verapamil (2.5- to 5-mg increments) (see Chapter 36).

   b. **Rapid ventricular rate with unstable hemodynamics** requires synchronized cardioversion starting with 50 J (see Chapter 36).

4. **Atrial flutter** is usually a regular rhythm with an atrial rate of 250 to 350 beats/min and a characteristic sawtooth configuration. It is seen with underlying heart disease (i.e., rheumatic heart disease and mitral stenosis). A 1:1 or 2:1 block will result in a rapid ventricular rate (usually 150 beats/min). Treatment usually includes β-adrenergic or calcium channel blockade or synchronized cardioversion (see Chapter 36).

5. **Paroxysmal supraventricular tachycardia** is a tachyarrhythmia (atrial and ventricular rates of 150 to 250 beats/min) with reentry usually through the AV node. This rhythm may be associated with **Wolff-Parkinson-White syndrome**, thyrotoxicosis, or mitral valve prolapse. Patients without heart disease may develop this arrhythmia due to stress, caffeine, or excess catecholamines. Treatment includes **adenosine** (6 to 18 mg IV), carotid sinus massage, or propranolol (1 to 2 mg IV). Synchronized cardioversion may be required for the hemodynamically unstable patient (also see Chapter 36).

E. **Ventricular arrhythmias**

   1. **Ventricular premature contractions (VPCs)** are bizarre widened QRS complexes. When coupled alternately with normal beats, ventricular bigeminy exists. VPCs are occasionally seen in normal individuals. Under anesthesia, they frequently occur during states of catecholamine excess, hypoxia, or hypercarbia. They may also signify myocardial ischemia or infarction, digitalis toxicity, or hypokalemia. **VPCs may require therapy when they are multifocal, occur in runs, increase in frequency, or occur on or near the preceding T wave (R-on-T phenomenon)**; these situations may precede the development of ventricular tachycardia, ventricular fibrillation, and cardiac arrest. Treatment in an otherwise healthy individual may include deepening anesthesia and ensuring adequate oxygenation and ventilation. Patients with coronary artery disease who continue to have ventricular irritability should have the ischemia treated. If the ectopy continues, then **lidocaine** may be given, 1 mg/kg IV, followed by a lidocaine infusion at 1 to 2 mg/min. Refractory ventricular ectopy may require further treatment (see Chapter 36).

2. Ventricular tachycardia is a wide-complex tachyarrhythmia at a rate of 150 to 250 beats/min. Unstable patients should be treated with synchronized cardioversion (100, 200, 300, and 360 J). For stable patients the first-line treatment depends on whether the ventricular tachycardia is monomorphic or polymorphic. In addition, the treatment depends on the ejection fraction (see Chapter 36 for specific recommendations).

3. Ventricular fibrillation is chaotic ventricular activity resulting in ineffective ventricular contractions. Defibrillation and cardiopulmonary resuscitation are required (see Chapter 36 for specific recommendations).

4. Ventricular preexcitation. Wolff-Parkinson-White syndrome is due to an accessory pathway connecting the atria and ventricle. The most common mechanism is characterized by antegrade conduction through the normal AV conduction system and retrograde conduction through the accessory pathway. Characteristic electrocardiographic (ECG) findings include a short PR interval and a slurred delta wave at the onset of the QRS. Tachyarrhythmias are common. Treatment depends on whether the patient is hemodynamically stable (see Chapter 36). Unstable patients should receive synchronized cardioversion starting at 50 J. These patients are at high risk for ventricular fibrillation.

IV. Hypoxia occurs when oxygen delivery to the tissues is insufficient to meet their metabolic demands.
  A. Intraoperative etiologies
    1. Inadequate oxygen supply
      a. Empty reserve oxygen tanks with loss of the main pipeline supply.
      b. An oxygen flowmeter that is leaking or not turned to a sufficient flow.
      c. Breathing system disconnection.
      d. Large leaks in the anesthesia machine, ventilator, carbon dioxide absorber, or breathing circuit or around the endotracheal tube. This may be managed acutely by using an self-inflating (Ambu) bag to deliver oxygen to the patient.
      e. Obstructed endotracheal tube.
      f. Malpositioned endotracheal tubes (e.g., esophageal or mainstem bronchial intubation).
    2. Hypoventilation (see section V)
    3. Ventilation-perfusion inequalities are seen with atelectasis, pneumonia, pulmonary edema, pneumothorax, and other

parenchymal pathologic states. Other causes include compression from packs and retractors and endobronchial intubation. In some cases, ventilation-perfusion inequalities may be corrected by increasing mean airway pressure or applying PEEP.

4. Right-to-left cardiac shunt

5. Reduction in oxygen-carrying capacity. Oxygen-carrying capacity is reduced with anemia, carbon monoxide poisoning, methemoglobinemia, and hemoglobinopathies despite a normal oxygen saturation as measured by pulse oximetry.

6. Leftward shift of the hemoglobin-oxygen dissociation curve results from hypothermia, decreased 2,3-diphosphoglycerate concentration, alkalosis, hypocarbia, and carbon monoxide poisoning.

B. Treatment

1. If the patient is being mechanically ventilated, manual ventilation with 100% oxygen should be begun to assess pulmonary compliance. Breath sounds should be evaluated, the surgical field checked for mechanical pressure on the airway, the endotracheal tube examined for obstruction or dislodgement, and adequate movement of the chest wall or diaphragm confirmed.

2. The breathing circuit, ventilator, and anesthesia machine should be checked for leaks. If present, ventilation should be started with 100% oxygen via an alternate source such as a self-inflating bag until the problem is rectified.

3. Adequate oxygen delivery to the patient should be confirmed with an in-line oxygen analyzer.

4. Further treatment is outline in Chapter 35.

V. Hypercarbia is due either to inadequate ventilation or to increased carbon dioxide production and can lead to increased pulmonary artery and intracranial pressures.

A. Inadequate ventilation

1. Central depression of the medullary respiratory center can be caused by opioids, barbiturates, benzodiazepines, volatile agents, or primary central nervous system pathology (e.g., tumor, ischemia, edema). Controlled ventilation or reversal agents (e.g., naloxone and flumazenil) may be required.

2. Neuromuscular depression may be seen with high spinal and epidural anesthesia, phrenic nerve paralysis, and muscle relaxants.

3. Inappropriate ventilator settings may result in a low minute ventilation.

4. Increased airway resistance may occur with bronchospasm, upper airway obstruction, mainstem intubation, kinked endotracheal tubes, severe chronic obstructive lung disease, congestive heart failure, and hemothorax or pneumothorax. Depending on the etiology, treatment may include the intravenous administration of sympathomimetics, repositioning of the endotracheal tube, suctioning, diuresis, or the placement of a chest tube.

5. Rebreathing of exhaled gases from an exhausted carbon dioxide absorber, inspiratory or expiratory valve failure, or inadequate fresh gas flows in nonrebreathing systems may occur.

B. Increased carbon dioxide production results from exogenous carbon dioxide (e.g., absorption of carbon dioxide from insufflation during laparoscopy), reperfusion, and hypermetabolic states (e.g., malignant hyperthermia).

VI. Abnormal urine output

A. Oliguria is defined as urine output less than 0.5 mL/kg/h. Prerenal, intrarenal, and postrenal causes are described in Chapter 4.

 1. Treatment includes ruling out mechanical causes (e.g., malpositioned or kinked Foley catheter).

 2. Hypotension should be corrected to improve renal perfusion pressure.

 3. Volume status should be assessed. A fluid bolus may be given if hypovolemia is suspected. If oliguria persists, central venous pressure measurement may help guide further fluid management. Patients with reduced ventricular function may require placement of a pulmonary artery catheter.

 4. If oliguria persists despite an adequate volume status, urine output can be increased with:

  a. Furosemide, 2 to 20 mg IV.

  b. Dopamine infusion, 1 to 3 µg/kg/min IV.

  c. Mannitol, 12.5 to 25.0 g IV.

 5. Intraoperative diuretics may be required to preserve urine output in patients on chronic diuretic therapy.

B. Anuria is a rare occurrence in the perioperative period. Mechanical causes, including Foley catheter malfunction or ureteral damage or transection, must be excluded and hemodynamic instability must be treated.

C. High urine output may occur in response to vigorous fluid administration, but other causes must be considered, including hyperglycemia, diabetes insipidus, and exogenous diuretic administration. High urine output is not a problem unless associated with hypovolemia or electrolyte abnormalities. Treatment should be directed at the underlying cause, maintaining volume status, and correcting electrolyte abnormalities.

VII. Hypothermia is a common problem in the operative period.

A. Heat loss may occur from any of the following mechanisms:

 1. Redistribution of heat from core areas (brain, heart, etc.) to peripheral tissues (limbs, skin, etc.). Redistribution results in a reduction in the core temperature with maintenance of the mean body temperature.

 2. Radiation. Radiant heat loss depends on cutaneous blood flow and exposed body surface area.

 3. Evaporation. Energy is lost as liquid vaporizes from mucosal and serosal surfaces, skin, and lungs. Evaporative losses depend on the exposed surface area and the relative humidity of ambient gas.

 4. Conduction, which is heat transfer from a warm to a cool object. This heat loss is proportional to the area exposed, difference in temperature, and thermal conductivity.

 5. Convection, which is the loss of heat by conduction to a moving gas. High air flow rates in the operating rooms (10 to 15 room volume changes per hour) may result in significant heat loss.

B. Pediatric patients are particularly susceptible to intraoperative hypothermia (see Chapter 28).

C.   Geriatric patients are also more prone to hypothermia (see Chapter 26).

D.   Anesthetic effects. Volatile anesthetics impair the thermoregulatory center located in the posterior hypothalamus and predispose to heat loss due to their vasodilatory properties. Opioids will reduce the vasoconstriction mechanism for heat conservation because of their sympatholytic properties. Muscle relaxants reduce muscle tone and prevent shivering. Regional anesthesia produces sympathetic blockade, muscle relaxation, and sensory blockade of thermal receptors, which inhibit compensatory responses.

E.   Hypothermia is associated with a number of physiologic changes:

1.   Cardiovascular. Increased SVR, ventricular arrhythmias, and myocardial depression may occur with severe hypothermia.

2.   Metabolic. Decreased metabolic rate and decreased tissue perfusion (from catecholamine response) may occur.

3.   Hematologic. Increased blood viscosity, leftward shift of the hemoglobin dissociation curve, impaired coagulation, and thrombocytopenia occur.

4.   Neurologic. Decreased cerebral blood flow, increased cerebrovascular resistance, decreased minimum alveolar concentration, delayed emergence from anesthesia, drowsiness, and confusion may occur.

5.   Drug disposition. Decreased hepatic blood flow and metabolism coupled with decreased renal blood flow and clearance result in decreased anesthetic requirement.

6.   Shivering can increase heat production by 100% to 300% but with a concomitant increase in oxygen consumption of up to 500% and increased carbon dioxide production.

F.   Prevention and treatment of hypothermia

1.   Maintain or increase ambient temperature. Anesthetized patients frequently become hypothermic if the room temperature is below 21°C.

2.   Covering exposed surfaces will minimize conductive and convective losses. Forced warmed air blankets (e.g., Bair Hugger and others) placed over the patient can provide both insulation and active cutaneous warming.

3.   Warming transfused fluids and blood is essential in cases with large fluid requirements (see Chapter 14).

4.   Use of closed or low-flow semiclosed circuit anesthesia will decrease evaporative losses and modestly reduce heat loss.

5.   Heated humidifiers added to the anesthetic circuit when high gas flow rates are required will warm and humidify inspired gas, minimizing evaporative loss from the lungs. The temperature of inspired gas must be monitored and kept below 105°F; otherwise, there is potential for airway burns. Alternatively, "artificial noses" (**passive heat and moisture exchangers**) can be placed between the endotracheal tube and breathing circuit. These are hygroscopic membrane filters with large surface areas that trap the humidity of expired air.

6.   Warming blankets placed beneath the patient can increase body temperature by conduction from warm water pumped through the blanket. This method is most effective in children less than 10 kg. The temperature should be kept below 40°C to avoid burns.

7. Radiant warmers and heating lamps warm patients by infrared radiation and are only useful for infants. The warming lamps should be kept at least 70 cm from the patient to avoid burns.

8. Warming irrigation solutions will reduce heat loss.

VIII. Hyperthermia is an increase in temperature of 2°C/h or 0.5°C/15 min. It is uncommon for a patient to become hyperthermic because of maneuvers to conserve body heat in the operating room. Because a decrease in temperature during anesthesia is usually the rule, any increase in temperature must be investigated. Hyperthermia and its accompanying hypermetabolic state produce an increase in oxygen consumption, cardiac work, glucose demand, and compensatory minute ventilation. Sweating and vasodilation will result in decreased intravascular volume and venous return.

A. Etiologies

1. Malignant hyperthermia must be considered during any perioperative temperature increase (see section XVII).

2. Inflammation, infection, and sepsis with release of inflammatory mediators may cause hyperthermia.

3. Hypermetabolic states such as thyrotoxicosis and pheochromocytoma may cause hyperthermia.

4. Injury to the hypothalamic thermoregulatory center from anoxia, edema, trauma, or tumor may affect temperature set points in the hypothalamus.

5. Neuroleptic malignant syndrome (NMS) from neuroleptics such as phenothiazines is a rare cause.

6. Sympathomimetics such as monoamine oxidase inhibitors, amphetamines, cocaine, and tricyclic antidepressants may produce a hypermetabolic state.

7. Anticholinergics, such as atropine and glycopyrrolate, may promote unopposed sympathetic vasoconstriction and suppress sweating.

B. Treatment

1. If malignant hyperthermia is suspected, dantrolene treatment must be initiated (see section XVII).

2. Severe hyperthermia can be treated by cooling exposed body surfaces (skin) with ice, cooling blankets, and reduced ambient temperature or by performing internal lavage (stomach, bladder, bowel, and peritoneum) using cold saline. Volatile liquids such as alcohol and Freon applied to the skin will promote evaporative heat loss. Conductive heat loss can be increased with vasodilators such as nitroprusside and nitroglycerin. Centrally active agents such as aspirin and acetaminophen can be given by nasogastric tube or rectally. Shivering can be prevented by maintaining neuromuscular blockade. When hyperthermia is profound, **extracorporeal cooling** can be used. Cooling should be stopped when body temperature reaches 38°C to avoid hypothermia.

IX. Diaphoresis (sweating) may occur in response to the sympathetic discharge caused by anxiety, pain, hypercarbia, or noxious stimuli in the presence of inadequate anesthesia. It may also be seen in conjunction with bradycardia, nausea, and hypotension as part of a generalized vagal reaction or as a thermoregulatory response to hyperthermia.

X. Laryngospasm

A. Laryngospasm is most commonly caused by an irritative stimulus to the airway during a light plane of anesthesia. Common noxious stimuli that may elicit this reflex include secretions, vomitus, blood, inhalation of pungent volatile anesthetics, oropharyngeal or nasopharyngeal airway placement, laryngoscopy, painful peripheral stimuli, and peritoneal traction during light anesthesia.

B. Reflex closure of the vocal cords, causing partial or total glottic obstruction, may be manifested in less severe cases by crowing respirations or stridor and, when complete, by a "rocking" obstructed pattern of breathing. In this situation, the abdominal wall rises with contraction of the diaphragm during inspiration, but because air entry is blocked the chest retracts or fails to expand. During expiration, the abdomen falls as the diaphragm relaxes and the chest returns to its original position. With complete obstruction, the anesthetist will not be able to ventilate the patient.

C. The hypoxia, hypercarbia, and acidosis that result can cause hypertension and tachycardia. Hypotension, bradycardia, and ventricular arrhythmias leading to cardiac arrest will ensue unless airway patency is restored within minutes. Children, because of their small functional residual capacity and relatively high oxygen consumption, are particularly prone to these complications.

D. Treatment. Deepening the anesthetic level and removing the stimulus (e.g., by suction, withdrawal of an artificial airway, or stopping peripheral stimulation) while administering 100% oxygen may be adequate to relieve laryngospasm. If laryngospasm is not relieved, **continuous positive pressure on the airway** with a good mask fit may "break" the spasm; if not, a small dose of **succinylcholine** (e.g., 10 to 20 mg IV in an adult) will relax the striated muscles of the larynx. The lungs should be ventilated with 100% oxygen, and either the anesthetic level should be deepened before the noxious stimulation is resumed or the patient may be allowed to awaken if laryngospasm has occurred during emergence.

XI. Bronchospasm

A. Reflex bronchiolar constriction may be centrally mediated or may be a local response to airway irritation. Bronchospasm is common in anaphylactoid drug and blood transfusion reactions, as well as in cigarette smokers and those with chronic bronchitis. Like laryngospasm, bronchospasm may be elicited by noxious stimuli such as secretions or endotracheal intubation.

B. Wheezing (usually more pronounced on expiration) characterizes bronchospasm and is associated with tachypnea and dyspnea in the awake patient. An anesthetized patient may be difficult to ventilate due to increased airway resistance. Decreased expiratory flow rates may produce air trapping and increase intrathoracic pressure, decreasing venous return, cardiac output, and blood pressure.

C. Histamine-releasing drugs (e.g., morphine, d-tubocurarine, atracurium) may exacerbate bronchoconstriction.

D. Treatment

1. The **endotracheal tube position** should be checked and withdrawn slightly, if carinal stimulation is the cause.

2.   Deepening the anesthetic level will frequently reverse bronchospasm that is secondary to "light anesthesia." This usually can be accomplished with an inhalation agent, but an intravenous agent may be necessary when ventilation is significantly impaired. Propofol produces fewer symptoms of bronchoconstriction than barbiturates and is usually preferable. Ketamine has the advantage of causing bronchodilatation by releasing endogenous catecholamines. The inspired oxygen concentration should be increased until adequate oxygenation is achieved.

3.   Medical treatment includes the administration of inhaled or intravenous β_2-adrenergic agonists and anticholinergics (see Chapter 3). Inhaled bronchodilators have limited systemic absorption, which may minimize cardiovascular side effects. Nebulized forms may contain large particles, which deposit to a large extent in tubing and upper airways. The dosage of metered dose inhalers should be titrated to effect when administered into a breathing circuit. Large doses (10 to 20 puffs) may be necessary.

4.   Adequate hydration and humidification of inspired gases will minimize inspissation of secretions and facilitate ventilation.

XII.   Aspiration. General anesthesia causes a depression of airway reflexes that predisposes patients to aspiration. Aspiration of gastric contents from vomiting or regurgitation may cause bronchospasm, hypoxemia, atelectasis, tachypnea, tachycardia, and hypotension. The severity of symptoms depends on the volume and pH of the gastric material aspirated. Conditions that predispose to aspiration include gastric outlet obstruction, gastroesophageal reflux, small-bowel obstruction, symptomatic hiatal hernia, pregnancy, severe obesity, and recent food ingestion.

A.   If vomiting or regurgitation occurs in an anesthetized patient whose airway is not protected by an endotracheal tube, the patient should be placed in the Trendelenburg position to minimize passive flow of gastric contents into the trachea, the head should be turned to the side, the upper airway suctioned, and an endotracheal tube placed. Suctioning the endotracheal tube before instituting positive-pressure ventilation avoids forcing gastric contents into the distal airways. Evidence of significant aspiration includes wheezing, decreased lung compliance, and hypoxemia. A chest radiograph should be obtained, but radiographic evidence of infiltrates may be delayed. Bronchodilators may be useful.

B.   Bronchoscopy should be performed if a clinically significant aspiration is suspected. The airways should be suctioned clear and foreign bodies such as teeth and food removed. Lavage with large volumes of saline is not helpful.

C.   Aspiration of blood, unless of large volume, is usually benign.

D.   The administration of antibiotics usually is not warranted unless the material aspirated contains a high bacterial load such as with bowel obstruction (see Chapter 7).

E.   A sputum specimen should be obtained for Gram stain and culture.

F.   Steroids are not useful for the treatment of aspiration.

G.   If significant aspiration has occurred, it is imperative that close postoperative observation be undertaken. This includes pulse oximetry and repeat chest radiography. Ventilatory support and supplemental oxygen may be necessary (see Chapter 35).

XIII.   Pneumothorax is the accumulation of gas within the pleural space.
   A.   Etiologies include the following:
      1.   Spontaneous rupture of blebs and bullae.
      2.   Blunt or penetrating chest trauma.
      3.   Surgical entrance into the pleural space during thoracic, upper abdominal, or retroperitoneal surgery, tracheostomy, or surgery of the chest wall or neck.
      4.   As a complication of procedures such as subclavian or internal jugular vein catheter placement, thoracentesis, pericardiocentesis, or intercostal nerve blockade.
      5.   During positive-pressure ventilation using high pressures and volumes, causing barotrauma and alveolar rupture. Patients with chronic obstructive pulmonary disease are at particularly high risk.
      6.   Malfunction of chest tubes.
   B.   Physiologic effects of pneumothoraces are largely a function of the gas volume and the rate of expansion. Small pneumothoraces may have no significant cardiopulmonary effect; larger ones may result in significant lung collapse and hypoxemia. A tension pneumothorax occurs when there is a one-way leak into the pleural space, causing a significant increase in intrapleural pressure. This can result in compression of major blood vessels and mediastinal shift with hypotension and a reduction in cardiac output.
   C.   The **diagnosis** of pneumothorax can be difficult. Signs of pneumothorax include decreased breath sounds, a reduction in lung compliance, an increase in peak inspiratory pressure, hypoxemia, and wheezing. Hypotension reflects the presence of a tension pneumothorax. A chest radiograph usually can confirm the diagnosis, but treatment of an unstable patient should not be delayed.
   D.   Treatment. Nitrous oxide should be discontinued, and the patient should be ventilated with 100% oxygen. Tension pneumothoraces require immediate evacuation. A large-bore catheter (14 to 16 gauge) on a 10-mL syringe can be inserted into the pleural space at the second or third intercostal space in the mid-clavicular line and aspirated to confirm the presence of air. A chest tube then can be placed at the eighth intercostal space in the posterior axillary line.

XIV.   Myocardial ischemia
   A.   Etiology. Myocardial ischemia is the result of an imbalance between myocardial oxygen supply and consumption and, if untreated, may lead to MI.
   B.   Clinical features
      1.   In the awake patient, myocardial ischemia may manifest as **chest pain. Asymptomatic ischemia is common** in the perioperative period, however, particularly in diabetic patients. In patients under general anesthesia, hemodynamic instability and ECG changes may occur with ischemia.
      2.   ECG changes such as **ST segment depression** greater than 1 mm or T-wave inversion may indicate subendocardial ischemia. **ST segment elevation** is seen with transmural myo-

cardial ischemia. T-wave changes may also be seen with electrolyte abnormalities. Lead V_5 is the most sensitive lead for detecting ischemia (see Chapter 10).

3. Other indicators of ischemia include:
   a. Hypotension.
   b. Changes in central filling pressures or cardiac output.
   c. Regional wall motion abnormalities as detected with transesophageal echocardiography.

C. Treatment

1. Hypoxemia and anemia should be corrected to maximize myocardial oxygen delivery.

2. β-Adrenergic antagonists (propranolol in 0.5- to 1.0-mg increments IV or esmolol in 5- to 10-mg increments IV) decrease myocardial oxygen consumption by decreasing heart rate and contractility.

3. Nitroglycerin (starting at 25 to 50 μg/kg/min IV or 0.15 mg sublingually) reduces ventricular diastolic pressure and volume through venodilation and thus decreases myocardial oxygen demand. Additionally, nitroglycerin may improve oxygen delivery by enhancing collateral coronary flow.

4. Myocardial ischemia occurring in the setting of hypotension may require a vasopressor such as phenylephrine (10 to 40 μg/min IV) or norepinephrine (2 to 20 μg/min IV) to improve myocardial perfusion pressure. Anesthetic depth may need to be decreased and intravascular volume optimized.

5. When myocardial ischemia results in a significant reduction in cardiac output and hypotension (cardiogenic shock), positive **inotropes** such as dopamine (5 to 20 μg/kg/min IV), dobutamine (5 to 20 μg/kg/min IV), or norepinephrine (2 to 20 μg/min IV) are indicated. Intraaortic balloon counterpulsation may be life saving. A pulmonary artery catheter may be helpful in assessing ventricular function and response to therapy.

6. Aspirin, heparinization, thrombolytic therapy, angioplasty, and coronary revascularization may be considered in selected patients.

XV. Pulmonary embolism is the obstruction of pulmonary blood flow by thrombus, air, fat, or amniotic fluid.

A. Thromboemboli most commonly arise from the deep venous system of the pelvis and lower extremities. Predisposing factors for the development of thrombi are stasis, hypercoagulability, and vascular wall abnormalities. Associated conditions include pregnancy, trauma, carcinoma, prolonged bed rest, and vasculitis.

1. Physical findings are nonspecific and include tachypnea and tachycardia, dyspnea, bronchospasm, and fever.

2. Laboratory studies. The ECG reveals a nonspecific tachycardia unless embolization is severe, in which case right-axis deviation, right bundle branch block, and anterior T-wave changes may be seen. The chest radiograph may be unremarkable unless pulmonary infarction has occurred. Typically, hypoxemia is present. With a large embolism, the end-tidal carbon dioxide will be decreased. In spontaneously breathing patients, hypocapnia and respiratory alkalosis may result from the increased respiratory rate. Definitive diagnosis requires a pulmonary angiogram or high-resolution computed tomography of the chest.

3.   Intraoperative treatment of a suspected pulmonary embolism is supportive. Oxygenation is increased. Intraoperative heparinization or thrombolytic therapy is usually not an option because of the risk of hemorrhage. In patients who are severely hypoxic or hypotensive, cardiopulmonary bypass and pulmonary embolectomy may be considered.

B.   Air embolism occurs during entrainment of air into a vein or venous sinus. It occurs most commonly during intracranial surgery in the sitting position, where dural venous sinuses are stented open. Air embolism may also occur during liver transplantation, open cardiac procedures, and insufflation during laparoscopy.

1.   Early indicators include air seen by transesophageal echocardiography or heard with a precordial Doppler, a decrease in end-tidal carbon dioxide tension, and an increase in end-tidal nitrogen tension.

2.   Late indicators include increased central venous pressure, hypoxemia, hypotension, ventricular ectopy, and a continuous "mill-wheel" precordial murmur.

3.   Treatment begins with limiting the entrainment of additional air by flooding the surgical field with saline or repositioning the patient so that venous pressure is increased. Nitrous oxide should be discontinued to avoid enlarging the size of bubbles within the circulation. Placing the patient in left lateral decubitus position may help to reduce air lock. If a central venous catheter is in place, it should be aspirated in an attempt to remove air. Fluid and vasopressors are used to maintain blood pressure.

4.   The use of PEEP in the setting of air embolism is controversial. It will limit the entrainment of air by raising central venous pressure but at the expense of reducing venous return and possibly cardiac output. **Hyperbaric oxygen** may decrease the side effects of the bubbles.

C.   Fat embolism occurs after trauma or surgery involving the long bones, pelvis, or ribs.

1.   Clinical features are related to mechanical obstruction of the pulmonary circulation and are similar to those found with pulmonary thromboembolism. The release of free fatty acids may lead to diminished mental status, worsening hypoxemia, fat globules in the urine, and petechial hemorrhages.

2.   Treatment is supportive, with the administration of supplemental oxygen and ventilation as necessary.

D.   Amniotic fluid emboli (see Chapter 29).

XVI.   Cardiac tamponade. Accumulation of blood or other fluid within the pericardial sac may prevent adequate ventricular filling and reduce stroke volume and cardiac output. When the accumulation is rapid, cardiovascular collapse may occur within minutes.

A.   Cardiac tamponade may be associated with:

1.   Chest trauma.

2.   Cardiac or thoracic surgery.

3.   Pericardial tumor.

4.   Pericarditis (acute viral, pyogenic, uremic, or postradiation).

5.   Myocardial perforation by a central venous or pulmonary artery catheter.

6.   Aortic dissection.

B.   Clinical features include tachycardia, hypotension, jugular venous distention, muffled heart sounds, and a decrease in pulse pressure. An ECG may reveal **electrical alternans** and diffusely low voltage. A **paradoxical pulse** (greater than a 10 mm Hg inspiratory decrease in systolic blood pressure) may be appreciated. There is **equalization of right and left heart pressures** as reflected in identical central venous, right ventricular end diastolic pressure, pulmonary artery diastolic pressure, and pulmonary capillary wedge pressures. Radiographic findings may include an enlarged cardiac silhouette. An **echocardiogram** is diagnostic.

C. The **treatment** of a hemodynamically unstable patient with suspected cardiac tamponade is pericardiocentesis. Intravascular volume should be augmented and vasopressors that maintain chronotropy and inotropy (e.g., dopamine) are administered to maintain blood pressure. A long needle (i.e., 22-gauge spinal needle) is inserted between the xiphoid process and the left costal margin and directed toward the left shoulder. If the precordial lead of the ECG is attached to the needle, an injury current (ST segment elevation) will be observed when the needle contacts the epicardium. The needle should be withdrawn slightly and aspirated. **Complications of pericardiocentesis** include pneumothorax, coronary artery laceration, and myocardial perforation.

XVII. Malignant hyperthermia

A. Etiology. Malignant hyperthermia is a hypermetabolic syndrome occurring in genetically susceptible patients after exposure to an anesthetic triggering agent. **Triggering anesthetics** include halothane, enflurane, isoflurane, desflurane, sevoflurane, and succinylcholine. The syndrome is thought to be due to a reduction in the reuptake of Ca^{2+} by the sarcoplasmic reticulum necessary for termination of muscle contraction. Consequently, muscle contraction is sustained, resulting in signs of hypermetabolism, including tachycardia, acidosis, hypercarbia, hypoxemia, and hyperthermia. The first signs of malignant hyperthermia usually occur in the operating room but may be delayed until the patient reaches the postanesthesia care unit or even the postoperative floor.

B. Clinical features

1. Unexplained tachycardia.

2. Hypercarbia or tachypnea in the spontaneously breathing patient.

3. Acidosis.

4. Muscle rigidity even in the presence of neuromuscular blockade. Masseter spasm after giving succinylcholine is associated with malignant hyperthermia. However, not all patients who develop masseter spasm will develop malignant hyperthermia.

5. Hypoxemia.

6. Ventricular arrhythmias.

7. Hyperkalemia.

8. Fever is a late sign.

9. Myoglobinuria.

10. The presence of a large difference between mixed venous and arterial carbon dioxide tensions confirms the diagnosis of malignant hyperthermia.

C. Treatment

1. Summon help as soon as malignant hyperthermia is suspected. Discontinue all triggering anesthetics, and hyperventilate with 100% oxygen. Surgery should be concluded as quickly as possible and the anesthesia machine changed when feasible.

2. Administer dantrolene (Dantrium), 3 mg/kg IV initially and repeated to a total of 10 mg/kg or more if signs of malignant hyperthermia persist. Dantrolene is the only known specific treatment for malignant hyperthermia. Its efficacy is due to its ability to inhibit Ca^{2+} release from the sarcoplasmic reticulum. Each ampule contains 20 mg of dantrolene and 3 g of mannitol and should be reconstituted with 50 mL of warm sterile water.

3. Sodium bicarbonate administration should be guided by pH and partial pressure of carbon dioxide (P_{CO_2}) measurements.

4. Hyperkalemia may be corrected with insulin and glucose. However, hypokalemia may occur as the attack is brought under control. Calcium is avoided.

5. Arrhythmias generally subside with resolution of the hypermetabolic phase of malignant hyperthermia. Persistent arrhythmias can be treated with procainamide.

6. Hyperthermia is treated by a variety of methods (see section VIII).

7. Urine output ideally should be maintained at 2 mL/kg/min to avoid renal tubular damage from myoglobin. This is done by maintaining adequate central filling pressures and administering furosemide or mannitol.

8. Recrudescence, disseminated intravascular coagulation, and acute tubular necrosis may occur after an acute episode of malignant hyperthermia. Therefore, dantrolene therapy (1 mg/kg IV or orally every 6 hours) and observation should be continued for 48 to 72 hours after an episode of malignant hyperthermia.

D. Anesthesia for malignant hyperthermia-susceptible patients

1. A **family history** of anesthetic problems suggesting susceptibility, such as unexplained fevers or death during anesthesia, should be sought in every patient.

2. Malignant hyperthermia may be triggered in susceptible patients who have had previous uneventful exposures to triggering agents.

3. Pretreatment with dantrolene generally is not recommended for malignant hyperthermia-susceptible patients. A malignant hyperthermia cart or other dantrolene supply, however, should be immediately available.

4. The anesthesia machine should be prepared by changing the carbon dioxide absorbent and fresh gas tubing, disconnecting the vaporizers, using a disposable breathing circuit, and flushing the machine with oxygen at a rate of 10 L/min for 5 minutes.

5. Local or regional anesthesia should be considered, but general anesthesia with nontriggering agents is acceptable. **Safe drugs** for induction and maintenance of general anesthesia include barbiturates, propofol, benzodiazepines, opioids, and nitrous oxide. Nondepolarizing neuromuscular blockers may be used and safely reversed.

6. Close monitoring for early signs of malignant hyperthermia such as unexplained hypercarbia or tachycardia is crucial.

E. Associated syndromes. An increased risk of malignant hyperthermia has been reported in association with a number of disorders. In many of these cases, the association is not well established. However, patients with the following disorders should be treated as though they are susceptible to malignant hyperthermia:

1. Duchenne muscular dystrophy and other **muscular dystrophies**.

2. King-Denborough syndrome, characterized by dwarfism, mental retardation, and musculoskeletal abnormalities.

3. Central core disease, a rare myopathy.

4. NMS, which is associated with the administration of neuroleptic drugs and shares many of the features of malignant hyperthermia.

   a. Clinical features. NMS typically develops over 24 to 72 hours and is clinically similar to malignant hyperthermia, presenting as a hypermetabolic episode consisting of hyperthermia, autonomic nervous system instability, pronounced muscle rigidity, and rhabdomyolysis. Creatine kinase and hepatic transaminases often are increased, and mortality approaches 30%.

   b. Treatment of NMS is with dantrolene, although benzodiazepines, dopamine antagonists like bromocriptine, and nondepolarizing muscle relaxants will also decrease muscle rigidity.

   c. Anesthetic implications. The exact relationship between NMS and malignant hyperthermia is unclear. Some patients with a history of NMS may be at risk for malignant hyperthermia, and a conservative approach may be warranted (e.g., avoidance of known triggering agents). Patients with NMS must be appropriately monitored for malignant hyperthermia during all anesthetics (e.g., temperature, end-tidal carbon dioxide). They should not be pretreated with dantrolene.

XVIII. Anaphylactic and anaphylactoid reactions

A. Anaphylaxis is a life-threatening allergic reaction. It is initiated by antigen binding to IgE antibodies on the surface of mast cells and basophils, which causes release of pharmacologically active substances. These include histamine, leukotrienes, prostaglandins, kinins, and platelet-activating factor.

B. Anaphylactoid reactions are clinically similar to anaphylactic reactions, but they are not mediated by IgE and do not require prior sensitization to an antigen.

C. Clinical features of anaphylactic or anaphylactoid reactions include:

1. Urticaria and flushing.

2. Bronchospasm or airway edema, which can produce respiratory failure.

3. Hypotension and shock due to peripheral vasodilation and increased capillary permeability.

4. Pulmonary edema.

D. Treatment

1. Discontinue anesthetic agents if circulatory collapse is present.

2. Administer 100% oxygen. Assess the need to intubate and support ventilation.

3. Treat hypotension with intravascular volume expansion.

4.   Give epinephrine, 50 to 100 µg IV. For overt cardiovascular collapse, epinephrine, 0.5 to 1.0 mg IV, is indicated, followed by an infusion if hypotension persists. Other catecholamines such as norepinephrine may be useful.

5.   Steroids (hydrocortisone, 250 mg to 1.0 g IV, or methylprednisolone, 1 to 2 g IV) may reduce the inflammatory response.

6.   Histamine antagonists (diphenhydramine, 50 mg IV, and ranitidine, 50 mg IV in the adult) may be useful as second-line therapy.

E.   Prophylaxis for drug hypersensitivity reactions

1.   Histamine (H_1) antagonists. Diphenhydramine (0.5 to 1.0 mg/kg or 50 mg IV in the adult) the night before and morning of exposure.

2. H_2 antagonists. Cimetidine (150 to 300 mg IV or orally in the adult) or ranitidine (50 mg IV or 150 mg orally in the adult) the night before and morning of exposure.

3.   Corticosteroids. Prednisone (1 mg/kg or 50 mg for adults) every 6 hours for four doses before exposure.

XIX.   Fire and electrical hazards in the operating room

A.   Fire in the operating room is a rare event that requires the presence of an ignition source, fuel, and an oxidizing agent.

1.   Lasers and electrocautery devices are the most common ignition sources.

2.   Fuels include alcohol, solvents, sheets, drapes, and plastic or rubber materials (including endotracheal tubes). Unlike diethyl ether and cyclopropane, modern inhalation anesthetics are not fuels. During an electrical fire, it is important to remember to unplug the electrical source.

3.   Oxygen is by far the most common oxidizing agent, although nitrous oxide will also support combustion. Materials that are only marginally combustible in air can produce a massive flame in the presence of a high oxygen concentration. Supplemental oxygen can accumulate under surgical drapes and should only be administered when medically indicated.

4.   Fire extinguishers should be readily available in all anesthetizing locations. Carbon dioxide or Halon fire extinguishers offer the advantage of efficacy against a variety of fires without producing the particulate contamination associated with dry chemical extinguishers.

B.   Electrical safety

1.   Macroshock is an electrical injury caused when a current passes through intact skin. It may produce a thermal injury, or it may disrupt normal physiologic function and cause cardiac or respiratory arrest. An alternating current of 60 cycles/sec will barely be perceptible at a current of 1 mA. A current of 10 to 20 mA results in a sustained muscular contraction referred to as the "let go current." At this current, a person is unable to let go of an electrical wire. Currents exceeding 100 mA may cause ventricular fibrillation.

2.   Conventional electrical circuits are grounded. They consist of three wires referred to as "hot," "neutral," and "ground." The danger of such circuits is that contact between the hot wire and an instrument's metal case (fault) can cause shock if a person contacts the case and ground. Fortunately, an intact ground wire provides a low-resistance pathway for current flow, which significantly reduces the current that passes through the case. An added measure of safety is provided by using an ungrounded electrical circuit in the operating room. This system uses an **isolation transformer** that isolates the power from ground. In such a system, an individual would have to contact both conductors simultaneously to be at risk of a shock. **In an ungrounded electrical circuit, a single fault does not result in shock hazard or power disruption.** A single fault simply converts an ungrounded system into a grounded system. All equipment will continue to function normally. The integrity of the circuit is monitored with a **line isolation monitor**. It alarms when a single fault capable of producing a "ground-seeking current" of more than 5 mA occurs. When this occurs, the offending piece of equipment should be sought out and removed, because a second fault may result in a shock hazard.

3. Microshock occurs when current passes directly to the heart. Commonly used guidewires and pacing wires provide electrical conduits to the heart. Ventricular fibrillation can be produced by as little as 100 μA of current applied to the myocardium. This is well below the 5 mA required before a line isolation monitor alarms. Line isolation monitors therefore do not protect a patient from microshock. To minimize the likelihood of microshock, all equipment should be properly grounded with a three-prong plug, and connections to the patient should be electrically isolated. Battery operation does not ensure electrical isolation.

4. Burns from electrosurgical units (Bovie) may result from poor contact between the dispersive electrode (grounding pad) and the patient, because electrical power dissipation is proportional to the resistance at the skin. Under such conditions, anything that is grounded may provide an alternate pathway for current to flow, resulting in burns at sites distant from the dispersive electrode. The risk of burn can be minimized by ensuring that the electrode gel is adequate, that the dispersive electrode is placed near the surgical site, and that the patient is insulated from possible alternative pathways for current flow.

SUGGESTED READING

Beebe JJ, Sessler DI. Preparation of anesthesia machines for patients susceptible to malignant hyperthermia. *Anesthesiology* 1988;69: 395–400.

Gravenstein N, Kirby RR. *Complications in anesthesiology*. Philadelphia: Lippincott, 1995.

Levy JH. Allergic reactions during anesthesia. *J Clin Anesth* 1988;1: 39–46.

Litt L, Ehrenwerth J. Electrical safety in the operating room: important old wine, disguised new bottles. *Anesth Analg* 1994;78:417–419.

Marik PE. Aspiration pneumonitis and aspiration pneumonia. *N Engl J Med* 2001;344:665–671.

Sessler DI. Complications and treatment of mild hypothermia. *Anesthesiology* 2001;95:531–543.

Stoelting RK, Dierdorf SF. *Anesthesia and co-existing disease*. New York: Churchill Livingstone, 1993.

19

Perioperative Hemodynamic Control

Vilma E. Ortiz and Robert R. Morgan, Jr.

I. **Blood flow.** Systemic blood pressure is monitored as a reflection of local tissue perfusion. This is because pressure is much easier to measure clinically than flow. Organs, however, require an adequate blood flow rather than a minimal blood pressure to meet their metabolic needs.

A. **Ohm's Law**: Pressure (i.e., blood pressure) = Flow (i.e., cardiac output) × Resistance

Organ blood flow = (mean arterial pressure [MAP] − organ venous pressure) / organ vascular resistance

B. **Cardiac output** is influenced by heart rate, preload, afterload, and myocardial compliance and contractility. These variables are separate yet intimately interdependent and controlled by the autonomic nervous system and humoral mechanisms.

II. **Autoregulation.** The ability of an organ or vascular bed to maintain adequate blood flow despite varying blood pressure is termed autoregulation. Metabolic regulation controls about 75% of all local blood flow in the body. Organs have differing ability (autoregulatory reserve) to increase or decrease their vascular resistance to provide tight coupling between metabolic demand and organ blood flow. In general, anesthetics inhibit autoregulation, making organ perfusion more pressure dependent. The most important of these organs are the brain, kidneys, heart, and lungs (see appropriate chapters for detailed discussions on each).

III. **Adrenergic receptor physiology.** Adrenergic receptors can be distinguished by their response to a series of catecholamines. Receptors that demonstrate an order of potency such that norepinephrine > epinephrine > isoproterenol are termed **α receptors**. Those receptors that respond with an order of potency isoproterenol > epinephrine > norepinephrine are termed **β receptors**. Receptors that interact exclusively with dopamine are termed **dopaminergic**. Adrenergic receptors can be further subdivided based on their pharmacology and anatomic location.

A. **α_1 Receptors** are located postsynaptically in vascular smooth muscle and in the smooth muscle of the coronary arteries, uterus, skin, intestinal mucosa, iris, and splanchnic bed. Activation causes arteriolar and venous constriction, mydriasis, and relaxation of the intestinal tract. Cardiac α_1 receptors increase inotropy and decrease heart rate.

B. **α_2 Receptors**

1. **Presynaptic α_2 receptors** are located within the central nervous system (CNS), specifically the locus ceruleus and substantia gelatinosa. Activation causes inhibition of norepineph-

rine, acetylcholine, serotonin, dopamine, and substance P release. Activation has been associated with hypnotic and sedative effects, antinociceptive action, hypotension, and bradycardia.

2. **Postsynaptic α_2 receptors** are located peripherally in vascular smooth muscle, the gastrointestinal tract, pancreatic beta cells, and within the CNS. Activation of peripheral postsynaptic α_2 receptors causes vasoconstriction and a hypertensive (pressor) response, decreased salivation, and decreased insulin release. Activation of the central receptors is associated with analgesia and an anesthesia-sparing effect.

C. **β_1 Receptors** are located in the myocardium, the sinoatrial node, the ventricular conduction system, adipose tissue, and renal tissue. Activation causes an increase in inotropy, chronotropy, myocardial conduction velocity, renin release, and lipolysis.

D. **β_2 Receptors** are located in vascular, bronchial, uterine smooth muscle, and the smooth muscle in skin. Stimulation leads to vasodilation, bronchodilation, and uterine relaxation. β_2 Receptor activation also promotes gluconeogenesis, insulin release, and potassium uptake by cells.

E. **β_3 Receptors** are involved in lipolysis and regulation of metabolic rate.

F. **Dopaminergic receptors**

    1. **Dopaminergic-1 receptors** are located postsynaptically on renal and mesenteric vascular smooth muscle and mediate vasodilation.

    2. **Dopaminergic-2 receptors** are presynaptic and inhibit norepinephrine release.

G. **Receptor regulation**. There is an inverse relationship between receptor number and the concentration of circulating adrenergic agonist and the duration of exposure to that agonist. This is termed receptor up-regulation and down-regulation. Sudden cessation of beta-blockade therapy may be associated with rebound hypertension and tachycardia with resulting myocardial ischemia. This is a result of β-receptor proliferation (up-regulation) and consequent hypersensitivity to endogenous catecholamines.

IV. **Adrenergic pharmacology** (Table 19-1)

A. **α Agonists**

    1. **Phenylephrine** is a direct-acting α_1 agonist at normal clinical doses, with some β-receptor activity at extremely high concentrations. Phenylephrine causes both arterial and venous vasoconstriction. This dual action increases venous return (preload) and mean arterial blood pressure (afterload). Phenylephrine maintains cardiac output in patients with a normal heart but may decrease cardiac performance in an ischemic heart. Phenylephrine has a short duration of action that makes it easily titratable.

    2. **Clonidine** is a centrally acting antihypertensive with relative selectivity for α_2 adrenoreceptors. Its actions include reducing sympathetic tone, increasing parasympathetic activity, reducing anesthetic and analgesic requirements, causing sedation, and decreasing salivation. It can be administered intravenously, intramuscularly, orally, transcutaneously, and into the intrathecal and epidural spaces.

Table 19-1. Commonly used vasopressors and inotropes

Drug Name (Trade Name)	IV Bolus	IV Infusion	Dose	Adrenergic Effects			
				α	β	DA	V
Dopamine (Inotropin)	NR	a. 200 mg/250 mL b. 800 µg/mL c. 1–20 µg/kg/min d. 5–10 min	Low High	 ++	 ++	+++ +++	
Dobutamine (Dobutrex)	NR	a. 250 mg/250 mL b. 1,000 µg/mL c. 2–20 µg/kg/min d. 5–10 min		+	+++		
Ephedrine	5–10 mg	NR 5–10 min duration		+	++		
Epinephrine (Adrenalin)	20–100 mg (hypotension); 0.5–1 mg (cardiac arrest)	a. 1 mg/250 mL b. 4 µg/mL c. 0.5–5 µg/min d. 1–2 min	Low High	+ +++	+++ ++++		

Drug	Bolus	IV infusion		α	β₁	β₂	V	Nonsympathomimetic
Inamrinone	NR	0.75–1.5 mg/kg IV load, then 5–10 µg/kg/min; 2.5–12 h duration						+++
Isoproterenol (Isuprel)	NR	a. 1 mg/250 mL b. 4 µg/mL c. 2–10 µg/min d. 5–10 min			++++	++++		
Norepinephrine (Levophed)	NR	a. 4 mg/250 mL b. 16 µg/mL c. 1–30 µg/min d. 1–2 min	Low High	++++	++++	+ ++		
Phenylephrine (Neo-Synephrine)	40–100 µg	a. 10 mg/250 mL b. 40 µg/mL c. 10–150 µg/min d. 5–10 min		++++				
Vasopressin (Pitressin)	40 U (cardiac arrest)	a. 50 U/250 mL b. 0.2 U/mL c. 0.01–0.1 U/min d. 10–20 min					+++	+++

a, mix in 5% dextrose in water; b, concentration; c, common IV dosage range; d, duration; DA, dopaminergic; IV, intravenous; NR, not recommended; V, vasopressin.

B.   β Agonists. Isoproterenol is a direct-acting β-adrenergic agonist. It causes an increase in heart rate and contractility while reducing systemic vascular resistance (SVR). It is also a pulmonary vasodilator and a bronchodilator.

1.   Indications

a.   Hemodynamically significant, atropine-resistant brady-cardia.

b.   Atrioventricular block until temporary pacing can be instituted.

c.   Low cardiac output states requiring fast heart rates (pediatric patients who have a fixed stroke volume, cardiac transplant recipients).

d.   Status asthmaticus.

e.   Beta-blockade overdose.

2.   Continuous electrocardiographic monitoring is recommended with intravenous administration, which may be through a peripheral intravenous line.

3.   Side effects include vasodilation, hypotension, and tachyarrhythmias.

C.   Mixed agonists

1.   Epinephrine is a direct-acting α- and β-receptor agonist produced by the adrenal medulla.

a.   Indications

(1)   Cardiac arrest.

(2)   Anaphylaxis.

(3)   Bronchospasm.

(4)   Cardiogenic shock.

(5)   Prolongation of regional anesthesia.

b.   The clinical effect of epinephrine is the sum of its α- and β-receptor activation on various tissue beds, with β effects predominating at lower doses. At lower doses, epinephrine causes bronchodilation, vasodilation, increased cardiac output, and tachycardia. As the dose of epinephrine increases, α effects predominate, and stroke volume may fall as SVR (afterload) increases. Significant tachycardia, arrhythmias, and myocardial ischemia may limit the usefulness of epinephrine in the clinical setting. Volatile anesthetics (especially halothane) can sensitize the myocardium to circulating catecholamines to produce potentially life-threatening arrhythmias. Epinephrine should be administered through a central intravenous line, because severe tissue necrosis can occur if it extravasates.

2.   Norepinephrine, the neurotransmitter of the sympathetic nervous system, is the biosynthetic precursor of epinephrine. Norepinephrine is a potent α- and β_1-receptor agonist, with α effects predominating at lower doses. Compared with epinephrine, it has minimal effects on β_2 receptors. Norepinephrine increases blood pressure by increasing SVR (afterload), whereas cardiac output remains relatively unchanged. Myocardial performance may improve, if the increased blood pressure improves coronary blood flow and relieves myocardial ischemia. Norepinephrine increases the vascular resistance of most organs, thereby diminishing organ blood flow despite increases in MAP. It is useful in the setting of hypotension that is associated with mild myocardial depression. As with most vasoactive drugs, electrocardiogram and invasive monitoring are recommended to follow clinical effectiveness, and the drug should be administered centrally.

3. Dopamine, the immediate precursor of norepinephrine, produces a dose-related combination of α-, β-, and dopamine-receptor effects. It is a neurotransmitter in the basal ganglia and chemoreceptor trigger zone. At lower doses (approximately < 4 μg/kg/min), renal and splanchnic vessel dopamine receptors are activated primarily, resulting in increased renal blood flow, glomerular filtration, and sodium (Na^+) excretion. As the concentration of dopamine is increased, β effects become apparent, leading to increases in myocardial contractility, heart rate, and arterial blood pressure. At high doses (>10 μg/kg/min), α_1 effects predominate, leading to marked increases in arterial and venous blood pressure and decreases in renal blood flow. Dopamine also causes release of norepinephrine from nerve terminals. Dopamine administration often increases urine output but does not prevent renal injury or alter its course. Dopamine may be indicated in states of shock associated with a failing myocardium, but tachycardia (often seen even at lower doses), increased myocardial oxygen consumption, and profound vasoconstriction frequently limit its clinical usefulness.

4. Dobutamine is a synthetic catecholamine that has β_1-, β_2-, and α_1-adrenergic receptor activity. Dobutamine is a mixture of stereoisomers; the L(−)-isomer stimulates α_1 receptors and the D(+)-isomer has β_1- and β_2-receptor activity. Dobutamine increases myocardial contractility through its effect on cardiac α_1 and β_1 receptors. In the peripheral vasculature, dobutamine is a vasodilator, because its β_2 effect overshadows its α_1 properties. Dobutamine may increase heart rate secondary to the positive chronotropic effects of β_1 activation. It is a useful agent for the treatment of low output states caused by myocardial dysfunction secondary to acute infarction, cardiomyopathy, or myocardial depression after cardiac surgery. Hemodynamic effects of dobutamine are similar to those of a combination of dopamine and nitroprusside. Dobutamine typically increases cardiac output and decreases SVR with minimal effects on arterial blood pressure and heart rate. Pulmonary vascular resistance (PVR) decreases, making dobutamine beneficial for patients with right heart failure. Systemic hypotension (dobutamine is an inotrope, not a pressor), increased myocardial oxygen consumption, and arrhythmias are the most common side effects.

5. Ephedrine is a plant-derived, noncatecholamine, direct, and indirect adrenergic agonist. Ephedrine causes the release of norepinephrine and other endogenous catecholamines stored within nerve terminals. Tachyphylaxis limits ephedrine use to bolus administration for the temporary treatment of hypotension associated with hypovolemia, sympathetic blockade, myocardial depression due to anesthetic overdose, or bradycardia.

D. Nonadrenergic sympathomimetic agents

1. Inamrinone (previously known as amrinone) and milrinone are synthetic, noncatecholamine, nonglycosidic, bipyridine derivatives. They act by inhibiting type III phosphodiesterase, thereby increasing cyclic adenosine monophosphate levels and causing increased contractility and peripheral vasodilation. Their action is independent of adrenergic receptors, and as such their effects are additive to that of adrenergic agents.

a.   **Inamrinone** produces a dose-dependent improvement in cardiac index, left ventricular work index, and ejection fraction. Heart rate and MAP remain constant. Time to peak effect is about 5 minutes, and hepatic elimination occurs with a half-life of 5 to 12 hours depending on the severity of cardiac disease. Side effects are uncommon and include dose-dependent but reversible hypotension, thrombocytopenia, liver function test abnormalities, fever, and gastrointestinal distress.

b.   **Milrinone** is a derivative of inamrinone and shares the same hemodynamic profile. Milrinone is 20 times more potent than inamrinone and lacks many of the side effects associated with its parent compound.

2.   **Arginine vasopressin (AVP)** is a synthetic analogue of antidiuretic hormone, which is produced by the posterior pituitary. AVP causes vasoconstriction by direct stimulation of smooth muscle V-1 receptors. It is a recommended alternative to epinephrine in the treatment of adult shock-refractory ventricular fibrillation as a one-time bolus (40 units IV). It may also be beneficial as a low dose (0.04 units/min) intravenous infusion in the setting of vasodilatory shock. AVP has a rapid onset with a duration of action of 10 to 20 minutes. Administration through a central line is recommended.

V.   β-Adrenergic antagonists (Table 19-2)

A.   **Propranolol** is a nonselective β_1- and β_2-adrenergic receptor antagonist available in both intravenous and oral forms. Propranolol is the prototype β-adrenergic antagonist against which other drugs in this class are judged. Propranolol is highly lipophilic, is almost entirely absorbed after oral administration, and undergoes up to 75% first-pass clearance by the liver. Hemodynamic effects of propranolol and other β-adrenergic antagonists are secondary to a reduction of cardiac output and suppression of the renin-angiotensin system. β-Adrenergic antagonists can be distinguished by their relative β_1 selectivity, their intrinsic sympathomimetic activity, and their pharmacologic half-lives.

B.   **Metoprolol** is a selective β_1-adrenergic receptor antagonist available in both oral and intravenous forms. It may be used perioperatively to treat supraventricular tachycardias. It is also effective in the treatment of angina pectoris, reducing mortality from myocardial infarction, and in treating mild to moderate hypertension. Metoprolol has an oral to intravenous beta-blockade ratio of 2.5:1.

C.   **Esmolol** is a selective β_1-adrenergic receptor antagonist that is metabolized rapidly by an esterase located in the cytoplasm of red blood cells. The time to its peak effect is 5 minutes and its elimination half-life is 9 minutes. Esmolol is valuable perioperatively because it can be administered intravenously, has a fast onset, has a very short duration of action, and can be given to patients with asthma, chronic obstructive pulmonary disease, or myocardial dysfunction. The red blood cell esterase is different from plasma pseudocholinesterase and is not affected by anticholinesterases. Rapid administration of esmolol in large boluses has

Table 19-2. β-Adrenergic antagonists

Drug Name (Trade Name)	β₁ Selectivity	Bioavailability (%)	Beta Half-Life[a]	Elimination	Usual Oral Dose	IV Dose
Atenolol (Tenormin)	++	55	6–9 h	R (85%)	50–100 mg qd	5-mg increments
Esmolol (Brevibloc)	++	—	9 min	Red blood cell esterase		10–20-mg bolus; 0.25–0.5-mg/kg load, then 50–200 μg/kg/min
Labetalol (Trandate, Normodyne)	0	25	3–8 h	H	100 mg bid	5–10-mg bolus; 10–40 mg/h titrated upward
Metoprolol (Lopressor)	++	50	3–6 h	H	25–100 mg qd–qid	5–25-mg increments
Nadolol (Corgard)	0	20	14–24 h	R (75%)	40–240 mg qd	NR
Propranolol (Inderal)	0	33	3–4 h	H	10–40 mg bid–qid	0.25–1-mg increments
Timolol (Blocadren)	0	75	4–5 h	H (80%) R (20%)	5–15 mg qd–bid	NR

H, hepatic elimination; IV, intravenous; NR, not recommended; R, renal elimination.
[a]Beta half-life may not be predictive of clinical duration of action.

Table 19-3.   Vasodilator drugs

Drug Name (Trade Name)	IV Bolus	IV Infusion	Mechanisms of Action
Fenoldopam (Corlopam)	NR	a. 10 mg/250 mL b. 40 μg/mL c. 0.05–1.5 μg/kg/min d. 1–4 h	D1-receptor agonist; moderate α_2-receptor affinity
Hydralazine (Apresoline)	2.5–5 mg q15 min, 20–40 mg IV q4–6 h	NR	Direct-acting vascular smooth muscle dilation
Labetalol (Trandate, Normodyne)	5–10 mg q5 min	a. 200 mg/250 mL b. 0.8 mg/mL c. 10–40 mg/h d. 15 min	Alpha receptor and beta receptor blockade
Nitroglycerin	50–100 μg	a. 50 mg/250 mL b. 200 μg/mL c. 0.5–15 μg/kg/min d. 4 min	Venous vasodilator

Drug		Dosage	Mechanism
Nitroprusside (Nipride)	NR	a. 50 mg/250 mL b. 200 μg/mL c. 0.2 μg/kg/min[a] d. 4 min	Arterial > venous vasodilator
Phentolamine (Regitine)	1–5 mg	NR	Alpha receptor blockade
Prostaglandin E1 (Alprostadil)	NR	a. 1–2 mg/250 mL b. 4–8 μg/mL c. 0.05 μg/kg/min[a] d. 1 min	Direct vasodilator via prostaglandin receptors in vascular smooth muscle
Trimethaphan (Arfonad)	0.5–2 mg; begin with 1 mg bolus	a. 500 mg/500 mL b. 1 mg/mL c. 0.5–6 mg/min d. 5–10 min	Ganglionic blockade and histamine release

a, mix in 5% dextrose in water; b, concentration; c, usual IV dosage range; d, duration; IV, intravenous; NR, not recommended.
[a]Dose may be titrated higher to desired effect.

been associated with severe hypotension and cardiac depression, leading to cardiac arrest in some situations.

D. **Labetalol** is a mixed α- and β-adrenergic receptor antagonist with a β- to α-adrenergic receptor blockade ratio of 3:1 when given orally and 7:1 when administered intravenously. Labetalol decreases PVR, blunts the reflex increase in heart rate, and minimally affects cardiac output. Labetalol is useful intraoperatively to blunt the sympathetic response to tracheal intubation and to control hypertensive episodes. Labetalol is also used in the management of patients with pheochromocytomas and the clonidine withdrawal syndrome.

VI. Vasodilators (Table 19-3)

A. **Sodium nitroprusside** is a direct-acting vasodilator that acts on arterial and venous vascular smooth muscle.

1. The mechanism of action of sodium nitroprusside is common to all nitrates. The nitroso moiety decomposes to release nitric oxide. Nitric oxide is an unstable short-lived free radical that activates guanylate cyclase. This results in an increase in the concentration of cyclic guanosine monophosphate, which causes smooth muscle relaxation.

2. The hemodynamic effects of sodium nitroprusside are principally afterload reduction by arterial vasodilation and some preload reduction by increasing venous capacitance. These effects typically cause a reflex increase in heart rate and myocardial contractility, an increase in cardiac output, and marked decreases in SVR and PVR. Sodium nitroprusside dilates cerebral blood vessels and should be used with caution in patients with decreased intracranial compliance.

3. Sodium nitroprusside dilates all vascular beds equally, increasing overall blood flow. A vascular steal phenomenon may be created where blood flow to an ischemic region that is maximally vasodilated may be shunted to nonischemic regions that can vasodilate further. This is especially important in the coronary vasculature, where ischemia may be exacerbated with the use of sodium nitroprusside even though overall myocardial oxygen consumption has been reduced by afterload reduction.

4. Sodium nitroprusside is useful perioperatively because it has a fast onset time (1 to 2 minutes) and its effects dissipate within 2 minutes of discontinuation.

5. **Cyanide toxicity.** *In vivo*, sodium nitroprusside reacts nonenzymatically with the sulfhydryl groups in hemoglobin to release five cyanide radicals per molecule. Some of these can be converted to **thiocyanate** by tissue and liver rhodanese and excreted in urine. Thiocyanate has a half-life of 4 days and will accumulate in the presence of renal failure. Cyanide radicals may also bind to intracellular cytochrome oxidase and disrupt the electron transport chain. This can lead to cell hypoxia and death even in the face of adequate oxygen tensions. In addition, cyanide can bind to methemoglobin, resulting in cyanmethemoglobin.

a. **Clinical features**. Tachyphylaxis, metabolic acidosis, and elevated mixed venous oxygen tensions are early signs of cyanide toxicity, which typically occurs when more than 1 mg/kg has been administered within 2.5 hours or when the blood concentration of cyanide ion is greater than 100 μg/dL.

Symptoms of cyanide toxicity include fatigue, nausea, muscle spasm, angina, and mental confusion.

b. Treatment. Cyanide toxicity is treated by discontinuation of sodium nitroprusside and the administration of 100% oxygen and **sodium thiosulfate** (a sulfur donor in the rhodanese reaction) 150 mg/kg dissolved in 50 mL of water, over 15 minutes. Severe cyanide toxicity (base deficit > 10 mEq, hemodynamic instability) may require the additional administration of **amyl nitrate** (0.3 mL by inhalation) or **sodium nitrate**, 5 mg/kg IV over 5 minutes. These two compounds create methemoglobin, which will bind to the cyanide ion and form inactive cyanmethemoglobin.

B. Nitroglycerin is a potent venodilator that also relaxes arterial, pulmonary, ureteral, uterine, gastrointestinal, and bronchial smooth muscle. Nitroglycerin has a greater effect on venous capacitance than on arteriolar tone. This is nitroglycerin's major mechanism of decreasing MAP.

1. Indications. Nitroglycerin is useful for treating congestive heart failure and myocardial ischemia by increasing coronary flow and improving left ventricular performance. Nitroglycerin increases venous capacitance, decreases venous return, and consequently decreases ventricular end-diastolic volume. By the law of Laplace (tension = pressure × radius), a decrease in end-diastolic volume is associated with a decrease in pressure and subsequently a decrease in ventricular wall tension, which reduces myocardial oxygen consumption.

2. Reflex tachycardia frequently occurs and must be treated with beta-blockade to avoid increasing myocardial consumption and negating nitroglycerin's beneficial effects.

3. Tachyphylaxis develops with continuous infusion.

4. Complications. Nitroglycerin is metabolized by the liver and has no known toxicity in the clinical dose range. Extremely high doses and prolonged continuous use produce methemoglobinemia. Nitroglycerin produces cerebral vasodilation and should be used with caution in patients with low intracranial compliance.

C. Hydralazine is a direct-acting arterial vasodilator. It decreases MAP by a reduction of arteriolar tone and vascular resistance of the coronary, cerebral, renal, uterine, and splanchnic beds. This helps preserve blood flow to these organs. The vasodilation induced by hydralazine triggers a reflex increase in heart rate and causes activation of the renin-angiotensin system. These effects can be attenuated by the concomitant use of a beta-blocker. Hydralazine can be administered by an intravenous bolus to treat hypertensive emergencies or to augment other hypotensive agents. The time to peak effect of intravenous hydralazine is 15 to 20 minutes with an elimination half-life of 4 hours. Long-term use has been associated with a lupus-like syndrome, skin rash, drug fever, pancytopenia, and peripheral neuropathy.

D. Calcium channel antagonists (verapamil, diltiazem, nifedipine) alter calcium flux across cell membranes and cause varying degrees of arterial vasodilation with minimal effect on venous capacitance. They decrease vascular resistance of peripheral organs and cause coronary artery vasodilation. They are also myocardial depressants and verapamil and diltiazem depress atrioventricular nodal conduction (see Chapter 36). Nifedipine is limited to oral administration for the treatment of hypertension. **Verapamil** and **diltiazem** additionally are indicated for the treatment of hemodynamically stable narrow-complex supraventricular tachyarrhythmias. The initial verapamil dose is 2.5 to 5.0 mg IV, with subsequent doses of 5 to 10 mg IV administered every 15 to 30 minutes. Diltiazem is given as an initial bolus of 20 mg. An additional dose of 25 mg and an infusion of 5 to 15 mg/h can be administered if needed. Oral diltiazem is commonly use for chronic therapy of myocardial ischemia. Their vasodilator and negative inotrope properties can cause hypotension, exacerbation of congestive heart failure, bradycardia, and enhancement of accessory conduction in patients with Wolff-Parkinson-White (WPW) syndrome.

E.   Enalaprilat is currently the only angiotensin-converting enzyme inhibitor available for intravenous use. It reduces systolic and diastolic blood pressure by inhibiting the conversion of angiotensin I to angiotensin II. Enalaprilat may be used to treat perioperative hypertension. It has an onset of action of approximately 15 minutes, peak effect of 1 to 4 hours, and overall duration of action of about 4 hours. Elimination is primarily renal and caution is recommended when used in the setting of renal dysfunction.

F.   Fenoldopam is a synthetic dopamine (DA-1) receptor agonist. A continuous intravenous infusion may be used perioperatively for the management of severe hypertension in patients with impaired renal function. Fenoldopam acts by dilation of selective arterial beds while maintaining renal perfusion. It also has diuretic and natriuretic properties. Initial hemodynamic response occurs within 5 to 15 minutes. The dose should be adjusted every 15 to 20 minutes until optimal blood pressure control is achieved. Side effects include dose-dependent tachycardia and occasional hypokalemia. Bolus administration is not recommended, and hypotension may occur with concomitant use of β-adrenergic receptor blockade.

G.   Adenosine is an endogenous nucleotide that, in high doses, has inhibitory effects on cardiac impulse conduction through the atrioventricular node. Adenosine dilates cerebral blood vessels, impairs autoregulation, and is metabolized to uric acid. Its ability to slow conduction through the atrioventricular node has led to its use in diagnosing and treating supraventricular tachyarrhythmias, including those with an aberrant pathway (e.g., WPW syndrome; see Chapter 36).

H.   Prostaglandin E_1 (PGE$_1$) is a stable metabolite of arachidonic acid that causes peripheral and pulmonary vasodilation. It is used to dilate the ductus arteriosus in neonates and infants with ductal-dependent congenital heart disease (e.g., transposition of the great arteries). PGE_1 also has been used to treat pulmonary hypertension after mitral valve replacement and in patients with severe right heart failure.

I.   Phentolamine is a short-acting selective α-adrenergic receptor antagonist that causes predominantly arterial and some venous vasodilation. Phentolamine is used mainly for states of norepinephrine excess (e.g., pheochromocytoma), as an adjuvant for induced hypotension, and for infiltration into skin where norepinephrine has been accidentally extravasated (5 to 10 mg diluted in 10 mL of saline).

J.   Trimethaphan decreases MAP through ganglionic blockade (both sympathetic and parasympathetic) and also by some direct vasodilator and histamine-releasing properties. It has a fast onset (1 to 2 minutes) and short duration of action (5 to 10 minutes) and can reduce MAP without decreasing cardiac output or causing reflex tachycardia. Disadvantages that limit its use include the rapid occurrence of tachyphylaxis, histamine release, and the side effects of ganglionic blockade such as mydriasis and cycloplegia.

VII.   Induced hypotension is a technique used when control of bleeding improves operating conditions and facilitates surgical technique (e.g., middle ear microsurgery, cerebral aneurysm clipping, plastic surgery) or reduces or eliminates the need for transfusion (e.g., orthopedic surgery, patients with rare blood groups, religious constraints). It is also useful when reduction in MAP decreases the risk of vessel rupture (e.g., aortic dissection, resection of intracranial aneurysms, arteriovenous malformation surgery). This technique is not appropriate for patients with a history of vascular insufficiency to the heart, brain, or kidneys; cardiac instability (unless afterload reduction improves performance); uncontrolled hypertension; anemia; or hypovolemia. Hypotension can be achieved by neuraxial blockade, high concentrations of volatile anesthetics, peripheral vasodilation (e.g., with nitroprusside or nitroglycerin), and/or ganglionic blockade (with trimethaphan).

VIII.   Drug dosage calculations. Drug dosages frequently require conversion between units of measurement before bolus or continuous infusion administration to the patient.

A.   A drug concentration expressed as $Z\%$ contains

$$Z \text{ mg/dL} = Z \text{ g/100 mL} = (10 \times Z) \text{ g/L} = (10 \times Z) \text{ mg/mL}$$

Example: A 2.5% solution of sodium thiopental is equivalent to 25 g/L or 25 mg/mL.

B.   A drug concentration that is expressed as a ratio is converted as follows:

$$1{:}1{,}000 = 1 \text{ g/1,000 mL} = 1 \text{ mg/mL}$$

$$1{:}10{,}000 = 1 \text{ g/10,000 mL} = 0.1 \text{ mg/mL}$$

$$1{:}100{,}000 = 1 \text{ g/100,000 mL} = 0.01 \text{ mg/mL}$$

C.   Continuous drug infusions are calculated based on a simple formula:

$Z \text{ mg/250 mL} =$

$Z \text{ μg/min at an infusion rate of 15 mL/h or 15 drops/min}$

Standard drug mixes in use at the Massachusetts General Hospital are shown in Table 19-1. The desired rate of infusion for any drug is easily calculated as either a fraction or multiple of 15 mL/h or 15 drops/min.

Example: An 80-kg patient needs dopamine at 5 μg/kg/min:

$5 \times 80 = 400$

400/200 (number of milligrams in 250-mL solution) $\times$ 15 mL/h

$= 30$ mL/h

SUGGESTED READING

Barnes P. β-Adrenergic receptors and their regulation. *Am J Respir Crit Care Med* 1995;152:838–860.

Frishman W, Hotchkiss H. Selective and nonselective dopamine receptor agonists: an innovative approach to cardiovascular disease treatment. *Am Heart J* 1996;132:861–870.

Gazmuri R, Ayoub I. Pressors for cardiopulmonary resuscitation: is there a new kid on the block? *Crit Care Med* 2000;28:1236–1238.

International Consensus on Science. Agents to optimize cardiac output and blood pressure. *Circulation* 2000;102[Suppl I]: I129–I135.

Kamibayashi T, Maze M. Clinical uses of α2-adrenergic agonists. *Anesthesiology* 2000;93:1345–1349.

Lawson N, Meyer D. Autonomic nervous system: physiology and pharmacology. In: Barash PG, Cullen BF, Stoelting RK, eds. *Clinical anesthesia*, 3rd ed. Philadelphia: Lippincott-Raven Publishers, 1997:243–309.

Rozenfeld V, Cheng J. The role of vasopressin in the treatment of vasodilation in shock states. *Ann Pharmacother* 2000;34:250–254.

Varon J, Marik P. The diagnosis and management of hypertensive crises. *Chest* 2000;118:214–227.

Anesthesia for Abdominal Surgery

Jean Kwo and John J. A. Marota

I. Preanesthetic considerations

Patients undergoing abdominal surgery should undergo a complete history and physical examination as outlined in Chapter 1. As well, the following issues should be considered.

A. Assessment of preoperative fluid status. Surgical pathology may cause severe derangements in volume homeostasis, producing both hypovolemia and anemia. The main sources of fluid deficits are inadequate intake, sequestration of water and electrolytes into abdominal structures, and fluid loss.

1. History of fluid losses

a. Patients may have had decreased or no oral intake for varying periods of time before surgery. Gastrointestinal tract obstruction may prevent adequate oral intake. Chronically ill patients may not be able to take adequate oral intake for a prolonged period due to anorexia.

b. Emesis or gastric drainage may produce significant losses, especially in patients with bowel obstruction. Quantity, quality (presence of blood), and frequency of emesis should be assessed.

c. Sequestration of fluid either in bowel lumen from ileus or interstitium from peritonitis.

d. Bleeding from gastrointestinal sources include ulcers, neoplasms, esophageal varices, diverticula, angiodysplasia, or hemorrhoids.

e. Diarrhea from intestinal disease, infection, or cathartic bowel preparation can cause significant extracellular fluid loss.

f. Fever increases insensible fluid loss.

2. Physical signs of hypovolemia. Postural changes in vital signs (increased heart rate and decreased blood pressure) may reveal mild to moderate hypovolemia; severe hypovolemia will produce tachycardia and hypotension. Dry mucous membranes, skin mottling, and decreased skin turgor and temperature indicate decreased peripheral perfusion secondary to hypovolemia.

3. Laboratory analysis including hematocrit, serum osmolality, blood urea nitrogen-creatinine ratio, serum and urine electrolyte concentrations, and urine output is sometimes helpful in estimating volume deficits. **No definitive laboratory test indicates intravascular volume status.**

4. If the intravascular volume status of a patient cannot be determined by clinical assessment alone, then **invasive monitoring** such as central venous pressure (CVP) and pulmonary artery pressure measurements may be necessary.

B.   Metabolic and hematologic derangements occur frequently in patients requiring emergency abdominal surgery. Hypokalemic metabolic alkalosis is common in patients with large gastric losses (emesis or nasogastric [NG] tube drainage); large diarrheal losses or septicemia can cause metabolic acidosis. Sepsis can also produce coagulopathy from disseminated intravascular coagulopathy (DIC).

C.   Length of surgery is influenced by history of previous abdominal surgery, intraabdominal infection, radiation therapy, and steroid use.

D.   All patients for emergency abdominal procedures are considered to have full stomachs. Premedication may include a histamine (H_2) antagonist and an oral nonparticulate antacid; metoclopramide should not be used in cases of bowel obstruction.

II.   Anesthetic techniques

A.   General anesthesia (GA) is the most commonly employed technique.

1.   Advantages include protection of the airway, assurance of adequate ventilation, and rapid induction of anesthesia with controlled depth and duration.

2.   Disadvantages include loss of airway reflexes, which increases the risk of aspiration during routine or emergency surgery, and the potential adverse hemodynamic consequences of general anesthetics.

B.   Regional anesthetic techniques for abdominal surgery include spinal, epidural, and caudal anesthesia and nerve blocks.

1.   Lower abdominal procedures (e.g., inguinal hernia repair) can be performed with regional anesthesia techniques that produce a sensory level to T4-6.

a.   Epidural anesthesia usually is performed by a continuous catheter technique. A "single-dose" technique is applicable for surgery less than 3 hours' duration.

b.   Spinal anesthesia with a single-dose technique.

c.   Nerve blocks can also provide adequate anesthesia for abdominal surgery.

(1) Bilateral blockade of T8-12 intercostal nerves provides somatic sensory anesthesia, whereas celiac plexus block provides visceral anesthesia.

(2) Blockade of the ilioinguinal, iliohypogastric, and genitofemoral nerves produces a field block satisfactory for herniorrhaphy. These nerve blocks are easily performed by the anesthesiologist but may require direct supplementation of spermatic cord structures by the surgeon.

2.   Upper abdominal procedures (above the umbilicus) usually are not tolerated under regional anesthesia alone.

a.   Spinal or epidural anesthesia for upper abdominal procedures may require a sensory level to T2-4. Paralysis of the intercostal muscles from a high thoracic level impairs deep breathing; although minute ventilation is maintained, patients often complain of dyspnea. Intraperitoneal air or high abdominal exploration produces a dull pain referred to a C-5 distribution (usually over the shoulders).

b.   Celiac plexus blockade alone incompletely blocks upper abdominal sensation, and visceral traction is poorly tolerated.

3. **Advantages**
   a. Maintenance of a patient's ability to communicate symptoms (e.g., chest pain).
   b. Maintenance of airway reflexes.
   c. Profound muscle relaxation and bowel contraction provide optimal surgical exposure.
   d. Bowel blood flow increases from complete sympathectomy.
   e. Postoperative analgesia can be provided with continuous-catheter techniques.
4. **Disadvantages**
   a. Local anesthetic toxicity with intravenous (IV) injection.
   b. Patient cooperation is necessary for institution of block and positioning during surgery.
   c. Failure necessitates intraoperative conversion to GA.
   d. Regional nerve blockade may be contraindicated in patients with abnormal bleeding profile or localized infection at site of injection.
   e. Sympathectomy produces venodilation and bradycardia; these can precipitate profound hypotension. Unopposed parasympathetic activity causes bowel to contract and may make construction of bowel anastomoses more difficult; this can be reversed with glycopyrrolate, 0.2 to 0.4 mg IV.
   f. High-level thoracic blocks may compromise pulmonary function.

C. **A combined technique** uses an epidural anesthetic along with a light general anesthetic. This technique is commonly used for extensive upper abdominal surgeries.
   1. **Advantages**
      a. Epidural anesthesia reduces the requirement for GA; this minimizes myocardial depression and may decrease emergence time and nausea.
      b. Combined techniques may be useful in reducing postoperative ventilatory depression and improving pulmonary function early after upper abdominal surgery, especially in patients at high risk for postoperative pulmonary complications (e.g., obese patients).
   2. **Disadvantages**
      a. In addition to the disadvantages listed in section II.B.4., sympathectomy produced by regional anesthesia can complicate the differential diagnosis of intraoperative hypotension.
      b. Epidural catheter placement and testing adds to preparation time and may not be appropriate in emergencies.

III. **Management of anesthesia**
   A. **Standard monitors** are used as described in Chapter 10.
   B. **Induction of anesthesia**
      1. Restoration of volume deficits before induction and careful titration of sedative premedications provide more hemodynamic stability.
      2. **Rapid sequence induction** or sometimes awake intubation (see Chapter 13, section VII.A) is required for all patients considered "full stomachs." Indications include:
         a. Trauma; gastric emptying is delayed.
         b. Bowel obstruction and ileus.

    c. Symptomatic hiatal hernias and gastroesophageal reflux disease.

    d. Second or third trimester of pregnancy.

    e. Significant obesity.

    f. Ascites.

C. Maintenance of anesthesia

  1. Fluid management requires appropriate administration of maintenance fluids and replacement of both deficits and ongoing losses.

    a. Bleeding should be estimated both by direct observation of the surgical field and suction traps and by weighing sponges. Blood loss concealed beneath drapes or within the patient may be impossible to estimate.

    b. Bowel and mesenteric edema can result from surgical manipulation or intestinal pathology.

    c. Evaporative losses from peritoneal surfaces are directly related to the area exposed. Fluid replacement is guided by clinical judgment or invasive monitoring; as a rough estimate, 10 to 15 mL/kg/h may be required.

    d. Abrupt drainage of ascitic fluid with surgical entry into the peritoneum can produce acute hypotension from sudden decreases of intraabdominal pressure and pooling of blood in mesenteric vessels. Postoperative reaccumulation of ascitic fluid can produce significant fluid losses.

    e. NG and other enteric drainage should be quantified and replaced appropriately.

  2. Fluid losses can be replaced with crystalloids, colloids, or blood products.

    a. Initially, fluid should be replaced through the administration of an **isotonic salt solution**. There is no formula for calculating the amount of saline required to correct extracellular fluid depletion. The adequacy of repletion must be assessed clinically; blood pressure, pulse, urine output, and hematocrit should be monitored. Further management of electrolyte and acid-base abnormalities should be based on laboratory studies. When a crystalloid solution containing a concentration of sodium isotonic with plasma is used to replace blood loss, about three-fourths of the solution will pass into the interstitial space and one-fourth will remain in the intravascular space.

    b. Colloids are fluids containing particles that are large enough to exert an oncotic pressure. Compared with crystalloids, they remain in the intravascular space longer. Multiple studies comparing fluid resuscitation with crystalloids to colloids have reported no benefit (and perhaps poorer outcome) with colloids. Colloids solutions are considerably more expensive than crystalloids; thus, their routine use is not justified.

    c. The use of **blood products** should be guided by laboratory measurements of hematocrit, platelet count, and coagulation parameters (see Chapter 33).

  3. Muscle relaxation is required for all but the most superficial intraperitoneal operations; sufficient relaxation is critical during abdominal closure because bowel distention, edema, or organ transplantation increases the volume of abdominal contents.

   a. Titrating relaxants to obtain a single twitch by train-of-four monitoring should provide enough relaxation for surgical closure yet allow reversibility of relaxation for extubation.

   b. Potent inhalational agents block neuromuscular conduction and are synergistic with relaxants.

   c. Epidural and spinal anesthesia with local anesthetics provide excellent muscle relaxation through the blockade of nerve fibers to abdominal muscles.

   d. Flexing the operating table may decrease tension on transverse abdominal and subcostal incisions.

4. Use of nitrous oxide (N_2O) may cause bowel distention. Because N_2O is more soluble in blood than nitrogen, it diffuses into the bowel lumen faster than nitrogen can diffuse out; the amount of distention depends on the concentration of N_2O delivered, the blood flow to the bowel, and the duration of N_2O administration. Under normal conditions, the initial volume of bowel gas is small. Therefore, doubling or tripling of this volume is not problematic. The use of N_2O is relatively contraindicated in bowel obstruction, however, in which the initial volume of bowel gas can be large. Bowel distention can make closure difficult and increased intraluminal pressures may impair bowel perfusion.

5. NG tubes are frequently placed in the perioperative period.

   a. Preoperative placement is indicated for decompression of the stomach, especially in trauma victims or patients with obstructed bowel. Although suction via a large-bore NG tube can reduce the volume of gastric contents, it does not completely evacuate the stomach. NG tubes may compromise mask fit and provide a route for the reflux of gastric contents past the lower esophageal sphincter. Before induction, suction should be applied to NG tubes; during induction, tubes should be allowed to drain. Cricoid pressure may help to prevent passive reflux when an NG tube is present.

   b. Intraoperative placement is required to drain gastric fluid and air during abdominal surgery. NG and orogastric tubes should never be placed with excessive force; lubrication and head flexion facilitate insertion. Tubes can be directed into the esophagus using a finger within the oropharynx or with Magill forceps under direct visualization with a laryngoscope. If these methods fail, a large endotracheal tube (9.5 mm or larger), split lengthwise, can be used as an introducer. The split endotracheal tube is introduced orally into the esophagus and the NG tube passed through the lubricated lumen of the tube into the stomach; the split tube is then removed while stabilizing the NG tube.

   c. Complications of NG tube insertion include bleeding, submucosal dissection in the retropharynx, or placement in the trachea. Intracranial placement has been described in patients with basilar skull fracture. The NG tube should be secured carefully to avoid excessive pressure on the nasal septum or nares, which may cause ischemic necrosis.

6. Common intraoperative problems associated with abdominal surgery include the following:

    a. Pulmonary compromise can be caused by surgical retraction of abdominal viscera to improve exposure (insertion of soft packs or rigid retractors), insufflation of gas during laparoscopy, or Trendelenburg positioning. These maneuvers may elevate the diaphragm, decrease functional residual capacity (FRC), and produce hypoxemia. Application of positive end-expiratory pressure (PEEP) may counter these effects.

    b. Temperature control. Heat loss in open abdominal procedures is common. Potential sources and treatment are discussed in Chapter 18, section VII.

    c. Hemodynamic changes as a result of bowel manipulation (i.e., hypotension, tachycardia, and facial flushing). Studies have implicated prostaglandin $F_{1\alpha}$, a prostanoid found in vascular endothelial cells and luminal cells of the bowel.

    d. Opioids may aggravate biliary tract spasm. Although uncommon, opioids may produce painful biliary spasm in some patients when administered as a premedication or epidurally. Intraoperative spasm rarely can complicate surgical repair or the interpretation of a cholangiogram. Spasm can be reversed with naloxone. Nitroglycerin and glucagon also relieve spasm by nonspecific smooth muscle relaxation.

    e. Fecal contamination from perforation of the gastrointestinal tract can cause infection and sepsis.

    f. Hiccups are episodic diaphragmatic spasms that may occur spontaneously or in response to stimulation of the diaphragm or abdominal viscera. Potential therapies include the following:

        (1) Increasing depth of anesthesia to ameliorate the reaction to endotracheal, visceral, or diaphragmatic stimulation.

        (2) Removal of the source of diaphragmatic irritation, such as gastric distention.

        (3) Increasing the degree of neuromuscular blockade; this may decrease the strength of spasms. Complete diaphragmatic paralysis is difficult to achieve and may be possible only with doses of relaxants in excess of those required for relaxation of abdominal musculature.

        (4) Chlorpromazine can be titrated in 5-mg IV increments.

IV. Anesthetic considerations for specific abdominal procedures

    A. Laparoscopic surgery. Due to advances in instrumentation and surgical techniques, laparoscopic approaches are applied to an increasing number of surgical procedures, including cholecystectomy, hernia repair, fundoplication, nephrectomy, and colon resection. Benefits of laparoscopic surgery include a smaller incision, reduced postoperative pain, decreased postoperative ileus, early ambulation, a shorter hospital stay, and earlier return to work and normal activities.

    1. The **operative technique** involves the intraperitoneal insufflation of carbon dioxide (CO_2) through a needle inserted into the abdomen via a small infraumbilical incision until an intraabdominal pressure of 12 to15 mm Hg has been reached.

Patient positioning is used to facilitate operative exposure; steep reverse Trendelenburg is used to improve visualization of upper abdominal structures, whereas the Trendelenburg position is used to visualize lower abdominal structures.

2. **Anesthetic considerations**

   a. The **hemodynamic changes** associated with laparoscopy are influenced by the intraabdominal pressure needed for the creation of pneumoperitoneum, the volume of CO_2 absorbed, the patient's intravascular status, the patient's positioning, and the anesthetic agents used. Intraabdominal pressures of 12 to 15 mm Hg generally are well tolerated in healthy patients. Mean arterial pressure and systemic vascular resistance usually increase with the creation of pneumoperitoneum in healthy patients; cardiac output is unaffected. Patients with coexisting cardiac disease may have a decreased cardiac output and hypotension associated with the creation of pneumoperitoneum. Absorption of CO_2 across the peritoneal surface can cause hypercarbia, resulting in sympathetic nervous system stimulation and increased blood pressure, heart rate, and cardiac output.

   b. The **reduction in FRC** associated with the GA is compounded by the creation of pneumoperitoneum. The FRC may be further compromised by the Trendelenburg position because of the increased weight of the abdominal viscera on the diaphragm. PEEP may be needed to treat alveolar collapse. Pneumoperitoneum may also decrease abdominal and chest wall compliance, leading to **decreased respiratory system compliance** and increased peak airway pressures. Because CO_2 is absorbed across the peritoneal surface, an increase in minute ventilation usually is needed to maintain normocarbia.

   c. The patient may be placed in steep Trendelenburg or reverse Trendelenburg position to optimize surgical exposure. Besides monitoring the expected changes in venous return caused by the changes in position, frequent attention to the patient's arms is needed to prevent **injury to the brachial plexus**.

   d. **Temperature control.** Heat loss may occur due to intraperitoneal insufflation of cold gas.

   e. Embryonic channels of communication between the peritoneal and pleural/pericardial cavities may open up with increased intraperitoneal pressure, leading to **pneumomediastinum**, **pneumopericardium**, and **pneumothorax**. Diffusion of gas cephalad from the mediastinum can lead to **subcutaneous emphysema** of the face and neck.

   f. **Vascular injuries** secondary to introduction of the needle or trocar can produce sudden blood loss and necessitate conversion to an open procedure to control the bleeding.

   g. **Venous gas embolism** is rare but may occur on induction of pneumoperitoneum if the needle or trocar is placed into a vessel or an abdominal organ or if gas is trapped in the portal circulation. The high carriage capacity of blood for CO_2 and its rapid elimination increases the margin of safety in case of IV injection of CO_2. Insufflation of gas under high pressure can lead to a "gas lock" in the vena cava and right atrium, which will decrease venous return and cardiac output and produce circulatory collapse. Embolization of gas into the pulmonary circulation leads to increased dead space, ventilation/perfusion mismatch, and hypoxemia. Systemic gas embolization (with occasionally devastating effects on the cerebral and coronary circulation) can occur with massive gas entrainment or via a patent foramen ovale. Treatment consists of stopping the gas insufflation, placing the patient on 100% O_2 to relieve hypoxemia, and placing the patient in a steep head-down left lateral decubitus position to displace the gas from the right ventricular outflow tract (see Chapter 18, section XV.B). Hyperventilation will increase CO_2 excretion.

   3. Anesthetic management. GA is usually required for laparoscopy. The creation of pneumoperitoneum and steep Trendelenburg positioning can compromise ventilatory function; thus controlled ventilation is necessary to prevent hypercarbia. A urinary bladder catheter and an NG tube usually are placed after the induction of anesthesia to reduce the risk of trauma to the bladder and stomach with trocar insertion and to improve visualization.

B. Esophageal surgery for gastroesophageal reflux disease can be performed via an intraabdominal approach.

   1. The Nissen fundoplication is the most common procedure performed and involves wrapping the fundus of the stomach around the lower part of the esophagus. This creates a collar in which any excess intragastric pressure serves to constrict the wrapped esophagus rather than pushing the gastric contents into the esophagus. Hiatal hernias, if present, are repaired at the time of surgery. This procedure is often performed using laparoscopic techniques to decrease the duration of postsurgical hospitalization.

      a. Anesthetic considerations: This procedure is usually performed with GA or combined GA–epidural (for open procedures). Patients who come to surgery often have been treated medically with proton pump inhibitors, H_2-receptor antagonists, or prokinetic agents. These should be continued until the day of surgery. A rapid sequence induction or awake intubation is indicated because of the high risk of aspiration.

      b. An esophageal bougie may be placed to calibrate the fundoplication and thereby ensure an adequate esophageal lumen and minimize postoperative dysphagia. Perforation of the stomach or esophagus by passage of the bougie or NG tube can occur. With the laparoscopic method, the bougie is directed into the stomach by observation alone. Correct angulation of the esophagus or stomach during this maneuver is extremely important in preventing this injury. The dilator or NG tube should be passed slowly and should be directly visualized. Particular attention must be paid to patients with esophageal strictures.

C. Gastric surgery is usually performed with GA or combined GA–epidural. The high likelihood of aspiration in these patients necessitates a rapid sequence or awake intubation. Large third-space losses and the potential for hemorrhage should be anticipated.

   1. Gastrectomy or **hemigastrectomy with gastroduodenostomy** (Billroth I) or **gastrojejunostomy** (Billroth II) is usually performed for gastric adenocarcinoma or intractable bleeding from gastric or duodenal ulcers; rarely, it is necessary to control Zollinger-Ellison syndrome.

2. Gastrostomy can be performed through a small upper abdominal incision or percutaneously with an endoscope. Local anesthesia with sedation is often adequate in the debilitated elderly patient, although some require GA.

D. Intestinal and peritoneal surgery

1. Indications for **small bowel resection** include penetrating trauma, Crohn disease, obstructing adhesions, Meckel diverticulum, carcinoma, or infarction (from volvulus, intussusception, or thromboemboli). Patients are usually hypovolemic (see section I.A.1) and are at risk for having a full stomach.

2. Appendectomy is performed through a small lower abdominal incision or via laparoscopy. Fever, poor oral intake, and vomiting may produce hypovolemia; IV hydration before induction is indicated. In rare cases where sepsis and dehydration are absent, a regional anesthetic may be appropriate; otherwise, GA with rapid-sequence or awake intubation is necessary.

3. Colectomy or hemicolectomy is used to treat colon cancer, diverticular disease, Crohn disease, ulcerative colitis, trauma, ischemic colitis, and abscess. Emergency colectomy on unprepared bowel carries a high risk of peritonitis from fecal contamination. Some emergencies involving the colon are treated with an initial diverting colostomy, followed later by bowel preparation and elective colectomy. Patients must be evaluated for hypovolemia, anemia, and sepsis. All emergency colectomies and colostomies should be treated as if at risk for full stomach. Combination general/regional anesthetics are preferable.

4. Perirectal abscess drainage, **hemorrhoidectomy**, and **pilonidal cystectomy** are relatively noninvasive and brief procedures. Pilonidal cysts are usually excised with the patient in the prone position; abscess drainage and hemorrhoidectomy can be done either prone or in lithotomy position. If GA is used, deep planes of anesthesia or use of muscle relaxants may be necessary to achieve adequate sphincter relaxation. Intubation is required to provide GA for prone patients. Hyperbaric spinal anesthesia is used for procedures in lithotomy position, whereas a hypobaric technique is useful for the flexed prone (jackknife) or knee–chest position; caudal block is applicable with either position.

5. Inguinal, femoral, or ventral herniorrhaphies can be performed under local anesthesia, regional anesthesia (spinal, epidural, caudal, or nerve block), or GA. Maximum stimulation and a profound vagal response may occur during spermatic cord or peritoneal retraction. If GA is selected, either a mask technique (e.g., laryngeal mask airway) or deep extubation should be considered to decrease coughing on emergence, which can strain the hernia repair.

E. Hepatic surgery

1. Partial hepatectomy is used to treat hepatoma, unilobar metastasis of a carcinoma, arteriovenous malformation, or echinococcal cysts. Because extensive hemorrhage is anticipated, standard monitors are supplemented with placement of arterial and central venous catheters and large-bore IV access. Blood loss during hepatic parenchymal division can be reduced by temporarily occluding the portal and arterial inflow at the level of the hepatic pedicle (Pringle maneuver). The normal liver has considerable reserve, and extensive resection must be performed before drug metabolism is clinically impaired. The effects of liver disease on anesthetic management are discussed in Chapter 5. Epidural catheters can be placed in patients with normal coagulation studies.

2. Patients with **portal hypertension** may present with the stigmata of liver failure, and some may be awaiting liver transplantation. Most patients are treat conservatively with pharmacotherapy (e.g., β-adrenergic blockers, vasodilators), endoscopy and sclerotherapy for acute esophageal variceal bleeding, and interventional radiology (transjugular intrahepatic portosystemic shunts). Surgery may be required for the palliation of variceal bleeding and ascites. Surgery is associated with an increased risk of encephalopathy, however, and does not significantly improve long-term outcome.

a. Portacaval shunts relieve portal hypertension by shunting blood to the inferior vena cava (IVC) through a surgically created anastomosis. Because complete diversion of portal venous flow through the IVC can lead to rapid hepatic failure, incomplete "H"-type shunts are usually constructed to permit partial decompression of the portal venous system. Shunting can significantly increase ventricular preload and precipitate heart failure.

b. Splenorenal shunting between the splenic and renal veins decompresses esophageal variceal collaterals and may be performed when variceal bleeding is refractory to sclerotherapy. Because surgery requires complete dissection of the splenic vein as it crosses the pancreatic bed, bleeding may be extensive and difficult to control in the setting of coagulopathy.

c. Peritoneovenous shunting is performed for the treatment of intractable ascites. Valved conduits, such as **the LeVeen and Denver shunts**, allow ascitic fluid to leave the peritoneal cavity and enter the venous system. These procedures can be performed with the infiltration of local anesthetic and superficial cervical plexus block. Shunting is rarely performed because it is associated with severe complications (i.e., superior vena cava thrombosis and fibrous peritonitis) and a high rate of shunt obstruction requiring reoperation. DIC precipitated by shunting is a rare complication and requires prompt removal of the device. Postoperative care is directed toward preventing circulatory overload and requires aggressive diuretic management.

F. Biliary tract procedures

1. Cholecystectomy is a common procedure performed either as open laparotomy or by laparoscopic technique. GA is required for either technique. During laparoscopic cholecystectomy, the patient is placed in steep reverse Trendelenburg position and the gallbladder is dissected from the liver bed using either cautery or laser. Muscle relaxants are required to provide adequate abdominal wall relaxation. The amount of hemorrhage is difficult to assess because of the limited field of view and high magnification of the laparoscope; heavy bleeding from the cystic or hepatic artery may occur. The advantages of laparoscopic cholecystectomy are minimal postoperative pain and a faster recovery. Most patients are discharged on the first postoperative day.

2. Biliary drainage procedures include **transduodenal sphincteroplasty** for extensive choledocholithiasis, **cholecystojejunostomy** for obstruction of the distal common bile duct from pancreatic cancer, and **choledochojejunostomy** for chronic pancreatitis, stone disease, and benign strictures of the distal bile duct. Endoscopic and transhepatic techniques are increasingly common, but open surgical drainage is occasionally required. Blood loss is usually minimal but fluid loss may be significant.

G. Pancreatic surgery

1. Although the initial treatment of acute pancreatitis is supportive, surgical intervention may be necessary for the **complications of pancreatitis**. Surgical debridement is indicated for infected pancreatic necrosis. Hemorrhagic pancreatitis unresponsive to resuscitation with blood products and correction of coagulopathy requires surgical intervention. Pancreatic pseudocysts may require drainage; the cyst may be anastomosed to a Roux-en-Y limb of the jejunum, to the posterior wall of the stomach, or to the duodenum. Surgical intervention can result in significant bleeding and third-space fluid losses. In severe acute pancreatitis, activation of inflammatory mediators can produce sepsis and multiple organ dysfunction, which require fluid resuscitation, mechanical ventilation, and vasopressor support.

2. Pancreatojejunostomy with gastrojejunostomy and choledochojejunostomy (Whipple procedure) is performed for resection of adenocarcinoma of the pancreas, malignant cystadenoma, or refractory pancreatitis confined to the head of the pancreas. These procedures are long and surgically difficult with a high potential for hemorrhage and fluid loss.

H. Splenectomy may be performed emergently after blunt or penetrating trauma or electively for treatment of idiopathic thrombocytopenic purpura or staging Hodgkin lymphoma. GA and muscle relaxation are required. Large-bore IV access is necessary because major blood loss requiring transfusion can be encountered. A combined epidural and general anesthetic technique is appropriate with the caveat that significant hemorrhage in a patient with a sympathectomy may potentiate hypotension. Occasionally, a transthoracic approach to gain control of the hilar vessels of a very large spleen may be necessary. Splenectomy patients should receive polyvalent pneumococcal vaccine in the postoperative period.

I. Orthotopic liver transplantation is a curative procedure for end-stage liver disease. Common etiologies include hepatoma, sclerosing cholangitis, Wilson disease, α_1-antitrypsin deficiency, primary biliary cirrhosis, and alcoholic cirrhosis. Unfortunately, because of a limited supply of donor livers, many patients who require transplants do not receive them. The supply of donor livers for children is even more scarce because of their need for size-matched organs; the size of the liver from an adult donor can be reduced for transplantation into a child. Currently, two strategies are used to expand the supply of liver grafts for children without affecting the supply for adults. The first strategy consists of removal of the left lateral liver segment from a **living-related donor** for transplantation into the child. The second strategy is **split-liver transplantation**; two grafts are obtained by dividing one liver from a cadaveric donor. Because the splitting of the liver allograft on the bench is a lengthy procedure, the prolonged ischemia time results in graft injury, which predisposes it to a high incidence of graft dysfunction unless it is placed in a favorable environment. Therefore, proper patient selection is of primary importance in decreasing the incidence of poor graft function. There is growing experience with grafts that are split *in situ* in a donor with a beating heart; patients who receive these grafts have similar survival rates as patients who received whole or reduced-sized grafts.

1. **Preanesthetic considerations** for the patient with liver disease are discussed in Chapter 5.

2. **Surgery for hepatic transplantation** proceeds in three distinct stages.

   a.   **Recipient hepatectomy**, including resection of the gallbladder, hepatic veins, and sometimes a section of the IVC.

   b.   **Anhepatic phase** marked by decreased venous return from interruption of the IVC. Venovenous bypass (typically left femoral and portal to left axillary vein) can often improve venous return.

   c.   **Postanhepatic phase** marked by reperfusion of the donor liver; this delivers hyperkalemic, hypothermic, and acidic solution to the central circulation. The patient's condition usually stabilizes after completion of vascular anastomoses. After the biliary anastomoses are completed, donor cholecystectomy, choledochojejunostomy, and placement of a choledochal tube complete the surgery.

3. **Anesthetic considerations**

   a.   **Hemorrhage** in the presence of a baseline coagulopathy can produce dramatic blood loss (multiple blood volumes); recipient hepatectomy is usually the period of greatest hemorrhage. Fibrinolysis during the anhepatic phase may worsen a preexisting coagulopathy. **Aminocaproic acid** (Amicar) and/or **aprotinin** may be helpful (see Chapter 33).

   b.   Measures to prevent **hypothermia** should be taken from the time of induction (see Chapter 18, section VII).

   c.   Metabolic derangements are common.

   (1)   **Oliguria** secondary to hypovolemia and hypoperfusion may produce renal failure and hyperkalemia.

   (2)   **Large-volume transfusion of citrated blood products** may lead to hypocalcemia and hyperkalemia.

   (3)   During the anhepatic phase there is a theoretical risk of **hypoglycemia**, although more typically **hyperglycemia** from administration of dextrose-containing solutions is seen. This phase of surgery is often marked by a progressive **metabolic acidosis**.

   d.   **Hypoxia** can occur from intrapulmonary shunting, thoracic restriction from surgical retraction, and Trendelenburg position. Adequate oxygenation may require high fraction of inspired oxygen (FIO_2) and application of PEEP.

e. Hypotension from hypovolemia or cardiac dysfunction should be anticipated. Vasopressors and inotropes are necessary until the underlying problem is corrected.

4. **Anesthetic management**

a. **Standard monitors**, a urinary catheter, and a radial arterial catheter are essential. Most patients also require pulmonary artery catheter placement via the internal jugular vein. **Venous access** should include a large-bore (12-gauge) catheter and a size 8.5 French catheter placed in a jugular vein. A **rapid transfusion system** capable of delivering 1.0 to 1.5 L/min at 38°C should supply the largest catheter.

b. **Rapid-sequence induction** of anesthesia is advised because these patients are at risk of reflux from a full stomach, ascites, or obtundation. Ketamine may be useful as an induction agent in unstable patients.

c. **Maintenance** of anesthesia usually is accomplished with a balanced technique including moderate- to high-dose opioids and isoflurane. Halothane is avoided because it can decrease hepatic blood flow; N_2O is avoided because of potential air embolism during venovenous bypass and to minimize bowel distention.

d. **Intraoperative laboratory studies** include arterial blood gas tensions, glucose, electrolytes, hematocrit, platelets, and coagulation profiles.

e. **Transfusion therapy** rests upon both autologous transfusion of salvaged blood from the surgical field and banked products. Laboratory and clinical assessment of coagulation will determine need for packed red blood cells, fresh frozen plasma, or other blood products. If possible, transfusion of platelets is delayed until after completion of venovenous bypass. Cryoprecipitate and aminocaproic acid are potential therapeutic adjuncts.

f. **Resuscitation from cardiac collapse** may be necessary during reperfusion. Malignant arrhythmias or cardiac arrest can result from the cold, hyperkalemic, acidemic washout of the donor organ, hypoperfused gut, and lower extremities. Normalization of serum potassium and acid-base status before reperfusion is helpful; administration of volume, sodium bicarbonate, diuretics, insulin, dextrose, and small doses of epinephrine (50 to 100 µg IV) may be necessary. Hyperventilation is useful.

g. **After surgery** the donor liver resumes function, coagulopathy generally improves and ongoing fluid requirements diminish. Patients require additional opioids for analgesia and sedation.

J. Renal transplantation (see Chapter 26).

K. Heterotopic pancreatic transplantation is usually performed in conjunction with heterotopic renal transplantation. Although recipients may undergo a nephrectomy, their native pancreas is left intact. Anesthetic considerations are primarily related to renal transplantation and management of diabetes (see Chapters 6 and 26).

1. Surgery often entails anastomosis of the donor pancreas to the recipient's bladder via a portion of duodenum; this permits exocrine pancreatic secretions to drain into the bladder. Blood glucose should be determined frequently, because it rapidly falls to normal with perfusion of the pancreas. Because there is no pepsin present, trypsinogen and chymotrypsinogen are not activated. Gram-negative urinary tract infection can activate these enzymes and lead to bladder damage requiring emergency removal of the transplanted pancreas. The pancreas secretes bicarbonate that is lost in the urine; severe metabolic acidosis can occur during renal failure.

2. Pancreatic islet cell transplantation remains an experimental procedure but holds promise for the treatment of diabetes. The procedure consists of purifying islets from cadaveric donors and injecting these into the liver via the portal vein. Transplantation can be performed percutaneously using local anesthesia.

L.   Intraoperative radiation therapy for pancreatic or colonic adenocarcinoma can accompany exploratory laparotomy with either a primary resection or a debulking procedure. Specially designed operating rooms have been constructed to accommodate intraoperative radiotherapy. If transport to a separate radiation therapy suite is necessary, however, the anesthetized patient is transported before wound closure. The patient requires continuous monitoring and ventilation with 100% oxygen during transport; medications and resuscitation equipment must accompany the patient. Anesthesia can be maintained by IV agents (e.g., propofol). A previously prepared anesthesia machine must be available in the radiation therapy suite. Patients are positioned so that monitor screens, and ventilation can be observed by remote television outside of the radiation area. Aortic or IVC compression may occur when the sterile cone of the treatment machine is positioned in the abdominal wound. Ventilation with 100% oxygen maximizes sensitivity of the tumor to radiation therapy. Treatments usually require 5 to 20 minutes but can be interrupted if difficulties with hemodynamics or ventilation occur. Wound closure may be performed either in the radiation suite or after transport back to the operating room.

M.   Surgery for the obese. With at least 50% of the U.S. population considered overweight, obesity is a major health issue. The **body mass index** (BMI) is correlated to the relative amount of adipose tissue and is calculated as:

$$BMI = body\ weight\ (kilograms)/height^2\ (meters)$$

Patients are considered overweight if their BMI is greater than 25, obese if their BMI is greater than 30, and morbidly obese if their BMI is greater than 35 to 40.

1.   Preanesthetic considerations

a.   Obese people have an **increased circulating blood volume** and **increased cardiac output** to meet their **increased oxygen consumption**. Depressed left ventricular function can be found even in young asymptomatic patients, and it is correlated to the degree of obesity. **Hypertension** is also significantly correlated with obesity.

b. Obese individuals are at higher risk for **hypercholesterolemia**, a risk factor for the development of atherosclerosis and coronary artery disease. Patients with several cardiac risk factors may require a cardiology consultation to optimize medical therapy in the perioperative period and to determine whether further cardiac testing is necessary.

c. Patients who have used the **appetite suppressants** dexfenfluramine or fenfluramine for more than 4 months have an increased risk of cardiac valve disorders, particularly aortic regurgitation. Pulmonary hypertension has also been associated with the use these drugs. A perioperative echocardiogram may be indicated to evaluate valve function.

d. The **compliance of the respiratory system** is decreased in obesity; this is mainly due to decreased chest wall compliance. There is a slight decrease in lung compliance due to increased pulmonary blood volume. Because of the decreased lung compliance, FRC is reduced. In the supine position, FRC may fall within the closing volume, leading to airway closure, ventilation perfusion mismatch, and hypoxemia. The higher metabolic demand of the obese person results in increased oxygen consumption and increased carbon dioxide production; an increased minute ventilation is required to maintain a normocapneic state.

e. Increased submucosal fat in the pharynx can cause severe collapse of the hypopharynx during sleep leading to **obstructive sleep apnea**. Long-standing hypoxemia can produce pulmonary hypertension and right heart failure. The presence of polycythemia suggests long-standing hypoxemia. Patients with severe sleep apnea may benefit from staying in a monitored setting in the immediate postoperative period.

f. Increased gastric emptying time and elevated intraabdominal pressure and volume predispose to a higher incidence of symptomatic **gastroesophageal reflux**.

g. Increased blood sugar levels, hyperinsulinemia, and insulin resistance may occur in obese individuals, leading to the development of type II **diabetes**. Because perfusion of adipose tissue is variable, an IV insulin infusion may be needed to control hyperglycemia. Guidelines for the management of glucose and insulin are covered in Chapter 6.

h. **Airway management** has traditionally been considered a challenge in obese patients because of the large size of the neck and face. A careful assessment of the mobility of the neck and jaw, inspection of the oropharynx, and examination of the dental status should be made. If the tracheal intubation is expected to be difficult, an awake intubation should be considered and discussed with the patient.

i. Significant **psychological problems**, such as depression and low self-esteem, may occur in many of these patients.

2. **Bariatric surgery** is currently the most effective treatment of morbid obesity. Patients with a BMI of 35 or greater with obesity-related comorbidities or patients with a BMI of 40 or greater are candidates for surgery. Surgery is associated with a loss of at least 50% of excess body weight; a decreased rate of hypertension, diabetes, and sleep apnea; and increased physical activity. Currently, two basic types of bariatric surgery are performed.

   a. The **vertical banded gastroplasty** results in the formation of a small gastric pouch that restricts the volume of food that can be ingested. Long-term weight loss may be limited by maladaptive eating patterns (liquids with high caloric content) or by staple line disruption.

   b. The **Roux-en-Y gastric bypass** surgery consists of formation of a small gastric pouch and the anastomosis of the pouch to the proximal jejunum. This combines a restrictive anatomy with a dumping physiology. Ingestion of liquids of high energy density leads to nausea, abdominal cramping, and diarrhea, which may serve as an impetus for behavioral modification. The Roux-en-Y gastric bypass can also be performed laparoscopically.

3. Anesthetic management

   a. Standard operating tables are often unable to accommodate the size and weight of the obese patient; tables designed for obese patients should be used. Extra padding and skin protection are required for even the shortest procedures.

   b. Standard noninvasive monitoring, with a urinary catheter, should be used in patients who are generally healthy. An appropriately sized blood pressure cuff should be used. A regular sized cuff placed on the forearm may be more effective than an oversized cuff on the arm. Intraarterial blood pressure monitoring should be used if strict blood pressure control is necessary or if frequent blood sampling is required. IV access may be challenging because of difficulty identifying veins.

   c. The **clinical evaluation of hydration and blood volume** in the obese patient may be difficult. They have an increased total circulating blood volume; however, it is less than normal when calculated on a per weight basis. Furthermore, technical difficulties with surgery can lead to increased blood and fluid losses. Although fluid replacement guided by hemodynamics and urine output is generally safe in healthy individuals, invasive monitoring to guide fluid management may be necessary in some patients. The interpretation of CVPs may be difficult because increased intraabdominal pressures can be transmitted to the thoracic cavity and may falsely elevate the CVP. A pulmonary artery catheter may be indicated for monitoring the volume status of patients with congestive heart failure or valvular disease. Again, transmitted intraabdominal pressures can increase falsely increase the pressure readings. However, increased intrathoracic pressures would not affect the validity of cardiac output and stroke volume measurements.

   d. Regional anesthesia techniques can be challenging because of difficulties in identifying anatomic landmarks. Nevertheless, the use of epidural anesthesia in combination with a light general anesthetic may be advantageous. The quality of postoperative analgesia is superior, and it avoids the risks of oversedation with opioids, which can lead to hypoxemia and hypercarbia in patients with a marginal respiratory status. Placement of the epidural catheter may be easier with the patient in the sitting position because the midline of the spine may not be readily evident when the patient is in the lateral decubitus position. Long epidural needles (5 inches) may be necessary. The local anesthetic dose requirements are decreased in the patient with morbid obesity; the volume of the epidural space is decreased because of fatty infiltration and increased blood volume in the epidural venous system.

e. The morbidly obese require either a **rapid-sequence induction** or an awake intubation for several reasons:

(1) Obese patients are at increased risk for aspiration because of delayed gastric emptying and gastroesophageal reflux disease.

(2) The combination of an increased metabolic demand and decreased FRC leads to **rapid desaturation** when morbidly obese patients become apneic. Preoxygenation for 3 to 5 minutes is recommended.

(3) **Mask ventilation** is often difficult and is associated with the loss of the small O_2 reserve established by preoxygenation.

f. **Tracheal intubation may be difficult** in the morbidly obese patient because of the increased size of the tongue and posterior pharyngeal structures. Awake fiberoptic intubation is recommended when difficult intubation is anticipated. Proper positioning with full atlanto-occipital extension (sniffing position) may require padding under both the chest and head and can significantly improve the view of the glottis with laryngoscopy. Different types and sizes of laryngoscope blades, stylets, laryngeal mask airways, and fiberoptic instruments should be available for intubation.

g. Morbidly obese patients have a greater reduction in lung volume than nonobese patients during GA, leading to greater **atelectasis**, **airway closure**, and **hypoxemia**. The alveolar collapse may be treated with PEEP and by higher tidal volumes. High airway pressures may be caused in part by decreased chest wall compliance and may not reflect true transpulmonary pressures.

h. **Drug doses** in the obese patient may differ from that used in the nonobese patient because of changes associated with obesity (e.g., increased cardiac output) as well as pharmacokinetic changes (e.g., volume of distribution, renal and hepatic clearances). Drug doses based on actual body weight may be excessive; however, the dosage required may be greater than that estimated by ideal body weight. Because of this, in general, short-acting drugs such as propofol, fentanyl, and cisatracurium are recommended. Both overdosage and underdosage of muscle relaxants may occur. Excessive dosages may be administered because of low chest wall compliance or to overcome technical difficulties by the surgeon. The need for relaxation may be underestimated by nerve stimulators, however, because of the thickness of the subcutaneous tissues at the monitoring site.

i. The patient should be **extubated** in the operating room when awake, with adequate cough reflexes, and after confirmation of adequate reversal of muscle relaxation. Because of their decreased FRC in the supine position, obese patients should be placed in a sitting position as soon as possible. Patients who use positive airway pressure by mask (noninvasive ventilation) to treat sleep apnea can resume this treatment as soon as necessary; gastric distention does not appear to be problematic.

j.   Admission to an intensive care unit postoperatively should be considered for patients with severe coronary artery disease, patients with diabetes that is hard to control, and patients with severe sleep apnea.

N.   Recovery of organs for transplantation after brain death

1. With the success of organ transplantation in treating end-stage kidney, liver, lung, and heart failure, many patients who need transplants do not receive them because of a gap between the supply of donated organs and the demand for these organs. To increase the donor pool, strict exclusion criteria such as age or coexisting illnesses are no longer used. **A transplant coordinator from an organ-procurement organization should screen all potential donors.**

2.   Organs may be deemed unsuitable based on donor age, organ injury, disease, or gross abnormalities.

3.   Organ-specific considerations

a.   Lung/heart–lung. Packed red blood cells are preferred for volume expansion. The partial pressure of oxygen (Pa_{O_2}) is maintained above 100 mm Hg with an $F_{I_{O_2}}$ less than or equal to 0.4 and PEEP of 5 cm H_2O.

b.   Heart. Low systemic vascular resistance is treated with a vasoconstrictor.

c.   Liver/pancreas. Dopamine is preferred for the treatment of hypotension. Excessive crystalloid infusions are avoided.

d.   Kidney. Dopamine is preferred for the treatment of hypotension. A brisk diuresis is preferred.

4.   Specific management problems

a.   Poikilothermia is common and hypothermia should be anticipated and treated early.

b.   Hypertension is infrequent. Nitroprusside can be used to treat severe, persistent hypertension.

c.   Hypotension is common. Central venous or pulmonary artery catheterization may be necessary. Hypovolemia can be treated with crystalloid and colloid solutions and blood products as necessary. After restoration of intravascular volume, vasopressors such as dopamine, epinephrine, or norepinephrine may be used. Depressed myocardial function may be treated with dopamine or dobutamine.

d.   Polyuria may be secondary to volume overload, osmotic diuresis, or diabetes insipidus (DI) and treated accordingly. An IV infusion of vasopressin or desmopressin may be titrated to treat severe DI (see Chapter 6, section VII.B.2).

e.   Hypoxemia may be caused by atelectasis, pulmonary edema, aspiration, or pneumonia. The $F_{I_{O_2}}$ and minute ventilation should be adjusted to maintain a Pa_{O_2} greater than 100 mmHg and a Pa_{CO_2} from 35 to 45. High levels of PEEP should be avoided to preserve cardiac output and avoid barotrauma. High $F_{I_{O_2}}$ should be avoided in potential lung donors to minimize possible oxygen toxicity.

5.   Anesthetic management for the harvesting of organs should focus on optimizing organ perfusion and oxygenation. A number of surgical teams are involved; effective communication among the surgical teams, the anesthetist, and the operating room staff is essential and is facilitated by the organ and tissue donation coordinator. Specific protocols are usually required and depend on the circumstances of the donation.

   a. **Dissection** of organs usually occurs in the following order: heart (30 minutes), lungs (1 to 1.5 hours), liver (1 to 1.5 hours), pancreas (1 to 1.5 hours), and kidneys (30 minutes to 1 hour).

   b. **Heparin** (20,000 to 30,000 units IV in adult donors) is administered. Simultaneously, the aorta is cross-clamped, the distal aorta and IVC are cannulated, and the harvested organs are perfused *in situ*, topically cooled, and exsanguinated via the IVC.

   c. **Ventilatory support** is discontinued when the aorta is cross-clamped.

SUGGESTED READING

Ballantyne JC, Carr DB, deFerranti S, et al. The comparative effects of postoperative analgesic therapies on pulmonary outcome: cumulative meta-analyses of randomized, controlled trials. *Anesth Analg* 1998;86: 598–612.

Carton EG, Plevak DJ, Kranner PW, et al. Perioperative care of the liver transplant patient. Part 2. *Anesth Analg* 1994;78:382–399.

Carton EG, Rettke SR, Plevak DJ, et al. Perioperative care of the liver transplant patient. Part 1. *Anesth Analg* 1994;78:120–133.

Choi PT, Yip G, Quinonez LG, Cook DJ. Crystalloids vs. colloids in fluid resuscitation: a systematic review. *Crit Care Med* 1999;27:200–210.

Gridelli B, Remuzzi G. Strategies for making more organs available for transplantation. *N Engl J Med* 2000;343:404–410.

Jaffe RA, Samuels SI. *Anesthesiologist's manual of surgical procedures*, 2nd edition. Philadelphia: Lippincott Williams & Wilkins, 1999.

Lowham AS, Filipi CJ, Hinder RA, et al. Mechanisms and avoidance of esophageal perforation by anesthesia personnel during laparoscopic foregut surgery. *Surg Endosc* 1996;10:979–982.

Patel T. Surgery in the patient with liver disease. *Mayo Clin Proc* 1999; 74:593–599.

Pelosi P, Ravagnan I, Giurati G, et al. Positive end-expiratory pressure improves respiratory function in obese but not in normal subjects during anesthesia and paralysis. *Anesthesiology* 1999;91:1221–1231.

Robertson KM, Cook DR. Perioperative management of the multiorgan donor. *Anesth Analg* 1990;70:546–556.

Shenkman Z, Shir Y, Brodsky JB. Perioperative management of the obese patient. *Br J Anaesth* 1993;70:349–359.

21

Anesthesia for Thoracic Surgery

Paul H. Alfille

I. Preoperative evaluation

A. Patients for thoracic surgery should undergo the usual preoperative assessment as detailed in Chapter 1.

    1. Any patient undergoing elective thoracic surgery should be carefully screened for underlying bronchitis or pneumonia and treated appropriately before surgery.

        a. Diagnostic procedures such as bronchoscopy and lung biopsy may be intended for persistent infection.

        b. Infection beyond an obstructing lesion may not resolve without surgery.

    2. In patients with **tracheal stenosis**, the history should focus on symptoms or signs of positional dyspnea, static versus dynamic airway collapse, and evidence of hypoxemia. The history may also suggest the probable location of the lesion.

B. Arterial blood gas (ABG) determinations may help to clarify the severity of underlying pulmonary disease but are not routinely necessary.

C. Pulmonary function tests are useful in assessing the pulmonary risk of lung resection. Both exercise function (maximal oxygen uptake [$\dot{V}o_{2max}$]) and spirometry (forced expiratory volume in 1 second) have been used to stratify risks of resection. In marginal cases, split-function radionuclide scans and ventilation/perfusion ($\dot{V}/\dot{Q}$) scans can determine the relative contribution of each lung and individual lung regions.

D. Cardiac function should be assessed if there is question of the relative contribution of cardiac and pulmonary disease in the patient's functional impairment. **Echocardiography** can estimate pulmonary artery pressure and right ventricular function.

E. Imaging studies, such as chest radiography, computed tomography (CT), and magnetic resonance imaging, are useful to determine the presence of tracheal deviation, the location of pulmonary infiltrates, effusion or pneumothorax, and the involvement of adjacent structures in the disease.

F. Tracheal tomography or three-dimensional reconstruction from CT is used to assess the caliber of stenotic airways and can be used to predict the size and length of the endotracheal tube that will be appropriate for the patient. Severe airway stenosis observed preoperatively may change the anesthetist's plans for induction and intubation.

II. Preoperative preparation

A. Preoperative sedation should be given carefully to patients with tracheal or pulmonary disease.

    1. Heavy sedation may impair postoperative deep breathing, coughing, and airway protection.

2. Patients with poor pulmonary function will be more prone to hypoxemia when their respiratory drive is suppressed. When sedating these patients, it is wise to monitor oxygenation and administer supplemental oxygen.

3. In the presence of airway obstruction, sedation must be carefully balanced. Oversedation may profoundly suppress ventilation, but an anxious patient may make exaggerated respiratory efforts. In this case, the increased turbulence may cause worsened airway obstruction, leading to increased anxiety. Benzodiazepines, reassuring words, careful monitoring, and an expeditious start to the procedure is the best approach. In patients with airway stenosis, heliox (a mixture of helium and oxygen) will lower the density of the respiratory gas and reduce airway resistance.

B. Aspiration prophylaxis, with an oral histamine-2 receptor antagonist and metoclopramide, should be considered in patients undergoing major thoracic surgery. Patients with esophageal disease should be considered at high risk for aspiration.

C. Glycopyrrolate (0.2 mg intravenously) may be given to decrease oral secretions.

III. Monitoring

A. Standard monitoring should be used as described in Chapter 10.

B. A **radial arterial catheter** should be placed in any patient undergoing major thoracic surgery.

1. Surgical exposure during thoracotomy and esophageal or pulmonary resection often compresses the heart and great vessels. Having continuous blood pressure readings allows for immediate feedback.

2. Peripheral thoracic surgery, such as thoracoscopic wedge resection, is less likely to rapidly impair cardiac function.

3. ABG measurements are helpful for tracheal surgery, especially in the postoperative period.

4. In the lateral position it is possible for blood flow to the dependent arm to be impaired. Pulsatile flow to the dependent arm should be monitored with an arterial catheter or a pulse oximeter.

5. During mediastinal surgery (e.g., tracheal reconstruction or mediastinoscopy) it is possible for the innominate artery to be compressed, stopping flow to the right carotid and brachial arteries. Perfusion to the right arm should be monitored by an arterial line or pulse oximeter.

C. Further invasive monitoring is dictated by the patient's condition. If a pulmonary artery catheter is placed,

1. It is customarily inserted from the nondependent side of the neck. If the catheter interferes with the surgical resection, it can be retracted into the main pulmonary artery and readvanced when artery on the operative side is clamped. Use of a long sterile sheath facilitates repositioning of the catheter during surgery.

2. Pressure measurements referenced to the atmosphere may be affected by lateral positioning and opening the chest. Trends in central venous pressure, pulmonary artery pressure, and pulmonary artery occlusion pressure can be followed, and cardiac output and stroke volume measurements remain accurate.

IV.   Endoscopic procedures include direct or indirect visualization of the pharynx, larynx, esophagus, trachea, and bronchi. Endoscopy may be undertaken to obtain biopsy samples, delineate upper airway anatomy, remove obstructing foreign bodies, assess hemoptysis, place stents and guidewires, position radiation catheters, apply photodynamic therapy, and perform laser surgery.

A.   Flexible bronchoscopy permits visualization from the larynx to the segmental bronchi.

1.   A "working lumen" is used for suction, administering drugs, and passing wire instruments.

2.   Ventilation must be around the flexible bronchoscope. Bronchoscopes range in diameter from around 5 mm for a standard adult size to 2 mm diameter neonatal bronchoscopes that lack a working lumen.

3.   Topical anesthesia, sometimes with the assistance of an anesthetist for monitoring and sedation, is the most common anesthetic approach.

a.   The patient should meet fasting (nothing by mouth) guidelines.

b.   Lidocaine (4% spray) is applied to the oro- or nasopharynx, larynx, and vocal cords. The trachea can be sprayed with anesthetic through the bronchoscope or by transtracheal injection. If this is done patiently, no further anesthesia is required.

c.   Premedication with atropine or glycopyrrolate will limit salivary dilution of the anesthetic and may improve the onset and efficacy of the anesthetic.

d.   Nerve blocks may be used to supplement airway anesthesia (see Chapter 13).

e.   The patient should have nothing by mouth until tracheal reflexes return (2 to 3 hours).

4.   General anesthesia may be indicated in anxious, compromised, or uncooperative patients or if bronchoscopy is part of a larger surgical procedure.

a.   Bronchoscopy is very stimulating but does not cause postoperative pain, so a potent short-acting anesthetic is preferable.

b.   Muscle relaxation or topical anesthesia to the trachea generally is needed to prevent coughing during the procedure.

c.   The endotracheal tube used should be sufficiently large (7 mm inner diameter or larger) to permit ventilation in the annular space around the scope.

d.   A laryngeal mask airway (LMA) has the advantage of allowing easy view of the cords and proximal trachea.

B.   Rigid bronchoscopy permits visualization of the larynx to the mainstem bronchi.

1.   A rigid bronchoscope has better optics and a larger working channel than a flexible bronchoscope and can be used to dilate a stenotic airway, easing subsequent airway management.

2.   Ventilation is accomplished through the lumen of the scope itself, allowing better control of a marginal airway.

3.   General anesthesia is required for rigid bronchoscopy. Either deep inhalation anesthesia or muscle relaxation is required to prevent movement and coughing.

4.   Conventional ventilation can be used, with the anesthesia circuit attached to a side arm of the rigid bronchoscope. The proximal end of the bronchoscope is closed by a clear lens, of instruments, or by a rubber gasket through which telescopes may be passed.

   a. A variable but potentially large leak requires an anesthesia machine capable of delivering high oxygen flows.

   b. Either an intravenous or potent inhalational anesthetic technique can be used.

   c. Close coordination between the surgeon and anesthetist is needed, because ventilation may need to be interrupted for instrumentation and surgery may in turn be interrupted by the need to ventilate.

5. In cases of severely compromised airways (e.g., severe airway stenosis or airway disruption), maintenance of spontaneous ventilation is indicated. The patient may be induced with an inhalational induction with sevoflurane and the rigid bronchoscope introduced under a deep plane of anesthesia.

6. Ventilating gas may leak out around the bronchoscope, so that measurements of end-tidal carbon dioxide may be inaccurate. Adequacy of ventilation should be assessed by observation of chest excursion, pulse oximetry, and, if necessary, blood gas analysis.

7. **Sanders rigid bronchoscopes** are designed for jet ventilation through a special small side lumen.

   a. The central lumen remains open. Severe barotrauma may occur if gas is not allowed to escape. Observation of chest movement during the expiratory phase is critical.

   b. An intravenous anesthetic technique (see Chapter 14) must be used. Muscle relaxation is required for the jet to inflate the lungs adequately.

   c. Additional gas is added to the inspired gas by the Venturi effect. The inspired oxygen concentration is uncertain, because the amount of room air entrained cannot be controlled.

   d. During laser surgery, the inspired oxygen concentration should be reduced to below 0.4, either by jetting air or using a gas blender for the jet intake.

   e. The advantage of the jet technique is that ventilation is not interrupted by suctioning or surgical manipulations, because the proximal end of the bronchoscope is always open. This makes the Sanders bronchoscope suitable for use during laser surgery of the larynx, vocal cords, or proximal trachea.

8. **Complications** of bronchoscopy include dental and laryngeal damage from intubation, injuries to the eyes or lips, airway rupture, pneumothorax, and hemorrhage. Airway obstruction may be caused by hemorrhage, a foreign body, or a dislodged mass.

C. **Flexible esophagoscopy** may be performed under local anesthesia as described for flexible bronchoscopy (see section IV.A) or after the induction of general anesthesia and endotracheal intubation. Use of a smaller caliber endotracheal tube will allow the surgeon more room to work in the pharynx and proximal esophagus.

D. **Rigid esophagoscopy** is commonly performed under general anesthesia with muscle relaxation. As with flexible esophagoscopy, a smaller endotracheal tube is used.

V. Mediastinal operations

A. Mediastinoscopy is indicated to determine the extrapulmonary spread of pulmonary tumors and to diagnose mediastinal masses. Mediastinoscopy is performed through an incision just superior to the manubrium. A rigid endoscope is then introduced beneath the sternum, and the anterior surfaces of the trachea and the hilum are examined.

1. Any general anesthetic technique may be used, provided the patient remains immobile. Although the procedure is not very painful, intermittent stimulation of the trachea, carina, and mainstem bronchi occurs.

2. **Complications** include pneumothorax, rupture of the great vessels, and damage to the airways. Blood pressures measured in the right arm may demonstrate intermittent occlusion if the innominate artery is compressed between the mediastinoscope and the posterior surface of the sternum. The trachea may be intermittently compressed by the mediastinoscope, and the position of the patient and surgeon increases the chance of accidental disconnection of the breathing circuit.

B. A Chamberlain procedure uses an anterior parasternal incision to obtain lung tissue for biopsy or to drain abscesses.

1. The procedure is performed with the patient in the supine position after induction of general anesthesia. If no ribs are resected, the procedure usually is not very painful. Infiltration of the incision with local anesthetic or administration of small doses of opioids usually is sufficient for analgesia.

2. One-lung ventilation is not required for lung biopsy, but manual ventilation in cooperation with the surgeon(s) can facilitate the procedure.

3. If the pleural space is evacuated as it is closed, a chest tube generally is not required postoperatively, although the patient should be monitored carefully for any signs of pneumothorax.

C. Mediastinal surgery

1. **Median sternotomy** is performed for resection of mediastinal tumors and for bilateral pulmonary resections. In descending order of frequency, mediastinal masses include neurogenic tumors, cysts, teratodermoids, lymphomas, thymomas, parathyroid tumors, and retrosternal thyroids.

2. **Thymectomy** is performed by median sternotomy and may be performed to treat myasthenia gravis. Anesthetic considerations for the patient with myasthenia gravis are detailed in Chapter 12, section VI.C.

3. **General anesthesia** may be induced and maintained with any technique.

   a. Muscle relaxants are not required to maintain surgical exposure but may be a useful adjunct to general anesthesia. Relaxants should be used with great caution or avoided in the myasthenic patient.

   b. During the actual sternotomy, the patient's lungs should be deflated and motionless. Even so, complications of sternotomy include laceration of the right ventricle, atrium, or great vessels (particularly the innominate artery) and unrecognized pneumothorax in either side of the chest.

c. Postoperative pain from a median sternotomy is significantly less than from a thoracotomy and may be managed with epidural or parenteral opioids.

VI. Pulmonary resection

A. Lateral or posterolateral thoracotomy is the most common approach for the resection of pulmonary neoplasms or abscesses. Thoracotomy may be preceded by staging procedures such as bronchoscopy, mediastinoscopy, or thoracoscopy. If the staging procedures are performed at the same sitting, the anesthetic should be planned to accommodate the possibility of a shortened procedure.

B. Endobronchial tubes. Placement of a double-lumen tube is indicated for lung protection (for significant hemoptysis or unilateral infection), bronchoalveolar lavage, or surgical exposure.

1. Choice

a. Double-lumen tubes range in size from 28 to 41 French. In general, a 39 or 41 French tube is chosen for adult males; a 35 or 37 French is chosen for adult females. Selection is also based on the patient's size.

b. Right- and left-sided double lumen tubes are available and are designed to conform to either the right or left main stem bronchus. Each tube has separate channels for independent ventilation of the distal bronchus and the trachea. Right-sided tubes have a separate opening to permit ventilation of the right upper lobe.

c. The choice of a left- or right-sided tube depends on the type and side of operation. If a mainstem bronchus is absent, stenotic, disrupted, or obstructed, the double-lumen tube must be placed on the opposite side, preferably under direct fiberoptic guidance. In most cases the choice of a left-versus right-sided tube is not so absolute. Most surgical procedures can be performed with a left-sided double-lumen tube. It is our practice, however, to selectively intubate the dependent (nonoperative) bronchus. This ensures that the endobronchial tube will not interfere with resection of the main stem bronchus, if this is necessary. Also, if the nondependent lung is intubated, ventilation of the dependent lung through the tracheal lumen may be compromised by mediastinal pressure pushing the tube against the tracheal wall and creating a "ball-valve" obstruction.

2. Insertion

a. The endobronchial tube, including both cuffs and all necessary connectors, should be carefully checked before placement. The tube may be lubricated, and a stylet should be placed in the bronchial lumen.

b. After laryngoscopy, the endobronchial tube should be inserted initially with the distal curve facing anteriorly. Once in the trachea, the stylet should be removed and the tube rotated so that the bronchial lumen is toward the appropriate side. The tube is then advanced to an average depth of 29 cm (27 cm in females), or less if resistance is met.

c. Alternatively, a fiberoptic bronchoscope can be passed down the bronchial lumen as soon as the tube is in the trachea and then used to guide the tube into the correct main stem bronchus.

d. Once the tube has been inserted and connected to the anesthesia circuit, the tracheal cuff is inflated, and manual ventilation is begun. Both lungs should expand evenly with bilateral breath sounds and no detectable air leak. The tracheal side of the adapter is then clamped and the distal tracheal lumen opened to room air via the access port. The bronchial cuff is inflated to a point just sufficient to eliminate air leak from the tracheal lumen, and the chest is auscultated. Breath sounds should now be limited to the nonoperative side of the chest. Moving the clamp to the bronchial side of the adapter and closing the tracheal access port should cause only the operative lung to be ventilated.

e. Once adequate lung isolation is achieved, the fiberoptic bronchoscope may be used to confirm position, because physical examination may be difficult or misleading. When passed down the tracheal lumen, the bronchoscope should reveal the carina with the top edge of the blue bronchial cuff just visible in the main stem bronchus. Passing the bronchoscope down the bronchial lumen should reveal either the left main stem bronchus or the bronchus intermedius depending on whether a left- or right-sided tube is being placed. The orifice of the right upper lobe should be visible through the side lumen of a right-sided tube. A bronchoscope should be kept available throughout the case.

3. Table 21-1 illustrates common errors with endobronchial tube placement. The most common error is positioning the tube too far into the bronchus so that the distal lumen is ventilating a single lobe.

4. The procedure for passing an endobronchial tube through an existing tracheostomy stoma is identical. Bronchoscopy will help to determine how far the tube should be advanced once it is in the trachea.

C. **Univent tubes** are large-caliber endotracheal tubes encompassing a small integrated channel for a built-in bronchial blocker.

　1. **Insertion**. The Univent tube is inserted into the trachea in the usual fashion and rotated toward the operative lung. After

Table 21-1.   Results of auscultation with both cuffs inflated and one lumen clamped

Bronchial Side Ventilated	Tracheal Side Ventilated	Problem
Clear unilateral breath sounds, high pressures	Clear breath sounds or no breath sounds	Tube in too far
Bilateral breath sounds	No breath sounds	Tube not in far enough
Unilateral breath sounds on wrong side	No breath sounds or breath sounds on wrong side	Tube in wrong side

inflation of the tracheal cuff, the bronchial blocker is advanced into the operative main stem bronchus under fiberoptic guidance, and the cuff is inflated. Because the Univent tube is made of Silastic rather than polyvinyl chloride, thorough lubrication of the bronchoscope is required.

2. Collapse of the operative lung occurs through both exhalation via the small distal opening in the blocker and by progressive absorption of oxygen from the lung, which will produce alveolar collapse. This is a slow process but may be hastened by deflating the blocker and disconnecting the anesthesia circuit while observing the lung. Once collapse has occurred, the blocker can be reinflated and the circuit reconnected.

D. Bronchial blockers may be used in situations in which it is not possible to place an endobronchial tube, typically in pediatric patients, in those with difficult airway anatomy or where satisfactory lung isolation cannot be achieved by other means.

1. Insertion. An appropriately sized Fogarty catheter (8 to 14 French venous occlusion catheter with a 10 mL balloon) is selected and placed into the trachea before endotracheal intubation. After intubation, the balloon tip is positioned with a fiberoptic bronchoscope in the appropriate main stem bronchus and inflated. Lung collapse occurs slowly, via absorption of gases. The ability to suction or perform maneuvers such as continuous positive airway pressure (CPAP) to the nonventilated lung is lost.

2. The **Arndt blocker** is a bronchial blocker especially designed for lung isolation. Placement is facilitated by the looped suture that can be snared with a bronchoscope. The airway connector is well designed, allowing a seal for the blocker, bronchoscope, and ventilation. Like the Univent tube, the blocker has a small central lumen that can be used for lung collapse or CPAP.

3. A blocker can be placed either intraluminal or extraluminal to the endotracheal tube. Generally, if an endotracheal tube is already in place, only the intraluminal approach is possible. Placing the blocker via the bronchoscope adapter through the tube is relatively easy, provided the lumen of the tube will accommodate both blocker and bronchoscope.

E. Complications of lung isolation techniques include collapse of obstructed segments of the lung, airway trauma, bleeding, and aspiration during prolonged efforts at intubation. Hypoxia and hypoventilation may occur both during placement efforts and as a result of malpositioning.

F. Positioning. Thoracotomies for lung resection are most commonly performed in the lateral decubitus position with the bed sharply flexed and the surgical field parallel to the floor.

1. The arms are usually extended in front of the patient and must be carefully padded to avoid compression on the radial and ulnar nerves or obstruction of arterial and venous cannulas. The dependent brachial plexus must be checked for excessive tension. Various devices exist for supporting the upper arm securely above the lower, leaving the anesthetist with good access to the lower arm. Neither arm should be abducted more than 90 degrees.

2. The neck should remain in a neutral position, and the dependent eye and ear should be carefully checked to ensure that they are not under any direct pressure.

3. The lower extremities should be padded appropriately to avoid compression injuries. In male patients, the scrotum should be carefully positioned.

4. During the positioning process, the vital signs should be closely observed, because pooling of blood in dependent extremities may cause hypotension.

5. Changes in position can move the endobronchial tube or blocker and change $\dot{V}/\dot{Q}$ relationships. Lung compliance, lung isolation, and oxygenation should be reassessed after any change in position.

G. One-lung ventilation. General anesthesia, the lateral position, an open chest, surgical manipulations, and one-lung ventilation all alter ventilation and perfusion.

1. Oxygenation

a. The amount of pulmonary blood flow passing through the unventilated lung (pulmonary shunt) is the most important factor determining arterial oxygenation during one-lung ventilation.

b. Diseased lungs often have reduced perfusion secondary to vascular occlusion or vasoconstriction. This may limit shunting of blood through the nonventilated operative lung during one-lung ventilation.

c. Perfusion of the unventilated lung is also reduced by hypoxic pulmonary vasoconstriction.

d. The lateral position tends to reduce pulmonary shunting, because gravity decreases blood flowing to the nondependent lung.

e. Oxygenation should be continuously monitored by pulse oximetry.

2. Ventilation

a. Arterial carbon dioxide tension generally is maintained on one-lung ventilation at the same level as on two lungs. This should not be at the expense of hyperinflating or overdistending the ventilated lung.

b. Controlled ventilation is mandatory during open-chest operations.

c. Plateau (or end-inspiratory) airway pressure generally should be maintained below 30 cm H_2O to avoid overdistention of the lung. The occurrence of high airway pressure should be investigated immediately and usually is due to malposition of the tube or the presence of secretions.

d. A moderate increase of partial pressure of carbon dioxide in arterial blood is usually well tolerated. Respiratory rate can be increased to maintain minute ventilation if necessary, as long as intrinsic positive end-expiratory pressure (PEEP) and air trapping are minimal.

e. When switching from two-lung to one-lung ventilation, manual ventilation allows instantaneous adaptation to the expected changes in compliance and facilitates assessment of lung isolation. Once tidal volume and compliance have been assessed by hand and lung collapse confirmed visually, mechanical ventilation can be reinstituted.

H. Management of one-lung ventilation

1. Anesthetic management. During one-lung ventilation, the use of nitrous oxide is limited or discontinued if there is any evidence of a significant decrease in partial pressure of oxygen in arterial blood (i.e., a decrease in oxygen saturation).

2. Difficulties with oxygenation during one-lung ventilation may be treated with a variety of maneuvers, which are directed at decreasing blood flow to the nonventilated lung (decreasing shunt fraction), minimizing atelectasis in the ventilated lung, or providing additional oxygen to the operative lung.

   a. Tube position should be reassessed by fiberoptic bronchoscopy and repositioned if necessary.

   b. The tube should be suctioned to clear secretions and ensure patency.

   c. PEEP may be added to the ventilated lung to treat atelectasis, but this may lower arterial oxygen saturation if a greater proportion of blood flow is forced into the unventilated lung as a result.

   d. CPAP can be applied to the nonventilated lung using a separate circuit. Under direct visualization, the collapsed lung is inflated and then allowed to deflate and maintained at a volume that will not interfere with surgical exposure (usually 2 to 5 cm H_2O CPAP).

   e. Apneic oxygenation may be provided to the nonventilated lung by briefly inflating it with 100% oxygen and then capping the exhalation port. In this way, a motionless partially collapsed lung is maintained. Reinflation of the lung with oxygen will be necessary every 10 to 20 minutes.

   f. In the event of persistent hypoxemia that is uncorrectable by combinations of the above therapies or a sudden precipitous desaturation, the surgeon must be notified and the operative lung reinflated with 100% oxygen. Two-lung ventilation should be maintained until the situation has stabilized, after which the operative lung can be allowed to collapse again. Periodic reinflations or manual two-lung ventilation may be required to maintain an adequate arterial oxygen saturation throughout some procedures.

   g. If hypoxemia persists, the surgeon can improve $\dot{V}/\dot{Q}$ matching by compressing or clamping the pulmonary artery of the surgical lung or any of its available lobes.

   h. Cardiopulmonary bypass can be instituted to provide oxygenation (see Chapter 23) in extreme situations.

3. When switching from one-lung back to two-lung ventilation, a few manual breaths with a prolonged inspiratory hold will help to reexpand collapsed alveoli.

I. Anesthetic technique. General anesthesia, in combination with epidural anesthesia, is the preferred technique. Thoracic epidural catheters are usually placed (see Chapter 16 for technique).

1. General anesthesia typically is induced with propofol and a muscle relaxant (such as cisatracurium) and maintained with a volatile agent in oxygen.

   a. Nitrous oxide may be used during the procedure to reduce the requirement for volatile agents.

   (1) During one-lung ventilation, shunting and hypoxemia may limit the use of nitrous oxide in some patients.

(2) At the conclusion of the procedure with both lungs ventilated, nitrous oxide, in concentrations up to 70%, will provide a smoother emergence than a volatile agent alone. It is essential that the chest tubes are functioning.

b. Muscle relaxants are useful adjuncts to general anesthesia. Although surgical exposure does not require muscle relaxation, movement and coughing carries some risk.

2. Epidural analgesia is an effective method for postoperative pain relief after thoracotomy.

a. Intraoperative use of the epidural can be either with a local anesthetic, opioid, or an anesthetic–opioid mixture. Phenylephrine should be used to counteract hypotension associated with epidural blockade.

b. Stimulation caused by lung reexpansion, bronchoscopy, and bronchial dissection is not blunted by epidural analgesia and may provoke a sudden response in an otherwise well-anesthetized patient.

J. Emergence and extubation. The goal of the anesthetic technique selected is to have an awake, comfortable, and extubated patient at the end of the procedure.

1. Before closing the chest, the lungs are inflated to 30 cm H_2O pressure to reinflate atelectatic areas and check for significant air leaks.

2. Chest tubes are inserted to drain the pleural cavity and promote lung expansion. Chest tubes usually are placed under water seal and 20 cm H_2O suction, except after a pneumonectomy. After pneumonectomy, a chest tube, if used, should be placed under water seal only. Applying suction could shift the mediastinum to the draining side and reduce venous return.

3. Prompt extubation avoids the potential disruptive effects of endotracheal intubation and positive-pressure ventilation on fresh suture lines. If postoperative mechanical ventilation is required, the double-lumen tube should be exchanged for a conventional endotracheal tube with a high-volume low-pressure cuff. Inspiratory pressures should be kept as low as possible.

K. Postoperative analgesia. Lateral thoracotomy is a painful incision, involving multiple muscle layers, rib resection, and continuous motion as the patient breathes. Therapy for postoperative pain should begin before the patient emerges from general anesthesia.

1. Epidural analgesia has become the preferred approach for postthoracotomy pain management (see Chapter 37). Shoulder pain that thoracotomy patients commonly note is referred pain from diaphragmatic irritation and is not covered by epidural analgesia but is well treated with nonsteroidal analgesics.

2. Intercostal nerve blocks

a. Intercostal nerve blocks may be used in situations where epidural analgesia is impractical or ineffective.

b. Five interspaces are usually blocked: two above, two below, and one at the site of the incision.

c. Technique. Under sterile conditions, a 22-gauge needle is inserted perpendicular to the skin in the posterior axillary line over the lower edge of the rib. The needle then is "walked" off the rib inferiorly until it just slips off the rib. After a negative aspiration for blood, 4 to 5 mL of 0.5% bupivacaine with

1:200,000 epinephrine is injected. The procedure is repeated at each interspace to be blocked. In addition, subcutaneous infiltration with bupivacaine is performed in a V-shaped pattern around each chest tube site to reduce the discomfort of chest tube movement.

 d. If a chest tube is not in place, the risk of pneumothorax from the block needs to be considered.

 3. Parenteral narcotics, if required, should be administered judiciously.

 4. Nonsteroidal anti-inflammatory agents. Ketorolac has proved effective as a supplemental analgesic but should be used with caution in the elderly, patients with renal insufficiency, or those with a history of gastric bleeding.

VII. Tracheal resection and reconstruction

 A. General considerations. Surgery of the trachea and major airways involves significant anesthetic risks, including interruption of airway continuity and the potential for total obstruction of an already stenotic airway.

  1. The surgical approach depends on the location and extent of the lesion. Lesions of the cervical trachea are approached through a transverse neck incision. Lower lesions necessitate a manubrial split. Lesions of the distal trachea and carina may require a median sternotomy and/or single or bilateral thoracotomy.

  2. Extubation at the conclusion of the surgical procedure is the goal of the anesthetic, because it will put less strain on the fresh tracheal anastomosis.

 B. Induction

  1. The anesthetic techniquemust include a plan for preserving airway patency throughout induction and intubation and emergency plans and equipment for dealing with any sudden loss of airway control.

  2. If the airway is critically stenotic, spontaneous ventilation should be maintained throughout the induction, because it may not be possible to ventilate the lungs by mask ventilation if apnea occurs. A volatile agent in oxygen is the preferred anesthetic and no muscle relaxants are used. Sevoflurane, with its lack of airway irritability, is suitable for inhalational induction. A deep plane of anesthesia must be achieved before instrumentation, and this may require 15 to 20 minutes in a patient with small tidal volumes and a large functional residual capacity. Hemodynamic support with phenylephrine may be required for an elderly or debilitated patient to tolerate the necessary high concentration of volatile agent.

  3. Patients with preexisting mature tracheostomies may be induced with intravenous agents, allowing cannulation of the tracheostomy with a cuffed, flexible, armored endotracheal tube. The surgical field around the tube is prepared, and the tube is removed and replaced with a sterile one by the surgeon.

 C. Intraoperative management is complicated by periodic interruption of airway continuity by the surgical procedure.

  1. Rigid bronchoscopy is commonly performed before the surgical incision to delineate tracheal anatomy and caliber.

   a. If the surgeon determines that an endotracheal tube can be placed through the stenotic segment, this should be done as soon as the bronchoscope is withdrawn. Controlled ventilation can then be used safely.

b. If the stenotic segment is too narrow or friable to allow intubation, spontaneous ventilation and anesthesia must continue through the bronchoscope until surgical access to the distal trachea is achieved. Alternatives include having the surgeon "core out" the tracheal lesion with the rigid bronchoscope, placing a tracheostomy distal to the stenotic segment, intubating the trachea above the lesion or placing a LMA and allowing spontaneous ventilation to continue, or using a jet ventilation system to ventilate the patient from above the lesion.

2. Whenever the airway is in jeopardy or ventilation is intermittent, 100% oxygen should be administered.

3. For lower tracheal or carinal resections, a long endotracheal tube with a flexible armored wall can be used. This allows the surgeon to position the tip in the trachea or either main stem bronchus and to operate around it without interrupting ventilation.

4. When the trachea is surgically divided, the endotracheal tube must be retracted above the division and a sterile armored tube placed into the distal trachea by the surgeon. A suture may be placed in the endotracheal tube before pulling it back into the pharynx to facilitate replacing it in the trachea at the end of the procedure.

a. The tube may be frequently removed and reinserted by the surgeons as they work around it. Manual ventilation during this portion of the procedure will help avoid leakage of gas from the circuit.

b. Once the stenotic segment has been removed and the posterior tracheal reanastomosis completed, the transtracheal tube is removed and the endotracheal tube is readvanced from above. The distal trachea should be suctioned to remove accumulated blood and secretions. The patient's neck is then flexed forward, reducing tension on the trachea, and the anterior portion of the anastomosis is completed.

5. Jet ventilation through a catheter held by one of the surgeons may be required during carinal resection if the distal airways are too small to accommodate an endotracheal tube.

a. It is difficult to administer volatile agents by a jet ventilator, so intravenous agents will be needed during this portion of the surgery.

b. Jet ventilation rate and pressure should be carefully titrated by direct observation of the surgical field. Obstruction of exhalation will lead to "stacking" of breaths, increased airway pressure, and barotrauma.

6. At the conclusion of the procedure, a single large suture is placed from the chin to the anterior chest to preserve neck flexion and thereby minimize tension on the tracheal suture line. Several blankets under the head will help maintain flexion. Close attention during emergence, extubation, and transfer is essential.

D. Emergence and extubation

1. Spontaneous ventilation should be resumed as soon as possible after the procedure to minimize trauma to the tracheal suture line. Most patients may be safely extubated, but in those where difficult anatomy or copious secretions make this undesirable, a small tracheostomy may be placed below the tracheal repair.

   a. The patient should be awake enough to maintain spontaneous ventilation and avoid aspiration but should be extubated before excessive head movement can damage the surgical repair.

   b. If tracheal collapse, airway edema, or secretions cause respiratory distress after extubation, the patient should be reintubated fiberoptically with a small uncuffed endotracheal tube, preferably with the head maintained in forward flexion.

2. Frequent bronchoscopies at the bedside under local anesthesia may be required to remove secretions from the lungs in the postoperative period.

3. Only relatively small amounts of intravenous opioids are usually needed to treat the mild pain from the neck incision. Analgesia usually is administered after the patient is wide awake and responsive and while monitoring for undesirable respiratory depression.

E. **Tracheal disruption** may be caused by airway instrumentation or thoracic trauma and may be signaled by hypoxia, dyspnea, subcutaneous emphysema, pneumomediastinum, or pneumothorax.

   1. **The point of injury** is commonly at the cricoid, mid-trachea, carina, or either mainstem bronchus. Several mechanisms of injury have been proposed, including high airway pressures, lateral stretch of the thoracic cavity, and deceleration injury.

   2. **Positive-pressure ventilation** will exacerbate the air leak and rapidly worsen symptoms from pneumothorax or pneumomediastinum. If possible, the patient should be allowed to breathe spontaneously, following the protocol for the patient with critical tracheal stenosis.

   3. **Tracheal damage** in the already anesthetized patient may be treated initially by advancement of a small endotracheal tube past the point of injury. In the case of a difficult airway where the tube itself causes the injury, an immediate surgical tracheostomy must be performed and access to the distal trachea secured.

   4. Once a tube has been placed across or distal to the site of tracheal disruption, controlled positive-pressure ventilation can begin. Further management is as for the patient undergoing elective airway surgery.

VIII. **Intrapulmonary hemorrhage.** Massive hemoptysis may be caused by thoracic trauma, pulmonary artery rupture secondary to catheterization, or erosion into a vessel by a tracheostomy, abscess, or airway tumor.

   A. The trachea must be immediately intubated and the lungs ventilated with 100% oxygen.

   B. An attempt should be made to suction the airway clear, ideally by rigid bronchoscopy.

   C. **If a unilateral source is identified,** lung isolation may be undertaken to protect the uninvolved lung and facilitate corrective surgery. Techniques for lung isolation are described in section

VI.B. Obstruction of the endotracheal tube is an ever present danger, and frequent suctioning may be necessary.

1.   Lung isolation may be achieved either by placing an endobronchial blocker or double-lumen endobronchial tube. Choice of technique will depend on experience, equipment at hand, and the extent of active bleeding. Active bleeding may obscure airway visualization during flexible bronchoscopy.

2.   In an emergency, the existing endotracheal tube can be advanced into the mainstem bronchus of the uninvolved lung and the cuff inflated.

3.   Fiberoptic bronchoscopy is essential for suctioning blood and confirming isolation.

D.   Frequently, the source of bleeding is from the bronchial circulation. **Embolization** in the radiology suite will often be attempted if the patient is stable.

E.   Definitive treatment may require a thoracotomy and surgical repair.

IX.   Esophageal surgery includes procedures for resection of esophageal neoplasms, antireflux procedures, and repair of traumatic or congenital lesions.

A.   General considerations

1.   Patients may be chronically malnourished, both from systemic illness (carcinoma) and anatomic interference with swallowing. Enteral or parenteral nutrition may have been begun preoperatively.

2.   Both esophageal carcinoma and traumatic disruption of the distal esophagus are associated with ethanol abuse; patients may have impaired liver function, elevated portal pressures, anemia, cardiomyopathy, and bleeding disorders.

3.   Patients who have difficulty swallowing may be significantly hypovolemic. Cardiovascular instability may be further exacerbated by preoperative chemotherapy with cardiotoxins such as adriamycin.

4.   Most patients presenting for esophageal procedures will be at risk for aspiration. Appropriate preoperative prophylaxis should be given, and rapid sequence induction or awake intubation should be planned.

5.   Monitors should include a radial artery and urinary catheters. Central venous access may be desirable.

6.   Temperature conservation measures should be aggressively pursued. The use of a warmed air blanket over the lower body is routine.

B.   Operative approach and anesthesia

1.   Upper esophageal diverticula are approached through a lateral cervical incision, similar to that for carotid surgery. This incision may also be used for upper esophageal myotomies for swallowing disorders.

a.   Positioning. The patient is positioned supine with the neck extended and the head turned to the contralateral side.

b.   General anesthesia may be induced and maintained with any technique after rapid sequence intubation. Postoperative pain and fluid shifts are usually minimal with a cervical incision, and patients may be safely extubated at the conclusion of the procedure. The surgeons may or may not elect to leave a nasogastric tube in place.

2. Carcinoma

   a. Lesions of the upper esophagus are approached through a transverse cervical incision, allowing for a proximal anastomosis in the neck. A right-sided thoracic incision and a midline abdominal incision may also be required to complete the resection and reattach the proximal and distal ends.

   b. Lesions of the middle esophagus are commonly approached through a right-sided thoracotomy, which allows for a proximal anastomosis above the level of the aortic arch. Mobilization of the stomach or jejunum is accomplished through a midline abdominal incision. This combination is known as an **Ivor-Lewis procedure**.

   c. Lower esophageal lesions are approached through an extended left thoracoabdominal incision. After resection, the surgeon will either perform a primarily anastomosis of the esophagus or the esophagus and stomach or bring up a roux-en-Y loop of jejunum.

   d. Postoperative endotracheal extubation is performed when the patient can protect the his or her airway from aspiration and they are fully awake. Immediate postoperative extubation can be considered in healthier patients after uncomplicated procedures.

   e. Virtually any anesthetic technique may be used. Epidural analgesia is commonly used in the postoperative period.

   f. It is often necessary to change from a double-lumen to a conventional endotracheal tube at the conclusion of an esophageal resection. Dependent tissue edema may significantly narrow the airway, rendering reintubation difficult.

3. Traumatic damage to the entire esophagus (as with lye ingestion) or extensive cancers may necessitate a total esophagectomy with subsequent interposition of a segment of colon or jejunum to serve as a conduit between the pharynx and stomach.

   a. Surgical exposure may require two or three incisions. In some cases, the esophagus can be dissected bluntly from the posterior mediastinum through cervical and abdominal incisions, and no thoracotomy is necessary.

   b. These patients may have a prolonged postoperative course with significant fluid shifts and nutritional depletion and are at risk for aspiration pneumonia. The trachea should remain intubated at the conclusion of the surgical procedure.

4. Fundoplication (e.g., Belsey Mark IV, Hill, or Nissen) is performed for relief of gastroesophageal reflux, the specific procedure depending on the preference of the surgeon and the patient's anatomy.

   a. The surgical approach is transabdominal for the Hill and Nissen procedures and transthoracic for the Belsey. Collapse of the left lung is required for the latter procedure.

   b. Fluid shifts are usually less than after other esophageal surgeries, and these patients may be safely extubated at the conclusion of the procedure. Postoperative analgesic requirements will be determined by the specific incision made; most patients will benefit from epidural medications.

X. Lung transplantation is performed for several reasons (e.g., α_1-antitrypsin deficiency, cystic fibrosis, emphysema, or idiopathic pulmonary hypertension). Specific operations include living-donor single lobe, single and double lung, sequential single lung, and combined heart–lung transplantation. Patients will have undergone preoperative counseling, exercise and cardiac testing, and a conditioning program along with other assessments outlined in section I. Recipients are considered to have a "full stomach." Because the patients will be immunosuppressed, sterile technique for all procedures is paramount. Because the optimal donor ischemic time is less than 4 hours, time is of the essence.

A.   Monitors and equipment

1.   In addition to the usual monitoring for pulmonary resection, a pulmonary artery catheter is placed, incorporating a long sterile protective sheath.

2.   Medications should be immediately available to treat bronchospasm, pulmonary hypertension, and right ventricular failure.

3.   An epidural catheter should be placed for postoperative pain management, unless there is a strong possibility that the patient will need cardiopulmonary bypass and full heparinization.

4.   An additional mechanical ventilator may be required to optimally ventilate each lung.

5.   Equipment should be available for peripheral arteriovenous or venovenous bypass through an oxygenator if hypoxemia becomes a significant problem.

B.   Anesthetic technique. Any technique that provides cardiovascular stability is appropriate. A high-dose opioid technique with muscle relaxation and small doses of benzodiazepines or volatile anesthetic agents offer excellent analgesia and amnesia.

1.   Lung isolation is best achieved with a contralateral endobronchial tube. In the event of a double-lung transplant, a left-sided tube is used with the left-sided bronchial anastomosis performed distal to the tip.

2.   Capnography may be misleading because of severe mismatching of ventilation to perfusion. Frequent measurement of ABG tensions are warranted to assess ventilation.

3.   Full cardiopulmonary bypass may be necessary for the patient with pulmonary hypertension who cannot tolerate unilateral pulmonary artery clamping. Indications for bypass include arterial oxygen saturation less than 90% after clamping of the pulmonary artery, cardiac index less than 3.0 L/min/m^2 despite therapy with dopamine and nitroglycerin, or a systolic blood pressure less than 90 mm Hg. Continuous cardiac output monitors may be used to assess cardiac function. Management of cardiopulmonary bypass is discussed in Chapter 23.

4.   The surgical approach is via a standard posterolateral incision or a bilateral subcostal thoracotomy, extended toward the side of the transplant.

C.   After surgery, the trachea remains intubated, the lungs ventilated, and the patient sedated until the transplanted lung begins to function well and symptoms of reperfusion edema and acute rejection are controlled. The trachea is extubated only when the patient is hemodynamically stable and breathing comfortably.

1.   Serial ABGs are followed to document the function of the transplanted lung. Acute rejection may manifest as decreasing pulmonary compliance with worsening arterial oxygenation.

2. The patient must be observed for signs of toxicity from the immunosuppressive regimen, including acute renal failure.

D. Repeated bronchoscopies and biopsies of the transplanted lung are necessary after surgery and are managed under local anesthesia with intravenous sedation.

XI. Lung volume reduction surgery is performed on patients with severe bullous emphysema who experience incapacitating dyspnea despite maximal medical therapy. The goal is to relieve thoracic distention and improve ventilation. Patients are selected under strict criteria and undergo a period of cardiopulmonary conditioning before surgery.

A. The surgical approach is via thoracotomy or median sternotomy. The least functional part of the lung as determined by CT and intraoperative observation is resected with staples that are buttressed with bovine pericardium to reduce air leaks.

B. The anesthetic technique is similar to lung resection (see section VI). Postoperatively, epidural analgesia is essential.

C. Postoperative course. The trachea should be extubated postoperatively and the patients admitted to an intensive care unit. It is not infrequent that the lungs have air leaks postoperatively. If intubation and mechanical ventilation is required, it is imperative to minimize stress on the lung and suture lines by using low tidal volumes and airway pressures.

SUGGESTED READING

Benumof JL. *Anesthesia for thoracic surgery*, 2nd ed. Philadephia: WB Saunders, 1995.

Bernard A, Deschamps C, Allen MS, et al. Pneumonectomy for malignant disease: factors affecting early morbidity and mortality. *J Thorac Cardiovasc Surg* 2001;121:1076–1082.

Bolliger CT, Perruchoud AP. Functional evaluation of the lung resection candidate. *Eur Respir J* 1998;11:198–212.

Bracken CA, Gurkowski MA, Naples JJ. Lung transplantation: historical perspective, current concepts, and anesthetic considerations. *J Cardiothorac Vasc Anesth* 1997;11:220–241.

Cicala RS, Kudsk KA, Butts A, et al. Initial evaluation and management of upper airway injuries in trauma patients. *J Clin Anesth* 1991;3:91–98.

Devitt JH, Boulanger BR. Lower airway injuries and anaesthesia. *Can J Anaesth* 1996;43:148–159.

Grillo HC, Austen WG, Wilkins EW, et al. *Current therapy in cardiothoracic surgery.* Toronto: BC Decker, 1989.

Kaplan JA. *Thoracic anesthesia*, 3rd ed. New York: Churchill Livingstone, 1991.

Sandberg W. Anesthesia and airway management for tracheal resection and reconstruction. *Int Anesthesiol Clin* 2000;38:55–75.

Anesthesia for Vascular Surgery

Edward Bittner and Peter F. Dunn

I. Preoperative assessment and management should be aimed at identifying coexisting disease, optimizing specific therapies, and anticipating intra- and postoperative problems.

A. Cardiovascular system. Coronary artery disease is present in 40% to 80% of vascular surgery patients, and is a major source of morbidity and mortality. Myocardial infarction (MI) accounts for about one-half of early postoperative deaths. Cardiac risk factors include congestive heart failure, MI, hypertension, valvular heart disease, angina, and arrhythmias (see Chapter 2).

1. Coexisting medical conditions, such as claudication, disability from a prior stroke, and emphysema limit the utility of exercise tolerance as a tool for assessing cardiac function.

2. Specialized cardiac testing, such as exercise stress testing, dipyridamole-thallium stress testing, echocardiography, and cardiac catheterization help to stratify cardiac risk, as discussed in Chapter 2.

3. Due to the widespread nature of **atherosclerosis**, the presence of major differences in blood pressure readings between arms is relatively common and should be determined preoperatively.

4. Risk stratification may help with decisions regarding perioperative management. High-risk patients may benefit from additional preoperative medical therapy, coronary revascularization, and/or minimization of surgical procedures.

B. Respiratory system. Many vascular patients have a significant smoking history, which compromises their pulmonary function (see Chapter 3).

C. Renal system. Renal insufficiency is common. Important causes include atherosclerosis, hypertension, diabetes, inadequate perfusion, volume depletion, and angiographic, dye-related, acute tubular necrosis (see Chapter 4).

D. Central nervous system. Patients should be examined for carotid bruits and questioned for a history of transient ischemic attacks (TIAs) and cerebrovascular accidents. Their presence warrants further evaluation prior to major vascular surgery.

E. Endocrine system. Diabetics may manifest diffuse, accelerated atherosclerosis, as well as distal small-vessel disease. Longstanding diabetics may have autonomic neuropathy, silent ischemia, diabetic nephropathy, and reduced resistance to infection. Preoperative insulin orders and related management are discussed in Chapter 6. Patients receiving **metformin** (Glucophage) should have the drug discontinued 48 hours before receiving intravenous contrast dye, because of the potential for the development of severe lactic acidosis.

F. Hematologic system. Vascular surgical patients are often treated with anticoagulants (unfractionated or low molecular-weight heparin; warfarin; dipyridamole, clopidogrel; ticlodipine; or aspirin). A history of easy bruising, petechiae, or ecchymosis should be sought and evaluated with a prothrombin time, partial thromboplastin time, and platelet count where appropriate. Underlying coagulopathies may impact on choice of anesthetic technique and intraoperative blood loss.

G. Infection. There is a high mortality rate associated with infection in patients with vascular grafts. Patients with any evidence of infection should receive appropriate antibiotics preoperatively, and consideration should be given to postponing cases where heterologous graft materials will be used.

II. Preoperative medication

A. Cardiac medications should be continued up to the morning of surgery (see Chapter 2).

B. Anticoagulation. For patients on chronic anticoagulation therapy, warfarin should be discontinued at least 3 days prior to surgery, and, if indicated, heparin therapy started. If regional anesthesia is planned, unfractionated heparin generally is withheld 4 hours prior to surgery, in consultation with surgical staff. Low-molecular-weight heparin should be withheld for 24 hours prior to a regional anesthetic. **Clopidogrel** should be withheld for 1 week prior to surgery and **ticlodipine** for 10 to 14 days prior to elective surgery.

C. Sedatives. The goals and regimens for sedative premedication generally are the same as for elderly patients undergoing other major procedures (see Chapter 1).

III. Carotid endarterectomy

A. General considerations. Carotid endarterectomy is performed in patients with stenotic or ulcerative lesions of the common carotid artery and its internal and external branches. These lesions often present as carotid bruits and may produce TIAs or strokes.

1. Widespread atherosclerotic disease (especially coronary vessels) is often present.

2. The baseline blood pressure and heart rate should be determined by reviewing the medical record.

3. Preexisting neurologic deficits should be documented so that new deficits can be determined postoperatively. Patients may exhibit neurologic symptoms with extreme neck motion, necessitating careful positioning for surgery.

B. Monitoring

1. An arterial catheter, in addition to standard monitors, is used. In rare cases, a pulmonary artery (PA) catheter may be placed when needed (see Chapter 10). Sites for placement include the subclavian, antecubital, and contralateral internal jugular veins.

2. An electroencephalogram (EEG) is used during general anesthesia to ensure adequate perfusion during carotid cross-clamping and to identify patients who may require shunting to preserve cerebral blood flow (see Chapter 24).

C. Anesthetic technique

1. Regional anesthesia

a. Regional anesthesia may be performed with superficial and deep cervical plexus blocks (see Chapter17); both have potential complications.

b.   This technique requires an alert, cooperative patient who is able to tolerate lateral head positioning under the surgical drapes. It is important to properly position and drape the patient to provide access to the head and control of the airway, which may be necessary at any time. An appropriately sized laryngeal mask airway should be readily available.

c.   Continuous neurologic assessment is facilitated with an awake patient.

d.   Our preference is to use a superficial block with supplementation by the surgeons as needed. This minimizes the potential complications associated with the deep block, especially phrenic nerve paralysis.

2.   General anesthesia

a.   General anesthesia provides control of ventilation, oxygenation, and reduced cerebral metabolic demand.

b.   A baseline EEG is obtained in the preinduction period.

c.   Blood pressure should be maintained at the patient's high-normal range and may require a vasopressor such as phenylephrine.

d.   Induction requires the slow titration of anesthetic drugs to preserve cerebral perfusion while minimizing hemodynamic alterations. Ventilation should be adjusted to avoid hypocapnic cerebral vasoconstriction. Hypercarbia has no clinical benefit.

e.   A steady state of "light" anesthesia generally does not interfere with EEG monitoring and facilitates early postoperative neurologic examination. Muscle relaxants should be carefully titrated to minimize movement that can interfere with EEG interpretation.

D.   Carotid cross-clamping

1.   Surgical traction on the carotid sinus may cause an intense vagal stimulus, leading to hypotension and bradycardia. Infiltration with local anesthetic may abolish the response. Release of traction and administration of anticholinergics may be required.

2.   Heparin (5,000 units IV) is administered prior to cross-clamping.

3.   A shunt is placed if the patient's neurologic exam changes while under regional anesthesia, if EEG changes occur or, routinely, in cases without neurological monitoring.

4.   Blood pressure may be temporarily increased by use of a vasopressor, which may increase cerebral perfusion via the circle of Willis.

5.   Unclamping may produce reflex vasodilation and bradycardia. Vasopressors may be required as the baroreceptors adapt. Their use may also be required in the postoperative period.

E.   Postoperative neurologic deficits may occur from hypoperfusion or emboli (from shunts or ulcerated plaques). Minor neurologic changes usually resolve, but sudden major changes require immediate evaluation and possible re-exploration.

F.   Postoperative management. Patients are monitored during transport to the postanesthesia care unit, where they remain for observation. Major concerns include neurologic status, control of blood pressure and heart rate, and evidence of postoperative hemorrhage, which may lead to rapid airway obstruction.

IV. Peripheral vascular (arterial) surgery

A. General considerations. Peripheral vascular surgery is performed to bypass occlusive disease or aneurysms, remove emboli, and repair pseudoaneurysms and catheter injuries. Although peripheral vascular surgery is less of a physiologic insult than aortic surgery, their perioperative cardiac risks are comparable.

B. Femoral-popliteal and distal lower extremity bypass grafting. Lower-extremity, occlusive arterial disease is most often bypassed with an autologous saphenous vein graft. If this is not available or of unacceptable quality, arm vein or cryopreserved cadaveric vein may be used. The preparation of the vein and subsequent anastomoses to the arterial circulation may be time-consuming, but rarely place significant hemodynamic stress on the patient. The use of synthetic grafts (e.g., Gore-Tex) in selected patients may shorten these procedures. Although blood loss is usually minimal, revision of previous peripheral vascular procedures and surgically difficult cases may result in significant blood loss.

1. Monitoring. Most types of peripheral vascular procedures require similar monitoring, unless noted otherwise. In relatively healthy patients undergoing limited surgery, routine monitoring, as outlined in Chapter 10, is sufficient. As a case proceeds, hemodynamic lability, excessive blood loss, low urine output, or cardiac ischemia may dictate placement of invasive monitors (arterial, central venous, or PA catheters). A Foley catheter is placed routinely.

2. Regional anesthesia. A continuous lumbar epidural catheter is commonly used. It provides excellent anesthesia and a route to administer postoperative analgesia. Spinal anesthesia is appropriate if the length of the procedure can be predicted with some assurance. A continuous spinal technique is useful during prolonged procedures for patients in whom epidural anesthesia proves technically difficult or unsatisfactory. For procedures limited to a single limb, combined lumbar plexus and sciatic nerve block may be used.

    a. An α-adrenergic agent (e.g., phenylephrine) should be available to treat the hypotension associated with sympathetic blockade.

    b. Anticoagulation

        (1) The anticoagulated patient must either have his or her clotting abnormality corrected (with fresh-frozen plasma, vitamin K, or protamine) prior to catheter insertion or receive a general anesthetic.

        (2) There is no evidence that heparinization after epidural catheter placement increases the risk of epidural hematoma formation. If postoperative warfarin therapy is needed, the epidural should be removed prior to the onset of the anticoagulant effect (within 24 hours of the administration of the first dose).

    c. Regional anesthesia may help detect myocardial ischemia, since the patient can complain of chest pain or other symptoms.

    d. Attention to patient comfort is particularly important when using regional techniques during long procedures. Appropriate back and shoulder padding and freedom of the neck and arms should be provided. Sedation should reduce patient anxiety without producing confusion, respiratory depression, or unresponsiveness. Blankets and other warming measures are important, since heat loss from vasodilated extremities is significant. Shivering is not only unpleasant but may also be detrimental.

   3. General anesthesia. Any technique is appropriate provided hemodynamic stability is maintained.

C. Iliofemoral and iliodistal bypass grafting may be performed with spinal or epidural anesthesia. A higher anesthetic level is needed (i.e., T-8) because of proximal extension of the incision and peritoneal retraction for exposure of the iliac artery.

D. Peripheral embolectomy and femoral pseudoaneurysm repair frequently involve patients with unstable cardiovascular disease (e.g., recent MI). Some of these patients are anticoagulated or recently have received thrombolytic agents, thus precluding regional anesthesia. If not, lumbar plexus blockade provides adequate coverage. Field blocks with local anesthesia are sometimes appropriate. Surgical embolectomy and flushing of the thrombi from an obstructed artery may be associated with significant blood loss and hypotension.

E. Femoral-femoral bypass grafting is used to treat symptomatic unilateral iliac occlusive disease.

F. Peripheral aneurysms, such as popliteal aneurysms, rarely rupture but are associated with a high rate of thrombosis and embolism.

G. Axillofemoral bypass grafting provides arterial blood flow to the lower extremities. This approach is chosen when there is an active abdominal infection or an infected aortic bypass graft, or when a patient is medically unfit for abdominal aortic surgery. Routine monitoring is supplemented by an arterial catheter, which should be placed in the arm opposite the surgery. Central venous and PA lines are used as necessary.

H. Vascular surgery of the upper extremity usually includes distal embolectomy and repair of traumatic injuries. The surgery is localized, but there may be a need to harvest a vein graft at a site distant from the vascular repair. Possible anesthetic techniques include field block, regional, or general anesthesia. Proximal vascular surgical procedures (e.g., thoracic outlet syndrome and vertebral stenosis) may require an intrathoracic approach and/or temporary interruption of carotid blood flow.

I. Postoperative care. These patients require careful hemodynamic control and adequate analgesia. Graft occlusion in the immediate postoperative period may occur, requiring reexploration. Epidural catheters are left in place for the postoperative period.

V. Abdominal aortic surgery

A. Infrarenal aortic surgery

   1. Abdominal aortic surgery may be required for atherosclerotic occlusive disease or aneurysmal dilation. These processes can involve any portion of the aorta and its major branches, and lead to ischemia, rupture, and exsanguination. Ninety-five percent of all abdominal aortic aneurysms (AAAs) occur below the level of the renal arteries. Patients with AAAs over 5 cm in diameter, especially those shown to be expanding, have a better prognosis if they undergo elective resection. The annual risk of rupture of an expanding 5-cm aneurysm is about 4%. The operative mortality for elective AAA resection is less than 2%, while the overall mortality of aneurysm rupture is 70% to 80%.

2. Surgical technique. Compared with a transabdominal approach, the retroperitoneal approach may result in a lower incidence of postoperative ileus, pulmonary complications, cardiovascular complications, and fluid shifts. The approach is technically advantageous in morbidly obese patients or those who have had previous abdominal procedures.

3. Monitoring. A large peripheral IV (14 gauge), ECG (leads II and V5), a central venous catheter, arterial line, and Foley catheter, in addition to the usual monitoring, are required. PA catheters are employed when indicated, as outlined in Chapter 10. All monitoring catheters (except the Foley) are inserted prior to induction, and initial baseline values are obtained to guide anesthetic management. Vasoactive agents (e.g., nitroglycerin and phenylephrine) must be available for every case.

4. Anesthetic technique

   a. General considerations. Most patients receive combined general and epidural anesthesia using a midthoracic epidural catheter. Although general anesthesia alone is acceptable, a combined technique reduces anesthetic requirements, facilitates immediate extubation, and provides for postoperative analgesia.

   b. Induction. The epidural catheter is injected with 2% lidocaine and a sensory level is confirmed prior to administration of general anesthesia. Reduced blood pressure associated with the onset of epidural anesthesia is treated with phenylephrine. General anesthesia is induced in a slow and controlled fashion, titrating drugs to the desired hemodynamic and anesthetic effect. Since immediate postoperative extubation is usually planned, high-dose opioid techniques are generally avoided.

   c. Maintenance

      (1) Anesthesia is provided primarily by epidural blockade with 2% lidocaine. This is supplemented by nitrous oxide, muscle relaxants, and a low inspired concentration of a volatile anesthetic. A continuous epidural infusion of dilute 0.1% bupivacaine with an opioid (dilaudid or fentanyl) is begun during the procedure.

      (2) Heat conservation. Heat loss during aortic procedures may be considerable. Strategies for heat conservation are discussed in Chapter 14.

      (3) Bowel manipulation is necessary to gain access to the aorta during a transabdominal approach and may be accompanied by skin flushing, decreased systemic vascular resistance, and profound hypotension. These changes may be caused by release of prostaglandins and vasoactive peptides from the bowel and last for approximately 20 to 30 minutes. Treatment consists of IV phenylephrine, volume expansion, and reducing anesthetic depth.

      (4) Fluid management. Intravascular volume is depleted by hemorrhage, insensible losses into the bowel and peritoneal cavity, and evaporative losses associated with large abdominal incisions.

    (a) **Crystalloid solutions** are used for volume replacement at an approximate rate of 10 to 15 mL/kg per hour.

    (b) **Colloid solutions** are rarely necessary and are reserved for patients who are unresponsive or intolerant of large amounts of crystalloid.

    (c) The **hematocrit** should be maintained above the 30% range. With blood losses greater than 2,000 mL, coagulation profiles should be monitored, and platelets, clotting factors, and calcium replaced, guided by laboratory evaluation.

    (d) **Autotransfusion devices** should be used intraoperatively to scavenge shed blood. Autotransfused blood is deficient in plasma, clotting factors, and platelets.

(5) **Aortic cross-clamping**

    (a) **Heparin** (5,000 units IV) is given several minutes prior to applying an aortic cross-clamp.

    (b) **Increased afterload following aortic cross-clamping** is well tolerated by patients with normal hearts. Those with compromised left ventricular function may exhibit a decreased cardiac output and/or myocardial ischemia. The use of nitroglycerin or, rarely, nitroprusside may improve myocardial oxygen supply–demand balance.

(6) **Renal preservation.** The incidence of renal failure is 1% to 2% for infrarenal aortic surgery. Preoperative angiographic dye studies and preexisting renal disease increase this risk. Patients with chronically elevated creatinine levels (more than 2 mg/dL) have substantially greater morbidity and mortality after vascular surgery. Renal cortical blood flow and urine output may decrease with infrarenal aortic cross-clamping, possibly because of circulatory derangements, effects on the renin-angiotensin system, and microembolization. Maintenance of adequate hydration and urine flow is extremely important. If the urine output falls in spite of adequate hydration, intravenous mannitol, furosemide, dopamine infusion (1 to 2 µg/kg per minute), or fenoldopam (3 µg/kg per minute) may be given.

(7) **Aortic unclamping.** Intravascular volume must be maintained in the normal to hypervolemic range, anticipating a fall in systemic vascular resistance and venous return following release of the aortic cross-clamp. Volume loading, decreasing anesthetic depth, discontinuing vasodilators, infusing a vasopressor, and a slow, controlled release of the aortic cross-clamp will minimize hypotension. Reperfusion of the lower extremities, resulting in washout of anaerobic products and systemic acidosis, may produce a negative inotropic effect, which is related to the duration of cross-clamp time and degree of collateral flow. Sodium bicarbonate administration is rarely necessary.

(8) **Emergence.** Most patients are extubated at the end of the procedure. Patients with unstable cardiac or pulmonary function, ongoing bleeding, or severe hypothermia

(less than 33°C) are left intubated. Hypertension, tachycardia, pain, and shivering should be anticipated and treated.
(9) Transport. All patients should receive supplemental oxygen and continuous monitoring of blood pressure and ECG.

B. Suprarenal abdominal aortic surgery. The surgical procedure may involve cross-clamping of the aorta at various levels above the renal arteries. Anesthetic considerations are similar to those for infrarenal aortic surgery (see section V.A), with the following caveats:

  1. PA catheters are used more frequently.

  2. Blood loss is potentially greater.

  3. Renal perfusion is at greater risk because of longer cross-clamp times and potential for cholesterol embolization.

  4. Cross-clamping above the celiac and superior mesenteric arteries can produce visceral ischemia and profound acidosis. Sodium bicarbonate is given routinely prior to unclamping.

  5. Intravenous mannitol, lasix, dopamine, or fenoldopam may be administered prior to cross-clamping with the aim of minimizing ischemic renal injury.

C. Renal artery surgery. Renal artery stenoses or aneurysms are repaired with a variety of techniques. Aortorenal bypass and transaortic endarterectomy require aortic cross-clamping; hepatorenal (right) and splenorenal (left) bypass procedures avoid cross-clamping. The anesthetic considerations are the same as for abdominal aortic surgery (see section V.A). Postoperative concerns include ongoing hypertension and deterioration in renal function.

D. Endovascular abdominal aneurysm repair (EVR) (Fig. 22-1)

  1. EVR of an AAA involves deployment of a an expandable, prosthetic graft within the lumen of the aneurysm, thus excluding the aneurysm from the circulation and reducing the risk of its rupture. The graft usually is deployed, under fluoroscopic guidance, from sheaths placed in the femoral arteries via cutdown arteriotomies. Compared with conventional AAA repair, EVR involves less blood loss and a lower incidence of perioperative morbidity, including pulmonary, cardiovascular, and renal complications. The use of EVR has resulted in fewer postoperative intensive care unit (ICU) admissions, earlier ambulation, and shorter hospital stays.

  2. Patient selection and stent graft sizing depend on detailed preoperative imaging. Up to 60% of patients with known infrarenal AAAs may be amenable to EVR. Current devices require at least a 1.5 cm neck of normal aorta for proximal deployment of the graft between the renal arteries and the aneurysm. A short or extremely angulated neck of the normal aorta is the most common reason why patients are not candidates for EVR.

  3. Monitoring. In addition to standard monitors (Chapter 10), a large peripheral IV (14 to 16 gauge), arterial catheter, and Foley catheter are used. Conversion to an open procedure is relatively rare, but each case should be set up for the possibility of an emergent AAA repair (see below).

  4. Anesthetic technique. Most patients receive an epidural or combined spinal and epidural anesthetic. Intravenous seda-

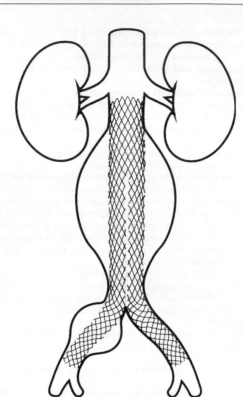

Fig. 22-1.   Endovascular graft repair of an infrarenal abdominal aortic aneurysm. From Kaufman JA, Geller SC, Brewster DC, *et al.* Endovascular repair of abdominal aortic aneurysm: current status and future directions. *Am J Roentgenol* 2000;175:289–302, with permission.

tion with propofol and/or benzodiazepines is titrated to patient comfort.

5.   Complications of EVR include failure to exclude the AAA from the arterial system (endoleak), embolism, arterial injury, graft kinking, limb ischemia, and infection.

E.   Emergency abdominal aortic surgery. Patients present with a wide spectrum of signs and symptoms and can be divided into two groups:

1.   The hemodynamically stable patient with an expanding contained rupture has the same anesthetic considerations as described above (see section V.A), but the preoperative preparation must proceed expeditiously.

a.   Foley catheter and nasogastric tube insertion should be delayed until after induction, to avoid Valsalva maneuvers (or hypertension) that may aggravate bleeding or cause frank rupture.

b.   Induction proceeds after preoxygenation, using placement of cricoid pressure and careful titration of hypnotic agents, opioids, and muscle relaxants. Hypertension must be avoided and anesthesia may be supplemented with vasoactive drugs.

2. **The hemodynamically unstable patient** (ruptured aneurysm) requires resuscitative measures. Mortality can be limited by restoration of intravascular volume, judicious use of vasoconstrictors, and rapid surgical control. Under the best of situations, there is a 40% to 50% mortality, usually resulting from the physiologic consequences of hypotension and massive blood transfusion. The incidence of MI, acute renal failure, respiratory failure, and coagulopathy is high.

   a. **General considerations**

      (1) **Large-bore intravenous access** is paramount.

      (2) **Blood samples** should be sent immediately for cross-matching and any other pertinent laboratory studies. Blood components should be ordered immediately, but universal donor-type blood (type O-negative in women of child bearing age, type O-positive in all others) should be obtained if type-specific blood is unavailable. Colloid solutions should be available. The autotransfusion team should be notified and equipment set up.

   b. **Surgical technique.** The immediate surgical priority will be to control bleeding by cross-clamping the aorta in the chest or abdomen.

   c. **Monitoring.** Minimum monitoring standards (see Chapter 10) should be applied during the initial volume resuscitation, followed by placement of invasive monitors as time and hemodynamics permit. Placement of monitors and fluid resuscitation should not delay definitive surgical control of a rupture in an unstable patient.

   d. **Anesthetic technique**

      (1) **Induction**

         (a) In **moribund patients**, endotracheal intubation should be performed immediately.

         (b) In **hypotensive patients**, a rapid careful induction is indicated, but the patient may only be able to tolerate small doses of scopolamine, ketamine, etomidate, and/or a benzodiazepine and a relaxant.

      (2) **Maintenance**

         (a) Once the aorta has been clamped to control bleeding, resuscitative efforts should continue until hemodynamic stability is achieved. Incremental doses of opioid and supplemental anesthetics are given as tolerated.

         (b) **Blood products** (including fresh-frozen plasma and platelets) are administered when available. Serial laboratory studies should guide further management.

         (c) **Hypothermia** is common and contributes to the acidosis, coagulopathy, and myocardial dysfunction that complicate aortic aneurysm repair. Methods of heat conservation and warming are discussed in Chapter 14.

         (d) **To prevent renal failure**, aggressive efforts should be made to preserve urine output with volume replacement, mannitol, furosemide, low-dose dopamine, or fenoldopam. Mortality in patients developing renal failure following ruptured a AAA is high.

(3) Emergence. Large fluid shifts; hypothermia; and acid-base, electrolyte, and coagulation abnormalities make the immediate postoperative period complex. Most patients remain endotracheally intubated and mechanically ventilated at the end of the procedure.

VI. Thoracic aortic surgery. Causes of thoracic aorta disease include atherosclerosis, degenerative disorders of connective tissue (e.g., Marfan and Ehlers-Danlos syndromes, and cystic necrosis), infection (e.g., syphilis), congenital defects (e.g., coarctation or congenital aneurysms of the sinus of Valsalva), trauma (e.g., penetrating and deceleration injuries), and inflammatory processes (e.g., Takayasu aortitis).

The most common problem affecting the thoracic aorta is **atherosclerotic aneurysm** of the descending portion, accounting for about 20% of all aortic aneurysms. When such aneurysms dissect proximally, they may involve the aortic valve or coronary ostia. Distal dissection may involve the abdominal aorta, or renal or mesenteric branches. The next most frequent problem is **traumatic disruption** of the thoracic aorta. Adventitial false aneurysms may form distal to the left subclavian artery at the insertion of the ligamentum arteriosum, because of penetrating or deceleration injuries. These false aneurysms may dissect anterograde and involve the arch and its major branches.

A. Ascending aortic aneurysms are approached by median sternotomy and require cardiopulmonary bypass with arterial cannulation through the femoral artery, the distal ascending aorta, or the aortic arch.

B. Transverse aortic arch repair requires median sternotomy, cardiopulmonary bypass, and hypothermic total circulatory arrest.

C. Descending thoracic aortic aneurysms often are approached by a left lateral thoracotomy with the cross-clamp placed distal to the left subclavian artery.

D. Thoracoabdominal aneurysms are approached by a thoracoabdominal incision.

1. Crawford classification of thoracoabdominal aneurysms (Fig. 22-2).

a. Type I. Aneurysm of the descending thoracic aorta distal to the subclavian artery, ending at or above the origin of the visceral vessels.

b. Type II. Aneurysm from the origin of the subclavian artery to the distal abdominal aorta.

c. Type III. Aneurysm from the mid-descending thoracic aorta to the distal abdominal aorta.

d. Type IV. Aneurysm from the diaphragm down to the distal aorta.

2. Associated findings

a. Airway deviation or compression, particularly of the left main stem bronchus, producing atelectasis.

b. Tracheal displacement or disruption, producing difficulties with endotracheal intubation and ventilation. Longstanding aneurysms may damage the recurrent laryngeal nerves, resulting in vocal cord paralysis and hoarseness.

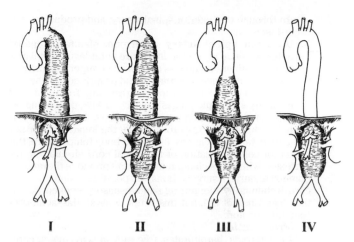

Fig. 22-2. Crawford classification of descending thoracic aortic aneurysms.

c. Hemoptysis, because of erosion of the aneurysm into an adjacent bronchus.

d. Esophageal compression with dysphagia and an increased risk of aspiration.

e. Distortion and compression of central venous and arterial anatomy, producing markedly asymmetric pulses and difficult internal jugular vein cannulation.

f. Hemothorax and mediastinal shift from rupture or leakage, producing respiratory and circulatory compromise.

g. Reduced distal perfusion secondary to aortic branch vessel occlusion, producing renal, mesenteric, spinal cord, or extremity ischemia.

3. Surgical technique. During repair of the aneurysm, the affected aortic segment is isolated, and an interposition graft is inserted. Proximal blood flow to collateral vessels provides the only distal perfusion. Additional distal perfusion may be provided via a heparin-bonded Gott shunt or pump-assisted bypass. The **inclusion technique** involves using the portion of native aorta containing the celiac, superior mesenteric, and renal ostia as a component of the bypass graft.

4. Spinal cord protection

a. Anatomic concerns

(1) The anterior spinal artery arises from the vertebral arteries at the base of the skull and anastomoses with aortic radicular arteries. The latter arise segmentally (a few in the lumbar and lower thoracic regions, but none or one in the upper thoracic region).

(2) The dominant vessel is the **artery of Adamkiewicz** (usually found between T-8 and T-12); cross-clamping of the aorta may compromise flow through this vessel, and in turn through the anterior spinal artery, and produce spinal cord ischemia.

b. **Anterior spinal artery syndrome.** Manifestations of the anterior spinal artery syndrome are paraplegia, rectal and urinary incontinence, and loss of pain and temperature sensation with maintenance of vibratory and proprioceptive sensation. The incidence of paraplegia resulting from anterior spinal artery syndrome ranges from 1% to 41%, depending on the type of aneurysm, among other factors. Risk factors include the duration of the cross-clamp, the location of proximal and distal cross-clamps, increased body temperature, the degree of collateralization of the spinal cord circulation, reperfusion with cross-clamp removal, and previous thoracoabdominal aneurysm surgery. It may be possible to detect spinal cord ischemia by monitoring somatosensory evoked potentials (see Chapter 24), but this is not done at Massachusetts General Hospital.

c. **Preservation**

(1) Steroids, barbiturates, free radical scavengers, cerebrospinal fluid (CSF) drainage, intrathecal papaverine, magnesium, naloxone, thiopental, and reanastomosis of intercostal vessels have all been tried without convincing evidence that any technique reduces the incidence of paraplegia.

(2) **Hypothermia** has been shown to be protective. Using a protocol developed at Massachusetts General Hospital (see Davison et al. 1994 in "Suggested Readings"), regional spinal cord cooling is begun before cross-clamping and continued until the graft is reperfused.

(3) **Lowering CSF pressure** may promote spinal cord perfusion. Therefore, a lumbar CSF catheter is inserted to monitor and control CSF pressure.

(4) **Glucose-containing solutions are avoided**, since experimental evidence suggests that hyperglycemia is detrimental during ischemia and may worsen neurologic outcome.

(5) **Monitoring.** Routine monitoring is supplemented with the following:

(a) Right radial arterial catheter (a high cross-clamp may compromise left subclavian artery flow).

(b) PA catheter.

(c) No. 8.5 French (Fr) introducer used for volume infusions.

(d) No. 4 Fr epidural cooling catheter at spinal level T-12 to L-1.

(e) No. 4 Fr subarachnoid catheter, with thermistor, at spinal level L-2, L-3.

(f) Foley catheter.

(6) **Anesthetic technique**

(a) **Vasopressors** (e.g., phenylephrine and norepinephrine), **vasodilators** (nitroglycerin and nitroprusside), and **diuretics** (mannitol, furosemide, and dopamine/fenoldopam) should be available prior to induction.

(b) **A thoracic epidural and a lumbar subarachnoid**

catheter are inserted preoperatively, and a sensory level is achieved with 2% lidocaine via the epidural catheter.

(c) **General anesthesia** is induced as detailed in section V.A.4.b.

(d) **A right-sided, double-lumen endobronchial tube** is placed to facilitate surgical access and protect the left lung from trauma during left thoracotomy (see Chapter 21).

(e) **Muscle relaxation** is usually provided by a cis-atracurium infusion.

(7) **Positioning.** The patient is turned to the right lateral decubitus position and prepared for incision.

(8) **Maintenance**

(a) **Anesthesia** is continued as in section V.A.4.c, and one-lung ventilation is begun as described in Chapter 21.

(b) **Fluid management** is limited to fresh-frozen plasma, red blood cells, platelets, and colloids after induction, in an attempt to limit the development of a coagulopathy and excessive edema. An autotransfusion device and a blood warmer capable of high flow rates (e.g., Level 1 D300) are used.

(9) **Aortic cross-clamping**

(a) Before cross-clamping, CSF pressure is adjusted and the spinal cord is cooled according to protocol.

(b) **Marked hypertension** is universal with a proximal aortic cross-clamp and is treated with epidural anesthesia, nitroglycerin, and nitroprusside.

(c) **Renal function** is preserved by infusion of iced saline solution through a catheter placed by the surgical team into the orifices of the renal arteries.

(10) **Aortic unclamping** produces hypotension by the mechanism discussed in section V.A.4.c.(7). Volume administration before and during unclamping, slow release of the cross-clamp, and use of vasopressors are continued until myocardial function and vascular tone have returned to normal.

(11) **Systemic acidosis** is universal following release of the aortic cross-clamp. An infusion of bicarbonate during the cross-clamping period will help prevent severe acidosis during reperfusion.

(12) **Emergence.** The patient is asked to move all four extremities, and once a satisfactory neurologic examination has been completed, the patient is again sedated and the double-lumen tube is replaced with a standard endotracheal tube. Dependent tissue edema may significantly narrow the airway, making reintubation difficult.

(13) **Transport.** The patient remains sedated for transport to the ICU. Both ECG and blood pressure are monitored.

VII. Postoperative considerations. Intensive care is required following most vascular surgical procedures. Attention to urine output, cardiac output, distal extremity perfusion, respiratory adequacy, hematocrit, and hemostasis is required. Postoperative complications include MI, renal failure, bowel ischemia or infarction, pancreatitis, sepsis, disseminated intravascular coagulation, peripheral embolization, respiratory insufficiency, and paraplegia. Hypotension in the postoperative period increases the risk of delayed onset paraplegia and should be avoided.

SUGGESTED READING

Barnett HJM, Taylor DW, Eliasziw M, et al. Benefit of carotid endarterectomy in patients with symptomatic moderate or severe stenosis. *N Engl J Med* 1998;339:1415–1425.

Baron JF, Bertrand M, Barre E, et al. Combined epidural and general anesthesia versus general anesthesia for abdominal aortic surgery. *Anesthesiology* 1991;75:611–618.

Brewster DC, Kaufman JA, Geller SC, et al. Initial experience with endovascular repair: comparison of early results with conventional open repair. *J Vasc Surg* 1998;27:992–1005.

Cambria RP, Davison JK. Regional hypothermia with epidural cooling for spinal cord protection during thoracoabdominal aneurysm repair. *Sem Vasc Surg* 2000;13:315–324.

Christopherson R, Beattie C, Frank SM, et al. Perioperative morbidity in patients randomized to epidural or general anesthesia for lower extremity vascular surgery. *Anesthesiology* 1993;79:422–434.

Crawford ES, Crawford JL, Safi HJ, et al. Thoracoabdominal aortic aneurysms: preoperative and intraoperative factors determining immediate and long-term results of operations in 605 patients. *J Vasc Surg* 1985; 3:389–404.

Davison JK, Cambria RP, Vierra DJ, et al. Epidural cooling for regional spinal cord hypothermia during thoracoabdominal aneurysm repair. *J Vasc Surg* 1994;20:304–310.

Gelman S. The pathophysiology of aortic cross-clamping and unclamping. *Anesthesiology* 1995;82:1026–1060.

Isaacson IJ, Lowdon JD, Berry AS, et al. The value of pulmonary artery and central venous monitoring in patients undergoing abdominal aortic reconstructive surgery. *J Vasc Surg* 1990;12:754–760.

Kashyap VP, Cambria RP, Davison JK, et al. Renal failure after thoracoabdominal aortic surgery. *J Vasc Surg* 1997;26:949–955.

Kaufman JA, Geller SC, Brewster DC, et al. Endovascular repair of abdominal aortic aneurysm: current status and future directions. *AJR Am J Roentgenol* 2000;175:289–302.

Mangano ET, Layug EL, Wallace A, et al. Effect of atenolol on mortality and cardiovascular morbidity after noncardiac surgery. *N Engl J Med* 1996;335:1713–1720.

Pierce ET, Pomposelli FB, Stanley GD, et al. Anesthesia type does not influence early graft patency or limb salvage rates of lower extremity arterial bypass. *J Vasc Surg* 1997;25:226–233.

Raby KE, Goldman L, Creager M, et al. Correlation between preoperative ischemia and major cardiac events after peripheral vascular surgery. *N Engl J Med* 1989;321:1296–1300.

Rao TLK, El-Etr AA. Anticoagulation following placement of epidural and subarachnoid catheters: an evaluation of neurologic sequelae. *Anesthesiology* 1981;55:618–620.

Tuman KJ, McCarthy RJ, March RJ, et al. Effects of epidural anesthesia and analgesia on coagulation and outcome after major vascular surgery. *Anesth Analg* 1991;73:696–704.

Wallace A, Layug B, Tateo I, et al. Prophylactic atenolol reduces postoperative myocardial ischemia. *Anesthesiology* 1998;88:7–17.

Anesthesia for Cardiac Surgery

Scott C. Streckenbach and Derrick B. Willsey

I. Preanesthetic assessment

A. Issues pertinent to cardiac surgical procedures and the physiologic impact of cardiopulmonary bypass (CPB) and elective arrest include the following (see also Chapters 1 and 2):

1. Prior surgery on the thorax, heart, great vessels, or lungs technically complicates cardiac surgery.

2. Prior admissions for peripheral vascular disease, including transient ischemic attacks or cerebral vascular accidents, and the results of noninvasive and invasive vascular studies should be noted. Symptomatic or documented carotid arterial disease may warrant endarterectomy prior to or simultaneous with the cardiac operation.

3. A history of bleeding tendency may reveal a condition responsive to preoperative or intraoperative therapy.

4. Patients with a history of **heparin-induced thrombocytopenia** (HIT) may develop life-threatening thrombotic complications when exposed to heparin; a plan for anticoagulation during CPB should be determined preoperatively.

5. Renal insufficiency may indicate the need for intraoperative renal protective measures.

6. Post-CPB pulmonary dysfunction can be life threatening; patients with pulmonary disease may benefit from preoperative antibiotics, bronchodilators, steroids, or chest physical therapy.

B. Cardiac evaluation should determine the major anatomic and physiologic characteristics of the cardiovascular system; this allows one to predict the likelihood of intraoperative ischemia and to determine functional reserve of the heart.

1. Radionuclide imaging may demonstrate the regions and extent of myocardium at risk for ischemia.

2. Radionuclide ventriculography delineates cardiac chamber volume, ejection fraction, and right-to-left stroke volume ratios.

3. Echocardiography provides an assessment of ventricular function and valve function. Regional wall motion abnormalities may reflect ischemia or a prior myocardial infarction (MI).

4. Cardiac catheterization provides anatomic and functional data often not available from noninvasive studies.

a. Anatomic data. Coronary angiography reveals the location and extent of coronary stenoses, distal runoff, collateral flow, and coronary dominance. **Significant stenosis** implies a greater than 70% reduction in luminal diameter. The **dominant coronary artery** supplies the atrioventricular node and the posterior descending coronary artery.

b. Functional data. Ventriculography may demonstrate

Table 23-1. Normal intracardiac pressure and oxygen saturation

	Pressure (mm Hg)	O$_2$ Saturation (%)
Superior vena cava	—	71
Inferior vena cava	—	77
Right atrium (mean)	1–8	75
Right ventricle (systolic/diastolic)	15–30/0–8	75
Pulmonary artery (systolic/diastolic)	15–30/4–12	75
Pulmonary artery occlusion pressure (mean)	2–12	—
Left atrium (mean)	2–12	98
Left ventricle (systolic/ diastolic/end-diastolic)	100–140/0–8/2–12	98
Aorta (systolic/diastolic)	100–140/60–90	98

wall motion abnormalities, mitral regurgitation, and intracardiac shunts. Left ventricular (LV) ejection fraction is normally greater than 0.6. Impaired ventricular performance is a useful predictor of increased surgical risk.

   c.   Hemodynamic data are compiled from both right and left heart catheterization. Intracardiac and pulmonary vascular pressures reflect volume status, cardiac valve function, and the presence of pulmonary vascular disease (normal values are presented in Table 23-1). An elevated left-ventricular end-diastolic pressure (LVEDP) (measured at the base of the "a" wave) may be due to ventricular failure and dilation, volume overload (mitral or aortic regurgitation [AR]), poor compliance from ischemia or hypertrophy, or a constrictive process. The LVEDP may rise substantially in patients with coronary artery disease (CAD) after dye injection for ventriculography or coronary angiography, despite otherwise normal hemodynamic values.

   d.   Left-to-right intracardiac shunts are demonstrated by an arterial oxygen saturation (Sao$_2$) "step up" in the right heart. Systemic and pulmonary flow and flow ratios can be calculated by Fick principles (see section IV.C.1.d for equations).

   e.   Cardiac output is determined by thermodilution, and hemodynamic indices can be derived (Table 23-2).

C.   Laboratory studies. Routine studies for patients undergoing a cardiac operation include a complete blood count, prothrombin time, partial thromboplastin time, platelet count, electrolytes, blood urea nitrogen, creatinine, glucose, aspartate aminotransferase, lactate dehydrogenase, creatine kinase, urinalysis, chest radiograph, and a 12-lead electrocardiogram (ECG) with a rhythm

Table 23-2. Ventricular function indices

Formula	Units	Normal Value
$SV = \dfrac{CO}{HR} \times 1{,}000$	mL/beat	60–90
$SI = \dfrac{SV}{BSA}$	mL/beat/m^2	40–60
$LVSWI = \dfrac{1.36\,(MAP - PAOP)}{100} \times SI$	$\dfrac{gram\text{-}meters/m^2}{beat}$	45–60
$RVSWI = \dfrac{1.36\,(PAP - CVP)}{100} \times SI$	$\dfrac{gram\text{-}meters/m^2}{beat}$	5–10
$SVR = \dfrac{MAP - CVP}{CO} \times 80$	dynes-sec/cm^5	900–1,500
$PVR = \dfrac{PAP - PCWP}{CO} \times 80$	dynes-sec/cm^5	50–150

BSA, body surface area; CO, cardiac output; CVP, mean central venous pressure; HR, heart rate; LVSWI, left ventricular stroke work index; MAP, mean systemic arterial pressure; PAP, mean pulmonary artery pressure; PAOP, mean pulmonary artery occlusion pressure; PVR, pulmonary vascular resistance; RSWI, right ventricular stroke work index; SI, stroke index; SV, stroke volume; SVR, systemic vascular resistance.

strip. A HIT-antibody ELISA test should be considered for patients with a low or rapidly falling platelet count who are receiving heparin.

II. Anesthetic management

A. Patient education. Anxieties are often allayed by an explanation of what is to be expected, both immediately before and after surgery. Emphasis that the patient will be well-sedated and comfortable is important.

B. Premedication

1. **Cardiac medications**

   a. Beta-adrenergic antagonists, calcium channel blockers, and nitrates, including intravenous nitroglycerin, routinely are continued on schedule until arrival in the operating room (OR).

   b. Digitalis preparations are commonly held for 24 hours preoperatively because of inherent toxicity (especially in the presence of hypokalemia) and a long elimination half-life. When rate control is critical, however, as in mitral stenosis (MS), digitalis should be continued.

   c. Antihypertensives, including angiotensin-converting enzyme (ACE) inhibitors and diuretics, are usually held the morning of surgery. Patients with significant LV dysfunction are more likely to develop vasodilatory shock when they receive an ACE inhibitor preoperatively. If the patient's blood pressure is extremely labile, however, the antihypertensives may need to be continued.

   d. Antiarrhythmics are generally continued to the time of surgery. Type I agents (e.g., quinidine, procainamide, and disopyramide) may suppress automaticity and conduction, especially when patients are hyperkalemic. **Amiodarone** has a half-life of 30 days; discontinuation within a few days of surgery will have little effect on serum levels. Amiodarone use may be associated with pulmonary toxicity, decreased atrioventricular nodal conduction, atropine-resistant bradycardia, and myocardial depression in the perioperative period.

e. Aspirin has been discontinued 7 to 10 days prior to heart surgery in the past. Recent evidence suggests that aspirin does not increase perioperative bleeding. Moreover, aspirin has a positive effect on graft patency. It may be prudent to continue aspirin therapy in patients who have significant CAD. Patients, particularly those who have had a recent interventional cardiac catheterization, may be receiving other antiplatelet agents that may or may not be reversible (see Table 23-3).

f. Warfarin (Coumadin) should be held 2 to 3 days preoperatively. A normal prothrombin time should be documented prior to surgery. Vitamin K (10 mg subcutaneously) or 2 to 4 units of fresh-frozen plasma (FFP) may be used emergently to correct coagulopathy.

g. Heparin infusions initiated for unstable angina or for patients with left main coronary disease are routinely continued preoperatively.

2. Sedation and analgesia are warranted in almost all cardiac surgical patients. Combinations of benzodiazepines and morphine provide excellent amnesia and analgesia for preinduction catheter insertion, with an acceptable degree of cardiorespiratory depression in all but the most debilitated patients.

a. For full-size adults with good LV function, **lorazepam**, 1 to 2 mg orally, is given the night before and again 1 hour before arrival in the OR, and **morphine**, 0.1 to 0.15 mg/kg intramuscularly (or subcutaneously if patient is anticoagulated), is given at least 1 hour before induction.

b. Even a small amount of premedication-induced hypotension can be hazardous to patients with severe aortic stenosis (AS) or left main CAD. Drug dosages should be reduced in these patients.

c. Patients with MS may develop life-threatening pulmonary hypertension with sedation-induced hypoventilation and hypoxemia. Since these patients may also be extremely sensitive to the central effects of sedation, no or minimal premedication is administered until the patient arrives in the OR.

d. Patients requiring anesthesia transport to the OR may be given IV premedication by the transport team.

3. Supplemental oxygen therapy is given primarily to patients with severe LV dysfunction, valvular disease, and compromised pulmonary function.

C. Monitoring

1. Standard monitors (see Chapter 10).

a. ECG. Continuous display of both leads II and V_5 with ST segment trend analysis will facilitate the diagnosis of ischemia and rhythm disturbance.

b. Temperature monitoring includes measurement of the "core" temperature, measured in the nasopharynx and reflec-

Table 23-3. Commonly used antiplatelet agents

Antiplatelet Agent	Inhibits	Reversibility	Duration of Action	Drug Delivered
Aspirin	Cyclooxygenase	No	7 d	PO
Dipyridamole	cAMP PDE; Adenosine uptake	Yes	4–10 h	PO
Ticlopidine (Ticlid)	ADP receptor	No	7 d	PO
Clopidogrel (Plavix)	ADP receptor	No	7 d	PO
Abciximab (Reopro)	GP IIb/IIIa receptor	Slowly	48 h	IV
Eptifibatide (Integrilin)	GP IIb/IIIa receptor	Yes	4–8 h	IV
Tirofiban (Aggrastat)	GP IIb/IIIa receptor	Yes	4–8 h	IV

ADP, adenosine diphosphate; cAMP, cyclic adenosine monophosphate; GP, glycoprotein; IV, intravenous; PDE, phosphodiesterase; PO, oral.

tive of brain and other highly perfused tissues; the blood temperature, measured by the pulmonary artery catheter; and the "shell" temperature, measured in the rectum and reflective of less perfused regions.

2. **Central venous and pulmonary artery pressures**

   a. **Patients with normal ventricular function** undergoing cardiac surgery can be effectively managed with central venous pressure (CVP) monitoring. Cardiac output and filling pressure data obtained from a pulmonary artery (PA) catheter, however, facilitate rational drug and volume therapy throughout the perioperative period.

   b. **Pacing pulmonary artery catheter and Paceport catheters** provide pacing capability for the management of a variety of valvular lesions (aortic insufficiency [AI] and mitral regurgitation) and conduction disorders and for "redo" operations during which rapid access for epicardial pacing may not be possible. **Mixed venous oxygen saturation** ($Smvo_2$) monitoring is available continuously with PA catheters specially equipped with a fiberoptic-linked oximeter. A decrease in $Smvo_2$ is the result of either decreased cardiac output, decreased hemoglobin, increased oxygen consumption, or decreased arterial oxygen saturation (Sao_2).

3. **Intraoperative   transesophageal   echocardiography (TEE)** can be very helpful for:

   a. Preoperative evaluation of valve pathology to help the surgeon determine if a repair, rather than a replacement, is possible.

   b. Preoperative evaluation for intracardiac thrombi, intracardiac shunts, and intraaortic plaques. The combination of TEE and epiaortic echocardiography helps the surgeon determine the best location to cannulate the aorta in the presence of aortic plaque. In patients with severe atheromatous disease in the proximal aorta, the femoral artery or axillary artery may be cannulated or off bypass coronary artery bypass grafting (CABG) can be performed.

   c. Preoperative evaluation of aortic dissection.

   d. Perioperative evaluation of myocardial ischemia.

   e. Evaluation of intracardiac air prior to terminating CPB.

   f. Postoperative evaluation of valve repair or replacement and intracardiac shunt repair.

   g. There are many ways to perform a comprehensive TEE exam. The Society of Cardiovascular Anesthesiologists/American Society of Echocardiography TEE guidelines are very helpful in ensuring that all necessary views are obtained.

D. **Preinduction.** Upon the patient's arrival in the OR, vital signs are checked, an adequate Sao_2 is ensured, and additional premedication (1 to 2 mg of midazolam), if indicated, is titrated.

   1. **Peripheral venous access** is established. In adults, one large-bore (14-gauge) peripheral IV is usually sufficient. If excessive bleeding is expected (e.g., a redo operation or a patient with a preexisting coagulopathy), a second peripheral line will facilitate blood product administration.

   2. **Arterial cannulation** is performed with either an 18- or 20-gauge catheter.

      a. When possible, in patients undergoing left internal mammary dissection, the right radial artery is cannulated so that the left arm may be safely tucked.

b. Bilateral radial artery cannulation is often performed for complex aortic arch surgery, particularly in the setting of an aortic dissection.

c. Cannulation distal to a previous brachial artery cutdown site should be avoided. Pressure gradients may occur across arteriotomies, especially during and after CPB.

d. If blood pressure measurements are asymmetric, the arterial catheter should be placed on the side with the higher value.

e. Make sure to note whether the surgeon will use the radial artery as a conduit for CABG surgery. If so, the radial artery on the opposite side must be used.

f. Femoral artery cannulation is a safe and reliable alternative to radial artery cannulation. Preoperative femoral artery cannulation in patients with severe CAD and poor LV function provides a site for postoperative intraaortic balloon (IABP) insertion, if it becomes necessary. Brachial and axillary artery cannulations are third and fourth choices.

g. Intraaortic balloon lumen pressure can be transduced as a temporary monitor of central arterial pressure.

3. Central venous access may be established before or after induction, depending on the clinical situation.

4. A defibrillator and external pacemaker generator must be available, as should a magnet to regulate pacemakers or implantable cardioverter defibrillators (ICDs), if applicable.

5. Typed and cross-matched packed red blood cells (2 to 4 units) must be present and checked.

6. Baseline hemodynamics, including cardiac output, and a 7-lead ECG are recorded.

7. Readily available medications should include heparin, calcium chloride, lidocaine, inotropes, vasopressors, and nitroglycerin. Protamine should also be available but never drawn up until the patient is safely separated from CPB.

E. Induction is one of the more critical times in the anesthetic management of the cardiac surgical patient. A surgeon should be available, and the CPB pump should be ready in the event that a hemodynamic emergency occurs. The choice of agents and sequence of events are dependent on the specific cardiac lesions, the patient's underlying condition, and the surgical plan. A systematic, gradual induction with frequent assessment of the degree of cardiovascular depression and depth of anesthesia (as determined by hemodynamic response to graded stimuli including oral airway insertion and Foley catheterization) will minimize hemodynamic instability.

1. Agents useful in the induction and maintenance of anesthesia in the cardiac surgical patient include the following:

a. Intravenous opioids produce varying degrees of vasodilation and bradycardia without significant myocardial depression. A high-dose technique utilizes fentanyl (50 to 100 μg/kg) or sufentanil (10 to 20 μg/kg) as both the induction and primary maintenance agent. Alternatively, a smaller induction bolus (fentanyl 25 to 50 μg/kg) may be supplemented with a continuous narcotic infusion, or even lower doses (fentanyl,

10 to 25 μg/kg, or sufentanil, 1 to 5 μg/kg) may be used in conjunction with other central nervous system depressants as part of a "balanced technique."

b. **Sedative hypnotics and amnestics**, including thiopental, propofol, and etomidate may be useful as coinduction agents in particular situations. Of these drugs, etomidate appears to cause the least amount of myocardial depression.

c. **Volatile inhalation anesthetics** are useful supplementary agents, especially in the treatment of hypertension.

d. **Muscle relaxants** with minimal cardiovascular effects are commonly chosen (e.g., vecuronium, cisatracurium). Pretreatment with a "priming dose" and early relaxant administration help to counteract chest wall rigidity often encountered during narcotic inductions. **Succinylcholine** is used in modified rapid sequence inductions for patients with reflux or a full stomach. **Pancuronium** is used to counteract the bradycardic effects of opioids.

2. **Specific considerations for valvular heart disease** (see also Chapter 2).

a. **Aortic stenosis.** Hemodynamic goals include adequate intravascular volume, slow heart rate with sinus rhythm, and maintenance of contractility and systemic vascular tone. The thick left ventricle associated with AS often requires markedly higher filling pressures (LVEDP = 20 to 30 mm Hg) than a normal LV. Anesthetic agents that reduce vascular tone or myocardial contractility (e.g., thiopental) should be avoided. An infusion of a vasopressor (e.g., norepinephrine) can be started 1 to 2 minutes before induction to decrease the risk of developing significant induction-induced hypotension. Arrhythmias must be treated aggressively.

b. **Aortic regurgitation.** Hemodynamic goals include adequate intravascular volume, maintenance of an increased heart rate and contractile state, and decreased systemic vascular tone to facilitate forward flow. Patients with AR often are highly dependent on endogenous sympathetic tone. Patients with coexisting CAD may decompensate with significant bradycardia (very low diastolic perfusion pressure); a rapid method for pacing should be available.

c. **Mitral stenosis.** Hemodynamic goals mandate maintenance of a slow rhythm, preferably sinus, and adequate intravascular volume, contractility, and systemic resistance. Elevated pulmonary vascular resistance (PVR), often secondary to hypoventilation or positive end-expiratory pressure (PEEP), must be avoided. Patients with severe MS and elevated PVR are extremely challenging to induce. Insertion of a PA line before induction is highly recommended.

d. **Mitral regurgitation.** Hemodynamic goals include maintenance of adequate volume, contractility, a normal to elevated heart rate, and a reduction of systemic vascular tone. Increased PVR should be avoided. Anesthesia-induced decreases in peripheral vascular resistance are usually well tolerated.

e. **In patients with mixed valvular lesions**, the most hemodynamically significant lesion will predominate the management goals. The addition of CAD to mixed valve lesions makes planning even more complex (e.g., AS with AI and CAD). In all situations, determine the three most likely problems that could occur during induction and plan the management for each.

3. Specific considerations for emergent inductions

a. Pulmonary embolus. Induction and positive pressure ventilation can precipitate cardiovascular collapse. It is prudent to prepare and drape the unstable patient before induction.

b. Pericardial tamponade. Similar concerns are present for patients with pericardial tamponade. Adequate volume administration is essential. Starting an inotropic agent and a vasopressor prior to induction may be helpful.

c. Aortic dissection. Hypertension can precipitate aortic rupture. Blood must be available prior to induction. Proximal extension of the dissection can occur, which can cause coronary ischemia or tamponade.

d. Ventricular septal defect (VSD) and papillary muscle rupture after MI. Patients may present with extreme hypotension. Rapidity in establishing CPB is essential and may be lifesaving.

e. Blood pressure may fall precipitously during the induction of critically ill patients. Cardiopulmonary resuscitation should not be delayed while waiting for pharmacologic therapy to work. If the patient does not recover quickly with chest compressions and defibrillation, consider initiating CPB immediately.

F. The prebypass period is characterized by variable levels of stimulation during preparation for the initiation of CPB. Particularly stimulating periods include sternal splitting and retraction, pericardial incision, and aortic root dissection and cannulation. Spontaneous cooling should occur.

1. A blood sample should be obtained to check the baseline arterial blood gas (ABG) tensions and pH, hematocrit, and a control activated clotting time (ACT). Phlebotomy and hemodilution may be considered in otherwise healthy patients with a starting hematocrit of 40% or greater, thus providing fresh autologous whole blood for transfusion following CPB and heparin reversal.

2. The lungs are deflated during sternal splitting. Anatomic changes in chest wall configuration will produce ECG changes, especially T-wave changes, which should be noted to avoid confusion with ischemia-induced changes.

3. Left internal mammary artery dissection may produce significant occult blood loss into the left chest.

4. Anticoagulation for cannulation

a. Before induction of anesthesia, 300 IU/kg of heparin (400 IU/kg if the patient is on IV heparin) should be prepared in case emergency initiation of CPB is necessary. Administer the heparin through a centrally placed catheter, aspirating blood both before and after injection to confirm patency.

b. Vasodilation often follows a heparin bolus.

c. The **ACT**, determined approximately 5 minutes after heparin administration, is used to monitor the degree of anticoagulation. Control values are 80 to 150 seconds. Heparinization sufficient to prevent microthrombus formation during CPB correlates with an ACT of more than 400 seconds (at higher than 35°C). Patients on continuous IV heparin preoperatively may become relatively "heparin resistant." If an ACT longer than 400 seconds is not achieved with standard heparin dose regimens, an additional 200 to 300 IU/kg is administered (exchanging porcine for bovine heparin, or vice versa, may be helpful). If this fails, antithrombin III (500 to 1,000 IU) or FFP may be necessary to correct a probable antithrombin III deficiency.

d.   Patients with a diagnosis of HIT require special antico-agulation management during CPB. Alternatives to heparin exist (see Table 23-4); each has significant limitations that should be discussed with the surgeon and a hematologist prior to use. One technique for management of patients with HIT includes the following:

(1)   All forms of heparin are removed preoperatively. (Saline is used to flush pressure transducers.)

(2)   Dipyridamole 75 mg orally is administered the night before surgery and on call to the OR.

(3)   A heparin-free PA catheter is used.

(4)   Prostaglandin E_1 (PGE_1) is begun before heparinization. The dose is increased as tolerated to 2 to 4 μg per minute.

(5)   A bypass dose of porcine heparin is administered before aortic cannulation (to minimize the likelihood of a repeat dose of heparin).

(6)   The PGE_1 infusion is discontinued approximately 15 minutes after all of the heparin has been reversed with protamine. (Pump blood contains heparin unless processed with the cell saver.)

(7)   Aspirin is administered early in the postoperative period.

5.   Preparation for CPB begins with aortic cannulation. **Epi-aortic scanning** is used to direct the cannulation site in patients with known aortic atherosclerotic disease (by history or intraoperative TEE). Maintaining a systolic blood pressure near 100 mm Hg during aortic cannulation decreases the risk of dissection.

6.   Some surgeons will perform the proximal saphenous vein graft anastomoses prior to going on CPB. An improperly placed side-biting clamp may occlude more than 50% of the aortic lumen and markedly increase afterload, causing myocardial decompensation. The early signs are hypotension, elevation of PA pressures, and ST-segment changes.

7.   The venous return cannula is inserted into the right atrium (or two cannulas into the superior and inferior vena cavae individually). A catheter frequently is inserted into the proximal ascending aorta for antegrade cardioplegia delivery and into the coronary sinus for retrograde cardioplegia delivery as well.

G.   Cardiopulmonary bypass

1.   CPB circuit. In the typical primary CPB circuit, blood is transferred by gravity through plastic tubing from the right atrium to a venous reservoir. A pump (roller or centrifugal) propels the venous blood into a heat exchanger and an oxygenator that adds oxygen and removes carbon dioxide. The arterialized

Table 23-4. Alternatives to heparin for cardiopulmonary bypass

Drug	Mechanism	Onset of Action	Monitor	Reversal
Danaparoid (Orgaran)	Inhibits factor Xa	Immediate	Anti Xa-activity	None
Lepirudin (Refludan)	Inhibits thrombin	Immediate	aPTT	Hemofiltration
Ancrod	Degrades fibrinogen	12 hr	Fibrinogen level	FFP, cryoprecipitate

aPTT, activated partial thromboplastic time; FFP, fresh frozen plasma.

blood passes through a filter before entering the patient's ascending aorta via the aortic cannula. The CPB machine also includes a circuit for the delivery of cardioplegia and one or more for aspirating blood from the surgical field. Approximately 1,600 mL of crystalloid is added to "prime" the primary circuit. This will decrease the patient's Hct proportionately: Hct = [pt weight (kg) × 70 mL/kg × Hct] / [pt weight × 70 mL/kg + pump prime (mL)]. As a general rule, a cardiac anesthetist should be able to prepare the CPB machine in an emergency and to anticipate and manage potential CPB-related problems (e.g., clotted membrane oxygenator, inadequate pump occlusion, and air embolus).

2.   Initiation of CPB. After adequate heparinization is established (an ACT of 400 to 450 seconds), the bypass is initiated when the surgeon releases the clamp on the venous line. After the perfusionist is convinced that the venous return is adequate, he or she will turn on the pump and progressively increase the speed to a flow of 2.0 to 2.4 L per minute per m^2 or roughly 50 mL/kg per minute for adults. A mean arterial pressure (MAP) of 40 to 120 mm Hg may be achieved by such flow, depending on vascular resistance, intravascular volume, and blood viscosity changes. Observe the bright red blood entering the aorta during this initiation to confirm that the membrane oxygenator is working properly. Once adequate flows and venous drainage are established, volatile anesthetics from the anesthesia machine, intravenous fluids, and positive-pressure ventilation are discontinued, and oxygen flows are reduced to 200 mL per minute. Muscle relaxants are supplemented to prevent shivering, which increases oxygen consumption and may produce acidosis during cooling. Anesthesia is maintained by IV agents or by inhalation agents administered through a vaporizer in the fresh gas flow line of the circuit. It is advisable to pull the PA catheter back 1 to 5 cm to prevent migration of the catheter tip into wedge position during CPB. If two venous return lines are used and tourniquets are applied to achieve complete CPB, the CVP should be measured in the most proximal position possible (i.e., side arm of the PA-line introducer). Since cerebral perfusion pressure is equal to MAP minus the superior vena cava (SVC) pressure, obstruction of the SVC cannula and consequent increasing SVC pressures must be detected to avoid potentially disastrous neurologic injury. Following fibrillation or arrest, mean PA pressures are displayed. A vent cannula may be inserted into the left ventricle to prevent distention.

3.   Maintenance of CPB

    a.   Myocardial protection during the cross-clamp period is achieved primarily by reducing myocardial oxygen consumption through either hypothermia, hyperkalemic arrest, or both.

        (1)   Cardioplegia solutions may be delivered antegrade through the aortic root, coronary ostia, or vein graft, or retrograde through the coronary sinus.

        (2)   Intermittent cold cardioplegia currently is the most commonly used technique. Cold (4° to 6°C) hyperkalemic solution with or without blood is delivered to the coronary circulation approximately every 20 minutes (or sooner if cardiac electrical activity returns). Systemic cooling of the patient and topical cooling of the heart augment the protection.

(3) The **warm cardioplegia technique** delivers warm (32° to 37°C) hyperkalemic solution mixed with blood at approximately a 1:5 ratio. The solution is delivered continuously during the cross-clamp period with a few interruptions to allow visualization of the anastomotic sites. Mild systemic cooling to 32° to 34°C is frequently employed. Lidocaine or esmolol may be used to augment the protection. Serum glucose levels will increase dramatically.

(4) The **cold fibrillating technique** (no aortic cross-clamp) may be used for CABG procedures. This technique requires elevated systemic pressure (MAP greater than 80 mm Hg), continuous measurement of LV vent pressure, and a continuous nitroglycerin infusion to ensure adequate myocardial perfusion.

b. **Hypothermia** (20° to 34°C) is commonly employed during CPB. Oxygen consumption, and thereby flow requirements, are reduced while blood viscosity increases, thus counteracting prime-induced hypoviscosity. Adverse effects of hypothermia include impaired autoregulatory, enzymatic, and cellular membrane function, decreased oxygen delivery (leftward shift of the hemoglobin oxygen dissociation curve), and potentiation of coagulopathy.

c. **Hemodynamic monitoring** during CPB is the shared responsibility of the perfusionist, anesthetist, and surgeon.

(1) **Hypotension** during initiation of CPB usually is due to hemodilution and hypoviscosity. Other important causes include inadequate pump flow, vasodilation, acute aortic dissection, or incorrect placement of the aortic cannula (e.g., directing flow toward the innominate artery not supplying the cannulated radial artery). The PA pressure and LV vent flow rate should be inspected to ensure that aortic incompetence has not compromised forward pump flow. (The venous cannula can potentially increase AI by compressing the noncoronary cusp of the aortic valve.) A phenylephrine infusion may be required to treat transient hypotension. During the course of CPB, a pressure gradient (as high as 40 mmHg) may develop between the radial artery and the aorta. The lower radial artery pressure could lead to overtreatment if this is not recognized. In the presence of carotid stenosis, MAP should be maintained at a higher level than usual (e.g., 80 to 90 mm Hg), and hypocarbia should be avoided.

(2) **Hypertension** (MAP higher than 90 mm Hg) may be due to excessive flow rates or increased vascular resistance, which may be treated with vasodilators or anesthetics.

(3) **Elevated PA pressures** indicate left heart distention, which may be due to inadequate venting, AR, or inadequate isolation of venous return. Severe distention may result in irreversible myocardial damage.

d. **Metabolic acidosis and oliguria** suggest inadequate systemic perfusion. Additional volume (blood or crystalloid depending on hematocrit) may be required to achieve increased flow. Brisk urine output should be established during the first 10 minutes of CPB.

(1) Oliguria (less than 1 mL/kg per hour) should be treated with a trial of increased perfusion pressure and/or flow, mannitol (0.25 to 0.5 g/kg), or dopamine (1 to 5 µg/kg per minute). Patients on chronic furosemide therapy may require their usual dose during CPB to sustain diuresis.

(2) Hemolysis during CPB usually is due to physical trauma to red blood cells by the pump suction. Released pigments may cause acute renal failure postoperatively. For hemoglobinuria, diuresis is maintained with mannitol or furosemide, and when severe, the urine is alkalinized by administering 0.5 to 1.0 mEq/kg of sodium bicarbonate.

e. Additional heparin may be needed for prolonged CPB. A 100 IU/kg hourly reinforcement dose is given, beginning 2 hours after the initial dose. An artificially elevated ACT is seen during aprotinin therapy when using Celite ACT tubes and when blood temperature is lower than 35°C. The duration of heparin anticoagulation may be shorter in patients on chronic heparin therapy or during cases in which systemic hypothermia is not employed. The ACT is checked every 30 minutes when the patient is warmer than 32°C.

H. Discontinuing CPB implies transferring cardiopulmonary function from the bypass system back to the patient. In preparation for this transition, the anesthetist must examine and optimize the patient's metabolic, anesthetic, and cardiorespiratory status.

1. Preparation for discontinuing CPB begins during rewarming. The arterial perfusate is warmed. The core temperature should reach but not exceed 37°C, and the shell (rectal) temperature, reflective of less highly perfused tissues, should reach 34° to 35°C prior to discontinuation from CPB.

a. Laboratory data to acquire during rewarming include ABG tensions and pH, potassium, calcium, glucose, hematocrit, and ACT. ABG tensions and pH can be reported both at 37°C (the temperature of the sample in the blood gas machine) and corrected to the patient's temperature. Clinical decisions concerning pH usually are made according to the values measured at 37°C (**alpha stat** management). The topic remains controversial, and some anesthetists in the past acted on the values reported at the patient's temperature (**pH stat** management).

b. Adequate anticoagulation during rewarming and separation from CPB is ensured with additional heparin if necessary.

c. Metabolic acidosis should be treated with sodium bicarbonate, and appropriate ventilatory changes should be instituted by the perfusionist.

d. Hyperkalemia, commonly seen following the use of cardioplegia, frequently corrects spontaneously by redistribution and diuresis. If not, the administration of IV insulin, sodium bicarbonate, and glucose will lower serum potassium.

e. Severe hyperglycemia (blood glucose higher than 400 to 500 mg/dL), most commonly seen in diabetic patients following a warm cardioplegia technique, requires an insulin infusion.

f. A **hematocrit** over 20% should be achieved prior to separation, either by transfusion or hemoconcentration, as indicated by the CPB reservoir volume status. A higher or lower hematocrit may be appropriate, depending on the patient's age and condition.

g. **FFP** should be thawed before separation from bypass (takes 30 to 45 minutes) if the patient is at risk for postoperative bleeding.

2. **Anesthetic considerations** during rewarming include maintenance of adequate neuromuscular blockade, analgesia, and amnesia. Supplementary relaxants, narcotics, and benzodiazepines may be given. Pressure transducers are rezeroed. Volatile anesthetics in use on the CPB system are discontinued. If MAP is elevated, sodium nitroprusside may be used for blood pressure control, as well as to facilitate rewarming.

3. **Separation from CPB**

a. Following procedures where the heart has been opened (e.g., valve replacements), "**de-airing maneuvers**" under TEE guidance are used to prevent air embolism to the cerebral or coronary circulations. Sustained positive-pressure ventilation accompanied by clamping of the venous return lines will move air forward from the pulmonary veins. Air in the ventricular trabeculae can be liberated by shifting the OR table from side to side and lifting the apex of the heart; it can then be evacuated by needle aspiration of the apex. Direct aspiration of air bubbles visible within coronary artery vein grafts may help prevent ischemia.

b. **Aortic cross-clamp removal** reestablishes coronary perfusion. A lidocaine bolus is given followed by an infusion (1 mg per minute). Nitroglycerin is started in CABG patients.

c. **Defibrillation** may be spontaneous; ventricular fibrillation is treated with directly applied 10- to 30-joule DC countershock. (If using a device capable of delivering a biphasic waveform, 7 to 10 joules is usually adequate). Failure may indicate inadequate warming, graft problems, or inadequate myocardial protection. Additional lidocaine, magnesium (1 gram IV slowly), or amiodarone (150-mg bolus followed by infusion at 1 mg per minute IV for 6 hours, then 0.5 mg per minute) may be required.

d. **Rhythm is assessed.** With slow rhythms, atrial pacing is established through epicardial wires, but if the PR interval is prolonged or there is complete heart block, ventricular pacing is added. Hypothermia, hypocalcemia, hyperkalemia, and magnesium from cardioplegia solutions may contribute to a high incidence of reversible heart block immediately following CPB. Atrial tachycardia may indicate inadequate anesthesia and may be treated with fentanyl. Other atrial arrhythmias may be treated with overdrive pacing, cardioversion, and then, if necessary, antiarrhythmics (e.g., esmolol, propranolol, amiodarone, verapamil, or rarely digoxin; see Chapter 18, section III, and Chapter 36).

e. **The ECG should be inspected** for evidence of ischemia possibly related to intracoronary air or inadequate revascularization.

f.   LV filling may be guided during separation from CPB by mean PA, PA occlusion pressure, or a surgically placed left atrial line. Right ventricular (RV) filling is indicated by the CVP or direct RV visualization. The determination of target postbypass filling pressures should consider the patient's preoperative pressures, the degree of left ventricular hypertrophy (LVH), the adequacy of the myocardial revascularization, and so on. A normotensive patient without LVH probably needs a left atrial (LA) pressure of 10 mmHg or a mean PA pressure of 20 mmHg. A patient with severe LVH and inadequate revascularization may need an LA pressure of 20 mm Hg and a mean PA pressure of 30 mm Hg. TEE is particularly helpful in the assessment of LV filling.

g.   Comparison is made between central (aortic) and peripheral (radial) arterial pressures to ensure that no significant pressure gradient exists.

h.   Compliance and resistance of the lungs is tested with a few trial breaths (ventilation should be reestablished when LV ejection, even on bypass, occurs). To facilitate expansion of the lungs, the stomach is suctioned, and if previously opened, the pleural cavities are drained. If the lungs are difficult to ventilate, suctioning or bronchodilators may be indicated (see Chapter 18, section XI).

i.   Visual inspection of the heart confirms atrioventricular synchrony; contractility is assessed both by gross appearance and by systolic performance, as estimated by peak systolic and pulse pressure, taking into account pump flow and left atrial and PA pressure. If poor myocardial performance is demonstrated or anticipated (e.g., impaired preoperative function or intraoperative ischemia), initiation of inotropic support before separation from CPB may be indicated. Pump flow rate is checked and compared with the patient's preoperative cardiac output. Significantly higher flows indicate the need to increase vascular tone (using agents such as norepinephrine and phenylephrine).

j.   Ionized Ca^{2+} may be corrected slowly 15 minutes after cross-clamp removal. Rapid Ca^{2+} administration, especially in the presence of myocardial ischemia, is associated with Ca^{2+}-induced myocardial injury (Ca^{2+} paradox). Calcium will increase both contractility and systemic vascular resistance (SVR).

I.   At the time of actual separation from CPB, venous lines are slowly clamped, allowing the heart to gradually fill and eject with each contraction. Prolonged partial venous line occlusion allows for "**partial bypass**," during which time cardiopulmonary function is shared and hemodynamics are assessed. Following complete venous line occlusion, once adequate filling pressures are achieved, perfusion through the aortic cannula is stopped, and the heart alone provides systemic perfusion. Manual ventilation with full tidal volumes and short inspiratory times facilitates RV performance.

1.   Pressure maintenance. Transfusion from the CPB reservoir maintains the left atrial pressure or mean PA pressure at an optimal level. Care is taken not to overdistend the heart. Should overdistention occur, the surgeon may "empty" the heart by transiently unclamping a venous line.

2. **After bypass has been terminated, assess the following:** ECG, systemic BP (SBP), left-sided filling pressure (LFP), right-sided filling pressure (RFP), and the cardiac output. Compare these values to the target values for the patient. If the patient is not doing well, correct any pacing problems, ask the surgeon to assess the adequacy of the grafts, and use TEE to assess the valve replacement or repair. Assuming no surgically related cause, the unstable patient will usually fall into one of the following situations:

a. **SBP low, CO low, LFP low, RFP low: Hypovolemia.** Give volume from the bypass reservoir. If the patient cannot tolerate the low BP (e.g., a patient with severe LVH and distal coronary disease), use a pressor transiently until the volume resuscitation is adequate.

b. **SBP low, CO low, LFP high, RFP low: Left heart failure.** Give a positive inotrope. A common first-line agent is dopamine, started at 200 to 300 μg per minute IV and titrated as necessary. Milrinone, a phosphodiesterase III inhibitor, is added when additional support is necessary (load 25 to 50 μg/kg followed by an infusion at 0.375 to 0.750 μg/kg per minute). The patient may need to go back on CPB temporarily. If inotropes are ineffective, an IABP (see section V.A) is inserted. The final intervention is insertion of a LV assist device (LVAD) (see section V.B).

c. **SBP low, CO low, LFP low, RFP high: Right heart failure.** This situation can be caused by primary RV failure (inadequate myocardial protection or intracoronary air) or secondary RV failure (severe protamine reaction, inadequate ventilation, fixed elevation in PVR). Management includes the following:

(1) If achievable, a rapid increase in systemic perfusion pressure using norepinephrine or epinephrine may reverse primary RV failure.

(2) Treat known causes of elevated PVR: light anesthesia, hypercarbia, hypoxemia, and acidemia. Vasopressors and calcium chloride should be administered through a left atrial line if available.

(3) Vasodilator therapy, including nitroglycerin, sodium nitroprusside, or PGE_1 (begin 0.05 μg/kg per minute IV, titrate as necessary) through a right-sided line. Systemic vasodilatation often necessitates compensatory vasopressor support through a left atrial line. Alternatively, inhaled nitric oxide can be used to avoid the systemic hypotension.

(4) Inotropic support is maintained with milrinone, dobutamine, or rarely, isoproterenol, for maximal pulmonary vasodilatation. Mechanical support (IABP or RV assist devices [RVAD; see sections V.A and B]) may be necessary.

d. **SBP low, CO low, LFP high, RFP high: Biventricular failure.** Management includes maneuvers to treat left and right heart failure, as outlined above. Frequently, the patient will need to go back on bypass.

e. **SBP low, CO high, LFP low, RFP low: Low SVR.** Initial management consists of administration of a pressor such as norepinephrine or phenylephrine. Epinephrine may be necessary. In certain patients with vasodilatory shock (e.g., following heart transplant or LVAD insertion), arginine vasopressin is used starting with an infusion at 0.1 unit per minute.

f.   SBP high, CO low, LFP normal, RFP normal: High SVR. Hypertension with adequate cardiac output should be treated to prevent bleeding at suture lines and cannulation sites. Vasodilators (e.g., nitroprusside), narcotics, or volatile anesthetics may be appropriate.

g.   If a return to CPB is necessary in any of the above situations, adequate anticoagulation must be ensured, and a full heparinizing dose is indicated if any protamine has been given.

J.   Postbypass period

1.   Hemodynamic stability is the primary goal, since myocardial function has been impaired by CPB. Maintain adequate volume status, perfusion pressure, and appropriate rate and rhythm. Continuously monitor and reassess the surgical field.

2.   Hemostasis. Once cardiovascular stability has been achieved and the surgeon is confident that the bleeding is under control, protamine administration begins. Initially, 25 to 50 mg are given over 2 to 3 minutes, and the hemodynamic response is observed. Protamine often causes systemic vasodilation that depends on the rate of administration; hence, slow infusions are prudent. Rarely, an anaphylactic or anaphylactoid reaction or catastrophic pulmonary hypertension is encountered. Upon severe reaction, protamine is immediately discontinued, appropriate resuscitative measures are employed, and if necessary, the patient is reheparinized (with a full loading dose) and CPB is reinitiated. If forward flow is compromised, ask the surgeon to inject the heparin into the right atrium.

a.   It is advisable to monitor PA pressures while administering protamine (even if left atrial pressure is available).

b.   In general, 1 mg of protamine is administered for each milligram (100 IU) of heparin administered throughout the procedure.

c.   After protamine, the ACT is measured and compared to baseline. Further protamine is given to return the ACT toward control.

d.   During transfusion of blood obtained from the hemoconcentrator, additional protamine (25 to 50 mg) is given to reverse the heparin. Blood obtained from auto-transfusion devices (Cell Saver) is essentially devoid of heparin.

e.   Desmopressin, aminocaproic acid, aprotinin, and various blood products may be of value in the treatment of post-CPB coagulopathy. Strategies for the diagnosis and management of intraoperative bleeding diatheses are discussed in Chapter 33.

3.   Pulmonary dysfunction may follow CPB. Aggressive treatment of bronchospasm before sternal closure is imperative.

4.   Pulmonary hypertension may arise during the post-CPB period. See section II.I.2.c for approaches to management.

5.   Sternal closure may precipitate acute cardiovascular decompensation. **Cardiac tamponade** may develop from compression of the heart and great vessels in the mediastinum.

a. Volatile anesthetics and other negative inotropes are avoided in anticipation of sternal closure. Intravascular volume should be optimized.

b. Immediately after sternal closure the filling pressures and cardiac output are compared to preclosure values, and appropriate adjustments in volume or drug infusions are made.

c. Mediastinal and chest tubes are placed on suction to prevent tamponade and quantify blood loss. Blood drainage of greater than 300 mL in 30 minutes is worrisome and might necessitate surgical reexploration.

d. The left atrial waveform and the ability of pacemakers to capture are rechecked to verify that displacement has not occurred during sternal closure.

e. If the patient is hemodynamically unstable or ventilation is inadequate, management should begin with early reopening of the sternum. The patient may require transfer to the intensive care unit (ICU) with the sternum open.

K. Transfer to the ICU

1. Patients should always be hemodynamically stable prior to transport. Immediately after transferring the patient from the OR table to the bed, reassess vital signs and confirm that drug infusions are still infusing. The patient's bed should be equipped with a full cylinder of oxygen, an Ambu bag, mask, intubation equipment, defibrillator, and essential monitors. Drugs for resuscitation should accompany the patient during transport and include calcium chloride, lidocaine, and a vasopressor.

2. During transfer, the ECG, arterial and PA pressures, and oxygen saturation are monitored.

3. Upon arrival to the ICU, mediastinal and pleural drainage tubes are attached to suction. The ECG and pressure transducers are attached to the ICU monitors. The patient is placed on the ICU ventilator, and ventilation is ensured. An anteroposterior chest radiograph and a 12-lead ECG are obtained, and blood samples are sent for ABG, electrolytes, hematocrit, platelet count, prothrombin time, and partial thromboplastin time. A thorough report is provided to the ICU team, including pertinent hemodynamics, vasoactive drips and dosages, and the problems that are anticipated. Prior to leaving the ICU, the anesthetist should review the ECG and ABG and should check the chest radiograph for the presence of abnormal findings (e.g., atelectasis, pneumothorax, malpositioned tubes and catheters, widened mediastinum, or pleural effusion).

III. Postoperative care

A. Warming. Most cardiac surgical patients will be hypothermic upon arrival in the ICU, and their initial course is notable for warming and vasodilation. A temperature overshoot phenomenon is common, and patients will, on average, reach a maximal temperature at 6 to 12 hours into their ICU stay. Pressor and volume requirements should be anticipated. Adequate sedation, either by periodic bolus or continuous infusion, will prevent early waking and shivering during this period.

B. Extubation. Ventilatory support is withdrawn coincident with emergence from anesthesia; most patients are extubated 6 to 18 hours after arrival in the ICU. Intracardiac cannulas and chest tubes are removed, and hemodynamic support is then gradually withdrawn.

C. Complications

1. Arrhythmias and myocardial ischemia are common in the immediate postoperative period. Diagnosis and management are discussed in Chapter 18.

2. Unexplained profound hypotension, unresponsive to volume and pharmacologic resuscitation, is an indication for immediate reopening of the chest in the ICU. The OR should be notified and blood products requisitioned.

3. Cardiac tamponade may occur insidiously and may be difficult to diagnose. Most often, an accumulation of blood in the mediastinum and inadequate chest tube drainage secondary to clot are responsible. Placing mediastinal tubes on suction as soon as the sternum is closed and frequent tube "stripping" of the tubes will help to prevent the development of tamponade. Reopening the sternum may be lifesaving. The diagnosis is considered with hypotension or low-output syndrome. Equilibration of mean CVP, PA pressure, and PA occlusion pressure is rarely present because the pericardium is open.

IV. Pediatric cardiac anesthesia

A. Transition from fetal to adult circulation. The transition from fetal to adult circulation is a transformation from a parallel to a series circulation (see Chapter 27). In utero, there is right-to-left shunting of blood across the ductus arteriosus. After birth, as the lungs are expanded and alveolar oxygen tension rises, the PVR decreases. Simultaneously, the SVR increases in association with the loss of the low-resistance placental circulation. The net effect of the PVR falling beneath the SVR is a reversal of ductus flow. The ductus arteriosus will contract and functionally close in the first 10 to 15 hours of life. This is caused by a loss of placental-produced prostaglandins and an increase in neonatal blood oxygen tension. Accompanying the decrease in PVR is an increase in pulmonary blood flow, an improvement in RV compliance, and a decrease in right-sided pressures relative to the left. This drop in right atrial pressure results in the closure of the foramen ovale. With the closure of the ductus arteriosus and the foramen ovale, the circulation assumes an adult configuration. These changes in the neonatal period are transitional, however, and reversion to a fetal circulation can occur during periods of abnormal physiologic stress. Persistence of elements of fetal circulation is common in many cases of congenital heart disease (CHD) and can occasionally be lifesaving.

B. Differences between neonatal and adult cardiac physiology

1. In infants, there is **parasympathetic nervous system dominance** that reflects the relative immaturity of the sympathetic nervous system. Infant hearts are more responsive to circulating catecholamines than to sympathetic nervous stimulation.

2. Neonatal hearts have more inelastic membrane mass than elastic contractile mass. Consequently, infant hearts have less myocardial reserve, a greater sensitivity to drugs causing myocardial depression, and a greater sensitivity to volume overload.

The relatively noncompliant ventricles make stroke volume less responsive to increases in preload or demand. As such, **increases in cardiac output are largely dependent on increases in heart rate.**

3. The right and left ventricles are equal in muscle mass at birth. A left to right muscle mass ratio of 2:1 is not achieved until the age of 4 to 5 months.

C. Congenital heart disease. In CHD, the clinical presentation is dependent on both the anatomy and the physiologic changes secondary to intracardiac shunts and obstructive lesions (also see Chapter 2).

1. Shunt classification. A shunt is an abnormal communication between the systemic and pulmonary circulations.

a. Simple shunts are not associated with any additional anatomic obstruction to ventricular outflow. Pulmonary and systemic blood flow is determined by both the size of the shunt and the relative PVR/SVR ratio.

b. Complex shunts are accompanied by an anatomic obstruction to blood flow. The direction and magnitude of blood flow are largely determined by the presence of the obstructive lesion. Blood flow depends less on the PVR/SVR ratio and more on the resistance of the obstructive lesion.

c. Balanced shunts are characterized by right and/or LV output that can be directed to either the pulmonary or systemic circulations. The amount of pulmonary and systemic blood flow is solely dependent on the PVR/SVR ratio.

d. Shunt flow calculation. The amount of systemic arterial desaturation due to CHD is determined by the relative amount of pulmonary-to-systemic blood shunting ($\dot{Q}p/\dot{Q}s$) and the saturation of the venous blood.

$$\dot{Q}p/\dot{Q}s = (Sao_2 - Smvo_2)/(Spvo_2 - Spao_2)$$

$$\dot{Q}p/\dot{Q}s > 1 \text{ left-to-right shunt}$$

$$\dot{Q}p/\dot{Q}s < 1 \text{ right-to-left shunt}$$

where $\dot{Q}p$, is pulmonary blood flow; $Smvo_2$, mixed venous oxygen saturation; $\dot{Q}s$, systemic blood flow; $Spvo_2$, pulmonary venous oxygen saturation; Sao_2, systemic arterial oxygen saturation; and $Spao_2$, pulmonary artery oxygen saturation.

Since we are calculating the ratio of flows, oxygen saturation can be used instead of oxygen content. To simplify the calculation, if systemic blood is fully saturated, one can approximate that there is no significant right-to-left shunting and that pulmonary venous oxygen saturation is equal to systemic oxygen saturation ($Spvo_2 = Sao_2$).

2. The effect of left-to-right shunts on the cardiovascular system includes ventricular volume overload and dysfunction, increased pulmonary blood flow and PA pressures, and the potential for permanent increases in PVR. The net effect on the pulmonary system is pulmonary edema, with associated decreases in compliance and ventilatory reserve. **Right-to-left shunting** can produce hypoxemia.

3. Clinical presentation

a. **Cyanosis** due to CHD is caused by inadequate pulmonary blood flow. This may be caused by a simple shunt with right-to-left flow (e.g., VSD with Eisenmenger syndrome), a complex shunt with right-to-left flow (e.g., tetralogy of Fallot or tricuspid atresia), or balanced shunts complicated by inadequate pulmonary blood flow (e.g., single ventricle lesions or truncus arteriosus).

b. **Congestive heart failure** (CHF) and/or hypotension may be caused by either left-to-right shunting and excessive pulmonary blood flow (e.g., atrial septal defect [ASD], VSD, or patent ductus arteriosus [PDA]) or LV outflow obstruction and pressure overload (e.g., congenital subvalvular, valvular, or great-vessel obstruction).

c. **Balanced shunts** (e.g., truncus arteriosus or hypoplastic left heart syndrome) can cause a combination of cyanosis due to mixing and/or systemic hypotension from pulmonary overcirculation.

D. **Anesthetic management**

  1. **Preoperative evaluation**

  a. The **history** should provide an assessment of the extent of cardiopulmonary impairment (e.g., presence of cyanosis or CHF, exercise tolerance, cyanotic spells, activity level, feeding and growth patterns, associated syndromes, and anatomic abnormalities).

  b. **Physical examination** should make note of skin color, activity level, respiratory pattern and frequency, and appropriateness of development for given age. The heart and lungs should be auscultated and close attention given to the patient's airway and IV access. Peripheral pulses should be palpated and blood pressure obtained in both arms and the lower extremities if coarctation is suspected.

  c. The **chest radiograph** is examined for evidence of increased heart size, presence of CHF, decreased pulmonary blood flow, abnormalities in heart position, and the presence of any thoracic cage abnormalities.

  d. The **ECG** may be normal even in the presence of CHD. However, abnormalities can be important clues to underlying cardiac lesions.

  e. **Echocardiography** will show anatomic abnormalities and, with Doppler, provide information about flow patterns and pressure gradients.

  f. **Cardiac catheterization** is, at present, the best window into the patient's central circulatory system. Anatomy can be defined, pulmonary and systemic shunt flows and vascular resistances quantified, and intracardiac chamber pressures measured.

  2. **Premedication.** Infants younger than 6 months of age, cyanotic or dyspneic children, and patients who are critically ill generally receive no premedication. Older or more vigorous children may be given oral midazolam (0.5 to 1.0 mg/kg); oral ketamine (5 to 7 mg/kg) may be added for a deeper level of sedation. An alternate intramuscular regimen is ketamine (3 to 5 mg/kg) in combination with midazolam (0.5 to 1.0 mg) and glycopyrrolate (0.1 to 0.2 mg) given in the preanesthetic holding area. Dosages are reduced in cases where decreasing SVR would increase right-to-left shunting. Fasting guidelines must be adjusted based on the patient's age and cardiac condition (see Chapter 1, section VII, and Chapter 28). Cyanotic infants are usually polycythemic and may be prone to vital organ thrombi if not hydrated with IV fluids preoperatively.

3. Monitoring and equipment (Table 23-5). In addition to the standard monitoring required for all patients, a precordial or esophageal stethoscope and three temperature probes (tympanic membrane, esophageal, and rectal) should be available. Intraarterial pressure monitoring usually is necessary. (Note that previous surgical procedures [e.g., classic Blalock-Taussig shunt or coarctation repair] may influence the choice of site for radial artery cannulation.) Central venous catheters are inserted regularly for infusion of vasoactive drugs, CVP measurement, and volume administration; a 4 Fr double-lumen catheter can be used for infants weighing 10 kg or less and a 5-Fr, triple-lumen catheter used for larger children. A warming/cooling blanket, radiant heating lamps, and a heated humidifier are useful perioperatively. Increasingly, TEE has become an important diagnostic and perioperative management tool. Using suitably sized pediatric TEE probes, children as small as 3.5 kg may be safely studied.

4. Resuscitation drugs and infusions of inotropic medications appropriate for pediatric use must be available. **Air bubbles** must be meticulously removed from all IV lines and syringes. **Air filters** should be used whenever possible. Even in the absence of shunts, paradoxical air emboli may traverse a probe-patent foramen ovale under some conditions.

5. Induction. The choice between an inhalation and intravenous induction is based primarily on ventricular function and the degree of patient cooperation. A slow, carefully titrated induction by either technique usually provides for a safe and stable anesthetic. Theoretically, patients with right-to-left shunts may have a slower rate of induction with volatile anesthetics, since blood is shunted past the lungs. Similarly, blood concentrations of IV anesthetic may increase faster in patients with a significant right-to-left shunt. For the uncooperative child or a child surviving primarily on sympathetic stimulation, intramuscular ketamine (3 to 5 mg/kg) along with an antisialagogue such as atropine (0.02 mg/kg) or glycopyrrolate (0.01 mg/kg) may be used.

E. Cardiopulmonary bypass

1. Pump prime volume ranges between 150 and 1200 mL depending on the weight of the infant and CPB circuit design. Packed red blood cells frequently are added to the prime to yield an initial hematocrit of less than 25% when on bypass. For smaller children, the red cells may be washed first to remove potassium, acid, and citrate-phosphate-dextrose-adenine (CPD-A_1) preservative and may be leukocyte-depleted to decrease patient exposure to cytomegalovirus. Typical constituents of pump prime include sodium bicarbonate (to counteract acidosis), mannitol (to promote diuresis), heparin, and calcium (to offset the effects of the citrate in CPD-A_1-preserved blood). Albumin solutions and FFP may be added to the prime for neonates.

2. Infants and children generally lack vasoocclusive disease. Consequently, blood flow during CPB is more important than

Table 23-5.   Equipment and drug checklist for pediatric cardiac surgery

Equipment

Pediatric anesthesia machine with air tank (full) and extra oxygen tanks

Pediatric circle circuit (appropriate for children of all sizes)

500-mL, 1-L, 2-L, and 3-L breathing bags

Heated humidifier or in-line passive humidifier

Halothane, sevoflurane, and isoflurane vaporizers (full)

Full ECG and invasive hemodynamic monitoring display

Pediatric ECG leads

Appropriate pressure transducer and flush systems

Two noninvasive automatic blood pressure machines

Neonatal, infant, and pediatric blood pressure cuffs

Two pulse oximeters and probes (infant and pediatric sizes)

Appropriate size masks, airways, laryngoscope blade, ETT cuffed and uncuffed, adult and pediatric stylets, Magill forceps

Lidocaine/phenylephrine solution (for nasal ETT and nasogastric tube insertion)

Nasogastric tubes

Tympanic/esophageal temperature probe and monitor

Rectal/bladder temperature probe and monitor

Esophageal stethoscope with integral temperature probe

Hat

Padded head rest

Capnograph with agent analyzer

End-tidal capnograph connector

Precordial stethoscope and stickers (when appropriate)

Suction catheters

TEE machine

Pediatric and adult biplane or omniplane (if available) TEE probes

Drugs

Calcium gluconate (100 mg/mL)

Cisatracurium

Dopamine, dobutamine, epinephrine, milrinone, isoproterenol, nitroglycerin, and prostaglandin E_1 drips as needed)

Epinephrine (1, 10, and 100 µg/mL concentration syringes)

Fentanyl (up to 100 µg/kg)

Ketamine (50 or 100 mg/mL concentration for PO, IM, or IV use)

Midazolam (1 or 5 mg/mL concentration for PO, IM, or IV use)

Morphine sulfate

Pancuronium

Phenylephrine (1, 10, and 100 µg/mL concentration syringes)

Sodium bicarbonate

Succinylcholine (4 mg/kg for emergent IM use)

Thiopental

ECG, electrocardiographic; ETT, endotracheal tubes; TEE, transesophageal echocardiography.

arterial pressure. Flows as high as 150 mL/kg per minute may be used in infants weighing less than 5 kg, while MAP as low as 30 mm Hg is well tolerated provided that SVC pressure is low (indicating that venous drainage is adequate).

3. Deep hypothermic circulatory arrest (DHCA) is used extensively for infants weighing less than 10 kg. Up to 1 hour of circulatory arrest is tolerated without neurologic injury at a core and brain temperature of 15° to 20°C. Phentolamine (0.2 mg/kg) or sodium nitroprusside (1 to 2 μg/kg per minute) is frequently administered to encourage even cooling in preparation for DHCA. Where appropriate, low-flow CPB may offer advantages over circulatory arrest. Management points include:

    a. Adequate brain hypothermia (e.g., packing the head with ice packs).

    b. Hemodilution.

    c. Acid-base balance.

    d. Muscle relaxation.

    e. Avoidance of increased blood glucose.

F. Procedures not requiring CPB

    1. Closed-heart cases without the use of CPB include PDA ligation, coarctation of the aorta repair, PA banding, and most shunts designed to increase pulmonary blood flow (e.g., modified Blalock-Taussig shunt).

    2. Open-heart cases without CPB include those that can be accomplished through normothermic caval inflow obstruction, such as pulmonary valvotomy, aortic valvotomy, and creation of ASDs. Increasingly, these procedures can be accomplished utilizing transvenous techniques in the cardiac catheterization laboratory.

G. Management of specific CHD lesions (Table 23-6).

    1. Lesions with decreased pulmonary blood flow (cyanotic lesions) can occur via an anatomic obstruction to pulmonary blood flow and/or right-to-left shunting and include tetralogy of Fallot, tricuspid atresia, pulmonary atresia, and pulmonary hypertension.

        a. Management goals are to decrease PVR, increase pulmonary blood flow, maintain SVR, and maintain central volume.

        b. Anesthetic maneuvers include modest hypocarbia, increased inspired oxygen concentration, maintaining normal functional residual capacity, and avoiding acidosis.

        c. For tetralogy of Fallot, a negative inotrope (e.g., propranolol or halothane) may be used to relax dynamic infundibular stenosis and improve pulmonary blood flow. Adequate volume loading is critical in the management of a "tet spell." PGE_1 (0.1 μg/kg per minute IV) may be helpful in supporting ductus arteriosus patency (when possible), decreasing PVR, and increasing pulmonary blood flow. A peripheral vasoconstrictor should be available.

    2. Lesions with increased pulmonary blood flow and left-to-right shunting include ASD, VSD, and PDA.

        a. Management goals are to avoid myocardial depressants and excessive pulmonary blood flow.

        b. Anesthetic maneuvers include IV induction (e.g., opiates or ketamine), avoiding negative inotropes (e.g., inhala-

Table 23-6. Specific congenital cardiac lesions

Lesion	Anatomy	Pathophysiology	Surgical Correction	Anesthetic Considerations
Atrial septal defect	Three varieties: 1. Ostium secundum: defect in septum (most common). 2. Ostium primum: endocardial cushion defect. 3. Sinus venosus: caval-atrial defect often with partial anomalous pulmonary venous return.	L to R shunt. RV volume overload. Potential for R to L shunting (e.g., during valsalva maneuver) with paradoxical embolus risk. Minimal symptoms until later age, when CHF may develop.	Suture or patch closure. Percutaneous catheterization device closure.	Inhalation or intravenous induction. Potential extubation at end of procedure. Avoid air bubbles.

Ventricular septal defect	Supracristal, membranous canal, and muscular subtypes.	L to R shunt. Increased pulmonary blood flow. Pulmonary hypertension and reversal of shunt as a late effect (Eisenmenger syndrome).	Dacron patch closure of singular or multiple defects. Muscular defects may be difficult to locate. Selected defects may be amenable to percutaneous catheterization device closure.	Hypocarbia and low FIO_2 to decrease pulmonary blood flow. Avoid myocardial depressants. Avoid air bubbles. Potential for postoperative AV block and pacing requirement. Potential need for post-repair inotropic support.
Coarctation of the aorta	Narrowing usually distal to origin of left subclavian artery. May be pre- or post-ductal in location. Often associated with a VSD.	Increased blood flow to upper extremities and head. Systemic hypoperfusion. Pressure overload of LV.	L thoracotomy approach. Subclavian artery flap angioplasty or resection and end-to-end anastomosis.	Non-CPB case. Arterial line on right. Suitable for regional anesthesia supplementation. Potential for post-repair hypertension.

(continues)

Table 23-6. *Continued*

Lesion	Anatomy	Pathophysiology	Surgical Correction	Anesthetic Considerations
Patent ductus arteriosus	Patent ductus arteriosus.	R to L shunt when PVR is high. L to R shunt as PVR decreases. Necessary for survival with certain lesions (e.g., hypoplastic left heart syndrome).	L thoracotomy vs thoracoscopic approach. Ligation and occasional division of PDA. Potential for percutaneous catheterization coil embolization.	Usually premature infants with concomitant pulmonary disease. Avoid high F_{IO_2} (risk of retrolental fibroplasia). Risk of recurrent laryngeal nerve damage.
Tetralogy of Fallot	1. VSD. 2. Pulmonary outflow tract obstruction. 3. RV hypertrophy. 4. Overriding aorta.	R to L shunting through VSD into overriding aorta. Fixed (pulmonic stenosis) and dynamic (infundibular hypertrophy) RV outflow obstruction components. Systemic desaturation ("Tet" spell).	Patch closure of VSD. RV outflow tract reconstruction/ augmentation. Excision of infundibular muscle band (when appropriate).	Management of "Tet spell": augment intravascular volume, minimize PVR (increase F_{IO_2}, decrease Pa_{CO_2}), increase SVR (knee-chest position, phenylephrine), consider negative inotropes (halothane, beta-blockade). Potential need for postoperative pacing.

Transposition of the great arteries	Transposition of both the aorta to the RV and the PA to the LV resulting in isolation of pulmonary and systemic circulations.	ASD, VSD, and/or PDA required for pulmonary and systemic blood mixing and, hence, survival.	Atrial switch procedure (Mustard, Senning): rarely performed. Arterial switch procedure (Jatene). When associated with a VSD and pulmonic stenosis, a Rastelli procedure (LV to aorta baffle closure via the VSD, and RV to PA allograft conduit).	Ductus/mixing lesion dependent CHD lesion. PGE_1 to maintain ductus patency (when appropriate).
Truncus arteriosus	Single great artery that gives rise to the aorta, PA, and coronary arteries. Associated VSD.	Mixing of pulmonary and systemic blood. Most commonly presents with pulmonary overcirculation.	VSD closure. RV to PA valved conduit. Valvuloplasty of truncal valve.	Increase PVR/decrease pulmonary blood flow precorrection (based on degree of pulmonary over circulation). Normalize PVR postcorrection. Potential need for inotropic support post-repair.

(continues)

Table 23-6. *Continued*

Lesion	Anatomy	Pathophysiology	Surgical Correction	Anesthetic Considerations
Atrioventricular canal defect	Common AV valve. Deficiency of atrial and ventricular septae.	Mixing of blood at the atrial and ventricular level. Usually presents with pulmonary overcirculation.	Closure of ASD and VSD. Mitral/tricuspid valvuloplasty.	Manipulate PVR to balance/optimize pulmonary systemic blood flow. Anticipate need for inotropic support post-repair. Associated with Down's syndrome (potential airway issues).
Hypoplastic left heart syndrome	Atretic/hypoplastic mitral valve, aortic valve, LV, and ascending aorta.	L to R shunt (obligatory) at atrial or ventricular level for mixing. Ductus arteriosus dependent for R to L (i.e., systemic) perfusion.	Palliative, staged repair: 1. Norwood I: atrial septectomy, reconstruction of aortic arch, PA plasty, creation of systemic to pulmonary shunt.	Critically ill neonates. Preoperative (ICU) management will impact outcome. PGE_1 to maintain ductal patency. Inotropes often necessary pre- and post-repair.

2. Bidirectional Glenn: takedown of systemic to pulmonary shunt. creation of SVC to PA (cavopulmonary) shunt.
3. Modified Fontan procedure: creation of an IVC to PA anastomosis via an intra-atrial baffle; creates total cavopulmonary continuity. Alternatively, cardiac transplantation is an option.

Avoid myocardial depressants. Fentanyl >50 μg/kg prior to sternotomy. Manipulate PVR via adjustments in FIO_2 and PCO_2 to balance/optimize pulmonary vs systemic perfusion. Target goal: MAP = 40, pH = 7.40, PaO_2 = 40, $PaCO_2$ = 40.

ASD, atrial septal defect; AV, atrioventricular; CHD, congenital heart disease; CHF, congestive heart failure; CPB, cardiopulmonary bypass; FIO_2 fraction of inspired oxygen; ICU, intensive care unit; IVC, inferior vena cava; L, left; LV, left ventricle; MAP, mean arterial pressure; PA, pulmonary artery; PaO_2, partial pressure of oxygen; $PaCO_2$, partial pressure of carbon dioxide; PDA, patent ductus arteriosus; PVR, pulmonary vascular resistance; R, right; RV, right ventricle; SVC, superior vena cava; SVR, systemic vascular resistance; VSD, ventricular septal defect.

tion agents or pentothal), normocarbia to slight hypercarbia, limiting inspired oxygen concentration, and PEEP.

3.   Balanced shunts have the potential for a ventricle's output to be directed to either the pulmonary or systemic circulation and include hypoplastic left heart syndrome, truncus arteriosus, double-outlet RV, and complete AV canal defect. The direction of blood flow is governed by relative resistances (PVR to SVR ratio).

a.   Management goals are to manipulate pulmonary blood flow to maintain adequate systemic perfusion. Often both a low-normal blood pressure (i.e., MAP = 40 mm Hg) and a low PaO_2 (i.e., 40 mmHg) must be tolerated.

b.   Anesthetic maneuvers depend on the balance of systemic versus pulmonary blood flow. These include:

(1)   Normal to slightly elevated $PaCO_2$, consideration of PEEP and limiting inspired oxygen concentration to increase PVR, decrease pulmonary blood flow, and favor systemic blood flow.

(2)   Normal to slightly decreased $PaCO_2$ and increased inspired oxygen concentration to decrease PVR and increase pulmonary relative to systemic blood flow.

H.   Anesthesia for cardiac catheterization. The goal is to provide sufficient sedation to allow the procedure to be completed without excessive movement while avoiding sedative-induced hemodynamic changes and hypoventilation.

1.   An anesthesia machine (fitted with compressed air as well as oxygen) and all standard monitoring equipment, resuscitation drugs, airway management equipment, and a defibrillator (with appropriately sized paddles) must be present.

2.   Premedication is similar to that mentioned in section IV.D.2. Patients generally are well sedated and maintain a good airway with a continuous infusion of ketamine (2 mg/kg per hour) and midazolam (0.1 mg/kg per hour) supplemented with additional boluses as needed. Alternatively, a low-dose propofol infusion (25 to 100 μg/kg per minute) may be employed.

3.   General endotracheal anesthesia may be utilized in children prone to airway obstruction (Down syndrome or nasopharyngeal defects) and in children with suprasystemic RV pressures where cyanosis from pulmonary hypertension may improve after anesthesia reduces sympathetic tone. Intravenous techniques utilizing a combination of remifentanil (0.1 to 0.5 μg/kg per minute) and propofol (50 to 100 μg/kg per minute) for amnesia can provide a rapidly titratable anesthetic.

V.   Mechanical support devices.

A.   The **intraaortic balloon pump** provides circulatory assistance for the failing or ischemic heart by augmenting aortic diastolic pressure during inflation and driving blood toward the coronary ostia, and augmenting coronary perfusion, particularly to the LV, which receives most of its blood supply in diastole. Also, deflation of the balloon reduces the impedance to LV ejection and hence myocardial oxygen consumption. **Preoperative indications** include unstable angina that is refractory to medical therapy; LV failure due to MI, ruptured papillary muscle, or VSD; and prophylaxis for a high-risk patient with severe left main disease. **Postby-**

pass indications include refractory LV failure preventing successful termination of CPB and refractory ST-segment elevation.

1. The IABP is inserted through a femoral artery and advanced until the tip is 1 to 2 cm distal to the left subclavian artery in the descending thoracic aorta (positioning can be guided by TEE). It can be placed transthoracically if iliofemoral occlusive disease precludes use of a femoral artery.

2. Inflation of the IABP is synchronized with either the patient's ECG, a pacemaker potential, or the arterial blood pressure trace. Balloon inflation occurs early in diastole (at the dicrotic notch of the arterial pressure waveform). **Balloon deflation** occurs during isovolumic contraction. Intraoperative triggering directly from a pacemaker generator will eliminate interference otherwise caused by electrocautery or blood sampling.

3. Relative contraindications include severe AI, aortic aneurysm, and severe peripheral vascular disease.

4. Complications of IABPs include distal embolization (to extremities, kidneys, brain, and the gastrointestinal tract), aortic dissection or rupture, and lower extremity ischemia.

B. Ventricular assist devices (VAD) may be classified as either extracorporeal or implantable. Although both types of devices require cannulation of the heart, extracorporeal devices employ a pump that is positioned outside of the patient; implanted device pumps are inserted into the left upper quadrant of the abdomen.

1. Extracorporeal devices (e.g., ABIOMED BVS 5000 and Thoratec VAD).

    a. Indications include postcardiotomy support, cardiogenic shock, and bridge to transplant.

    b. These devices can provide biventricular support. Inflow cannulation sites include the LV or LA for left-sided support and the RV or right atrium for right-sided support. Corresponding outflow cannulas are inserted into the ascending aorta and main pulmonary artery. The cannulas (inflow and outflow) are then connected to an external pump. Surgical time and dissection are significantly less than with the implanted devices.

    c. Both the ABIOMED BVS 5000 and the Thoratec VAD utilize pneumatically driven pumping sacs. Whereas the ABIOMED BVS 5000 depends on gravity for venous drainage, the Thoratec VAD is equipped with vacuum-assisted drainage. The primary difference between the two devices is patient mobility. Patients with the ABIOMED BVS 5000 must lie supine; patients with the Thoratec may ambulate (albeit with a large and heavy console).

2. Implantable devices (e.g., Novacor V-E, HeartMate V-E, and HeartMate Pneumatic).

    a. These devices are typically used for patients who have cardiogenic shock and are candidates for transplantation.

    b. These devices are designed for LV support only. They consist of an inflow cannula (inserted into the LV apex), a pump, and an outflow cannula (inserted into the ascending aorta). A drive line that is tunneled through the skin connects the implanted pump to the external console. CPB is always necessary.

c. The Novacor V-E and the HeartMate V-E devices are electrically driven; the rechargeable power source fits into a backpack and allows the patient to leave the hospital.

3. Anesthetic considerations

a. Patients will have **marginal cardiac function**; extreme care is required during induction to minimize decreases in contractility and preload.

b. **Bleeding** can be problematic especially with the implanted devices. Establish adequate IV access for volume administration and consider using an antifibrinolytic drug.

c. If the patient is receiving the device as a bridge to transplant, transfuse with leukocyte-depleted cellular blood products to minimize HLA-antigen exposure.

d. **TEE is required.** Determine the degree of AI (if significant, a tissue valve may need to be inserted), the degree of tricuspid regurgitation, the presence of a patent foramen ovale, the degree of right heart dysfunction (the patient may require mechanical RV support), and the presence of thrombus. Postoperative TEE examination is used to assess whether the inflow cannula is properly inserted (look for the absence of turbulent flow) and ensure that any air is removed from the heart.

e. Patients receiving an LVAD frequently require RV support. Inotropes, nitric oxide, and occasionally an RVAD are required.

f. Most devices function best in the automatic mode after chest closure. The flow will then depend largely on venous return. Decreased venous return will be signaled by a decreased pumping rate since the devices will pump only when adequately filled. Volume administration or a pressor agent should be given.

VI. Other cardiac procedures

A. Off-bypass CABG is performed to avoid the complications associated with CPB and to minimize aortic manipulation. Proximal grafts are performed using a partial aortic cross-clamp technique. Distal grafts are performed using one of several heart stabilizing devices. Considerations for this procedure include:

1. Temperature management. Warm the room and consider using an active heating device (e.g., Bair Hugger).

2. Patients can be **extubated early** after the surgery, so the anesthetic should be tailored to allow early extubation (e.g., fentanyl 5 to 10 μg/kg, volatile anesthetic, then propofol infusion).

3. Heparin 3 mg/kg IV is given and the ACT is maintained above 400 seconds. This allows the patient to emergently go on CPB if necessary and has the theoretical benefit of less graft thrombosis. Antifibrinolytic therapy is avoided. A small dose of protamine (50 to 100 mg) is given following the procedure.

4. Drugs that might provide beneficial ischemic preconditioning to the myocardium are used including a nitroglycerin infusion, morphine (0.25 to 0.50 mg/kg), and isoflurane (0.5% to 1.0%). Hyperglycemia (>300 mg/dL) is avoided since it inhibits ischemic preconditioning.

5. Monitoring the ECG is difficult because the heart is placed in nonanatomical positions. Nonetheless, it is important to establish a baseline ECG (for each position) and to monitor the ST-segments.

6. Hemodynamic instability is common, particularly when the surgeon is performing the distal anastomoses to the right coronary and left circumflex coronary arteries. Grafts to vessels that have lesser disease tend to be associated with more instability than those to vessels that are occluded.

7. Intravenous volume requirements tend to be high. A full heart tends to tolerate the positioning better. A diuretic may be required at the end of the operation.

8. Patented immobilizers are used to stabilize the heart; they decrease the need for drug-induced heart rate slowing.

9. Arrhythmias may be a problem. Lidocaine and magnesium (0.5 g per hour) infusions are frequently used. Potassium is maintained above 4.0 mEq/dL.

B. "Redo" cardiac surgery

1. Mediastinal structures, including the heart, major vessels, vascular grafts, or lungs may be adherent to the underside of the sternum and can be lacerated during sternotomy. Preoperatively determine which grafts are patent since they could be transected during sternotomy. Blood must be in the OR and checked prior to sternotomy. An extra 14-gauge IV or a rapid infusion catheter should be placed to facilitate volume resuscitation. Because the patient may need to go on CPB emergently, heparin must be in a syringe ready to administer immediately. In emergency situations, venous return may be supplied from the pump suction line on the field ("sucker bypass").

2. Line insertion may be difficult at sites previously used for indwelling catheters.

3. Insertion of a PA line equipped with pacing capability is prudent since emergent epicardial pacing may not be possible during chest opening. Transcutaneous defibrillation pads should be applied to the lateral aspects of the patient's chest since the surgeon will not be able to use internal paddles before the heart is exposed.

4. Diffuse bleeding from extensive dissection of scar tissue may occur following CPB. Use of an antifibrinolytic drug is encouraged. Ascertain whether the patient has received aprotinin in the past, however, since reexposure is associated with 2% to 3% risk of anaphylaxis.

5. Careful ECG monitoring is imperative since manipulation of atheromatous grafts may send emboli to the coronary circulation. Because myocardial protection is more challenging in patients with previous coronary grafts, postbypass myocardial dysfunction is more likely.

C. Cardiac tamponade and constrictive pericarditis

1. The **major goals** are to avoid decreases in myocardial contractility, peripheral vascular resistance, and heart rate. **Pericardiocentesis** may be advisable before induction in patients with tamponade (unless associated with an aortic dissection).

2. Lines should include an arterial line, a large-bore IV, and preferably a PA line (if the patient can tolerate its insertion).

3. Useful induction agents include etomidate and ketamine.

A dopamine infusion during induction and the prepping phase is helpful.

4. A method for **backup atrial pacing** (transesophageal or transvenous) should be available.

5. **In severe cases**, consider an awake intubation and/or having the patient surgically prepped and draped prior to induction.

D. Cardiac transplantation

1. Management of the donor (see Chapter 20).

2. Anesthetic management of the recipient

a. The key to patient survival is minimizing the time that the donor heart is ischemic. Consequently, expeditious preparation of the recipient and direct communication with the surgeon is essential.

b. Preoperative evaluation of the recipient should determine if the patient had previous chest surgery (more time required), if the patient has elevated PVR, and if the patient is coagulopathic.

c. Invasive monitoring should include an arterial line and a triple lumen central venous catheter; a PA catheter is used when the patient has severe increases in PVR. **Sterility** is critical since the patient will be immunocompromised after the surgery.

d. Precautions for a full stomach may be necessary during induction. Etomidate and fentanyl are good choices to provide hypnosis and analgesia. If the patient is receiving inotropic infusions, consider empirically increasing their doses before induction. If a VAD is present, venous return must be maintained for the pump to maintain its flow rate.

e. Right heart failure and coagulopathy are common problems during the rewarming phase of bypass. Transfusion requirements should be anticipated; cellular blood products should be leukocyte-depleted to minimize foreign HLA-antigen exposure.

f. When weaning from CPB, the donor heart will be unresponsive to interventions mediated by the recipient's autonomic nervous system. The optimal heart rate is between 80 and 110 beats per minute. An isoproterenol infusion is used to achieve this pharmacologically since it also increases cardiac output and dilates pulmonary vessels.

g. Immunosuppressants will be necessary and are administered in consultation with the transplant cardiologist.

E. Circulatory arrest may be necessary for surgery on the distal ascending aorta or aortic arch (for an aneurysm or aortic dissection). Management issues include:

1. Systemic cooling to 18°C and application of ice around the head.

2. Supplemental administration of drugs such as pentothal, magnesium, ketamine, methylprednisolone, mannitol, and additional heparin before circulatory arrest.

3. Trendelenburg (head down) position.

4. Retrograde cerebral perfusion (with arterialized blood) through the SVC cannula with pressure monitoring through the sidearm of the PA-line introducer (pressure maintained at 25 mm Hg, and blood flow at 300 to 600 mL per minute).

F. Antiarrhythmia surgery may involve aneurysmectomy

(with or without electrophysiologic mapping), cryoablation, endo-cardial resection, or implantation of an ICD system.

1. Aneurysmectomy. It is crucial to prevent hyperdynamic responses; stress on the ventricular suture line is life-threaten-ing. Large resections may compromise ventricular stroke vol-ume. Thus, patients may be rendered highly rate dependent to achieve adequate cardiac output.

2. ICD surgery. Modern ICDs consist of an endocardial lead system and a pectoral pulse generator. Older systems used epi-cardial lead systems and abdominal generators.

    a. Most devices are now placed under local anesthesia in the electrophysiology (EP) laboratory. A brief period of general anesthesia is necessary for testing of the device once it is implanted; **intravenous propofol** and spontaneous ventila-tion with airway support are suitable. Patients with severe reflux, a difficult airway, or agitation may need endotracheal intubation. Standard monitoring is employed. Intubation equipment, a bag and mask, emergency drugs, oxygen, suc-tion, and a defibrillator must be present.

    b. Rarely, patients go to the OR for patch electrode place-ment. These patients are invariably hemodynamically com-promised; it is helpful to have a large-bore IV, an arterial line, and a line for vasoactive medications (either a separate IV or a central line). Emergency drugs, including epinephrine, must be immediately available.

VII. Anesthesia for cardioversion and electrophysiology pro-cedures

    A. Cardioversion. The patient will usually fall into one of three categories:

    1. Hemodynamically stable and fasting. After careful air-way assessment, propofol (or etomidate) can be given in small doses until the patient loses consciousness. A prolonged drug delivery time should be anticipated. Phenylephrine or ephed-rine, succinylcholine, airway equipment, and suction should be immediately available.

    2. Hemodynamically stable and a full stomach. The patient and cardiologist are given two choices: rapid sequence induc-tion with general endotracheal anesthesia or waiting until the patient has been fasting for 4 to 6 hours. Usually the decision is made to wait the necessary time for gastric emptying to occur.

    3. Hemodynamically unstable. The patient should be cardi-overted as soon as possible and administration of general anes-thesia may be risky. Provision of sedation and an amnestic should be considered for conscious patients.

    B. Noninvasive programmed stimulation is used to test the function of an ICD after it has been implanted. An ICD programmer is used to induce the irregular rhythm (ventricular fibrillation or tachycardia). The device then is checked for proper sensing and rhythm termination. Since this is an elective situation, the patient should be fasting and propofol anesthesia is used as described in section VI.F.2.a.

SUGGESTED READING

Argenziano M, Chen JM, Choudhri AF, et al. Management of vasodilatory shock after cardiac surgery: identification of predisposing factors and use of a novel pressor agent. *J Thorac Cardiovasc Surg* 1998;116: 973–980.

Dacey LJ, Munoz JJ, Johnson ER, et al: Effect of perioperative aspirin use on mortality in coronary artery bypass grafting patients. *Ann Thorac Surg* 2000;70:1986–1990.

D'Ambra MN, LaRaia PJ, Philbin DM, et al. Prostaglandin E1: a new therapy for refractory right heart failure and pulmonary hypertension after mitral valve replacement. *J Thorac Cardiovasc Surg* 1985;89: 567–572.

Dowling RD, Etoch SW. Clinically available extracorporeal assist devices. *Prog Cardiovasc Dis* 2000;43:27–36.

Ellenbogen KA. *Clinical cardiac pacing and defibrillation*. Philadelphia: WB Saunders, 2000.

Frederiksen JW. Cardiopulmonary bypass in humans: bypassing unfractionated heparin. *Ann Thorac Surg* 2000;70:1434–1443.

Hensley FA Jr, Martin DE. *The practical approach to cardiac anesthesia*, 2nd ed. Boston: Little Brown, 1995.

Kaplan JA. *Cardiac anesthesia*, 4th ed. New York: Grune & Stratton, 1999.

Lake CL. *Pediatric cardiac anesthesia*, 2nd ed. Norwalk, CT: Appleton and Lange, 1993.

Lichtenstein SV, Salerno TA, Slutsky AS. Pro: warm continuous cardioplegia is preferable to intermittent hypothermic cardioplegia for myocardial protection during cardiopulmonary bypass. *J Cardiothorac Anesth* 1990;4:279–281.

Lowenstein E, Johnston WE, Lappas DG, et al. Catastrophic pulmonary vasoconstriction associated with protamine reversal of heparin. *Anesthesiology* 1983;59:470–473.

McCarthy PM, Hoercher K. Clinically available intracorporeal left ventricular assist devices. *Prog Cardiovasc Dis* 2000;43:37–46.

Mets B. Anesthesia for left ventricular assist device placement. *J Cardiothorac Vasc Anesth* 2000;14:316–326.

Mora CT. *Cardiopulmonary bypass*. New York: Springer-Verlag, 1995.

Shanewise JS, Cheung AT, Aronson S, et al. ASE/SCA guidelines for performing a comprehensive intraoperative multiplane transesophageal echocardiography examination. *Anesth Analg* 1999;89:870–884.

Sharpe MD. Anaesthesia and the transplanted patient. *Can J Anaesth* 1996;43:R89–98.

Slaughter TF, Greenberg CS. Antifibrinolytic drugs and perioperative hemostasis. *Am J Hematol* 1997;56:32–36.

Anesthesia for Neurosurgery

Wolfgang Steudel and Michele Szabo

I. Physiology

A. Cerebral blood flow (CBF) is equal to cerebral perfusion pressure (defined as the difference between mean arterial pressure [MAP] and intracranial pressure [ICP] or central venous pressure, whichever is higher) divided by the cerebral vascular resistance. CBF averages 50 mL/100 g of brain tissue per minute in the normal brain and is affected by blood pressure, metabolic demands, $Paco_2$, Pao_2, and blood viscosity.

1. **CBF** is maintained at a constant level by constriction and dilation of arterioles (autoregulation) (Fig. 24-1) when the MAP is between 50 and 150 mm Hg. CBF varies directly with MAP beyond these limits. Chronic hypertension shifts the autoregulatory curve to the right, rendering patients susceptible to cerebral ischemia at blood pressures considered normal in healthy individuals. Chronic antihypertensive therapy may bring the autoregulatory range back toward normal. Cerebral ischemia, trauma, hypoxia, hypercarbia, edema, mass effect, and volatile anesthetics attenuate or abolish autoregulation and may make blood flow to the affected area dependent on MAP.

2. **$Paco_2$** has profound effects on CBF by its effect on the pH of brain extracellular fluid (ECF). CBF increases linearly with increasing $Paco_2$ in the range from 20 to 80 mm Hg, with an absolute change of 1 to 2 mL/100 g per minute for each mm Hg change in $Paco_2$. The effect of $Paco_2$ on CBF decreases over 6 to 24 hours, due to slow adaptive changes in brain ECF bicarbonate concentration. Sustained hyperventilation causes cerebrospinal fluid (CSF) HCO_3 production to decrease, allowing CSF pH to gradually return to normal. Rapid normalization of $Paco_2$ after a period of hyperventilation results in a significant CSF acidosis with vasodilation and increased ICP.

3. **Pao_2.** Hypoxia is a potent cerebral vasodilator; CBF increases markedly below a Pao_2 of 60 mm Hg. Pao_2's from 60 to more than 300 mm Hg have little influence on CBF.

B. Cerebral metabolic rate ($CMRO_2$) and CBF are coupled, since the brain requires a constant supply of substrate to meet its relatively high metabolic demands. Regional or global increases in $CMRO_2$ elicit a corresponding increase in CBF, probably mediated by metabolic factors such as nitric oxide. Other factors that affect $CMRO_2$ (and CBF through this mechanism) include:

1. **Anesthetics** (see sections II.A and B).

2. **Temperature.** Hypothermia decreases $CMRO_2$ 7% per 1°C, and hyperthermia increases it.

3. **Seizures**

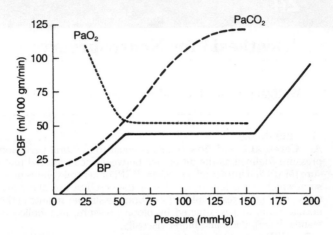

Fig. 24-1. Autoregulation maintains a constant level of cerebral blood flow (CBF) over a wide range of carotid artery mean blood pressures. Independent of this effect, CBF is elevated by hypercarbia (Paco$_2$) and hypoxemia (Pao$_2$); hypocarbia diminishes CBF.

C.   ICP reflects the relationship between the volume of the intracranial contents (brain, blood, and CSF) and the volume of the cranial vault. **Normal ICP is 5 to 15 mm Hg.**

   1.   **The cranial vault is rigid**, and its capacity to accommodate increases in intracranial volume is limited. A developing intracranial mass (e.g., tumor, edema, hematoma, and hydrocephalus) initially displaces one or more of the intracranial components and ICP remains relatively normal (Fig. 24-2). As intracranial volume increases further, intracranial compliance decreases, and ICP rises rapidly (Fig. 24-2). Thus, patients with decreased compliance may develop marked increases in ICP even with small increases in intracranial volume (i.e., cerebral vasodilation due to anesthesia, hypertension, or carbon dioxide retention) (Fig. 24-2).

   2.   **Methods commonly used to measure ICP:**

   a.   **A ventriculostomy catheter** is inserted through a burr hole into a lateral ventricle. It is the gold standard to which other devices are compared and can be used to drain CSF. When transporting a patient with a ventriculostomy, always monitor the CSF pressure and when appropriate clamp off the CSF drainage catheter to avoid inadvertent rapid changes in ICP.

   b.   **A subarachnoid bolt** is a hollow screw placed through a burr hole in direct communication with the intradural space. This is connected by saline-filled tubing to a pressure transducer. It is useful for the measurement of ICP, but does not allow for CSF drainage.

   c.   **A Camino catheter** is a solid-state intraparenchymal ICP monitor. It does not rely on a fluid column for pressure measurement, and cannot be used for CSF drainage.

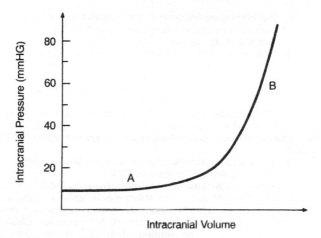

Fig. 24-2. **The intracranial compliance curve. In the normal intracranial pressure (ICP) range (A), increases in intracranial volume produce minimal changes in ICP. Further small increases in ICP after the "elbow" of the curve can produce abrupt increases in ICP (B).**

3. Clinical features of elevated ICP. ICP elevation decreases cerebral perfusion pressure and may cause ischemia in regions of the brain where autoregulation is defective and CBF is dependent on cerebral perfusion pressure. Early signs and symptoms of increased ICP include headache, nausea, vomiting, and decreased levels of consciousness. As ICP continues to increase, distortion and ischemia of the brainstem and/or brain herniation may occur and result in hypertension with brady- or tachyarrhythmias; irregular respiration; oculomotor (third cranial) nerve palsy leading to ipsilateral pupillary dilation with no light reflex; abducens (sixth cranial) nerve palsy; contralateral hemiparesis or hemiplegia; and ultimately coma and respiratory arrest.

4. Treatment of elevated ICP involves strategies aimed at decreasing the volume of the intracranial components:

    a. Hypoxia and hypercarbia cause cerebral vasodilation and should be avoided. Hyperventilation to a $Paco_2$ of 25 to 30 mm Hg produces cerebral vasoconstriction and is useful in acute management of increased ICP. Since there is little additional decrease in CBF below 20 to 25 mm Hg $Paco_2$ and biochemical evidence of cerebral ischemia may develop, excessive hyperventilation should be avoided.

    b. Elevating the head at least 30 degrees promotes venous drainage and decreases intracranial venous blood volume. Avoid excessive flexion or rotation of the neck and prevent increases in intrathoracic pressure (e.g., coughing and straining and elevated intrathoracic pressure). Positive end-expiratory pressure should be minimized to the lowest level that provides adequate lung recruitment.

   c.   Barbiturates are potent vasoconstrictors that decrease cerebral blood volume while decreasing $CMRO_2$.

   d.   Maintaining high serum osmolality (305 to 320 mOsm/kg) may reduce cerebral edema and decrease brain volume. Fluid management is designed to achieve this goal (see section V.D). In addition, **mannitol** (0.5 to 2.0 g/kg intravenous) and **furosemide** produce a hyperosmolar state and are effective in the acute reduction of ICP.

   e.   CSF volume can be reduced by draining CSF through a lumbar subarachnoid or ventriculostomy catheter.

II.   Pharmacology. Agents used in anesthesia may affect $CMRO_2$ and CBF.

   A.   Inhalation anesthetics produce a dose-related reduction in $CMRO_2$ while causing an increase in CBF.

   1.   The effect of **nitrous oxide** is controversial, but it probably is a cerebral vasodilator. This effect can be greatly attenuated or abolished when it is administered in conjunction with intravenous anesthetic agents. Nitrous oxide slightly increases $CMRO_2$. Nitrous oxide should be avoided when intracranial airspaces (e.g., pneumocephalus) exist, since it diffuses more rapidly into such spaces than nitrogen diffuses out and may produce an acute rise in ICP.

   2.   **Halothane, enflurane, isoflurane, sevoflurane, and desflurane** cause increases in CBF. Autoregulation can be attenuated or abolished by increasing the concentration of these drugs, but responsiveness to carbon dioxide seems to be preserved. Institution of hyperventilation prior to administration of the agent may attenuate the rise in ICP. Enflurane at concentrations greater than 1.5 times the minimum alveolar concentration (MAC) for anesthesia, when combined with hypocarbia ($Paco_2$ less than 30 mm Hg), can induce seizure-like activity on the electroencephalogram (EEG). The clinical significance of this has not been established.

   3.   Volatile anesthetics produce dose-dependent reductions in metabolism ($CMRO_2$), probably by depressing neuronal electrical activity. Isoflurane is the most potent in this respect and is the only volatile agent that induces an isoelectric EEG at clinically relevant concentrations ($2 \times$ MAC).

B.   Most **intravenous anesthetics** (e.g., barbiturates, benzodiazepines, opioids, etomidate, and propofol) cause coupled reduction in CBF and $CMRO_2$ in a dose-dependent manner. This is due to depression of cerebral metabolism. **Barbiturates** and **etomidate** markedly decrease CBF and $CMRO_2$ and can produce isoelectric EEGs. Etomidate has been associated with seizures and is best avoided in seizure-prone patients. **Ketamine** increases CBF and $CMRO_2$, and is used infrequently in neuroanesthesia. **Opioids** produce minimal changes in CBF and $CMRO_2$. **Lidocaine** in therapeutic doses decreases both CBF and $CMRO_2$. Autoregulation and carbon dioxide responsiveness appear to be preserved with these IV agents.

C.   **Muscle relaxants** have no direct effect on CBF and CMR_2 because they do not cross the blood–brain barrier. They may alter cerebral hemodynamics indirectly through their effects on blood pressure. **Succinylcholine** produces a transient increase in ICP, likely caused by arousal phenomena, which can be attenuated by

prior administration of a barbiturate or a defasciculating dose of a nondepolarizing muscle relaxant.
D. **Vasoactive drugs**
    1. **Adrenergic agonists.** Alpha-adrenergic agonists and low dose beta-adrenergic agonists have little influence on CBF. Larger doses of beta-adrenergic agonists can produce an increase in $CMRO_2$ and CBF that can be exaggerated in the setting of a defect in the blood–brain barrier. Dopamine causes an increase in CBF with little change in CMR.
    2. **Vasodilators.** Sodium nitroprusside, nitroglycerin, and hydralazine can increase CBF and ICP by direct cerebral vasodilation if arterial blood pressure is maintained. Beta-adrenergic blocking agents probably have minimal effects, if cerebral perfusion pressure is maintained. Despite these profiles, all of these agents have been used safely during neuroanesthesia.
E. **Cerebral protection**
    1. **Cerebral ischemia** can be classified into three types:
        a. **Focal**, characterized by the presence of surrounding non-ischemic brain and possible collateral blood flow to the ischemic region (e.g., stroke, arterial occlusion, embolization).
        b. **Incomplete global**, insufficient blood supply or oxygen delivery to the whole brain (e.g., hypotension or increased ICP).
        c. **Complete global**, characterized by absent CBF (e.g., cardiac arrest).
    2. **Agents**
        a. **Barbiturates** may slightly improve the neurologic recovery from focal or incomplete global ischemia, possibly by decreasing metabolic rate or by a direct pharmacologic effect. The protective benefit is likely achieved with an induction dose of barbiturate (thiopental 3 to 7 mg/kg IV). In contrast, barbiturates have been shown to be of no benefit following cardiac arrest. Propofol and etomidate have not been shown to confer any brain protection.
        b. **Isoflurane**, which can induce an isoelectric EEG and significantly lower CMR, has not been shown to be beneficial in the setting of global ischemia.
        c. **Hypothermia**, which can reduce metabolism for both neuronal and cellular functions, is the established protective technique for circulatory arrest procedures. Its use is limited by cardiovascular and respiratory depression, arrhythmias, tissue hypoperfusion, and coagulopathy. In the laboratory, mild hypothermia (a 2° to 4°C reduction) can confer significant cerebral protection during focal ischemia while minimizing associated risks.
        d. **Hyperthermia** worsens outcome from focal cerebral ischemia and should be avoided.
        e. **Hyperglycemia** may worsen neurologic outcome following ischemic insult, probably because anaerobic metabolism of glucose produces excessive lactate, which can lead to intracellular acidosis.
        f. **Nimodipine**, a calcium channel antagonist, has been shown in some studies to improve outcome after stroke and attenuate cerebral hypoperfusion following global ischemia, although with inconsistent neurologic recovery. Nimodipine's

beneficial effects on vasospasm after subarachnoid hemorrhage (SAH) are well established.

g.   Steroids have not been found to be beneficial after
stroke or severe head injury. High-dose methylprednisolone
has been shown to produce modest improvement in neurologic recovery following acute spinal cord injury if the treatment is started within 8 hours of injury.

III.   Electrophysiologic monitoring

A.   Electroencephalography (EEG) measures electrical activity of the neurons of the cerebral cortex and is thus used as a
threshold marker for the detection of ischemia due to inadequate
CBF. It is used frequently during procedures that jeopardize cerebral perfusion such as carotid endarterectomy or to assure electrical silence before circulatory arrest.

1.   When CBF decreases below 20 to 25 mL/100 g per minute
under nitrous oxide-oxygen-halothane anesthesia, EEG slowing
occurs; in the vicinity of 18 mL/100 g per minute, the EEG becomes isoelectric ("flat"). Sustained reduction of CBF to 8 to
10 mL/100 g per minute results in tissue infarction. Thus, EEG
changes can warn of ischemia before CBF becomes insufficient
to maintain tissue viability. **The critical level of CBF** is defined
as that degree of CBF below which signs of ischemia are seen
on EEG, and it is roughly correlated with the extent to which
each anesthetic depresses $CMRO_2$. The level of critical CBF varies with the anesthetic agents: 20 mL/100 g per minute for halothane, 18 mL/100 g per minute for enflurane, and 10 mL/100 g
per minute for isoflurane.

2.   The EEG may exhibit changes intraoperatively with no de-
monstrable neurologic deficit during postoperative examination. Cerebral ischemia can produce electrical dysfunction without causing neuronal cell damage because the blood flow
threshold for electrical failure is higher than that needed to
maintain cellular integrity.

3.   Factors other than anesthetics that may affect the EEG include hypothermia (which may limit the usefulness of EEG during cardiopulmonary bypass), hypotension, hypoxia, tumors,
vascular abnormalities, and epilepsy. An abnormal EEG in patients with preexisting neurologic deficits, strokes in evolution,
and recent reversible ischemic neurologic deficits can also make
it difficult to interpret new changes.

4.   Anesthetic effects on the EEG are generally global,
which often helps distinguish them from the focal changes of
ischemia. A predominance of slow activity is seen as the anesthetic depth increases. "Deep" anesthesia may cause marked
EEG slowing, making detection of superimposed ischemic
changes during critical periods difficult to interpret. Maintaining
a constant level of anesthesia during critical periods (e.g., carotid clamping) facilitates EEG interpretation.

B.   Evoked potential monitoring

1.   Sensory-evoked potentials (EPs) are electrical potentials
generated within the neuraxis in response to stimulation of a
peripheral or cranial nerve. As they travel from the periphery
to the brain, these potentials are recorded by electrodes placed
over the scalp and along the transmission pathway. EPs are
of lower voltage compared with background EEG activity, but
summation of hundreds of signals using computerized devices

makes it possible to extract them by averaging out the random background EEG. A normal response implies that the conduction pathway is intact. Damage to the pathway generally decreases the amplitude or prolongs latency (i.e., the time from peripheral stimulus to arrival of potentials at the recording site) of the peaks of a waveform. EPs are classified according to the nerve tract being evaluated. Intraoperative monitoring of evoked potentials does not guarantee the prevention of postoperative neurologic deficits, since false positives and false negatives do occur.

    a. Somatosensory-evoked potentials (SSEPs) are obtained by stimulating a peripheral nerve (e.g., median nerve at the wrist, or posterior tibial nerve at the ankle or in the popliteal fossa) and recording the elicited signals over the spinal cord (spinal SSEPs) or cerebral cortex (cortical SSEPs). SSEPs are used most commonly to monitor spinal cord function during spinal cord or vertebral column surgery (e.g., Harrington rod instrumentation) and may be used during peripheral nerve, brachial plexus, or thoracic aortic surgery (to detect spinal ischemia during aortic cross-clamping). Since SSEPs are conducted primarily by the posterior column in the spinal cord, there are concerns about the reliability of SSEP monitoring for detecting threatened motor function (i.e., anterior spinal cord ischemia). For this reason, the wake-up test is used in some centers (see section VII.A.2), and motor-evoked potential (MEP) monitoring has been developed recently.

    b. Brainstem–auditory-evoked potentials (BAEPs) are recorded by delivering a "clicking" sound to one ear through an ear-insert headphone. BAEPs reflect the transmission of electrical impulses along the auditory pathway and are monitored during posterior fossa surgery in an attempt to avoid brainstem or auditory (eighth cranial) nerve damage.

2. Motor-evoked potentials. Monitoring of the integrity of the motor tracts within the spinal cord may be more reliable than SSEP monitoring during spinal surgery. The vascular supply to the anterior motor columns of the spinal cord may be at greater risk from ischemia than the circulation of the posterior proprioceptive fibers. Motor impulses can be generated by transcranial magnetic or electrical stimulation, or by stimulation of the spinal cord above the surgical field. The evoked responses are measured as potential over the spinal cord below the surgical field, the peripheral nerve, and as movement of the muscle itself. Anesthetics substantially modify transcranially induced potentials, and less so if the stimulus is directly applied to the spinal cord. Measurement of spinal cord responses seems to be more reliable than muscle activity assessment during anesthesia. The measurement of spinal cord or peripheral nerve activity allows the use of muscle relaxants, which is not possible if the motor response must be assessed. The clinical value of MEP is still under discussion, since an improvement of neurological outcome by MEP monitoring has not been proved.

3. Electromyography (EMG) records muscle responses to stimulation of motor nerves. They are used frequently when there is risk of facial nerve injury during cerebellopontine angle surgery (e.g., posterior fossae surgery for meningioma). Since the EMG records motor responses to stimulation, neuromuscular blocking agents are limited during the periods of electrical stimulation.

4.   Confounding factors. Interpretation of EP changes are confounded by factors similar to those that affect the EEG (e.g., anesthetics, temperature, hypotension, hypoxia, anemia, preexisting neurologic lesions). Volatile anesthetics can depress EPs by reducing the amplitude or prolonging the latency of the EPs. Spinal SSEPs and BAEPs appear to be more resistant to the depressive effects of anesthetics than cortical SSEPs. Intravenous anesthetics have less of an effect; barbiturates, propofol, and fentanyl (up to 50µg/kg) are compatible with effective monitoring of cortical SSEPs and BAEPs.

5.   False positives. Changes in EPs occur frequently and often are not associated with postoperative neurologic complications. Further work is required to establish the nature, magnitude, and duration of EP changes associated with irreversible damage.

IV.   Preoperative considerations for neurosurgical procedures

A.   Intracranial compliance may be decreased by intracranial mass lesions (e.g., tumor, hematoma, or abscess). Surrounding normal brain tissue may be compressed, leading to brain edema and loss of autoregulation of cerebral vessels in that area. Signs and symptoms of increased ICP are discussed in section I.C.3.

B.   A computed tomography (CT) or magnetic resonance imaging (MRI) scan should be reviewed. Midline shift, and compressed ventricles or cisterns suggest the presence of diminished intracranial compliance. The degree of brain edema surrounding the mass and the site of the lesion in relation to major intracranial vessels and structures should be noted. Lesions near the dural venous sinuses may require exposure of the sinuses to the atmosphere and may be associated with a higher risk of venous air embolism (see section VI.D.3).

C.   The pathology of the mass is important in anticipating possible perioperative problems. Vascular lesions (e.g., meningiomas and some metastatic brain tumors) may bleed profusely. Infiltrating malignant tumors may render the patient particularly prone to postoperative brain edema.

D.   Preoperative fluid and electrolyte imbalances and glucose intolerance are common due to poor oral intake, use of diuretics and steroids, and centrally mediated endocrine abnormalities.

E.   Anticonvulsants may be required to control seizures. **Corticosteroids** may be necessary to treat edema. These drugs should be continued preoperatively.

F.   Premedication should be prescribed cautiously, since patients with intracranial disease may be extremely sensitive to the effects of central nervous system (CNS) depressants. Frequently, no premedication is given, and if sedation is needed, diazepam (0.1 to 0.2 mg/kg PO) can be used. Additional sedation can be given once the patient arrives in the operating room. Opioids should be avoided because of their respiratory depressant effects and the increases in CBF that occur with hypercarbia.

G.   Besides standard monitoring (see Chapter 10), arterial catheters are used in most patients undergoing craniotomy. Capnography is particularly useful when reducing ICP by hyperventilation. A urinary catheter is placed to aid fluid management and diuretic therapy. Invasive monitoring (e.g., pulmonary artery catheter) may be indicated for patients with severe cardiac, renal, or pulmonary disease in the face of marked diuretic-induced fluid shifts. Since access to the neck is limited during neurosurgery, placing central lines by brachial or subclavian approaches should be considered. A second IV catheter for drug administration is often useful.

V. Intraoperative management. Anesthetic goals for intracranial procedures include amnesia, immobility, control of ICP and cerebral perfusion pressure, and a "relaxed brain" (i.e., optimal surgical conditions). Whenever possible, the anesthetic plan should provide an awake, extubated patient who can be evaluated neurologically at the end of the procedure.

A.   Induction of anesthesia must be accomplished without increasing ICP or compromising CBF. Hypertension, hypotension, hypoxia, hypercarbia, and coughing should be avoided.

1.   While thiopental (3 to 7 mg/kg), propofol (2.0 to 2.5 mg/kg), midazolam (0.2 to 0.4 mg/kg), and etomidate (0.3 to 0.4 mg/kg) are all reasonable IV induction agents, the hemodynamic effects caused by these agents should be anticipated.

2.   An adequate mask airway is essential. Following induction, hyperventilation by mask is started with either a nitrous oxide–oxygen mixture or 100% oxygen.

3.   An intubating dose of muscle relaxant is given. Nondepolarizing agents are commonly chosen. Adequate relaxation should be obtained prior to laryngoscopy and intubation to avoid coughing and straining during these procedures.

4.   Opioids cause minimal changes in cerebral hemodynamics and are useful in blunting responses to intubation and craniotomy. Since intubation, placement of head pins, and craniotomy (skin incision and manipulation of the periosteum) represent the most stimulating periods during intracranial procedures, generous doses of narcotics are given prior to these manipulations. Fentanyl (5 to 10 µg/kg) and sufentanil (0.5 to 1.0 µg/kg) are most commonly used, since both have rapid onset and high potency. Lidocaine (1.5 mg/kg IV) can also be used to attenuate the cardiovascular and ICP responses to intubation.

5.   Low concentrations of a potent volatile agent occasionally are added to prevent hypertension during the initial surgical stimulation.

6.   Following intubation, the eyes are covered with watertight patches to prevent irritation from surgical preparation solutions, the head is carefully checked after final positioning to ensure good venous return, and close attention is paid to the airway, since access to the airway is limited during neurosurgical procedures. Breath sounds and ventilation should be checked after final positioning to ensure proper placement of the endotracheal tube, and all connections in the breathing circuit should be securely tightened.

B.   Maintenance

1.   Adequate brain relaxation is necessary prior to opening the dura. This is achieved by ensuring adequate oxygenation, venous return, muscle relaxation, anesthetic depth, hyperventilation to a $Paco_2$ of 25 to 30 mm Hg, and often the administration of furosemide (10 to 20 mg IV) and mannitol (0.5 to 1.5 g/kg IV) before the craniotomy is completed. The surgeon can assess the need for further brain relaxation by checking the tension of the dura. If necessary, additional IV thiopental can be administered or CSF drained through a previously placed lumbar subarachnoid catheter.

2. **Anesthetic requirements** are substantially lower after craniotomy and dural opening, since the brain parenchyma is devoid of sensation. If supplemental narcotics are needed, small doses of morphine, fentanyl, or sufentanil can be given. A continuous infusion of propofol (50 to 150 µg/kg per minute) and/or remifentanil (0.1 to 0.5 µg/kg per minute) produces a stable level of anesthesia and allows a rapid emergence. Long-acting narcotics and sedatives are usually avoided during the last 1 to 2 hours of the procedure to facilitate neurologic examination at the end of surgery and avoid potential drowsiness and hypoventilation.

3. **Muscle relaxants** frequently are continued throughout the procedure to prevent movement. Patients receiving anticonvulsants (e.g., phenytoin) may require more frequent administration of muscle relaxants.

4. **Hyperventilation** is continued.

C. **Emergence** should occur promptly without straining or coughing. Intravenous lidocaine may be administered to suppress the cough reflex, but may delay emergence. Toward the end of the procedure, Pa_{CO_2} is normalized gradually. Hypertension should be controlled to minimize bleeding; rapidly acting IV agents such as labetalol, esmolol, sodium nitroprusside, or nitroglycerin often are used. Muscle relaxation is usually maintained until the head dressing is completed and then reversal agents are administered. Before leaving the operating room, the patient should be awake so that a brief neurologic examination can be performed. The differential diagnosis of persisting unconsciousness after discontinuation of all anesthetics should include residual anesthesia, hypothermia, hypoxia, hypercapnia, partial neuromuscular blockade, and surgically induced increases in ICP (bleeding, edema, and hydrocephalus). Physostigmine (0.01 to 0.03 mg/kg IV) or naloxone (0.04 to 0.4 mg IV) may help antagonize pharmacologically induced CNS depression. The presence of new localized or generalized neurological deficits should be immediately addressed and may be evaluated by CT and/or surgical reexploration.

D. **Perioperative fluid management** is designed to decrease brain water content, thereby reducing ICP and providing adequate brain relaxation, while maintaining hemodynamic stability and cerebral perfusion pressure.

1. **The blood–brain barrier** is selectively permeable. Gradients for osmotically active substances ultimately determine the distribution of fluids between the brain and intravascular spaces.

a. **Water freely passes through the blood–brain barrier.** Intravascular infusion of free water may increase brain water content and may elevate ICP. Isosmotic glucose solutions (e.g., 5% dextrose in water) have the same effect, since the glucose is metabolized and free water remains. These are usually avoided during neurosurgery.

b. The blood–brain barrier is impermeable to most ions including Na^+. Unlike the peripheral vasculature, total osmolality, rather than colloid oncotic pressure, determines the osmotic pressure gradient across the blood–brain barrier. Consequently, maintenance of high-normal serum osmolality can decrease brain water content, while administration of a large amount of hyposmolar crystalloid solution may increase it.

c. Large, polar substances cross the blood–brain barrier poorly. Albumin has little effect on brain ECF, since the colloid oncotic pressure contributes to only a small portion of total plasma osmolality (approximately 1 mOsm/L).

d. If the blood–brain barrier is disrupted (e.g., by ischemia, head trauma, or tumor), permeability to mannitol, albumin, and saline increases such that these molecules have equal access to brain ECF. Under such circumstances, iso-osmolar colloid and crystalloid solutions seem to have similar effects on edema formation and ICP.

2. Severe fluid restriction can produce marked hypovolemia, leading to hypotension, reduced CBF, and ischemia of the brain and other organs, while only modestly decreasing brain water content. **Excessive hypervolemia** may cause hypertension and cerebral edema.

3. Specific treatment recommendations. The overall goal is to maintain normal intravascular volume and to produce a hyperosmolar state.

a. Fluid losses. The fluid deficit incurred by an overnight fast is usually not replaced. Physiologic maintenance fluids are given. Third-spacing of fluids during intracranial surgery is minimal and usually does not warrant replacement. Two-thirds to total intraoperative urine output is replaced with crystalloid. If signs of hypovolemia develop, additional fluid is administered.

b. Assessment of blood loss may be difficult during intracranial procedures because significant amounts can be hidden under the drapes. Also, irrigating solutions are used generously by the neurosurgeon.

c. The serum osmolality is increased to 305 to 320 mOsm/kg. If large fluids requirements are anticipated, iso-osmolar crystalloid solutions such as 0.9% normal saline (309 mOsm/kg) may be preferable to hyposmolar solutions such as lactated Ringer's (272 mOsm/kg). Mannitol (0.5 to 2.0 g/kg IV) and/or furosemide (5 to 20 mg IV) are also administered. The large diuresis produced by these agents demands close monitoring of intravascular volume and electrolytes.

d. Hypokalemia may develop from the use of steroids or potassium-wasting diuretics and is exacerbated by hyperventilation. Nevertheless, intraoperative administration of potassium is rarely necessary.

e. Hyponatremia may be produced by diuretics or inappropriate antidiuretic hormone secretion (SIADH).

f. Hyperglycemia may worsen neurologic outcome after ischemia (see section II.E.2.d). Glucose-containing solutions are avoided in patients at risk for CNS ischemia.

E.   Immediate postoperative care. Patients are observed closely in an intensive care setting following most intracranial neurosurgical procedures.

1.   The head of the bed should be elevated 30 degrees to promote venous drainage.

2.   Neurologic function, including the level of consciousness, orientation, pupillary size, and motor strength, should be assessed frequently. Deterioration of any of these may indicate development of brain edema, hematoma, hydrocephalus, or herniation.

3.   Adequate ventilation and oxygenation are essential in patients with reduced level of consciousness.

4.   Continuous monitoring of ICP may be indicated if intracranial hypertension exists at the time of dural closure or is anticipated in the postoperative period.

5.   Serum electrolytes and osmolarity should be checked.

6.   SIADH can be diagnosed by hyponatremia and serum hyposmolality with high urine osmolality and is treated by restricting free water intake.

7.   Diabetes insipidus may occur after any intracranial procedure, but is most common after pituitary surgery. **Polyuria** is associated with hypernatremia, serum hyperosmolality, and urine hyposmolality. Conscious patients can compensate by increasing their fluid intake; otherwise, adequate IV replacement is mandatory. **Aqueous vasopressin** (5 to 10 USP units subcutaneously or 3 units per hour by IV infusion) may be given. Larger doses may cause hypertension. Alternatively, **desmopressin** (DDAVP; 1 to 2 μg IV or subcutaneously q6 to 12h) can be used and is associated with a lower incidence of hypertension.

8.   Seizures may indicate the presence of an expanding intracranial hematoma or cerebral edema. If a seizure occurs, airway patency, oxygenation, and ventilation must be ensured. For acute therapy, thiopental (50 to 100 mg IV), midazolam (2 to 4 mg IV), or diazepam (5 to 20 mg IV for adults) may be used. Fosphenytoin (15 to 20 mg/kg IV, 100 to 150 mg per minute) or phenytoin (15 mg/kg IV over 20 minutes) can be administered to prevent recurrence.

9.   Tension pneumocephalus may occur and should be suspected after failure to awaken from anesthesia. Skull radiographs or head CT scans confirm the diagnosis; treatment consists of opening the dura to release the air.

VI.   Specific neurosurgical procedures

A.   Patients with **intracranial aneurysms** present for surgery electively or emergently following **SAH**.

1.   Preoperative evaluation of patients with SAH should include all components of a routine preoperative evaluation (see Chapter 1), with attention to known associated physiologic perturbations. These include the **neurologic grade** (Table 24-1); presence of **vasospasm** (and the hemodynamic parameters that have been effective in relieving clinical symptoms); degree of hydrocephalus; ICP elevation; and concurrent drug therapy such as calcium channel blockade with nimodipine, which may cause lower systemic pressures intraoperatively. **Electrocardiographic changes** are common following SAH and include ar-

Table 24-1.   **Classification of patients with intracranial aneurysms according to surgical risk (Hunt and Hess classification)**

Grade	Characteristics
I	Asymptomatic or minimal headache and slight nuchal rigidity
II	Moderate to severe headache, nuchal rigidity, no neurologic deficit other than cranial nerve palsy
III	Drowsiness, confusion, mild focal deficit
IV	Stupor, moderate to severe hemiparesis, possibly early decerebrate rigidity, vegetative disturbances
V	Deep coma, decerebrate rigidity, moribund

rhythmias and fluctuating ST-segment, QT-interval and T-wave changes. These are probably caused by subendocardial injury following the autonomic discharge that occurs in association with the initial SAH. Provided these are not associated with cardiac dysfunction, no modification of patient management is necessary.

2. Current practice is to intervene early during the first 72 hours after SAH for patients with neurologic grades I-III, which decreases the risk of rebleeding and facilitates the hypertensive management of vasospasm. Otherwise, surgery is delayed for 2 weeks or beyond the period of vasospasm risk.

3. Specific anesthetic considerations include:

a. Avoidance of hypertension, which may increase the risk of aneurysm rupture, prior to aneurysm clipping. Prophylactic use of agents such as fentanyl, beta-adrenergic blockers, lidocaine, or additional doses of barbiturates or propofol often will attenuate the blood pressure response to laryngoscopy and intubation.

b. Avoidance of hypotension to maintain adequate cerebral perfusion pressure.

c. Providing adequate brain relaxation to optimize surgical exposure. Rapid reductions in ICP may affect transmural pressure and increase the risk of aneurysm rupture. This should be done cautiously prior to dural opening.

d. Induced hypertension may be requested during temporary clipping to improve collateral blood flow to regions that were perfused by the clipped arteries. Often intravenous phenylephrine is used for this purpose.

e. Intraoperative aneurysm rupture can produce rapid and massive blood loss requiring large-bore intravenous access for volume resuscitation. Accurate estimation of blood loss is essential to guide volume repletion. Induced hypotension or, occasionally, manual pressure on the ipsilateral carotid artery in the neck may be helpful during an uncontrolled premature rupture.

f. Mild hypothermia (34°C) may be used as a protective

strategy for the brain during periods of cerebral ischemia. Hypothermic patients must be rewarmed adequately prior to emergence, in order to decrease cardiac and infectious complications.

g.   Once the permanent clips have been placed on the aneurysm, prevention of postoperative vasospasm becomes important. Blood pressure is increased moderately, and fluids are administered to achieve a mildly positive fluid balance.

C.   An arteriovenous malformation (AVM) is a direct communication between cerebral arteries and veins without an intervening capillary bed. Since an AVM is a high-flow, low-resistance system, surrounding brain regions may be hypoperfused by the diversion of blood (steal) through the AVM. The most common presentations of an AVM are SAH, seizures, headaches, and progressive neurologic deficits that are due to mass effect and focal cerebral ischemia.

1.   Patients with AVMs may require anesthetic care for either embolization procedures or surgical resection.

a.   Embolizations are usually done to decrease blood flow to the AVM prior to surgical resection. Embolization may decrease the risk of intraoperative bleeding and postoperative reperfusion hyperemia.

b.   Embolizations can be done under general anesthesia or sedation with monitored anesthesia care, which has the advantage of permitting continuous neurologic evaluation.

c.   The anesthetist should be prepared for adverse reactions to the contrast dye (anaphylaxis; osmotic load that may cause congestive heart failure), vessel perforation (sudden and rapid blood loss requiring immediate craniotomy), and neurologic changes.

2.   The anesthetic management for surgical resection of an AVM is similar to that for cerebral aneurysms.

a.   The primary focus is on tight blood pressure control, since hypotension can lead to ischemia of hypoperfused regions. Hypertension can exacerbate perfusion pressure breakthrough, a poorly understood phenomenon that is thought to be caused by abrupt diversion of the AVMs blood flow to adjacent, previously marginally perfused brain, and which produces sudden engorgement of the brain and hemorrhage.

b.   Postoperative angiography to confirm complete AVM resection is usually done immediately following surgery. Should any residual AVM be detected, the patient returns directly to the operating room for further resection.

D.   Posterior fossa surgery

1.   Posterior fossa tumors may cause cranial nerve palsies, cerebellar dysfunction, and hydrocephalus due to obstruction of the fourth ventricle. Tumors or surgery around the glossopharyngeal and vagus nerves may impair the gag reflex and increase the risk of aspiration. Tumor resection that results in edema in the floor of the fourth ventricle may damage respiratory centers and necessitate postoperative mechanical ventilation.

2.   Cardiovascular instability resulting from surgical manipulation is common. Sudden severe bradycardia and hypertension occur if the trigeminal nerve is stimulated. Bradycardia, asystole, or hypotension may follow stimulation of the glossopharyngeal or vagus nerve. In such cases, the surgeon should be notified immediately, since the instability usually resolves with cessation of the stimulus. Further treatment (e.g., atropine, glycopyrrolate, or ephedrine) rarely is necessary.

3. A **sitting position** is occasionally used for posterior fossa surgery. Its advantages include better surgical exposure; improved venous and CSF drainage; diminished bleeding due to lower venous pressures; and improved access to the airway, chest and extremities for the anesthetist. The sitting position also is associated with a higher incidence of venous air embolism and cardiovascular instability. Modified supine, prone, and three-quarter prone positioning may be substituted for the sitting position because of these concerns.

   a. **Venous air embolism** is a risk whenever the operative site is above the level of the heart. Under these circumstances, an open venous sinus can entrain air and produce hypoxia, hypercarbia, bronchoconstriction, hypotension, and ultimately cardiovascular collapse. Systemic arterial air embolism is a risk whenever right to left shunts occur and can cause myocardial and cerebral ischemia. Monitoring devices for the detection of air embolism and central venous catheters for aspiration of air often are placed when there is risk for venous air embolism.

   b. **Methods used to monitor for venous air embolism** include Doppler ultrasound, which detects a characteristic "mill wheel" murmur when air is entrained; capnography, which may reveal a sudden decrease in $ETCO_2$; mass spectroscopy; and transesophageal echocardiography.

   c. **If air is detected**, the surgeons are notified so they can eliminate the source of air (close the dural opening, place bone wax, or flood the surgical field), nitrous oxide is discontinued, and air is aspirated from the CVP catheter. If the patient remains stable, the prevention of further air entry may be all that is needed. If hypotension develops, Trendelenburg positioning, fluid administration, and inotropic support may be required.

4. At the end of surgery, the adequacy of the airway and respiration should be verified prior to extubation. Surgical manipulation may have caused damage to the cranial nerves or respiratory center in the brainstem with resulting pharyngeal or respiratory dysfunction. Postoperative infarction, edema, or hematoma formation in the posterior fossa can cause rapid clinical deterioration. Close observation and prompt support including intubation, mechanical ventilation, and circulatory management may be required.

E. **Transsphenoidal resection of the pituitary gland** is performed through either a nasal or labial incision.

1. Although nonfunctioning **pituitary adenomas** are the most common tumor type, some patients have endocrine deficiencies due to hypothalamopituitary compression. Various hyperpituitarism syndromes may accompany functioning adenomas, including Cushing's syndrome, acromegaly (and associated airway difficulties), and amenorrhea-galactorrhea (see Chapter 6).

2. ICP is not a concern as these tumors are usually small and unlikely to compromise intracranial compliance.

3.   Uncontrollable bleeding is rare but can be massive and catastrophic. Frontal craniotomy may ultimately be required to achieve hemostasis.

4.   Monitoring. Access to the patient's head is obstructed by the operating microscope, so the endotracheal tube must be firmly secured. Continuous monitoring of ventilation is essential. Arterial monitors are usually not indicated.

5.   Throat packs will prevent blood from accumulating in the stomach and may reduce postoperative vomiting. The throat pack must be removed prior to extubation.

6.   At the conclusion of surgery, nasal breathing will be obstructed by packs. Patients should be prepared for this preoperatively.

7.   Diabetes insipidus may occur after transsphenoidal hypophysectomy. Treatment with IV fluids or vasopressin may be necessary (see section V.E.7). Some patients may develop postoperative adrenal insufficiency and require corticosteroids postoperatively.

F.   Stereotactic surgery is performed through a burr hole, using a three-dimensional reference grid attached to the head with pins placed in the outer table of the skull. This approach allows localization of a discrete area of brain for biopsy or ablation. In most cases, the procedure can be performed under local anesthesia with IV sedation. Since the stereotactic apparatus precludes full access to the airway, sedation must be given with caution. If general anesthesia is needed after the frame is placed, the technique for securing the airway is selected based on the urgency of airway management and whether the stereotactic frame interferes with the mask airway. Since the frame may also prevent optimal head positioning for mask ventilation and direct laryngoscopy, laryngeal mask airways and equipment for awake intubation, preferably with a fiberoptic laryngoscope, should be available. The stereotactic frame can be removed in an emergency; newer models can be quickly removed to provide access to the airway.

G.   Epilepsy surgery is performed in patients with epilepsy of focal origin who are refractory to medical therapy or intolerant of the side effects of anticonvulsants. The procedures include excision of a seizure focus or interruption of epileptiform pathways. Electrophysiologic mapping of the epileptic focus and other cortical areas (e.g., language, memory, or sensorimotor) often is performed to maximize the resection of the epileptogenic lesion while minimizing the neurologic deficits. Awake craniotomy with IV sedation and local anesthesia of the scalp permits performance of the mapping procedure, which requires patient cooperation. General anesthesia offers the advantages of patient comfort, immobility, a secure airway, and ability to control $Paco_2$ and other variables. The anesthetic technique is chosen on its ability to augment (e.g., enflurane, methohexital, etomidate, or ketamine) or attenuate (e.g., benzodiazepines, barbiturates, or isoflurane) the seizure focus and its compatibility with intraoperative monitoring (see section III). Since there often is an initial increase in seizure activity postoperatively, anticonvulsants should be resumed promptly.

H.   Head trauma. Anesthetic management of the patient with head trauma is complicated by the challenging combination of a "tight" head, full stomach, and potentially unstable cervical spine.

While following the "ABCs" of resuscitation, the anesthesiologist should ascertain the mechanism and extent of injury. **Cervical spinal cord injury** must be suspected and the neck stabilized until cervical vertebral fracture is excluded.

1. Patients who are responsive and ventilating adequately should receive supplemental oxygen and be observed closely for evidence of neurologic deterioration.

2. Comatose patients require immediate endotracheal intubation for airway protection and to avoid hypercarbia and hypoxia, which can exacerbate increases in ICP and contribute to secondary brain injury.

3. Endotracheal intubation should be accomplished rapidly, with blood pressure stability and without coughing or straining.

   a. A rapid sequence induction is usually performed. If a cervical spine fracture has not been excluded, the neck should be immobilized with manual in-line stabilization. The anterior part of the cervical collar may be removed to apply gentle cricoid pressure (excessive pressure may displace a fracture) and obtain sufficient mouth opening. A short-acting induction agent such as propofol, thiopental, or etomidate is used to induce anesthesia, which is immediately followed by an intubating dose of muscle relaxant. Succinylcholine can be used safely unless contraindicated for other reasons (see section II.C and Chapter 12). Nondepolarizing relaxants also may be used. Hyperventilation via mask is started until sufficient muscle relaxation is obtained if its benefits (e.g., ICP reduction or maintenance of adequate Pao_2) are considered to outweigh the risk of aspiration.

   b. Awake intubation (e.g., blind nasal or fiberoptic) may be advocated because of full-stomach considerations, the potential for worsening neck injuries during manipulation of the airway, and anticipation of a difficult airway due to associated facial injuries. Awake approaches are often impractical or unwise in head-injured patients because of lack of cooperation, airway bleeding, and increases in ICP that can be induced by hypertension, coughing, and straining.

   c. Nasal intubation and nasogastric tube placement are relatively contraindicated in the presence of a basilar skull fracture (e.g., CSF rhinorrhea, otorrhea, or Le Fort III facial fracture).

4. Hypertension in head-injured patients may be the body's compensatory effort to maintain cerebral perfusion pressure in the face of increased ICP. **Hypotension can be detrimental** in patients with elevated ICP and when combined with tachycardia should lead one to suspect bleeding from other injuries. Interventions to stop bleeding and restore intravascular volume should precede or proceed in concert with surgical treatment of the head injury.

5. ICP monitoring can be performed if severe or progressive intracranial hypertension is suspected (see section I.C.2).

6. Seizures may accompany direct cerebral injury or signal the expansion of an intracranial hematoma.

7. Brain contusion is the most common type of head injury. Surgery usually is reserved for acute epidural hematomas and acute subdural hematomas. Subdural hematomas are much more common than epidural hematomas and carry a worse prognosis. Intracranial hypertension is frequently seen even after evacuation of hematomas because of severe brain swelling.

8.   Penetrating brain injuries require early debridement of injured tissue and removal of bone fragments and hematoma. Skull fractures may require debridement, cranioplasty, and repair of dural lacerations.

9.   Anesthetic management follows the general rules of maintaining cerebral perfusion pressure and reducing ICP and cerebral edema. Postoperative intubation and ventilatory support frequently are required for ICP control and airway protection in patients with prolonged loss of consciousness or an inadequate gag reflex. Preoperative alteration in the level of consciousness is helpful in predicting the need for postoperative intubation.

10.   Disseminated intravascular coagulation is a frequent complication of an acute head injury, particularly those associated with a subdural hematoma. Frequent monitoring of patient's coagulation status is recommended throughout the procedure.

VII.   Surgery on the spine and spinal cord is undertaken for a variety of conditions, including intervertebral disk diseases, spondylosis, stenosis, neoplasm, scoliosis, and trauma. The physiology of the spinal cord and brain is similar, even though absolute rates of blood flow and metabolism are lower in the spinal cord. Maintaining spinal cord perfusion pressure (which equals MAP minus extrinsic pressure on the cord) and reducing cord compression are clinical management objectives.

A.   The prone position is frequently used. Most patients can be anesthetized on a stretcher and "log rolled" onto the operating room table after endotracheal intubation. Awake intubation should be considered for patients with tenuous neurologic conditions that may be worsened by laryngoscopy/intubation or positioning (e.g., patients with unstable cervical or thoracic spine injuries). Under these circumstances, an abbreviated neurologic examination should be performed after intubation and transfer to ensure that injury has not occurred. The anesthetist should ensure that all pressure points are padded; neck and extremities are in neutral positions; eyes, ears, nose, and genitalia are free from pressure; and all monitors and lines are secured in place and functioning. Special attention should be paid to the endotracheal tube, since it can move or kink in the process of positioning.

B.   Surgery to correct scoliosis can be accompanied by significant blood loss. Various techniques can be used to reduce homologous blood transfusion, including preoperative autologous donation, intraoperative hemodilution, use of intraoperative blood-scavenging techniques, and meticulous patient positioning to prevent increased abdominal and intrathoracic pressures that can increase venous bleeding. Because of concern of neurologic sequelae, we do not employ induced hypotension in this procedure. Scoliosis surgery is accompanied by a 1% to 4% incidence of serious postoperative neurologic complications. Spinal instrumentation and distraction can cause spinal cord ischemia and result in paraplegia. Intraoperative monitoring of spinal cord function (e.g., the wake-up test and/or SSEP monitoring) is used frequently.

    1. **SSEP monitoring** provides continuous evaluation of posterior spinal cord function (see section III.B).

    2. **The wake-up test.** Intraoperatively, after spinal instrumentation and distraction are complete, the presence of neuromuscular function is assured and the patients are awakened briefly and asked to move their legs. If there is no leg movement, the spine distraction is released until movement is observed. Patients should be prepared for this event preoperatively. Wake-up tests can be performed in older children.

    3. **Nitrous oxide–narcotic-relaxant anesthesia** usually is selected because it usually provides a fast, smooth, and pain-free wake-up test and is less likely to interfere with SSEP monitoring than volatile anesthetics. Volatile inhalation agents may be added to a nitrous oxide–narcotic anesthetic to lower blood pressure and provide amnesia but should be maintained at a constant level during the crucial periods of surgery. Of the volatile agents, desflurane causes the least suppression of evoked potentials.

C. **After acute spinal cord injury**, surgery may be required to decompress and stabilize the spinal cord. The primary goal in the initial management of acute spinal cord injury is to prevent secondary damage to the injured cord. This is accomplished by stabilizing the spine and correcting circulatory and ventilatory abnormalities that can exacerbate the primary injury. The presence of cervical cord injury should lead one to suspect associated head, face, or tracheal trauma; thoracic and lumbar spine injuries often are associated with chest or intraabdominal trauma.

    1. **Spinal shock** is characterized by vasodilation and hypotension. If the lesion involves the cardiac accelerator nerves (T-1 to T-4), bradycardia, bradyarrhythmias, atrioventricular block, and cardiac arrest can occur due to unopposed vagal activity. Spinal shock occurs because of functional transection of sympathetic innervation below the level of the injury and may persist for days to weeks. Bradycardia can be treated by atropine. Hypotension can be treated by fluid, vasopressors, or both. A pulmonary artery catheter may be helpful when other injuries are present and volume status is uncertain. Patients with high spinal cord injury may be unusually sensitive to the cardiovascular depressant effects of anesthetics because of an inability to increase sympathetic tone.

    2. **Lesions above C-3 to C-4 necessitate intubation and mechanical ventilatory support** because of loss of innervation to the diaphragm (C-3 to C-5). Lesions below C-5 to C-6 may still cause as much as a 70% reduction in vital capacity and FEV_1 with impaired ventilation and oxygenation.

    3. **Atony of the gastrointestinal tract and urinary bladder** necessitates a nasogastric tube and indwelling urinary catheter, respectively. These patients are also **prone to heat loss** because of inability to vasoconstrict.

    4. **Methylprednisolone** (30 mg/kg IV loading dose, followed by an infusion of 5.4 mg/kg per hour for 23 hours) may improve the functional recovery of patients with acute spinal cord injuries if treatment is begun within the first 3 hours following injury. If corticosteroid therapy is initiated from 3 to 8 hours after injury, the infusion should be extended to 47 hours. Complications of corticosteroid therapy are discussed in Chapter 6.

5. Chronic spinal cord injuries are discussed in Chapter 26.

6. Airway management of patients with cervical spine injury is discussed in section VI.H.

VIII. Neuroradiological procedures are performed in suites often remote from the main operating room.

A. MRI scanning may require sedation or general anesthesia for uncooperative or claustrophobic adults, and smaller children. The space within the scanner is confining and the studies often last at least 1 hour. **The avoidance of all ferromagnetic objects** close to the strong magnetic field of the scanner is mandatory. MRI-compatible carts, airway instruments, oximeters, capnographs, noninvasive blood pressure monitors, and anesthesia machines are available. Additional details are provided in Chapter 31.

B. Interventional radiologic procedures are performed under guidance of conventional fluoroscopy, ultrasound, or CT. Aneurysms, AVM, and tumor devascularization with special balloons, coils, or glue introduced via a femoral arterial sheath and catheter constitute most elective procedures. Stenting of extracranial carotid lesions, intraarterial administration of thrombolytics after ischemic stroke, and papaverine instillation or balloon-dilation to treat recurrent vasospasm after SAH are procedures that frequently require sedation or general anesthesia. Frequent blood pressure monitoring (preferentially via a separate arterial line or via the femoral introducer) and pharmacologic control of blood pressure is required. The use of short-acting muscle relaxants and rapidly reversible anesthetics and analgesics should be considered since the length of the procedure often is not predictable. The radiologist may ask for the patient to awaken for neurologic evaluation as soon as the intervention is completed (see section V). Temperature monitoring and warming devices should be employed to maintain body temperature.

SUGGESTED READING

Cottrell JE, Smith DS, eds. *Anesthesia and neurosurgery*, 4th ed. St. Louis: Mosby, 2001.

Cucchiara RF, Black S, Michenfelder JD, eds. *Clinical neuroanesthesia*, 2nd ed. New York: Churchill Livingstone, 1998.

Drummond JC, Patel PM. *Neurosurgical anesthesia*. In Miller RD, ed. *Anesthesia*. New York: Churchill Livingstone, 2000;1895–1933.

Anesthesia for Head and Neck Surgery

Avinc Lydon and Martin Andrew Acquadro

I. Anesthesia for ophthalmic surgery
A. General considerations
1. **Intraocular pressure** (IOP; normal, 10 to 22 mm Hg; abnormal, more than 25 mm Hg) is determined mainly by the rate of production of aqueous humor in relation to its rate of drainage.

   a. **Factors that may increase IOP** include hypertension, hypercarbia, laryngoscopy and endotracheal intubation, venous congestion, vomiting, coughing, straining, succinylcholine, and ketamine.

   b. **Factors that may decrease IOP** include hyperventilation, hypothermia, central nervous system (CNS) depressants, ganglionic blockers, most volatile and intravenous anesthetics, nondepolarizing muscle relaxants, mannitol, and acetazolamide.

2. **Glaucoma**

   a. **Open-angle glaucoma** usually arises from chronic obstruction of aqueous humor drainage and is characterized by a progressive insidious course that may not be associated with pain.

   b. **Closed-angle glaucoma** results from acute aqueous outflow obstruction caused by a narrowing of the anterior chamber as a result of pupillary dilation or lens edema.

3. **Oculocardiac reflex**

   a. The oculocardiac reflex can be triggered by increased pressure on the globe or by traction on the extrinsic eye muscles, causing cardiac arrhythmias (e.g., bradycardia or asystole). Administration of ocular regional anesthesia may also elicit this response.

   b. The **afferent arc** of this reflex is mediated by the trigeminal (fifth cranial) nerve and the **efferent arc** by the vagus (tenth cranial) nerve. The oculocardiac reflex should be promptly treated by cessation of the stimulus. Atropine (0.010 mg/kg intravenously [IV]) administration minimizes these arrhythmias. Atropine prophylaxis does not always prevent the reflex. If the reflex persists, infiltration of local anesthetic near the extrinsic eye muscles is effective. The reflex fatigues quickly with repeated stimulation.

4. **Commonly used drugs**

   a. **Topical.** Most ophthalmic medications are highly concentrated solutions that are administered topically and may produce systemic effects.

   (1) **Mydriatics**

(a) **Phenylephrine** eye drops may cause hypertension, especially when administered as a 10% solution. For this reason, a 2.5% solution is commonly used.

(b) **Cyclopentolate** may produce CNS toxicity (e.g., confusion, seizures).

(2) **Miotics.** Cholinergic drugs (e.g., pilocarpine 0.25% to 4% solution) may produce bradycardia, salivation, bronchorrhea, and diaphoresis.

(3) **Drugs that decrease IOP**

(a) **Topical β-adrenergic antagonists** (e.g., timolol or betaxolol) may cause bradycardia, hypotension, congestive heart failure, and bronchospasm.

(b) **Anticholinesterases** such as echothiophate depress plasma cholinesterase activity for 2 to 4 weeks, and may prolong the recovery from succinylcholine and mivacurium.

b. **Systemic. Acetazolamide**, a carbonic anhydrase inhibitor, is administered systemically to control aqueous humor secretion. Chronic use can lead to the development of hyponatremia, hypokalemia, and metabolic acidosis.

B. **Anesthetic management**

1. **Preoperative evaluation.** Patients undergoing eye surgery often present with significant concomitant diseases that require careful evaluation (i.e., the formerly premature infant with bronchopulmonary dysplasia for retinal surgery or the elderly patient with cardiovascular disease for cataract excision).

2. **Premedication**

a. Visually impaired patients may be apprehensive about surgery and require constant verbal communication.

b. Ophthalmic procedures performed with ocular regional anesthesia require a calm and cooperative patient.

c. Common premedications do not increase IOP. There is no evidence that premedication with customary doses of parenteral atropine causes increased IOP, even in glaucoma patients.

d. **Benzodiazepines** are effective anxiolytics with amnestic properties. Diazepam, 5 to 10 mg orally or lorazepam, 0.5 to 2 mg orally, 1 hour preoperatively can be used. Alternatively, midazolam, 0.5 to 2 mg IV before the administration of anesthesia is very effective.

e. Opioids, if used, can be given in combination with an antiemetic such as metoclopramide, droperidol, or ondansetron. Use of antidopaminergic agents in elderly patients may be associated with confusion.

3. **The avoidance of coughing, sudden movement, or straining is essential.** Unexpected patient or eye movements during delicate microscopic intraocular surgery can lead to increased IOP, choroidal hemorrhage, expulsion of vitreous material, and loss of vision.

4. **Regional anesthesia (retrobulbar or peribulbar block)**

a. Ophthalmic procedures such as cataract extraction, corneal transplant, and anterior chamber irrigation can be performed using a regional anesthetic and light conscious sedation.

b. Patient cooperation and lack of head motion are important for the success of this technique. Patients who are unable to understand because of impaired hearing, senility, psychosis, or language barrier, or who are unable to maintain a relatively motionless position because of chronic cough, tremor, or arthritis may not be candidates for regional anesthesia for delicate eye surgery.

c.   The advantages of regional anesthesia include a lower incidence of coughing, straining, and emesis. The technique is useful for ambulatory patients and provides postoperative analgesia.

d.   **Intravenous sedation** may be used perioperatively. Midazolam (0.25 to 1 mg IV), fentanyl (10 to 50 µg IV), remifentanil (0.1 to 0.5 µg/kg IV), or propofol (5 to 20 mg IV) can be administered just before the regional injection. Patients should be monitored during regional block placement and receive supplemental oxygen if indicated.

e.   **Technique.** Intraocular surgery requires adequate sensory and motor block of the eye and often the eyelids as well. Anesthesia of the eye is accomplished by injecting local anesthetic into either the retrobulbar or peribulbar space, facilitating neural blockade of cranial nerves II through VI. The **retrobulbar block** is achieved by injecting 4 to 6 mL of a 50:50 mixture of 2% lidocaine and 0.75% bupivacaine (with 1:200,000 to 1:400,000 epinephrine) within the muscle cone formed by the four recti muscles and the two oblique muscles. With the eye in neutral position, a 23- or 25-gauge needle is inserted through the lower lid or conjunctiva at the level of the inferior orbital rim in the inferotemporal quadrant. The needle is first advanced slightly inferiorly and temporally approximately 1.5 cm; once past the equator of the eye, the needle is then directed superiorly and nasally towards the apex of the orbit to a depth of approximately 3.5 cm, while feeling for a "pop" as the needle penetrates through the muscle cone. With the **peribulbar block**, there is no attempt made to enter the muscle cone. The needle is advanced along the inferior orbital floor to a depth of approximately 2.5 cm. Eight to 10 mL of local anesthetic is required, and hyaluronidase (5 U/mL) frequently is added to help facilitate spread through the muscle cone. Careful aspiration before injection is required for both blocks, followed by gentle massage or orbital compression to decrease IOP and promote spread of the anesthetic. If desired, the facial nerve can also be blocked by infiltration of 2 to 4 mL of additional local anesthetic along the inferior and superior orbital rim to help prevent active squeezing. The retrobulbar block provides faster, more reliable anesthesia and akinesia but has a higher complication rate than the peribulbar block.

f.   **Complications** are infrequent but include direct optic nerve trauma, retrobulbar hemorrhage, transient globe compression with increased IOP, globe perforation, and stimulation of the oculocardiac reflex. Intravascular injection may cause seizures or myocardial depression. Rarely, the local anesthetic may dissect proximally along the neural sheath of the optic nerve and cause temporary (15 minutes) loss of consciousness without seizures. The patient may become apneic briefly; treatment is supportive.

g. During the procedure, **fresh air** at a flow rate of 10 to 15 L per minute is provided for the patient under the drapes using a large face mask. This helps to remove exhaled carbon dioxide and helps offset the sense of suffocation or claustrophobia some patients may experience. **Oxygen** may be used if indicated but the surgeon should be notified not to use electrocautery while oxygen is flowing. During supplementation of intravenous sedation the patient should not become unresponsive; undue restlessness may be a sign of oversedation in the elderly. End-tidal carbon dioxide monitoring through the face mask can be used or a precordial stethoscope can be applied since observation of ventilation can be obscured by drapes.

5. General anesthesia

a. The eye is a very sensitive, highly innervated organ. Eye surgery requires sufficient depth of general anesthesia to prevent eye motion, coughing, straining, or hypertension. General anesthesia using an inhalation agent, supplemented by a nondepolarizing muscle relaxant, is usually satisfactory. Coughing or straining with an open eye can lead to catastrophic choroidal hemorrhage.

b. The lack of access to the airway during the procedure necessitates endotracheal intubation or a laryngeal mask airway. If intubation is planned, intravenous lidocaine (1.0 to 1.5 mg/kg) or 4% lidocaine spray to the larynx and trachea may help to prevent straining. The endotracheal tube should be firmly supported and taped in place to prevent disconnection, extubation, and stimulation of a cough reflex by motion.

c. Ketamine can cause blepharospasm, nystagmus, increased arterial pressure, and vomiting, and may increase IOP. For these reasons, ketamine usually is a poor choice for most ophthalmic surgery. Low doses of ketamine, however, do not increase IOP and may be useful as a supplement to IV sedation for retrobulbar or peribulbar block.

d. Smooth emergence and extubation are particularly desirable following ophthalmic surgery. This may be facilitated by thorough posterior pharyngeal suctioning while the patient is still deeply anesthetized, administration of an opioid to reduce the cough reflex, and intravenous lidocaine (1 to 1.5 mg/kg) 5 minutes before planned extubation. The patient may then be extubated awake with intact airway reflexes. Deep extubation is also an option but does not guarantee a smooth emergence.

C. Specific procedures

1. Open-eye injury. Penetrating eye trauma is a surgical emergency, frequently occurring in patients who have recently eaten. It requires a carefully conducted anesthetic designed to prevent aspiration and favorably affect IOP (see section I.A.1). A sudden increase in IOP can result in extrusion of ocular contents and cause permanent vision loss. Trauma to the eye and orbit, length and complexity of the procedure, and a crying patient with a full stomach usually mandates a general endotracheal anesthetic. Orbital pressure from face masks should avoided.

   a. **Succinylcholine** administered during a rapid sequence induction causes an increase in IOP of approximately 10 mm Hg for 5 minutes. Pretreatment with nondepolarizing muscle relaxants may attenuate but does not ablate this response. Nevertheless, succinylcholine often is the drug of choice to quickly establish adequate intubating conditions in the eye surgery patient with a full stomach. Alternatively, nondepolarizing muscle relaxants can be used, but adequate intubating conditions may not be achieved for 60 to 90 seconds.

   b. An adequate depth of anesthesia and degree of neuromuscular blockade must be ensured prior to laryngoscopy and intubation to minimize increases in IOP (which may rise to 40 to 50 mm Hg) secondary to straining, coughing, and bucking.

   c. In children, if an IV cannot be placed, an inhalation induction using cricoid pressure and nonirritating volatile anesthetics (nitrous oxide, sevoflurane, or halothane) may be necessary.

2. **Strabismus repair** is a common pediatric operation whereby the lengths of the extraocular muscles are altered by recession or resection.

   a. **Succinylcholine administration** can interfere with the forced duction test for up to 20 minutes; therefore, laryngoscopy and intubation are facilitated by a nondepolarizing muscle relaxant or adequate inhalation anesthesia.

   b. Surgical manipulation frequently elicits **the oculocardiac reflex** (see section I.A.3).

   c. **Postoperative nausea and vomiting** are very common (80% incidence in untreated patients). Metoclopramide (0.1 to 0.15 mg/kg IV), droperidol (25 to 30 µg/kg IV), or ondansetron (0.15 mg/kg IV) often is administered approximately 30 minutes before conclusion of surgery, and the stomach is decompressed with an orogastric tube. Other strategies to decrease the incidence of postoperative vomiting include the omission of nitrous oxide and the continuous use of propofol.

   d. Patients with musculoskeletal abnormalities may be at increased risk for **malignant hyperthermia**. A thorough family history should be obtained and heart rate, end-tidal carbon dioxide, ventilatory parameters, and temperature should be carefully monitored for early detection of malignant hyperthermia.

3. **Retinal surgery for detachment and vitreous hemorrhage** often is performed on premature infants with retinopathy of prematurity. Concomitant medical problems are often present; meticulous attention to airway management, fluid status, normothermia, and postoperative transport is crucial (see Chapters 6, 28, and 33). Patients with diabetes or sickle cell anemia also may require retinal surgery.

   a. **Regional anesthesia** is suitable for short procedures (less than 2 hours) in cooperative patients, although unexpected movement during the delicate retinal repair may result in vision loss. If **general anesthesia** is administered, deep inhalational anesthesia, intravenous anesthesia with an opioid and/or propofol, use of a remifentanil infusion or a balanced technique with an adequate degree of neuromuscular blockade is recommended. Postoperative coughing, straining, and vomiting should be prevented (see section I.C.2).

b. An **intravitreal gas bubble** containing an inert, high-molecular-weight, low-diffusivity gas such as SF_6, C_3F_8, or C_4F_8, or air, may be injected at the conclusion of surgery to reduce intravitreal bleeding. Nitrous oxide should be discontinued at least 20 minutes prior to bubble injection. The presence of nitrous oxide will rapidly expand the bubble and increase IOP; cessation of nitrous oxide at the end of the procedure shrinks the bubble, with resulting loss of its mechanical advantage. Since these gas bubbles remain for varying periods of time, readministration of nitrous oxide should be avoided for 5 days following an air injection, 10 days following SF_6 injection, and 60 days following C_3F_8 injection.

II. Anesthesia for otorhinolaryngologic procedures
A. General considerations
1. Airway. For many otorhinolaryngologic (ORL) surgical procedures, the airway must be shared with the surgeon. Pathology, scarring from previous surgery or irradiation, congenital deformities, trauma, or manipulation can produce chronic or acute airway obstruction, bleeding, and a potentially difficult airway. Preoperative discussion with the surgeon and analysis of previous anesthetic records regarding perioperative airway management, endotracheal tube size and position, patient positioning, and use of nitrous oxide and muscle relaxants is essential. The patient may require an awake examination of the airway under sedation and topical anesthesia or an awake fiberoptic intubation before induction of general anesthesia.

2. Patients presenting for ORL surgery may have a history of heavy smoking, alcohol abuse, obstructive sleep apnea, and chronic upper respiratory tract infections. Preoperative laboratory testing, imaging, and evaluation of cardiac, hepatic, and pulmonary function may be necessary.

3. In addition to standard monitors, major procedures may require monitoring of intraarterial blood pressure and urine output.

4. Extubation following any upper airway surgery requires careful planning. Throat packs are removed, the pharynx is suctioned, the patient is oxygenated, and extubation performed when full protective laryngeal reflexes return. Excessive upper airway bleeding, edema, or pathology may preclude extubation in the operating room.

B. Ear surgery
1. Preoperative considerations

a. Ear surgery often involves dissecting and preserving the **facial (cranial nerve VII) nerve.**

b. The **middle ear** communicates with the oropharynx via the Eustachian tube. If Eustachian tube patency is compromised by trauma, edema, inflammation, or congenital deformity, normal venting of middle ear pressure cannot occur. In this situation, a high concentration of nitrous oxide can increase middle ear pressure to 300 to 400 mm Hg in 30 minutes. Conversely, acute cessation of nitrous oxide can result in rapid resorption and a net negative pressure in the middle ear. These changes may result in altered middle ear anatomy, tympanic membrane rupture, disarticulation of artificial stapes, disruption of surgical grafts, and postoperative nausea and vomiting.

    c. Positioning. During surgery, the patient's head often is elevated and turned to the side. Extremes of head position should be assessed preoperatively to determine limits of range of motion, especially in patients with arthritis or cerebrovascular disease. Eyes should be taped closed and padded.

2. Anesthesia is induced with a hypnotic and short-acting muscle relaxant or by inhalation and usually maintained with a volatile anesthetic. The use of nitrous oxide should be discussed with the surgeon; it should be discontinued at least 30 minutes prior to placement of a tympanic membrane graft.

    a. Delicate microsurgery of the ear requires adequate hemostasis. Volatile anesthetics and α- or β-adrenergic blocking agents work well to induce mean arterial pressures of 60 to 70 mm Hg. Elevation of the head to approximately 15 degrees to decrease venous congestion and local application of epinephrine usually improve operating conditions.

    b. Antiemetics should be given, since postoperative vomiting is very common with ear surgery (see section I.C.2).

C. Nasal surgery

1. Anesthetic technique. Nasal surgery can be performed with local or general anesthesia. With either technique, the surgeon may initially apply 4% cocaine to the nasal mucosa, followed by injection of 1% to 2% lidocaine with 1:100,000 to 1:200,000 epinephrine for hemostasis. These agents may cause tachycardia, hypertension, and arrhythmias, especially in the presence of halothane. In a healthy adult, the cocaine dose should not exceed 1.5 mg/kg. Smaller doses should be used when administered with epinephrine, in the presence of halothane, or in patients with cardiovascular disease. General anesthesia may be needed immobility, airway protections, or to provide amnesia.

2. Following **nasal cosmetic surgery**, the nose is unstable and application of a face mask is undesirable. Smooth emergence and extubation are important to decrease postoperative bleeding, and to avoid laryngospasm and the need for positive pressure ventilation by mask.

3. Blood loss during nasal surgery may be substantial and difficult to estimate. A throat pack may help decrease postoperative nausea and vomiting by preventing passage of blood into the stomach. The throat pack must always be removed prior to extubation. An orogastric tube may be placed to evacuate the stomach of any swallowed blood.

4. Patients with **severe epistaxis** presenting for internal maxillary artery ligation or embolization often are anxious, tired, hypertensive, tachycardic, and hypovolemic. These patients need reassurance, hydration, and prompt care. They are assumed to have a full stomach and induction of anesthesia and endotracheal intubation should be planned accordingly. Hypertension should be controlled to reduce blood loss. Posterior nasal packing, while helpful, can cause edema and hypoventilation. Since the extent of blood loss is difficult to assess, adequate intravenous access (14- or 16-gauge IV) and blood for transfusion should be available. Removal of the posterior packing can be associated with substantial blood loss.

D.   Upper airway surgery

1.   Tonsillectomy and adenoidectomy

a.   Preoperative evaluation should seek a history of bleeding disorders, obstructive sleep apnea, and loose teeth. Coagulation studies are performed. Many of these patients have chronic or recurrent upper respiratory tract infections; an acute infection would necessitate postponing the procedure. Obstructive sleep apnea patients tend to be obese, and may be difficult to ventilate and intubate.

b.   Most children receive an inhalation induction, followed by placement of an appropriately large IV. A technique consisting of a volatile agent, and an opioid (e.g., morphine 0.1 mg/kg IV) usually is preferred. Glycopyrrolate (5 to 10 μg/kg IV) sometimes is administered to decrease secretions, and antiemetics should be considered. Muscle relaxation facilitates intubation, but is not mandatory. Inadvertent endotracheal tube obstruction, disconnection, or dislodgment can occur during head and mouth gag manipulation.

c.   At the end of surgery, an orogastric tube should be placed to empty the stomach of any swallowed blood and the pharynx suctioned thoroughly. Extubation may be performed under deep anesthesia or when the patient is awake with intact airway reflexes. Coughing on the endotracheal tube may be attenuated by the administration of lidocaine (1 to 1.5 mg/kg IV) 5 minutes before planned extubation. The use of oropharyngeal airways following surgery should be avoided to prevent surgical wound disruption and bleeding. Nasal airways are a useful alternative.

d.   After extubation, patients are placed on their side and in slight Trendelenburg position, administered 100% oxygen, and observed for unobstructed ventilation. In the postanesthesia care unit (PACU), patients are given humidified oxygen by mask, monitored according to recovery room protocol, and checked for a dry pharynx before discharge.

2.   Bleeding tonsil

a.   Rebleeding following a pediatric tonsillectomy usually occurs within 24 hours after surgery, but may be delayed for 5 to 10 days. Hematemesis, tachycardia, frequent swallowing, pallor, and airway obstruction may be seen. The extent of blood loss is often underestimated because blood is swallowed.

b. The induction of anesthesia in a bleeding, hypovolemic child can result in severe hypotension or cardiac arrest. Adequate IV access is necessary and the patient should be adequately resuscitated (with blood products if necessary) before reoperation. Hematocrit, coagulation studies, and availability of blood products should be ascertained. Doses of anesthetic agents may need to be reduced in the setting of hypovolemia.

c. Since the stomach is full of blood, a **rapid-sequence induction** with cricoid pressure should be performed. Two working suctions and an additional styletted endotracheal tube one size smaller than anticipated should be available. The surgeon should be present.

3. A tonsillar or parapharyngeal abscess may present with trismus, dysphagia, and a distorted, compromised airway. The surgeon may be able to decompress the abscess with needle aspiration before induction of anesthesia. If appropriate, an awake fiberoptic intubation may be performed. Anesthetic management and extubation procedures are similar to those for tonsillectomy (see section II.D.1).

4. Direct laryngoscopy is indicated for diagnostic (biopsy) or therapeutic (vocal cord polyp removal) purposes, and may involve potentially compromised airways. Evaluation of imaging studies (magnetic resonance imaging or computed tomography) and laboratory studies (pulmonary flow-volume loops) may help identify airway abnormalities and potential perioperative problems. Many patients have a history of smoking and cardiopulmonary disease.

a. Anesthetic management is described in Chapter 21, section IV.

b. Postoperative airway edema may develop. If anticipated, dexamethasone, 4 to 8 mg IV, may be given. Additional treatment includes head elevation, humidified oxygen by mask, and nebulized epinephrine. Occasionally, cessation of nebulized epinephrine is associated with the return of airway edema.

5. Laser (light amplification by stimulated emission of radiation) produces a high-energy, high-density beam of coherent light that generates focused heat on contact with tissue. The emission media used to produce the monochromatic light determines the wavelength.

a. Short wavelength (1 μm) laser (argon gas, ruby, yttrium aluminum garnet [YAG]) emissions in the red–green visible part of the electromagnetic spectrum are poorly absorbed by water but well absorbed by pigmented tissues such as the retina and blood vessels.

b. Infrared (10 μm) carbon dioxide laser emissions are well absorbed by water and superficial surface cells, and commonly are used to treat laryngeal lesions. They cannot be transmitted through fiberoptics.

c. Eyes must be protected from the laser beam. Operating room personnel must wear appropriate safety goggles (green-tinted for argon, amber for YAG, and clear for carbon dioxide) and the patient's eyes should be taped closed and covered with wet gauze.

d. The most serious complication of laser airway surgery is fire. The likelihood of fire depends on the gas environment of the airway, the energy level of the laser, the manner in which the laser is used, the presence of moisture, and the type of endotracheal tube. Oxygen and nitrous oxide both support combustion. A safe gas mixture during laser upper airway surgery is oxygen/air or oxygen/helium to achieve an oxygen concentration of 25% to 30%.

e. Safe laser use. Lasers should be used intermittently, in the noncontinuous mode, and at moderate power (10 to 15 watts). Surgeons should not use the laser as a cautery and should share responsibility for fire prevention by limiting the energy input, allowing time for heat dispersal, packing aside nontarget tissue and endotracheal tube cuffs with moist gauze, and maintaining moisture (as a heat sink) in the field.

f. Airway options during laser surgery. Specially designed, fire-resistant, impregnated or shielded endotracheal tubes (e.g., Xomed-Treace Laser-Shield II endotracheal tube) are used and the cuff filled with saline. The use of a jet-Venturi technique eliminates the need for an endotracheal tube, but dry tissue can still spark and inflame, causing a blowtorch effect with jet oxygen. Jet ventilation should be accomplished with air, not oxygen, during laser use.

g. If an airway fire occurs, stop ventilation and immediately disconnect the endotracheal tube from the breathing circuit, remove the tube, pour saline in the pharynx to absorb the heat, suction, and reintubate with a new endotracheal tube. While ventilating with 100% oxygen, the airway is examined by bronchoscopy. **Complications** include airway edema, inhalation injury, tracheal and laryngeal granulation tissue formation, and airway stenosis.

h. The **anesthetic technique** for laser surgery is similar to that described for endoscopy (see Chapter 21). Goals include adequate surgical exposure, fire prevention, laryngeal and vocal cord immobility, and return of protective airway reflexes prior to extubation. Endotracheal intubation, jet ventilation, or intermittent mask/endotracheal tube ventilation may be used; regardless of the technique a mixture of oxygen/air is used (less than 30% oxygen). Since airway edema may occur, the patient is given humidified oxygen postoperatively and observed closely in the PACU. Corticosteroids or aerosolized epinephrine may be necessary.

III. Anesthesia for head and neck procedures

  A. **The primary anesthetic concern** during head and neck surgery is establishing and maintaining a secure airway.

    1. An **armored endotracheal tube** (e.g., Tovell) may be necessary to prevent kinking.

    2. An **elective tracheostomy** under local anesthesia may be performed before induction of general anesthesia for some extensive procedures or those with the potential for acute airway obstruction.

    3. Vocal cord paralysis. Injury to one recurrent laryngeal nerve may cause unilateral vocal cord paralysis, a benign condition limited to hoarseness and a weak voice. Bilateral vocal cord paralysis, however, usually leads to increasing upper airway obstruction and stridor, and the patient will be unable to phonate. Obstruction may be relieved by positive pressure ventilation while preparations are being made for reintubation.

    4. Bleeding at the operative site following thyroid or parathyroid surgery may compress the trachea and cause airway obstruction. Opening the wound by placing a sterile hemostat through the incision allows egress of trapped blood. If this maneuver fails, the obstruction may be secondary to acute lymphedema and necessitate immediate reintubation.

    5. Teflon injection of the vocal cords must be performed during awake laryngoscopy in order to continuously assess voice quality. The procedure should be performed with adequate local anesthesia and light sedation.

B. **Radical neck dissection**

1. **Patient condition.** These patients are often elderly, chronically debilitated, malnourished, and often have a history of tobacco and alcohol use. The severity of cardiac, pulmonary, and hepatic disease will determine the extent of preoperative evaluation and choice of perioperative monitoring. Radical neck dissection in previously irradiated patients may be associated with large blood loss.

2. **Anesthetic technique.** A volatile anesthetic without a muscle relaxant is preferred to allow the surgeon to identify nerves with a nerve stimulator. A 15- to 30-degree head up-tilt and mild hypotension (mean arterial pressure 60 to 70 mm Hg), facilitated by a volatile anesthetic, vasodilators, or β-adrenergic antagonists, may help reduce blood loss.

3. During dissection, traction or pressure on the carotid sinus can cause **arrhythmias** such as bradycardia or asystole. Treatment is immediate cessation of the stimulus. If necessary, the surgeon can infiltrate local anesthetic near the sinus. Atropine (0.07 mg/kg IV) or glycopyrrolate (0.01 mg/kg) can be given if arrhythmias persist.

4. The patient is at risk for pneumothorax and venous air embolism during surgical dissection.

5. If airway compromise is anticipated postoperatively, the endotracheal tube is left in place or elective tracheostomy is performed.

6. Avoidance of hypothermia and minimizing the use of vasoconstrictors are desirable during reconstructive flap transfer surgery.

C. **Dentistry and oral and maxillofacial surgery**

1. Patients requiring general anesthesia for dentistry may be young children, adults with severe phobias, or mentally or physically impaired, and require adequate sedation. Oral midazolam (0.5 to 1.0 mg/kg) or rectal methohexital (25 mg/kg as a 10% solution) is suitable for children less than five years old. Intramuscular ketamine (0.3 to 0.5 mg/kg) may be necessary for the agitated or uncooperative patient.

2. **Nasal intubation** is usually required; care must be taken not to damage the turbinates or adenoids. Prior administration of topical phenylephrine to the nasal mucosa, use of a lubricant, and warming/softening the endotracheal tube before intubation may help to reduce epistaxis. The endotracheal tube should be securely taped, pressure on the nose is avoided, and the eyes are protected and padded.

3. Patients with maxillo-mandibular skeletal anomalies, temporomandibular pathology, facial fractures, intermaxillary fixation, or trismus may require fiberoptic intubation.

4. **Hypotensive anesthesia** (mean arterial pressure 60 to 70 mm Hg) for orthognathic surgery may reduce blood loss and can be facilitated by volatile anesthetics, α- and β-adrenergic blockers, nitroprusside, and head elevation. The overall medical condition of the patient may preclude use of induced hypotension.

5. If intermaxillary fixation with wires is present, the endotra-

cheal tube is removed only when the patient is awake, edema has subsided, and bleeding is controlled. Administration of an antiemetic and decompression of the stomach with a nasogastric tube before extubation are recommended. Wire cutters are kept at the bedside should emergent access to the mouth be necessary.

SUGGESTED READING

Brimacombe J, Berry A. The laryngeal mask airway for dental surgery—a review. *Aust Dent J* 1995;40:10–14.

Ferrari LR, Vassallo SA. Anesthesia for otorhinolaryngology procedures and anesthesia for ophthalmology. Coté CJ, Todres ID, Ryan JF, Goudzousian N, eds. *A practice of anesthesia for infants and children*, 3rd ed. Philadelphia: WB Saunders, 2001:461–492.

Donlon JV Jr. Anesthesia for eye, ear, nose, and throat surgery. In: Miller RD, ed. *Anesthesia*, 5th ed. New York: Churchill Livingstone, 2000: 2173–2198.

McGoldrick KE, ed. *Anesthesia for ophthalmic and otolaryngologic surgery*. Philadelphia: WB Saunders, 1992.

Rampil IJ. Anesthesia for laser surgery. In: Miller RD, ed. *Anesthesia*, 5th ed. New York: Churchill Livingstone, 2000:2199–2212.

Supkis DE, Dougherty TB, Nguyen DT, et al. Anesthetic management of the patient undergoing head and neck cancer surgery. *Int Anesthesiol Clin* 1998;36:21–29.

Troll GF. Regional ophthalmic anesthesia: safe techniques and avoidance of complications. *J Clin Anesth* 1995;7:163–172.

26

Anesthesia for the Elderly and for Urologic Surgery

Harvey C. Shew and William Kimball

I. **Anesthesia for elderly patients.** Individuals over age 65 years comprise 12% of the population in the United States, but undergo about a third of all surgeries. These proportions will increase over the next few decades. Independent of overt disease, elderly persons have many physiologic and pharmacologic alterations.
   A. **Physiologic changes of aging**
      1. **Cardiovascular**
         a. **Arteries stiffen with age**, leading to faster propagation and reflection of the pulse pressure waveform. The reflected waveform augments the native pressure seen at the aortic root. With increasing age, the reflected energy arrives progressively earlier in the cardiac cycle, shifting from early diastole to late systole. Thus, aging causes decreased diastolic and increased systolic pressure (and pulse pressure), leading to ventricular thickening and prolonged ejection.
         b. **Slower myocardial relaxation and ventricular hypertrophy** lead to late diastolic filling and diastolic dysfunction. Atrial contraction is important to maintain late filling.
         c. **Reduced venous capacitance** decreases the "vascular reserve volume" available to buffer hemorrhage.
         d. **Reduced baroreceptor reflexes** result from increased sympathetic tone, decreased parasympathetic tone, decreased baroreceptor sensitivity, and decreased responsiveness to β-adrenergic stimulation. Thus, hypotension occurs quite frequently from changes in volume, position, anesthetic depth, or regional anesthetic-induced sympathetic blockade.
         e. **Maximal heart rate decreases with age while stroke volume remains constant**, but end-diastolic volume increases and ejection fraction decreases.
         f. **Maximal oxygen consumption decreases** because of reductions in arteriovenous oxygen tension difference and cardiac output.
      2. **Respiratory**
         a. **Parenchymal changes**: Approximately 30% of alveolar wall tissue is lost between ages 20 and 80, diminishing elastic recoil and parenchymal traction that maintain airway patency. This produces:
            (1) **Increased residual volume, closing volume, and functional residual capacity**; decreased vital capacity and forced expiratory volume in 1 second (FEV_1).
            (2) **Progressive mismatching of ventilation to perfusion**, with an age-dependent decrease in arterial oxygen tension.

(3) **Increased physiologic dead space** and reduced diffusing capacity.

b. Chest wall changes: Multiple factors lead to a stiffer chest wall, while respiratory muscle mass decreases.

c. Depressed ventilatory response to hypoxia and hypercarbia.

d. Decreased protective airway reflexes increase aspiration risk.

3. **Renal**

a. Serum creatinine remains stable with advancing age because age-associated decreases of creatinine clearance are offset by reduced creatinine production from skeletal muscle. A normal creatinine level in the elderly should not be interpreted as an absence of renal impairment. For example, a healthy 80-year-old patient is expected to have half the creatinine clearance of a 20-year-old patient, although they may have similar serum creatinine levels.

b. Progressive atrophy of renal parenchyma and sclerosis of vascular structures lead to **diminished renal blood flow and glomerular filtration rate**.

c. Reduced ability to correct alterations in electrolyte concentrations, intravascular volume, and free water.

d. Reduced glomerular filtration rate leads to delayed renal drug excretion.

4. **Central nervous system**

a. Progressive loss of large neurons and decreased neurotransmitter activity contribute to **decreased anesthetic requirements** for all agents.

b. Cerebral autoregulatory responses to blood pressure, CO_2, and O_2 are maintained.

5. **Hepatic**

a. Liver mass decreases significantly with proportional reductions in both splanchnic and hepatic blood flows, reducing hepatic drug clearance.

b. Activity of some cytochrome P-450 isoforms decreases with aging.

c. Phase 1 (oxidation and reduction) and phase 2 (conjugation) reactions may be depressed with aging.

6. **Body composition and thermoregulation**

a. Basal metabolism and heat production decrease because of skeletal muscle atrophy and variable replacement with adipose tissue.

b. The propensity for hypothermia increases because of blunted central thermoregulation and body compositional changes.

c. Decreases in muscle mass and total body water, coupled with increases in body fat, reduce the volume of distribution of water-soluble drugs and increase it for lipid-soluble drugs.

B. Pharmacologic implications of aging

1. The binding site for most lipophilic basic drugs, alpha$_1$-acid glycoprotein, increases in concentration with age.

2. Adverse drug reactions increase in frequency and severity in the elderly.

3. Drug sensitivity varies with type of drug. Responses to specific drugs are difficult to predict and may vary widely in the

elderly. For example, catecholamines require higher doses for equivalent effects, and benzodiazepines exert greater effects in the elderly.

4. The minimum alveolar concentration for inhalational anesthetics decreases with age, with up to a 30% reduction between the ages of 20 and 70 years. Requirements for all intravenous anesthetic agents are also decreased.

C. Anesthetic considerations in the elderly

1. Age-related coexisting disease is a major predictor for perioperative mortality and serious morbidity. Age alone is a minor predictor.

2. Major risk factors for serious adverse perioperative events in the elderly are emergency surgery, operative site within a major body cavity or vascular surgery, and American Society of Anesthesiologists physical status.

3. No significant difference in perioperative complications can be attributed to any specific anesthetic agent or to regional versus general anesthesia.

4. In general, the elderly have reduced functional reserves of all organ systems, which diminishes the therapeutic index of anesthetic interventions. This therapeutic diminution is highly variable and unpredictable, due to such factors as environmental effects, physical deconditioning, and undiagnosed diseases. These diminished functional reserves may be manifest only under severe stress, such as that of surgery. Thus, vigilance and preparation for contingencies are essential in the conduct of anesthesia for the elderly.

II. Anesthesia for specific urologic procedures

A. Ureteroscopy and **cystoscopy** are performed to evaluate the upper (ureter, kidney) and lower (bladder, prostate, urethra) urinary tracts and to diagnose and treat a variety conditions such as hematuria, pyuria, calculi, trauma, obstruction, and cancer.

1. Irrigation solutions are used to distend the urologic system, to couple surgical energy sources to targets, and to remove blood, tissue or stones from the surgeon's view. Irrigation solutions include:

   a. Electrolyte solutions, such as normal saline or lactated Ringer's solution, are inexpensive and well tolerated if absorbed in large volume, but their high degree of ionization disperses electrocautery current, excessively slowing surgery.

   b. Distilled water has the best visibility, is nonconductive, and is inexpensive. Since absorbing large quantities can lead to hyponatremia, water intoxication, and hemolysis, it is limited to procedures with minimal bleeding (e.g., cystoscopy and bladder tumor resections).

   c. Near isosmotic, nonelectrolyte solutions, such as **1.5% glycine** or **Cytal** (0.54% mannitol and 2.7% sorbitol), are relatively inexpensive, have good visibility, and are nonconductive.

      (1) Because they are nearly isosmotic with blood, hemolysis is minimal even if large volumes are absorbed.

      (2) Massive absorption causes dilutional hyponatremia, and may cause delayed hyposmolality. The resulting hyposmolality is less severe than that occurring with massive absorption of distilled water.

(3) **Glycine toxicity** is manifest as nausea, vomiting, visual disturbances, and transient blindness.

(4) Glycine is hepatically metabolized, and thus has the potential for causing high serum-ammonia levels, which in turn may be partly responsible for central nervous system toxicity.

2. **Anesthesia**

   a. Bladder and ureteral distention are usually quite painful and thus require regional or general anesthesia. Women often tolerate minor cystoscopic procedures under local anesthesia alone.

   b. If regional anesthesia is utilized, a T-6 vertebral level is required for upper tract instrumentation, whereas a T-10 level is adequate for lower tract surgery.

B. Transurethral resection of the prostate (TURP) is performed in men, typically over 60 years of age, to treat urinary obstruction because of benign prostatic hypertrophy. This procedure uses a modified cystoscope (resectoscope) with a wire loop connected to an electrocautery unit for resection of tissue and coagulation of bleeding vessels.

1. During surgery, large prostatic venous sinuses are opened, which absorb the irrigant. Excessive absorption can cause the TURP syndrome, described below. The quantity of fluid absorbed depends on the following factors:

   a. **Irrigant hydrostatic pressure**, proportional to the relative height of the irrigant above the patient (should be less than 70 cm).

   b. **Surgical technique,** duration of surgery, irrigation flow rate, and cystoscope size.

   c. Number and size of **venous sinuses** opened.

   d. **Peripheral venous pressure** (about 10 mm Hg in prostate).

2. **Anesthesia**

   a. If general anesthesia is used, anesthetic depth should be sufficient to prevent coughing or patient movement, which could cause increased bleeding or bladder/prostatic capsule perforation.

   b. Advantages of regional anesthesia may include:

      (1) An atonic bladder (increased capacity and improved surgical visualization).

      (2) Earlier detection of the TURP syndrome (via changed mentation of awake patients).

      (3) Elimination of bladder spasms (more rapid hemostasis postoperatively).

3. **Complications**

   a. **TURP syndrome** is a collection of symptoms caused by excessive irrigant absorption, leading to dilutional hyponatremia, with or without hypoosmolality. Hypervolemia initially occurs with fluid absorption, followed by rapid redistribution of the irrigant to the interstitium.

      (1) TURP syndrome may occur early (direct intravascular absorption) or several hours later (resorption of periprostatic fluid collections from the interstitium).

(**2**) Conscious patients may experience headache, dizziness, confusion, dyspnea, agitation, nausea, or visual disturbances. These may progress to stupor, coma, seizures, and cardiovascular collapse.

(**3**) Signs accompanying general anesthesia are less specific: an unexplained rise or fall in blood pressure, refractory bradycardia, and ECG changes such as widened QRS complex, ST segment elevations, and ventricular tachycardia or fibrillation.

(**4**) Treatment includes:

(**a**) Notifying the surgeon and discontinuing surgery as soon as possible.

(**b**) Diuresis.

(**c**) Administering sodium (normal saline if [Na$^+$] greater than 120 mmol/L, or possibly 3% saline if [Na$^+$] less than 120 mmol/L). Frequent sodium measurements should guide therapy.

b. **Perforation of bladder or urethra**

(**1**) **Extraperitoneal perforation** is more common and manifests as suprapubic fullness, abdominal spasm, or pain in the suprapubic, inguinal, or periumbilical region(s).

(**2**) **Intraperitoneal perforation** presents as upper abdominal pain or referred pain from the diaphragm to the shoulder, hypertension, tachycardia, and abdominal distention, followed by hypotension and cardiovascular collapse.

c. **Hypothermia** can occur when using cool irrigant.

d. **Bacteremia or septicemia**, due to absorption of bacteria through prostatic venous sinuses, is especially common with indwelling urinary catheters or with subclinical or partially treated prostatitis.

e. **Blood loss and coagulopathy**. Assessing blood loss is extremely difficult during TURP because of massive dilution of shed blood by the irrigant.

(**1**) Continuous postoperative bleeding may result from dilutional thrombocytopenia, disseminated intravascular coagulation, or the release of urokinase (plentiful in prostate).

(**2**) Concomitant platelet dysfunction may exist in patients with renal dysfunction.

(**3**) Hemodynamic responses to blood loss may be masked by hypervolemia from irrigant absorption.

f. **Myocardial infarction and pulmonary edema** are complications of TURP, and can be precipitated by volume overload from irrigant absorption.

C. **Open prostatic procedures** are performed for resection of large prostatic masses (greater than 60 g) or tumors. Laparoscopic approaches may be used at some centers.

1. **Anesthetic considerations**

a. May be performed under regional or general anesthesia depending on surgical positioning. Large-bore intravenous (IV) access is required.

b. **Diagnostic dyes** may be used during the procedure.

(**1**) **Methylene blue**, 1% (1 mL) bolus, may lead to hypotension. Methylene blue also may cause transient erroneous decreases in pulse oximetry readings (Sao_2) to as low as 65%, lasting 10 to 70 seconds.

(2) **Indigo carmine**, 0.8% (5 mL)—an α-adrenergic agonist—may cause hypertension.

2. **Complications** usually are related to blood loss, including hypothermia, anemia, and coagulopathy.

D. **Nephrectomy** usually is performed for neoplasm, transplantation, chronic infection, trauma, cystic, or calculous disease. Nephrectomy may be performed by an open or laparoscopic approach.

1. Patients undergoing nephrectomy for renal cell carcinoma require preoperative staging. If the tumor extends into the inferior vena cava (IVC) or right atrium, two potential complications need to be considered:

a. **The tumor may partially or fully occlude the IVC**, leading to poor venous return, hypotension, and an abnormal relationship between volume status and central venous pressure.

b. **Tumor fragments** can dislodge and cause **pulmonary emboli**. Occasionally, placement of pulmonary artery or central venous catheters may contact and dislodge tumor.

c. **Cardiopulmonary bypass** may be utilized to reduce the risk of pulmonary emboli.

d. Blood loss can be massive because of the size and vascularity of the tumor.

2. The patient is positioned supine for an abdominal incision or in the lateral decubitus position for a retroperitoneal approach. In the lateral position, the table is fully flexed and the kidney bar may be raised.

a. Hypotension can be produced by IVC compression.

b. Radical nephrectomy may require a thoracoabdominal incision.

c. Adequate hydration and preservation of renal blood flow are the key goals.

E. **Radical cystectomy and ileal/colonic conduit.** Patients with invasive bladder tumors may require cystectomy. Other patients with pelvic malignancies, neurogenic bladder dysfunction, chronic lower urinary tract obstruction, or postirradiation bladder dysfunction may require an ileal or colonic urinary diverting procedure.

1. **Anesthetic considerations**

a. **Large-bore IV access** is imperative as significant blood loss is may occur.

b. **Arterial or central venous access** may be indicated because large volume shifts occur while the ureters are disconnected.

2. **Combined epidural and general anesthesia** is used frequently. Surgeons may request that nitrous oxide be avoided to minimize bowel distention. An epidural at full anesthetic levels may offset this distention, however.

F. **Orchidopexy, orchiectomy, and urogenital plastic surgery procedures** are performed to treat congenital deformities, neoplasms, and impotence. Patients with torsion of the testicle may require emergency reduction and orchidopexy to prevent ischemia. A T-9 sensory level is required if regional anesthesia is used.

G. **Renal transplantation** is performed for patients with end-stage renal disease. The recipients commonly have hypertension, electrolyte and acid-base abnormalities, and anemia. Preoperative dialysis, if possible, should correct potassium and acid-base abnormalities. Anemia is common and well tolerated.

1. **Donor kidney preservation** is accomplished by continuous perfusion with a cold (4°C) preservative solution, commonly called University of Wisconsin (UW) solution. Its multiple additives can cause hypersensitivity reactions in recipients.

2. **Anesthetic considerations**

a. Intravenous access may be difficult and placement in extremities with fistulas or shunts should be avoided.

b. Patients frequently have poor gastric emptying because of gastroparesis from diabetes or renal failure.

c. Hyperkalemia may contraindicate succinylcholine.

d. Regional anesthesia may be contraindicated by coagulopathy or immunosuppression.

e. Normal saline solution may be preferred to lactated Ringer's solution when hyperkalemia is a concern.

f. Adequate hydration before vascular anastomosis is crucial, since the kidney needs to be well perfused immediately after removal from preservative.

g. Urine output provides an immediate gauge of renal function, which may be affected by acute rejection or vascular thrombosis. Methylprednisolone and diuretics (mannitol and/or furosemide) are also given at this time. Dopamine may be used to treat oliguria.

III. **Extracorporeal shock wave lithotripsy (ESWL)**

A. **ESWL** focuses acoustic shock waves at urinary or biliary stones. At interfaces between materials of differing density, such as between soft tissue and stones, reflections of these acoustic waves set up complex patterns of internal echoes resulting in stresses that cause the stones to fracture. All lithotriptors have four main features:

1. **Shock wave generator** (electrohydraulic, piezoelectric, or electromagnetic).

2. **Acoustic focusing mechanism**

3. **Coupling mechanism**. First-generation lithotriptors used an immersion tank, whereas newer units employ water-filled cushions or shock tubes.

4. **Stone localization and visualization system** (fluoroscopy or ultrasonography).

B. **Anesthetic considerations**

1. **Immersion into water baths** (first-generation lithotriptors) increases venous return and decreases functional residual capacity and vital capacity, which may be hazardous for patients with marginal cardiac or pulmonary function. Hypothermia and hyperthermia can occur. **General, spinal, or epidural anesthesia** is necessary for first-generation lithotriptors because of significant pain.

2. The patient is positioned supine, or prone if the stone is in the ureter. Lithotomy position may be necessary for cystoscopy or stent placement.

3.   Standard monitors are adequate unless significant coexisting disease is present.

4.   Monitored anesthesia care with IV sedation usually is adequate for newer lithotriptors, since they cause less pain. Various techniques, including local anesthetic skin infiltration over an approximately 10 × 10 cm area, 30 g of EMLA cream, and a variety of intravenous infusions, including propofol, alfentanil, midazolam, and remifentanil, have been used successfully.

5.   Adequate IV hydration with occasional diuretic supplementation may aid passage of stone fragments.

6.   Absolute contraindications are pregnancy, untreated infections, bleeding diatheses, and abdominal pacemakers.

7.   The shock waves are synchronized to the refractory period of the cardiac cycle to minimize the risk of causing ventricular arrhythmias.

C.   **Complications**

1.   Ureteral colic may manifest as nausea, vomiting, or bradycardia.

2.   Hematuria is common and treated with hydration and diuresis.

3.   Cardiac arrhythmias such as bradycardia, premature atrial contractions, and premature ventricular contractions can occur, primarily during the procedure, because of mechanical strains on the cardiac conduction system.

4.   Renal (subcapsular) hematoma from collateral damage to renal vasculature, especially in hypertensive patients.

5.   Hypertension occurs primarily with patients who have autonomic dysreflexia.

6.   Severe pulmonary or intestinal damage is rare, but can occur if the shock waves inadvertently are applied to the lung or intestines, which could occur with the patient movement during treatment.

IV.   **Patients with spinal cord pathology**

A.   **Altered physiology**

1.   Spinal cord injury frequently causes bladder dysfunction, which commonly leads to urinary tract infections, pyelonephritis, nephrolithiasis, vesico-ureteric reflux, and renal failure. Hence, such patients undergo frequent urological procedures.

2.   Pulmonary dysfunction

a.   Diaphragmatic paralysis may result if the lesion is above C-6.

b.   Due to loss of intercostal (and abdominal) muscle function, lesions above T-7 will result in significant alterations of pulmonary function, including: decreased vital capacity, expiratory reserve volume, and FEV_1.

3.   Gastric emptying is delayed, and, acutely, gastroparesis and paralytic ileus are common, thus increasing the risk of aspiration.

4.   Thermoregulation is lost below the level of the lesion. Patients, especially those with higher-level lesions, tend to be poikilothermic.

5.   Patients have overall reduced sympathetic tone, and peripheral α-adrenergic receptor hyperreactivity.

B.   **Spinal shock** usually occurs immediately after injury and may last from a few hours to several weeks. Spinal shock follows acute spinal cord injury and results from elimination of sympathetic tone below the level of injury. Spinal shock may cause a dramatic loss of vascular resistance, loss of the baroreceptor reflex, flaccid paralysis, paralytic ileus, and significant bradycardia from unopposed parasympathetic activity, if sympathetic cardiac accelerator (T-1 to T-4) fibers are lost. Bradycardia may manifest as sinus pauses or arrest, sick sinus syndrome, wandering atrial pacemaker, or junctional rhythm, and may require pacing.

C.   Autonomic dysreflexia is a common condition manifested by acute onset of sympathetic hyperreactivity in patients with cord lesions, usually at or above the T-4 to T-8 level (the level of the splanchnic outflow). The syndrome may appear at any time from a few weeks to many years after the injury.

1.   It is generally precipitated by bladder distention, lower urinary tract stimulation, or fecal impaction, but also can be secondary to other cutaneous or visceral stimuli below the level of the lesion.

2.   Sympathetic hyperreactivity occurs because of loss of descending inhibition of the autonomic response.

3.   Noxious stimuli can cause severe hypertension, reflex bradycardia, excessive sweating, facial flushing, nasal congestion, muscle spasms, and pounding headaches.

4.   Sequelae may include seizures, hemorrhagic or hypertensive cerebrovascular accidents, retinal hemorrhages, ventricular arrhythmias, and cardiac arrest.

5.   Treatment of autonomic dysreflexia includes:

a.   Removal of the inciting stimulus (e.g., bladder drainage, fecal disimpaction, or removal of pressure from ulcers).

b.   Raising level of regional anesthesia.

c.   Deepening general anesthesia.

d.   Sitting the patient upright.

e.   Pharmacologic agents with rapid onset and short duration of action are ideal to treat hypertension since episodes tend to be paroxysmal. Agents include:

(1)   Nifedipine 10 mg orally, either 20 minutes before stimulation or as a response to hypertension.

(2)   Nitroglycerin (0.15 to 0.6 mg sublingually or 0.2 to 10 μg per minute IV).

(3)   Sodium nitroprusside (0.5 to 1.5 mg per minute IV).

(4)   Hydralazine (20 to 40 mg IV).

D.   Indications for anesthesia

1.   Pain control for surgeries that cause stimulation above the level of spinal injury, and below the level of incomplete spinal injuries.

2.   Control of spasticity, which is often exacerbated by surgical stimuli.

3.   Hemodynamic stability for patients prone to autonomic dysreflexia.

E.   Anesthetic considerations

1.   Regional anesthesia has the advantage of blocking both limbs of the reflex arc and thereby avoids autonomic dysreflexia. Determining the level of anesthesia by cutaneous testing is difficult with a preexisting complete sensory deficit.

2.   Epidural anesthesia via catheter may be preferable to

spinal anesthesia since the level of anesthesia may be raised as necessary, but is subject to possible incomplete surgical block.
3. A low spinal "saddle" block frequently is adequate if the procedure only involves the perineal area.

SUGGESTED READING

Epstein M. Aging and the kidney. *J Am Soc Nephrol* 1996;7:1006–1022.

Gravenstein D. Transurethral resection of the prostate (TURP) syndrome: a review of the pathophysiology and management. *Anesth Analg* 1997;84:438–446.

Hambly PR, Martin B. Anaesthesia for chronic spinal cord lesions. *Anaesthesia* 1998;53:273–289.

Hosking MP, Warner MA, Lobdell CM, et al. Outcomes of surgery in patients 90 years of age and older. *JAMA* 1989;261:1909–1915.

Lakatta EG. Cardiovascular aging in health. *Clin Geriatr Med* 2000;16:419–44.

Podrazik PM, Schwartz JB. Cardiovascular pharmacology of aging. *Cardiol Clin* 1999;17:17–34.

Rossi A, Ganassini A, Tantucci C, et al. Aging and the respiratory system. *Aging (Milano)* 1996;8:143–161.

Anesthesia for Surgical Emergencies in the Neonate

Jesse D. Roberts Jr., Jonathan H. Cronin, and
Maria M. Zestos

I. **Development**

A. **Organogenesis** is virtually complete after the twelfth gestational week.

B. **Respiratory development**

   1. **Anatomic**

      a. **The lungs** begin as a bud on the embryonic gut in the fourth week of gestation. Failure of separation of the lung bud from the gut later results in the formation of a **tracheoesophageal fistula** (TEF).

      b. **The diaphragm** forms during the tenth week of gestation, dividing the abdominal and thoracic cavities. The posterior part of the diaphragm is the last part to close, and the left side closes after the right.

      (1) If the diaphragm is not completely formed when the midgut reenters the abdomen from the umbilical pouch, the abdominal contents can enter the thorax.

      (2) Although the mechanism is incompletely understood, the presence of abdominal contents within the thorax is associated with arrested lung growth.

      (3) The lungs from patients with **congenital diaphragmatic hernia** have a decreased number of arterioles in the hypoplastic lung. In addition, the pulmonary arteries of both lungs are abnormally thick and reactive, resulting in increased pulmonary vascular resistance.

   2. **Physiologic**

      a. **Lung development** is generally insufficient for survival at less than the twenty-third week of gestation. This may be related to an alveolar to pulmonary capillary distance that is too great for oxygen diffusion to take place.

      b. Secretion of **surfactant**, which reduces alveolar wall surface tension and promotes alveolar aeration, is inadequate until the last month of gestation.

      (1) Birth prior to 32 weeks gestation is associated with **respiratory distress syndrome** (RDS).

      (2) Because glucose metabolism affects lung maturation, babies from mothers with diabetes may have RDS if born later in gestation.

      (3) Antenatal treatment with steroids is associated with a decrease in the incidence of RDS in prematurely born newborns.

      c. Following birth, the first breath and the onset of postnatal breathing are stimulated by hypoxemia, hypercarbia, tactile stimulation, and a decrease in plasma prostaglandin E_2. Following aeration and distension of the lung, the pulmonary vascular resistance decreases, and pulmonary blood flow increases nearly ten-fold. Failure of the reduction of pulmonary vascular resistance following birth is associated with **persistent pulmonary hypertension in the newborn** (PPHN).

C.   Cardiovascular development

  1.   Anatomic

    a.   The primitive **cardiac tube** forms during the first month of gestation and consists of the sinoatrium, the primitive ventricle, the bulbus cordis (primitive right ventricle), and the truncus (primitive main pulmonary artery). During the second month of gestation, a heart with two parallel pumping systems develops out of this initial tubular system. During this process, various structures divide and migrate. Failure of structural maturation at this stage of development causes numerous cardiac malformations. For example:

      (1)   Failure of division of the sinoatrium into the two atria results in a single atrium. Improper closure results in an **atrial septal defect**.

      (2)   Failure of migration of the ventricular septum and atrioventricular valve between the primitive ventricle and the bulbus cordis results in a **double-outlet left ventricle** (single ventricle). Minor migrational defects result in a **ventriculoseptal defect**.

      (3)   Failure of division of the truncus into the pulmonary artery and the aorta results in **truncus arteriosus**.

    b.   The **aortic arch system** initially consists of six pairs of arches; only the third, fourth, and sixth aortic arches develop further.

      (1)   The **third arches** form the connections between the external and internal carotid arteries.

      (2)   The **left fourth arch** becomes the segment of aorta between the left carotid and the subclavian arteries. The **right fourth arch** becomes the proximal subclavian artery.

      (3)   The **sixth arches** produce the pulmonary arteries. The **ductus arteriosus** develops from the distal portion of the right sixth arch. Although the left proximal sixth arch usually degenerates, it can persist and form an aberrant left ductus arteriosus.

      (4)   Failure of regression of various portions of the aorta and arch system can result in aberrant vessels. For example, failure of regression causes a **double aortic arch**. Regression of the left-sided arches but not the right-sided ones can result in a **right-sided aortic arch**.

  2.   Physiologic

    a.   Fetal circulation. After the twelfth week, the circulatory system is in its final form. Oxygenated blood from the placenta passes through the umbilical vein, the ductus venosus, and returns to the heart. Subsequently, most of the blood bypasses the pulmonary circulation by passing right-to-left through the foramen ovale and the ductus arteriosus into the aorta.

    b.   At birth, umbilical placental circulation ceases. The blood flow through the ductus venosus decreases. The ductus venosus closes in 3 to 7 days. The decrease in venous return causes reduced right atrial pressure and functional closure of the foramen ovale. At the same time, the gas exchange is transferred from the placenta to the newly ventilated lungs. Pulmonary resistance decreases as the postnatal pulmonary circulation is established. With increasing arterial oxygen tension (Pao_2), constriction of the ductus arteriosus occurs. Cessation of ductal blood flow often occurs within several hours.

D. Body composition
   1. **Extracellular fluid** (ECF) decreases as the fetus grows. ECF is 90% of total body weight at 30 weeks, 85% at 36 weeks, and 75% at term.
   2. After birth, a physiologic diuresis occurs, with the infant losing about 5% to 10% of ECF in the first few days of life. Factors affecting the fluid requirements of a newborn include prematurity, use of phototherapy, and insensible water losses.
   3. Before 32 weeks of gestation, the **neonatal kidney is immature** and less able to concentrate urine or handle solute loads. Renal tubular function improves with postnatal age.

II. General assessment
A. History
   1. **Prenatal**. The history of the neonate begins in utero. Fetal growth and development are affected by maternal disorders, including hypertension, diabetes, and drug, cigarette, and alcohol use. Polyhydramnios, abnormal alpha-fetoprotein, maternal infections, and premature labor often are associated with neonatal problems.
   2. **Perinatal history** includes gestational age, time of onset of labor and rupture of membranes, use of tocolytics and fetal monitors, signs of fetal distress, type of anesthesia, mode of the newborn's delivery (spontaneous, forceps or vacuum assisted, or cesarean), condition of the infant at delivery, Apgar scores, and immediate resuscitation steps required. Ensure that vitamin K and ocular antibiotic ointment were given.
B. Physical examination
   1. **General inspection**. A careful, complete, systematic evaluation is needed. No assumptions concerning the development, location, or function of organ systems should be made. An abnormality in one system may be associated with abnormalities in another.
   2. **Vital signs** provide a useful physiologic screen of organ function. If cardiac abnormality is suspected, an electrocardiogram (ECG) and upper and lower extremity blood pressure measurements are required. In addition, an echocardiogram and pediatric cardiology consultation should be considered. Normal vital signs are summarized in Table 27-1.
   3. **The Apgar score** reflects the degree of intrapartum stress as well as the effectiveness of initial resuscitation (See Table 27-2). Points are awarded for each of the five criteria, with the maximum score being 10. Although the Apgar score at 1 minute correlates best with intrauterine conditions, the 5- and 10-minute Apgar scores correlate best with neonatal outcome.
   4. **Gestational age** influences care, management, and survival potential of the neonate. An infant is considered preterm if the gestational age is less than 37 weeks, term if 37 to 42

Table 27-1. Normal vital signs

Vital Sign	Term	Preterm
Pulse (beats/min)	110–120	140–180
Respiration (breaths/min)	35–40	50–70
Blood pressure (mmHg)	60–90/40–60	40–60/20–40
Temperature (°C)	37.5 (rectal)	37.5

weeks, and postterm if the gestational age is more than 42 weeks. Although the date of conception and ultrasound examination can be used to predict gestational age, a physical examination and Dubowitz scoring to determine gestational age should be performed. The **Dubowitz scoring system** involves evaluation of physical characteristics of the skin, external genitalia, ears, breasts, and neuromuscular behavior to assess gestational age.

5. **Weight determination**. Infants who are **small for gestational age (SGA)** often have had intrauterine growth retardation. This may be the result of chromosomal defects, maternal hypertension, chronic placental insufficiency, maternal cigarette or drug use, or congenital infection. These infants have a high incidence of hypoglycemia, hypocalcemia, and polycythemia. Infants who are **large for gestational age** (LGA) may have mothers with diabetes. In the immediate postnatal period, LGA newborns should be evaluated for hypoglycemia and polycythemia.

6. **Respiratory**. Signs of respiratory distress include tachypnea, grunting, nasal flaring, intercostal retractions, rales, rhonchi, asymmetry of breath sounds, and apneic periods. **Pulse oximetry** has become a standard noninvasive screen of oxygenation in neonates.

7. **Cardiovascular**. Central cyanosis and capillary refill should be assessed. Distal pulses should be palpated, noting whether they are bounding. A delay between brachial and femoral pulses is suggestive of **coarctation of the aorta**. Note the character and location of murmurs and splitting of the second heart sound. During the first 48 hours, murmurs may appear

Table 27-2. Apgar scores

Sign	Score		
	0	1	2
Heart rate	Absent	<100/min	>100/min
Respiratory effort	Absent	Irregular	Good, crying
Muscle tone	Limp	Some flexion	Active motion
Reflex irritability	Absent	Grimace	Cough or sneeze
Color	Blue	Acrocyanosis	Completely pink

as intracardiac pressure gradients change, or disappear as the ductus arteriosus closes.

8. Gastrointestinal. A scaphoid abdomen suggests **diaphragmatic hernia**. A normal umbilical cord has two arteries and one vein. Note the location and patency of the anus, the size of the liver, spleen, and kidney by palpation, as well as the presence of hernias or abdominal masses.

9. Neurologic. A thorough examination includes evaluation of motor activity, strength, symmetry, tone, and newborn reflexes (Moro, tonic neck, grasp, suck, and stepping reflexes). Full-term newborns should have an upgoing Babinski reflex and brisk deep tendon reflexes.

10. Genitourinary. The gonads may be differentiated or ambiguous, and the testes should be palpable. The location of the urethra should be determined, remembering that hypospadias precludes a circumcision.

11. Musculoskeletal. Any deformities, unusual posturing, or asymmetric limb movement should be noted, and the hips should be examined for possible dislocation. Clavicles may be fractured during a difficult delivery.

12. Craniofacial. One should determine head circumference, the location and size of the fontanelles, and the presence of hematoma or caput. A No. 8 suction catheter passed through each naris and into the posterior pharynx will exclude choanal atresia.

C. Laboratory studies. Routine laboratory studies may include an initial hematocrit and serum glucose. Additional studies should be guided by the individual problem. For example, blood type and Coombs' test may be indicated in infants at risk for hyperbilirubinemia. Special considerations for newborns are as follows:

D. Fluids

1. Initial volume requirements vary with birth weight.
   a. Less than 1.0 kg, use 100 mL/kg per day
   b. 1.0 to 1.5 kg, use 80 to 90 mL/kg per day
   c. 1.5 to 2.5 kg, use 80 mL/kg per day
   d. More than 2.5 kg, use 60 mL/kg per day

2. Isosmolar solutions should be used.
   a. Electrolyte supplementation is not required within the first day of life for maintenance fluids in full-term infants. For premature infants, check the electrolytes at 12 to 24 hours of life and consider adjusting the fluid infusion rate and/or adding electrolytes.
   b. Dextrose (5% to 10%) in water (D/W) may be used for babies under 1.0 kg and 10% D/W for those weighing more than 1.0 kg.

3. Additional fluids may be required for **insensible water losses**.
   a. Fluid requirements increase with lower birth weight, phototherapy, or radiant warmer use.
   b. These losses must be replaced, as well as those from pathologic causes (e.g., omphalocele). The electrolyte composition of the replacement fluid should match that of what is lost.
   c. Infants who are mechanically ventilated absorb free water from their respiratory system.

  4.   Several signs will determine adequacy of fluid infusions.
  a.   Urine output at 0.5 mL/kg per hour
  b.   Only a 1% loss in body weight per day for the first 10 days
  of life
  c.   Stable hemodynamics and good perfusion
E.   Electrolytes
  1.   The usual electrolyte requirements after the first 12 to 24
  hours of life are:
  a. Na^+, 2 to 4 mEq/kg per day
  b. K^+, 1 to 3 mEq/kg per day
  c. Ca^{2+}, 150 to 220 mEq/kg per day.
  2.   The frequency of laboratory tests for serum electrolyte levels will be determined by the rate of insensible losses.
F.   Glucose. Supplemental glucose should be given after birth
to keep blood glucose levels between 40 and 125 mg/dL.
  1.   In most infants 10% D/W at maintenance fluid infusion rates
  will provide adequate glucose. This infusion rate provides the 5
  to 8 mg/kg per minute of glucose required for basal metabolism.
  2.   Infants with hyperinsulinism or intrauterine growth retardation will require higher glucose infusion rates or 12 to 15 mg/
  kg per minute.
  3.   In peripheral intravenous (IV) lines, up to 12.5% D/W may
  be infused; 15% to 20% D/W may be infused via central lines.
  4.   Hypoglycemia (glucose ≤ 40 mg/dL) is treated with a bolus
  of glucose and increased glucose infusion rate.
  a.   200 mg/kg glucose IV is given over 1 minute (example: 2
  mL/kg of 10% D/W).
  b.   The glucose infusion rate is increased from the current
  level or started at 8 mg/kg per minute IV.
  c.   Serial blood tests are necessary to determine the effectiveness of the increased glucose.
G.   Nutrition. The gastrointestinal tract is functional after 28
weeks gestation but is of limited capacity. Requirements vary with
each neonate.
  1.   Caloric requirements are 100 to 130 kcal/kg per day.
  2.   Protein requirements are 2 to 4 g/kg per day.
  3.   Fat. Initiate at 1 g/kg per day and increase as tolerated so
  that the fat provides 40% of the calories.
  4.   Vitamins A, B, C, D, E, and K should be provided.
  5.   Iron requirements are 2 mg/kg per day of elemental iron.
  The adequacy of iron supplementation can be assessed by measuring the hemoglobin or hematocrit and the reticulocyte count.
  6.   Minerals. Calcium, phosphate, magnesium, zinc, copper,
  manganese, and iron need to be replaced.
  7.   Enteral feedings. A formula that simulates human milk
  with a high whey/casein ratio is preferred if breast milk is unavailable. Preterm infants often have lactose intolerance, for
  which nonlactose formulas are available. Infants under 32
  weeks gestation often have poor suck and swallow reflexes and
  require gavage feedings. With all premature infants or ill neonates, small feedings with a slowly advancing schedule should
  be used.
  8.   Parenteral feeding. When needed, parenteral nutrition
  should be started as soon as possible to promote positive nitrogen balance and growth. The infant should be followed closely

to adjust the solutions to the infant's needs and to identify signs of toxicity from hyperalimentation. Usual studies include serum glucose, electrolytes, osmolality, liver function tests, blood urea nitrogen (BUN), creatinine, lipid levels, and platelet count.

III. Respiratory disorders

A. Differential diagnosis. Many diseases share the same signs and symptoms with pulmonary parenchymal disease and should be considered when evaluating an infant with respiratory distress.

1. Airway obstruction. Choanal atresia, vocal cord palsy, laryngomalacia, tracheal stenosis, and obstruction of the trachea by external masses (e.g., cystic hygroma, hemangioma, and vascular ring).

2. Developmental anomalies. TEF, congenital diaphragmatic hernia, congenital emphysema, and lung cysts.

3. Nonpulmonary. Cyanotic heart disease, persistent pulmonary hypertension of the newborn, congestive heart failure, and metabolic disturbances (e.g., acidosis).

B. Laboratory studies for an infant in respiratory distress should include arterial blood gas (ABG) tensions and pH, pre- and post-ductal oxygen saturation (Sao_2) determined by pulse oximetry, hemoglobin or hematocrit, 12-lead ECG, and chest radiograph (CXR). Should these be abnormal, it would be important to consider obtaining an ABG during 100% oxygen breathing, an echocardiogram, and cardiology consultation.

C. Apnea

1. Etiology

a. Central apnea is due to immaturity or depression of the respiratory center (e.g., opioids). It is related to the degree of prematurity and is exacerbated by metabolic disturbances, such as hypoglycemia, hypocalcemia, hypothermia, hyperthermia, and sepsis. Central apnea is often treated with **methylxanthines** such as theophylline and caffeine.

b. Obstructive apnea is caused by inconsistent maintenance of a patent airway and may be associated with incomplete maturation and poor coordination of upper airway musculature. This form of apnea may respond to changes in head position, insertion of an oral or nasal airway, or placing the infant in a prone position. Occasionally, administration of **continuous positive airway pressure** (CPAP) may be beneficial.

c. Mixed apnea represents a combination of both central and obstructive apnea.

2. Postoperative apnea in the neonate

a. Apnea may be associated with anesthesia in formerly preterm infants. Although it has been associated with general anesthesia, some reports of apnea have been associated with local anesthesia.

b. If it is not possible to delay elective surgery, it is prudent to use **postoperative apnea monitoring** in neonates who undergo anesthesia at less than 45 weeks after conception.

D. Respiratory distress syndrome

1. Pathophysiology. RDS (formerly referred to as hyaline membrane disease) results from physiologic surfactant deficiency. This causes decreased lung compliance, alveolar instability, and progressive atelectasis, and hypoxemia because of intrapulmonary shunting of deoxygenated blood.

2. Infants at risk for RDS include premature infants, infants of diabetic mothers, and infants born by cesarean delivery. Infants at risk may be identified prenatally by amniocentesis and evaluation of the amniotic fluid phospholipid profile. Lung maturity is associated with a lecithin (phosphatidylcholine)/sphingomyelin ratio (L/S ratio) greater than 2, saturated phosphatidylcholine level greater than 500 $\mu g/dL$, or presence of phosphatidylglycerol in the specimen.

3. Glucocorticoid (betamethasone) treatment of the mother at least 2 days before delivery decreases the incidence and severity of RDS.

4. Clinical features include tachypnea, nasal flaring, grunting, retractions, and cyanosis that appears shortly after birth. Because of intrapulmonary shunt, the infants remain hypoxemic despite breathing at a high fraction of inspired oxygen (FIO_2).

5. The CXR will show low lung volumes. A "ground-glass" pattern of the lung fields, and air bronchograms may also be evident.

6. Initial treatment includes treating the patient with warmed, humidified oxygen administered by hood. The FIO_2 should be adjusted to maintain the PaO_2 between 50 and 80 mm Hg (SaO_2 less than 96%). If a FIO_2 greater than 60% is required to maintain adequate oxygenation, **nasal CPAP** can be administered. With more severe disease, or if the nasal CPAP is poorly tolerated, endotracheal intubation and mechanical ventilation with positive end-expiratory pressure may be required. Endotracheally administered exogenous **surfactant** decreases the severity, morbidity, and mortality of the disease. **High-frequency oscillatory ventilation** (HFOV) decreases the incidence of pneumothorax and chronic lung disease (CLD) in infants with severe RDS.

7. Broad-spectrum antibiotics often are begun after appropriate cultures are obtained, since the clinical signs and CXR of patients with RDS is indistinguishable from pneumonia.

8. In more mature newborns, RDS may be self-limited; clinical improvement after 2 to 3 days may be associated with a spontaneous diuresis. In extremely premature newborns, RDS may progress to CLD. Recent laboratory studies suggest that **inhaled nitric oxide** (NO) may decrease the evolution of pulmonary hypertension associated with CLD.

9. The morbidity and mortality of patients with RDS are directly related to the degree of prematurity, the perinatal resuscitation, and the coexistence of other problems (e.g., patent ductus arteriosus [PDA]). **Pneumothoraces** and **pulmonary interstitial emphysema** may complicate the recovery and may be associated with the evolution to CLD.

E. Chronic lung disease

1. Etiology. CLD, formally referred to as **bronchopulmonary dysplasia**, is defined as the continued need for respiratory support with oxygen therapy or mechanical ventilation beyond 36 weeks postconceptual age. CLD usually follows severe RDS, and is associated with oxygen toxicity, chronic inflammation, and mechanical injury in the lung. CLD can be worsened by the presence of a PDA and resultant pulmonary edema, or air leaks (pneumothorax).

2. Clinical features include retractions, rales, and areas of lung hyperinflation and underinflation. Because of nonhomogenous ventilation, an intrapulmonary shunt may produce hypoxemia in patients with CLD. Hypoxia may also be associated with bronchospasm in many patients with severe CLD. Most patients have growth retardation.

3. Treatment consists of supportive respiratory care, adequate nutrition, and diuretic therapy. Since patients with CLD may have lung segments with increased airways resistance and long expiratory time constants, a ventilatory pattern with low respiratory rates and increased inspiratory and expiratory time may decrease gas trapping and improve gas exchange. In addition, **bronchodilator therapy** may be lifesaving in patients with CLD and bronchospasm. Systemic or inhaled corticosteroids sometimes are used to treat patients with CLD. However, there is growing concern about the long-term safety of steroid therapy.

4. Recent data suggest that treatment with inhaled NO might prevent the pulmonary vascular disease that is associated with lung injury and CLD.

5. Prognosis varies with the severity of the disease. Of severely affected infants, 25% die within the first year. Most infants are asymptomatic by 2 years of age. It is rare for infants to have signs and symptoms of CLD beyond 5 years of age.

F. Pneumothorax

1. Etiology. Pneumothorax can occur in mechanically ventilated newborns. In addition, nonventilated, otherwise normal full-term infants can also have spontaneous pneumothoraces. Although the cause is unknown, uneven ventilation with overdistention of airways and alveoli may be associated with pneumothoraces. The incidence is 2% in patients born by cesarean deliveries, 10% in patients with meconium staining, and 5% to 10% in RDS.

2. Clinical features. The diagnosis should be considered in any neonate with respiratory distress or in the ventilated infant with an acute deterioration in clinical condition (e.g., sudden cyanosis and hypotension). Occasionally, asymmetric chest movement with ventilation and asymmetric breath sounds may be appreciated. An endobronchial intubation should be excluded.

3. Laboratory studies. Transillumination of the chest with a strong light usually will show a hyperlucent hemithorax. A CXR will confirm the diagnosis.

4. Treatment

    a. In otherwise stable and well-oxygenated infants with minimal respiratory distress, washout of nitrogen by breathing a high concentration of oxygen may cause resolution of the pneumothorax and may be the only therapy required.

    b. In the unstable infant, the pleural space should be immediately aspirated with an IV catheter. Reaccumulation of air after aspiration warrants placement of a chest tube.

G. **Meconium aspiration syndrome**
  1. **Meconium staining of amniotic fluid** occurs in 10% of all births and may be associated with fetal distress and asphyxia.
  2. To **decrease the effects of aspiration**, it is prudent to intubate and suction the airways of infants with meconium-stained fluid who are born with depressed respirations.
  3. **Meconium aspiration** may produce lung airspace disease by mechanical obstruction of the airways and pneumonitis. Complete obstruction of the airways by meconium results in distal atelectasis. Partial obstruction of the airway may produce overinflation of distal air spaces by a ball-valve effect, leading to pneumothorax. The bile in meconium may cause chemical pneumonitis and airway edema.
  4. **Meconium aspiration syndrome** has also been associated with PPHN (see section IV.E).
  5. **Respiratory support** for meconium aspiration is dependent on the etiology of the poor gas exchange. Obstruction of airways with meconium may require mechanical ventilation with long expiratory times to decrease gas trapping. Pneumothorax is treated by placement of a chest tube. Sometimes HFOV is useful to recruit closed lung segments and improve gas exchange. Alkalosis and inhaled nitric oxide have been useful to decrease pulmonary vasoconstriction in patients with meconium aspiration. Exogenous surfactant has been observed to be beneficial since meconium inhibits endogenous surfactant activity.

H. **Congenital diaphragmatic hernia**
  1. **Congenital diaphragmatic hernia** occurs in 1:5,000 live births. It has a high mortality, with 50% not surviving infancy. Seventy percent of the defects occur on the left. The embryology and pathophysiology are discussed in section I.B.
  2. **Clinical features**. The defect is often detected during the prenatal ultrasound. At birth, a scaphoid abdomen can be observed, and breath sounds are absent on the involved side. Rarely, bowel sounds are heard in the affected hemithorax. Although the clinical spectrum may vary, and is probably related to the degree of lung hypoplasia, often patients exhibit severe respiratory distress in the postnatal period.
  3. **The diagnosis** is confirmed by CXR. Often the intestine and stomach are observed in the thorax.
  4. **Treatment** consists of respiratory and cardiovascular support. Endotracheal intubation and mechanical ventilation often are used to decrease air entry into the stomach and intestines. Insufflation of the stomach and intestines is minimized by performing endotracheal intubation while the patients are spontaneously breathing. If the patient is apneic, ventilation with bag and mask should be accomplished using minimal airway pressures. Continuous gastric suction also decreases air insufflation. Treatment often is directed toward decreasing pulmonary vascular resistance and facilitating CO_2 elimination. Conventional ventilation or HFOV is used. Ventilation with inhaled NO has been observed to decrease pulmonary vasoconstriction and cyanosis in some patients. The main causes of mortality are respiratory insufficiency and PPHN (see section IV.E). Pneumothorax in the unaffected lung can occur and often is the cause of death

during resuscitation. Hypotension and shock can occur because of prolonged systemic hypoxemia, shifting of the mediastinal contents by the hernia, and gastrointestinal fluid losses.

5.   Surgical repair involves replacing the abdominal contents and repairing the diaphragm. In the past, this was performed urgently in the critically ill infant. Currently, many patients are first stabilized with medical and ventilatory treatment and extracorporeal membrane oxygenation (ECMO) before surgery (see section IV.E.4).

6.   Anesthetic considerations

a.   Decompression of the gut with continuous nasogastric (NG) suction

b.   Although **spontaneous ventilation** may prevent gastric inflation and lung compression, often mechanical ventilation support is needed. Nevertheless, use the **lowest effective inflating pressures** to reduce the risk of pneumothorax in the normal lung on the side opposite to the hernia.

c.   Nitrous oxide is avoided since it may distend the gut and compromise lung function.

d.   An arterial catheter is indicated for the frequent assessment of acid-base balance, oxygenation, and ventilation. Sodium bicarbonate and hyperventilation are used to treat metabolic and respiratory acidosis, respectively. Alkalosis and inhaled nitric oxide may decrease pulmonary vasoconstriction.

e.   Opioids, muscle relaxants, and **increased F_{IO_2}** often are used during anesthesia.

f.   Body temperature is maintained with warming lights, fluid warmer, and a warming mattress.

IV.   Cardiovascular disorders

A.   Laboratory studies. In the infant with signs and symptoms of cardiovascular disease, relevant studies include an ABG, pre- and post-ductal Sa_{O_2}, determination of ABG tensions during inhalation of pure oxygen (" **hyperoxia test**"), hemoglobin or hematocrit, CXR, and ECG. Two-dimensional echocardiography is frequently performed to detect potential structural heart lesions.

B.   Patent ductus arteriosus

1.   Clinical features. PDA is seen commonly in the premature infant and is characterized by a murmur at the left sternal border radiating to the back, bounding pulses, widened pulse pressure, evidence of increased pulmonary blood flow by CXR, and excessive weight gain. In some cases, cardiac dysfunction associated with a PDA may decrease systemic blood pressure, peripheral perfusion, and urine output, and may be associated with metabolic acidosis.

2.   Although **early treatment** of a PDA consists of fluid restriction and diuretic therapy, it is very important to maintain systemic perfusion. If the degree of shunt through the ductus arteriosus is significant, and renal and platelet function are adequate, pharmacological closure of the ductus with **indomethacin** may be attempted. **Surgical closure** of a PDA is used for the infant for whom indomethacin has not closed the ductus, or for those with decreased renal or platelet function, for whom indomethacin is contraindicated. In addition, surgery is often indicated for those with decreased systemic oxygenation because of extrapulmonary shunt associated with the open ductus arteriosus.

C.   **Cyanosis**

1.   Etiology. There are many causes of cyanosis, including diffusion abnormalities in the lung, intracardiac and extracardiac shunts, and polycythemia. These need to be considered when evaluating an infant with cyanosis. Additional causes of lung diffusion abnormalities are described above.

2.   Cardiac lesions may cause systemic hypoxemia by decreasing pulmonary blood flow, or causing mixture of systemic and pulmonary venous blood via shunts.

3. In the fetus and immediate postnatal period, **the ductus arteriosus may permit pulmonary blood flow** in patients with transposition of the great arteries, pulmonic stenosis or atresia, tetralogy of Fallot, and ventricular hypoplasia. Most of these infants become symptomatic as the ductus arteriosus closes at 2 to 3 days of life. If a ductal-dependent lesion exists, prevention of ductal closure is critical to maintain pulmonary blood flow. This may be accomplished with a **prostaglandin E_1** infusion. Side effects of this infusion include apnea, hypotension, and seizure activity.

4. Many patients with **septal defects** may be asymptomatic during the fetal and neonatal period. With increased pulmonary vascular resistance, however, right-to-left shunting of blood may produce systemic hypoxemia. Later in life, with decreased pulmonary vascular resistance, increased pulmonary blood flow may cause pulmonary vascular disease and pulmonary hypertension.

5.   A CXR and a hyperoxia test can confirm the diagnosis of an intracardiac shunt. The CXR may reveal decreased pulmonary blood flow. The Pao_2 remains below 150 mm Hg when an infant with a significant shunt breathes 100% oxygen. A echocardiogram is invaluable in determining the etiology of the intracardiac shunt.

D.   **Arrhythmias**

1.   Supraventricular tachycardia is the most frequent arrhythmia seen in neonates. This may be self-limited and well tolerated, but if hypotension or desaturation occurs, treatment is required.

2.   Treatment consists of vagal maneuvers such as nasopharyngeal stimulation or placement of cold on the face. Massage of the eye should be avoided, since this may disrupt the lens in neonates. **Adenosine** and **esophageal pacing** also are useful for acute management of **supraventricular tachycardia**.

3.   Digoxin will usually convert paroxysmal atrial tachycardia to sinus rhythm; maintenance therapy for 1 year is sometimes indicated. **Propranolol** and **quinidine** are second-line medications.

4.   Electrical cardioversion is indicated if the patient is hemodynamically unstable.

E.   **Persistent pulmonary hypertension of the newborn**

1.   Pathophysiology. PPHN, previously referred to as persistent fetal circulation, is manifested by an increase in pulmonary vascular resistance with resulting pulmonary arterial hypertension, right-to-left shunting across the foramen ovale and the ductus arteriosus, and profound cyanosis.

2. Etiology. It is suspected that many newborns with PPHN have abnormal pulmonary artery reactivity and structure. Although many infants with PPHN may have asphyxia, meconium aspiration, bacterial pneumonia, and sepsis, the role of these in causing the disease is unknown.

3. Clinical features. Newborns with PPHN have severe systemic hypoxemia unrelieved by breathing at high F_{IO_2}. They may have extrapulmonary shunting of blood evidenced by a higher Sa_{O_2} in the upper versus lower extremities. An ECG may reveal right-ventricular hypertrophy; CXR may show decreased pulmonary vascular markings. Echocardiography may show shunting of blood at the level of the PDA, PFO, or both.

4. Treatment of severe systemic hypoxemia:

    a. Endotracheal intubation and mechanical ventilation at high F_{IO_2}. Often treatment with opioids (e.g., fentanyl 1 to 2 μg/kg per hour) and neuromuscular blockade will facilitate ventilation.

    b. Induced respiratory and/or metabolic alkalosis .

    c. In many patients, **inhaled nitric oxide** rapidly decreases pulmonary vasoconstriction and extrapulmonary shunt and increases systemic oxygenation. In these infants, inhaled NO reverses PPHN and decreases the need for ECMO.

    d. ECMO may be lifesaving for some patients with PPHN refractory to ventilatory and medical therapy. Because it is quite expensive, ECMO is not available at all medical centers.

        (1) **The ECMO circuit** consists of tubing, a reservoir, pump, membrane oxygenator, and heat exchanger. The patient is heparinized to prevent clotting. Because of platelet consumption during ECMO, often platelet infusions are required.

        (2) **Access.** General anesthesia is required for cannulation via the right common carotid artery and the right internal jugular vein, or the femoral artery and vein may be used.

        (3) **Morbidity** may be related to ECMO. Heparinization can cause intracranial hemorrhage and bleeding from other sites. Right-sided cerebral injuries (focal left-sided seizures, left hemiparesis, and progressive right cerebral atrophy) are thought secondary to cannulation and ligation of the right internal carotid artery.

        (4) Because of the potential risks of ECMO, it is reserved for patients with severe systemic hypoxemia. In addition, infants with intraventricular hemorrhage are excluded because of their unacceptable risk of hemorrhage extension while heparinized. Also excluded are infants with multiple congenital anomalies, severe neurologic impairment, or cyanotic congenital heart disease (CHD). It is often technically difficult to obtain adequate ECMO circuit flows to increase systemic oxygenation in preterm infants.

V. Hematologic disorders

A. Hemolytic disease of the newborn (erythroblastosis fetalis)

    1. Isoimmune hemolytic anemia in the fetus is caused by

the transplacental passage of maternal antibody against fetal erythrocytes into the fetus. Only IgG can cross the placenta.

2.   Rh hemolytic disease is usually caused by the anti-D antibody, but can also be caused by antibodies to minor antigens including Kell, Duff, Kidd, or Ss antigens. The absence of D antigen, which makes an individual Rh negative, occurs in 15% of whites and 5% of blacks. A mother can be sensitized to fetal antigens by leakage of fetal blood into the maternal circulation during pregnancy, delivery, abortion, or amniocentesis. To prevent sensitization, an unsensitized Rh-negative mother is given **anti-D immune globulin (RhoGAM)** during pregnancy and after delivery. Once a mother is sensitized, immune prophylaxis is of no value. Even if treated with immune globulin, a mother can still be sensitized during pregnancy if a large fetomaternal transfusion occurs.

3.   ABO hemolytic disease can occur without maternal sensitization, since a mother with group O blood has naturally occurring anti-A and anti-B antibodies in her circulation. These are usually IgM antibodies, but some may be IgG. This disease tends to be milder than Rh disease, with little or no anemia, mild indirect hyperbilirubinemia, and rarely a need for exchange transfusion.

4.   An indirect Coombs test on maternal blood can detect the presence of IgG antibodies in her serum.

5.   A direct Coombs test on the infant's blood can detect cells already coated with antibody, thus indicating a risk for hemolysis.

6.   Hemolysis occurs when antibody crosses the placenta and attaches to the corresponding antigen on fetal erythrocytes. Hepatosplenomegaly results from increased hematopoiesis triggered by hemolysis.

7.   Clinical features include hepatosplenomegaly, edema, pallor, and jaundice.

8.   Laboratory studies often reveal anemia, thrombocytopenia, a positive direct Coombs test, indirect hyperbilirubinemia, hypoglycemia, hypoalbuminemia, and an elevated reticulocyte count that increases proportionally with the severity of the disease. Serial hematocrit and indirect bilirubin levels should be followed.

9.   Treatment consists of **phototherapy**. An exchange transfusion may be required if the level of bilirubin is high or the rate of rise of bilirubin exceeds 1 mg/dL per hour.

B.   **Hydrops fetalis**

1.   Hydrops fetalis is an excessive accumulation of fluid by the fetus and can range from mild peripheral edema to massive anasarca.

2.   Etiologies. Hydrops can be seen in hemolytic disease and is thought to be caused by increased capillary permeability secondary to anemia. Other etiologies of hydrops include anemias (e.g., fetomaternal hemorrhage or donor twin–twin transfusion), cardiac arrhythmias (e.g., complete heart block or supraventricular tachycardia), CHD, vascular or lymphatic malformation (e.g., hemangioma of the liver or cystic hygroma), or infection (e.g., viral, toxoplasmosis, or syphilis).

3.   Treatment goals include prevention of intrauterine or extrauterine death from anemia and hypoxia, restoration of intravascular volume, and avoidance of neurotoxicity from hyperbilirubinemia.

a. Survival of the unborn infant may be improved by in utero transfusion via the umbilical vein.

b. Care of the liveborn infant should include correction of hypovolemia and acidosis, as well as potential exchange transfusion.

c. Late complications include anemia; mild graft-versus-host reactions; inspissated bile syndrome (characterized by persistent icterus with elevated direct and indirect bilirubin); and portal vein thrombosis (as a complication of umbilical vein catheterization).

VI. Gastrointestinal disorders
A. Hyperbilirubinemia

1. Physiology. Bilirubin is formed from the breakdown of heme, then bound to albumin, transported to the liver (where it is conjugated with glucuronide), and delivered to the intestine in bile. In the intestine, it is either deconjugated by intestinal bacteria and reabsorbed or converted to excretory urobilinogen.

2. Etiology. Hyperbilirubinemia results from overproduction (e.g., hemolysis, absorption of sequestered blood, or polycythemia), underconjugation (e.g., immature or damaged liver), or underexcretion (e.g., biliary atresia). It is often seen in sepsis, asphyxia, and metabolic disorders (e.g., hypothyroidism, hypoglycemia, or galactosemia) as well as in healthy newborns and breast-fed infants.

3. Toxic effects. Unconjugated (indirect) bilirubin is lipid soluble and is capable of entering the central nervous system. Toxic levels produce bilirubin staining and necrosis of neurons in the basal ganglia, the hippocampus, and the subthalamic nuclei. This process, known as **bilirubin encephalopathy** or **kernicterus**, may have clinical symptoms ranging from mild lethargy and fever to convulsions. Infants with respiratory distress, sepsis, metabolic acidosis, hypoglycemia, hypoalbuminemia, or severe hemolytic disease are at increased risk for kernicterus. Survivors evaluated in childhood are found to have neurologic sequelae ranging from diminished cognitive function to mental retardation and choreoathetoid cerebral palsy.

4. Physiologic jaundice results from increased red cell turnover and an immature hepatic conjugation system. It occurs in 60% of newborns, and peak bilirubin levels occur by the second to fourth day of life. Premature infants have an increased incidence (80%) and later bilirubin peak (day 5 to 7).

5. Breast milk jaundice develops gradually, occurring in the second or third week of life, with peak bilirubin levels of 15 to 25 mg/dL, which may persist for 2 to 3 months. Other causes should be excluded before making this diagnosis. Interrupting nursing for a few days results in a marked decrease in serum levels, at which time nursing can be restarted. This is a benign type of jaundice without adverse sequelae.

6. Laboratory studies include total and direct bilirubin, direct Coombs test, reticulocyte count, blood smear for red cell morphology, electrolytes, BUN, creatinine, and appropriate cultures if sepsis is suspected. Since hyperbilirubinemia may be the presenting sign of a urinary tract infection, urinalysis and urine cultures should be considered.

7. Treatment

    a.   Management of physiologic or mild hemolytic jaundice consists of monitoring serial bilirubin levels and starting early feeding to reduce enterohepatic cycling of bilirubin.

    b.   Phototherapy is used if moderate indirect bilirubin levels or an accelerated rate of rise is noted (e.g., indirect bilirubin level greater than 5 mg/dL in a full-term infant on day 1 of life). Light therapy of 420- to 470-nm wavelength results in photoisomerization of bilirubin, making it water soluble. Eyes must be shielded to prevent retinal damage.

    c.   For severe hyperbilirubinemia, **exchange transfusion** is indicated (e.g., indirect bilirubin greater than 25 mg/dL in a full-term infant).

B.   Esophageal atresia and TEF

    1.   Esophageal atresia usually is associated with **TEF**. The location of the fistula is variable in these patients.

    2.   Pathophysiology. The proximal blind esophageal pouch has a small capacity, resulting in overflow aspiration. This produces the classic clinical triad of coughing, choking, and cyanosis. Occasionally, only drooling that requires frequent suctioning may be noted.

    3.   The diagnosis is confirmed by the inability to pass a NG tube into the stomach. A CXR with air or water-soluble contrast agents will confirm the existence of esophageal atresia.

    4.   Medical treatment is directed at reducing aspiration. Neonates should have nothing by mouth. A NG tube is positioned in the pouch and placed on continuous low suction. The head of the bed is elevated. Aspiration pneumonia should be treated with chest physiotherapy and antibiotics and oxygen as required. Endotracheal intubation and mechanical ventilation may be required for severe pneumonia. Ventilation can be difficult when a TEF exists.

    5.   Surgical treatment depends on the stability of the infant. In newborns with severe pneumonia, it often is prudent to delay surgery until the lungs improve. A gastrostomy tube may be placed under local anesthesia to decompress the stomach, if required. In stable patients, definitive repair of the esophagus and fistula can be performed.

    6.   Anesthesia. It is critical, and sometimes difficult, to establish an airway in patients with a TEF. Surgeons should be readily available during the induction should emergent decompression of the stomach be required. The patient should be fully monitored; a precordial stethoscope should be placed over the left thorax. If the patient has a gastrostomy tube, it should be placed to water seal. An inhalational induction or awake intubation should be performed. To facilitate placement of the tip of the endotracheal tube between the fistula and the carina, the tube first may be placed into the right mainstem bronchus. The tube then can be slowly withdrawn until breath sounds are heard over the left thorax. Decreased breath sounds and insufflation of the stomach or gas exiting from the gastrostomy tube suggest that the end of the endotracheal tube is above the fistula and that it should be advanced. Once the tube is in a good location, then it is critical to secure it in place. One person can be assigned to monitor the location of the tube throughout the surgery. Inhalation anesthesia with spontaneous ventilation should be maintained until a gastrostomy is performed. The adequacy of positive pressure ventilation should be assured before a muscle relaxant is administered.

C. **Duodenal atresia**
   1. **Clinical features**. Duodenal atresia usually presents with bile-stained emesis, upper abdominal distention, and increased volume of gastric aspirates. It is associated with trisomy 21 (Down syndrome) and can coexist with other intestinal malformations.
   2. **An abdominal radiograph** often reveals a "double bubble," representing air in the stomach and upper duodenum.
   3. **Treatment** includes avoiding oral feedings, use of NG suction, ensuring adequate hydration and serum electrolyte levels. Anesthesia consists of awake or rapid-sequence endotracheal intubation, avoidance of nitrous oxide, and often the use of muscle relaxants.

D. **Pyloric stenosis**
   1. Although usually presenting in the second or third week of life, pyloric stenosis may be present in the immediate newborn period.
   2. **Clinical features** include persistent nonbilious emesis and a metabolic alkalosis from prolonged gastric suctioning and removal of hydrochloric acid. With protracted vomiting, the patient may present with metabolic acidosis and shock. An abdominal mass consisting of the hypertrophic pylorus or "olive" is often palpable.
   3. **An abdominal radiograph** usually shows gastric dilatation. The diagnosis is confirmed by abdominal ultrasonography or by a barium swallow examination.
   4. **Treatment** consists of rehydration, correction of metabolic alkalosis, and NG drainage before surgical repair.
   5. **Intraoperative management**. It is critical to empty the stomach before induction of anesthesia. The patient's NG tube can be blocked with barium or other matter. We often replace the NG tube with a new one, and suction the patient while lying supine, lateral and prone before induction. A rapid-sequence induction or awake intubation may be performed. Inhalation anesthetics or muscle relaxants can be used as needed. The neonate should be fully awake and breathing adequately before the endotracheal tube is removed.

E. **Omphalocele and gastroschisis**
   1. An **omphalocele** is caused by failure of the migration of the intestine into the abdomen and subsequent closure of the abdominal wall at 6 to 8 weeks of gestation. The viscera remain outside the abdominal cavity, where they are covered with intact peritoneum. Omphaloceles may be associated with genetic abnormalities, cardiac lesions, extrophy of the bladder, and Beckwith–Wiedemann syndrome.
   2. **Gastroschisis** occurs later in fetal life (12 to 18 weeks gestation) from interruption of the omphalomesenteric artery. The resulting paraumbilical defect has no peritoneal coverage and

exposes the bowel to the intrauterine environment; bowel loops are often edematous and covered with an inflammatory exudate.

3.   Medical stabilization includes NG drainage, IV hydration, and protection of the viscera before imminent surgical repair. If the peritoneal sac is intact, the omphalocele should be covered with sterile, warm, saline-soaked gauze to decrease heat and water loss and the risk of infection. If the sac has ruptured or if the infant has gastroschisis, saline-soaked gauze should be used to wrap the exposed viscera; the infant then should be wrapped in warm sterile towels while awaiting surgical repair.

F.   Necrotizing enterocolitis

1.   Necrotizing enterocolitis is an acquired intestinal necrosis that appears in the absence of functional (e.g., Hirschsprung's disease) or anatomic (e.g., malrotation) lesions. It occurs predominantly (90%) in premature infants and may be endemic or epidemic in nature. It usually develops during the first few weeks of life, almost always after the institution of enteral feedings. Mortality may be as high as 40%. Clinical studies suggest that breast-milk feeding protects against necrotizing enterocolitis.

2.   Pathogenesis is unclear but involves critical stress of an immature gut by ischemic, infectious, or immunologic insults. Enteral feedings seem to potentiate mucosal injury.

3.   Clinical features include abdominal distention, ileus, increase in gastric aspirates, abdominal wall erythema, and bloody stool. The infant may demonstrate systemic signs such as temperature instability, lethargy, respiratory and circulatory instability, oliguria, and bleeding diatheses.

4.   Laboratory studies should include an abdominal radiograph (which may show pneumatosis intestinalis, fixed loops of bowel, portal air, or free intraperitoneal air), complete blood count (revealing leukocytosis, leukopenia, or thrombocytopenia), ABG (demonstrating acidosis), stool guaiac (often showing occult blood), and stool Clinitest (showing evidence of carbohydrate malabsorption). Since the differential diagnosis includes sepsis, cultures of blood, urine, and stool also should be obtained. If the patient is stable and disseminated intravascular coagulation is not evident, cerebrospinal fluid (CSF) should be obtained by lumbar puncture for Gram stain and culture.

5.   Treatment. When necrotizing enterocolitis is suspected, enteral feedings are discontinued, and the stomach is decompressed with a NG tube. Oral feedings are withheld for at least 2 weeks and the patient is supported with parenteral feedings. Broad-spectrum antibiotics (ampicillin, an aminoglycoside, and if perforation is suspected, metronidazole) are administered empirically.

6.   Surgical consultation is indicated, although laparotomy is usually reserved for intestinal perforation.

G.   Volvulus

1.   Volvulus may occur as a primary lesion or more commonly as the result of intestinal malrotation. If present in utero, intestinal necrosis may be present at birth, and immediate resection is indicated.

2.   Clinical features may include abdominal distention, bilious emesis, and signs of sepsis or shock.

3. **The diagnosis** of malrotation is made by barium enema, which demonstrates an abnormally positioned ligament of Treitz.

4. **Treatment** involves volume resuscitation, placement of a NG tube, and surgical repair.

5. **Intraoperative management**. After evacuation of the stomach, a rapid sequence induction should be performed, and anesthesia maintained with inhalation or intravenous anesthetics as tolerated. Nitrous oxide should be avoided. Oxygen should be diluted with air to minimize the risk of pulmonary or ocular toxicity.

VII. **Neurologic disorders**

  A. **Seizures**

   1. **Seizures** may be generalized, focal, or subtle. Even jitteriness may be a manifestation of a seizure disorder.

   2. **Etiologies** include birth trauma, intracranial hemorrhage, postasphyxial encephalopathy, metabolic disturbances (hypoglycemia or hypocalcemia), drug withdrawal, and infections.

   3. **Laboratory evaluation** should include:

     a. Initial evaluation includes electrolytes, glucose, calcium, magnesium, and ABG tensions and pH. If a metabolic disease is suspected, serum and urine amino acids should be obtained.

     b. Complete blood count with differential, platelet count, and the appropriate cultures, including CSF.

     c. Cranial ultrasound, computed tomography (CT) scan, or both.

     d. Electroencephalogram before and after pyridoxine administration.

   4. **Treatment** includes supportive care. Adequate oxygenation should be assured and underlying problems (e.g., hypoglycemia or hypocalcemia) corrected. Anticonvulsants are started, and if indicated, a test dose of pyridoxine is administered.

   5. **Anticonvulsants**

     a. **Acute medical treatments** include:

       (1) **Benzodiazepines** (e.g., lorazepam 0.1 to 0.3 mg/kg IV).

       (2) **Phenobarbital**, 20 mg/kg IV load over 10 minutes; maintenance dose of 2.5 mg/kg twice daily to maintain a serum level of 20 to 40 µg/mL.

       (3) **Fosphenytoin**, 15 to 20 mg/kg IV load over 15 minutes; maintenance dose of 2.5 mg/kg twice daily to maintain a therapeutic level of 15 to 30 µg/mL.

     b. **Chronic treatment** for seizures usually is with phenobarbital.

  B. **Intracranial hemorrhage**

   1. **Intraventricular hemorrhage** occurs in over 30% of infants with birth weights below 1,500 g. Subdural and subarachnoid hemorrhages are much less common.

   2. **Clinical features**. Intraventricular hemorrhage is often asymptomatic, although it may present with unexplained lethargy, apnea, and seizures. On examination, the head circumference is increased and the fontanelles may be bulging. Anemia and acidosis may be present. Diagnosis is made by cranial ultrasound or CT scan.

3. Grading of intraventricular hemorrhage

a. Grade I. Subependymal bleeding only.

b. Grade II. Intraventricular bleeding without dilation of ventricles.

c. Grade III. Intraventricular bleeding with dilation of ventricles.

d. Grade IV. Grade III with intraparenchymal blood.

4. The **major complication** of intraventricular hemorrhage is CSF obstruction resulting in posthemorrhagic **hydrocephalus**. This is followed by measuring daily head circumferences and by serial ultrasound examinations. Intraventricular shunting is often required.

5. Hypertonic agents (e.g., 25% dextrose in water) that had previously been advocated in the treatment of hypoglycemia have been implicated in the etiology of intraventricular hemorrhage and should be avoided.

C. Retinopathy of prematurity

1. Etiologies

a. The risk of retinopathy of prematurity (ROP) is increased in premature neonates requiring oxygen therapy. ROP is seen in infants with birth weights less than 1,700 g, with an 80% incidence in infants less than 1,000 g. To decrease the incidence of ROP, **hyperoxia should be avoided**.

b. Factors other than hyperoxic exposure and prematurity may produce ROP, as has been demonstrated in full-term infants, infants with cyanotic heart disease, stillborn infants, and infants with no hyperoxic exposure, as well as in a single eye. Factors that may increase risk include anemia, infection, intracranial hemorrhage, acidosis, and PDA.

2. Pathophysiology. ROP begins in the temporal peripheral retina, which is the last part of the retina to vascularize. An elevated ridge demarcating vascularized and nonvascularized retina is seen initially. **Fibrovascular proliferation** from this border extends posteriorly, and in 90% of patients, gradual resolution occurs from this stage. These patients may develop strabismus, amblyopia, myopia, or peripheral retinal detachment in later life.

3. In 10% of patients, fibrovascularization extends into the vitreous, resulting in vitreous hemorrhage, peripheral retinal scarring, temporal dragging of the disk and macula, and partial retinal detachment. In severe disease, extensive fibrovascular proliferation can produce a retrolental white mass (leukokoria), complete retinal detachment, and loss of vision.

4. All infants at risk are examined with indirect ophthalmoscopy after 1 month of postnatal age, or at 32-weeks–corrected gestational age. If ROP is identified, the infant is reexamined at 2-week intervals until spontaneous resolution occurs. New cases of ROP do not occur after 3 months of age.

5. Treatment for severe manifestations of ROP has included photocoagulation, diathermy, cryotherapy, and vitrectomy.

VIII. Infectious diseases

A. Environment

1. Neonates are particularly vulnerable to infection. They have decreased cellular and humoral immune defense systems and are at increased risk for colonization and nosocomial infection.

2. Prevention. Infectious transmission may be reduced by using separate equipment and isolettes for each infant, by hand washing before and after each contact, and by wearing gloves and cover gowns.

B. Risk factors for infection. Prolonged rupture of membranes is associated with a high incidence of amnionitis and subsequent ascending bacterial and viral infection in the neonate. Maternal fever, maternal leukocytosis, and fetal tachycardia are also associated with neonatal infection.

C. Laboratory studies include complete blood count with differential and blood cultures. A lumbar puncture for culture and analysis of CSF may be indicated. If appropriate, viral cultures are should be obtained.

D. Neonatal sepsis

1. Organisms responsible for infections soon after birth are usually acquired in utero or during passage through the birth canal. These can include group B β-hemolytic streptococcus, *Escherichia coli*, *Listeria*, and herpes. Later-onset infections may be caused by *Staphylococcus aureus*, *Staphylococcus epidermidis*, *Enterobacter cloacae*, and *Pseudomonas aeruginosa*.

2. The clinical features of sepsis include respiratory failure, seizures, and shock. Often subtle signs, including respiratory distress, apnea, irritability, or poor feeding, are seen first and warrant evaluation.

3. Laboratory studies should include cultures of blood, urine and CSF, complete blood count with platelet count, urinalysis, and CXR.

4. Antibiotic coverage with ampicillin and an aminoglycoside is begun and continued for 48 to 72 hours. If culture results are positive, treatment should continue as indicated by the severity and location of infection. Aminoglycoside serum levels should be monitored and dosages adjusted to prevent toxicity.

SUGGESTED READING

Barry JE, Auldist AW. The Vater association: one end of a spectrum of anomalies. *Am J Dis Child* 1974;128:769–771.

Bartlett RH, Roloff DW, Cornell RG, et al. Extracorporeal circulation in neonatal respiratory failure: a prospective randomized study. *Pediatrics* 1985;76:479–487.

Cloherty JP, Stark AR, eds. *Manual of neonatal care*. Philadelphia: Lippincott-Raven, 1998.

Cronin JH. High frequency ventilator therapy for newborns. *J Int Care Med* 1994;9:71–85.

Dennery PA, Seidman DS, Stevenson DK. Neonatal hyperbilirubinemia. *N Engl J Med* 2001;344:581–590.

Findlay RD, Taeusch HW, Walther FJ. Surfactant replacement therapy for meconium aspiration syndrome. *Pediatrics* 1996;97:48–52.

Gersony WM, Peckham GJ, Ellison RC, et al. Effects of indomethacin in premature infants with patent ductus arteriosus: results of a national collaborative study. *J Pediatr* 1983;102:895–906.

Gregory GA, Steward DJ. Life-threatening perioperative apnea in the ex-"premie". *Anesthesiology* 1983;59:495–498.

Insoft RM, Sanderson IR, Walker WA. Development of immune function in the intestine and its role in neonatal diseases. *Pediatr Clin North Am* 1996;43:551–571.

Jobe AH. Pulmonary surfactant therapy. *N Engl J Med* 1993;328:861–868.

Kurth CD, Spitzer AR, Broennle AM, et al. Postoperative apnea in preterm infants. *Anesthesiology* 1987;66:483–488.

Liu LM, Cote CJ, Goudsouzian NG, et al. Life-threatening apnea in infants recovering from anesthesia. *Anesthesiology* 1983;59:506–510.

Murphy BP, Inder TE, Huppi PS, et al. Impaired cerebral cortical gray matter growth after treatment with dexamethasone for neonatal CLD. *Pediatrics* 2001;107:217–221.

O'Rourke PP, Crone RK, Vacanti JP, et al. Extracorporeal membrane oxygenation and conventional medical therapy in neonates with persistent pulmonary hypertension of the newborn: a prospective randomized study. *Pediatrics* 1989;84:957–963.

Peckham GJ, Fox WW. Physiologic factors affecting pulmonary artery pressure in infants with persistent pulmonary hypertension. *J Pediatr* 1978;93:1005–1010.

Roberts JD Jr, Cronin JH, Todres ID. Neonatal emergencies. In: Coté C, Todres ID, Goudsouzian N, Ryan JF, eds. *A practice of anesthesia for infants and children*, 3rd ed. Philadelphia: WB Saunders, 2001: 294–314.

Roberts JD Jr. Neonatal pulmonary hypertension. In: Polin RA, Fox WW, eds. *Fetal and neonatal physiology*, 2nd ed. Philadelphia: WB Saunders, 1998:970–976.

Roberts JD Jr, Fineman JR, Morin FC 3rd, et al. Inhaled nitric oxide and persistent pulmonary hypertension of the newborn. *N Engl J Med* 1997; 336:605–610.

Shannon DC, Gotay F, Stein IM, et al. Prevention of apnea and bradycardia in low-birthweight infants. *Pediatrics* 1975;55:589–594.

Soll RF, Hoekstra RE, Fangman JJ, et al. Multicenter trial of single-dose modified bovine surfactant extract (Survanta) for prevention of respiratory distress syndrome. Ross Collaborative Surfactant Prevention Study Group. *Pediatrics* 1990;85:1092–1102.

Steward DJ. Preterm infants are more prone to complications following minor surgery than are term infants. *Anesthesiology* 1982;56:304–306.

Tobias JD, Burd RS, Helikson MA. Apnea following spinal anaesthesia in two former pre-term infants. *Can J Anaesth* 1998;45:985–989.

Volpe JJ. *Neurology of the newborn*, 3rd ed. Philadelphia: WB Saunders, 1995.

Anesthesia for Pediatric Surgery

Susan A. Vassallo

I. Anatomy and physiology
A. Upper airway
1. **Neonates are obligate nose breathers** because of weak oropharyngeal muscles. Their nares are relatively narrow, and a significant fraction of the work of breathing is needed to overcome their resistance. Occlusion of the nares by bilateral choanal atresia or tenacious secretions can cause complete airway obstruction. Placement of an oral airway, a laryngeal mask airway (LMA), or an endotracheal tube (ETT) may be necessary to reestablish airway patency during sedation or anesthesia.

2. **Infants have a relatively large tongue**, which makes mask ventilation and laryngoscopy challenging. The tongue can easily obstruct the airway if excessive submandibular pressure is applied during mask ventilation.

3. **Infants and children have a more cephalad glottis** (C-3 vertebral level in premature infants, C-4 in infants, C-5 in adults) and **a narrow, long, angulated epiglottis**, which can make laryngoscopy more difficult.

4. In infants and young children, **the narrowest part of the airway is at the cricoid cartilage**, rather than at the glottis (as in adults). An endotracheal tube that passes through the cords may still be too large distally.

5. **Deciduous teeth** erupt within the first year of age and are shed between ages 6 and 13 years. To avoid dislodging a loose tooth, it is safest to open the mandible directly, without introducing a finger or appliance into the oral cavity. Loose teeth should be documented on the preoperative evaluation. In some instances unstable teeth should be removed before laryngoscopy. Parents and patients should be informed of this possibility in advance.

6. **Airway resistance** in infants and children can be increased dramatically by subtle changes in an already small-caliber system. Even a small amount of edema can significantly increase airway resistance and cause airway compromise.

B. Pulmonary system
1. Neonates have **high metabolic rates**, resulting in an elevated oxygen consumption (6 to 9 mL/kg per minute) compared with adults (3 mL/kg per minute).

2. **Neonatal lungs have high closing volumes**, which fall within the lower range of their normal tidal volume. Below closing volume, alveolar collapse and shunting occurs.

3. To meet the higher oxygen demand, infants have a **higher respiratory rate and minute ventilation**. An infant's functional residual capacity (FRC), expressed as milliliters per kilogram, is nearly equivalent to adults (FRC of an infant,

25 mL/kg; adult, 40 mg/kg). Their higher minute ventilation to FRC ratio results in the rapid induction of anesthesia with inhalation agents. The tidal volume for infants and adults is equivalent (7 mL/kg).

4. Anatomic shunts including patent ductus arteriosus and patent foramen ovale may develop significant right-to-left flow with increases in pulmonary artery pressure (e.g., hypoxia, acidosis, or high positive airway pressure).

5. The characteristics of the infant's pulmonary system contribute to **rapid desaturation during apnea**. Profound desaturation can occur when an infant coughs or strains and alveoli collapse. Treatment may require deepening anesthesia with intravenous (IV) drugs or the use of neuromuscular relaxants.

6. The **diaphragm** is the infant's major muscle of ventilation. Compared with the adult diaphragm, the newborn has only half the number of Type I, slow-twitch, high-oxidative muscle fibers essential for sustained increased respiratory effort. Thus, the infant's diaphragm fatigues earlier than the adult's. By 2 years of age, the infant's diaphragm has attained mature levels of Type I fibers.

7. The **pliable rib cage** (compliant chest wall) of an infant cannot maintain negative intrathoracic pressure easily. This diminishes the efficacy of the infant's attempts to increase ventilation.

8. An infant's **dead space** is 2 to 2.5 mL/kg, equivalent to an adult's.

9. Infants' high baseline minute ventilation limits their ability to increase their ventilatory effort further. End-tidal CO_2 concentrations should be followed if spontaneous ventilation is permitted under anesthesia; assisted or controlled ventilation may be necessary.

10. Alveolar maturation occurs by 8 to 10 years of age when alveoli number and size reach adult ranges.

11. Retinopathy of prematurity. See Chapter 27, section VII.C.

12. Apnea and bradycardia following general anesthesia occur with increased frequency in infants who are premature and in infants who have anemia, sepsis, hypothermia, central nervous system (CNS) disease, hypoglycemia, hypothermia, or other metabolic derangements. These patients should have cardiorespiratory monitoring for a minimum of 24 hours postoperatively. Such infants are not candidates for ambulatory day surgery. The guidelines for discharge vary among institutions. Most hospitals agree that infants who are less than 45 to 55 weeks postconceptual age are monitored postoperatively. Any fullterm infant who displays apnea after general anesthesia is also monitored.

C. Cardiovascular system

1. Heart rate and **blood pressure** vary with age and should be maintained at age-appropriate levels perioperatively (Tables 28-1 and 28-2).

2. Cardiac output is 180 to 240 mL/kg per minute in newborns, which is two to three times that of adults. This higher cardiac output is necessary to meet the higher metabolic oxygen consumption demands.

Table 28-1. Age dependence of typical respiratory parameters

Variable	Newborn	1 Year	3 Years	5 Years	Adult
Respirations (breaths/min)	40–60	20–30	Gradual decrease to 18–25	18–25	12–20
Tidal volume (mL)	15	80	110	250	500
FRC (mL/kg)	25		35		40
Minute ventilation (L/min)	1	1.8	2.5	5.5	6.5
Hematocrit (%)	47–60	33.42	—	—	40–50
Arterial pH	7.30–7.40	7.35–7.45	—	—	—
$PaCO_2$ (mm Hg)	30–35	30–40	—	—	—
PaO_2 (mm Hg)	60–90	80–100	—	—	—

FRC, functional residual capacity.

Table 28-2.   Cardiovascular variables

| | Heart Rate (Beats/min) | Blood Pressure (mm Hg) | |
		Systolic	Diastolic
Age			
Preterm neonate	120–180	45–60	30
Term neonate	100–180	55–70	40
1 Year	100–140	70–100	60
3 Years	84–115	75–110	70
5 Years	80–100	80–120	70

3. The **ventricles** are less compliant and have a relatively smaller contractile muscle mass in newborns and infants. The ability to increase contractility is limited; increases in cardiac output occur by increasing heart rate rather than stroke volume. Bradycardia is the most deleterious arrhythmia in infants and hypoxemia is a frequent cause of bradycardia in infants and children.

D. Fluid and electrolyte balance

1. The **glomerular filtration rate** at birth is 15% to 30% of normal adult values. Adult values are reached by 1 year of age. Renal clearance of drugs and their metabolites is diminished during the first year of life.

2. Neonates have an intact renin-angiotensin aldosterone pathway, but the distal tubules resorb less sodium in response to aldosterone. Thus, newborns are "obligate sodium losers" and intravenous fluids should contain sodium.

3. The **total body water** in the preterm infant is 90% of body weight. In term infants, it is 80%; at 6 to 12 months, it is 60%. This increased percentage of total body water affects drug volumes of distribution. The dosages of some drugs (e.g., thiopental, propofol, succinylcholine, pancuronium, and rocuronium) are 20% to 30% greater than the equally effective dose for adults.

E. Hematologic system

1. Normal values for hematocrit are listed in Table 28-1. The nadir of physiologic anemia is at 3 months of age and the hematocrit may reach as low as 28% in an otherwise healthy infant. Premature infants may demonstrate a decrease in hemoglobin concentration as early as 4 to 6 weeks of age.

2. At birth, **fetal hemoglobin** (HbF) predominates, but β-chain synthesis shifts to the adult type (HbA) by 3 to 4 months of age. Fetal hemoglobin has a higher affinity for oxygen (the oxyhemoglobin dissociation curve is shifted to the left), but this is not clinically significant.

3. See section VII.B for calculations of blood volume and red cell mass.

F. Hepatobiliary system

1. Liver enzyme systems, particularly those involved in phase-II (conjugation) reactions, are immature in the infant.

Drugs metabolized by the P-450 system may have prolonged elimination times.

2. Jaundice is common in neonates and can be physiologic or have pathologic causes.

3. Hyperbilirubinemia and displacement of bilirubin from albumin by drugs can result in kernicterus. Premature infants develop kernicterus at lower levels of bilirubin than do term infants (see Chapter 27, section VI.A).

4. Plasma levels of albumin are lower at birth and this results in decreased protein binding of some drugs, and higher free drug concentration.

G. Endocrine system

1. Newborns, particularly premature babies and those small for gestational age, have decreased glycogen stores and are more susceptible to **hypoglycemia.** Infants of diabetic mothers have high insulin levels because of prolonged exposure to elevated maternal serum glucose levels and are prone to hypoglycemia. Infants who fall into these groups may have dextrose requirements as high as 5 to 15 mg/kg per minute. Normal glucose concentrations in the full-term infant is greater than or equal to 45 mg/dL (2.5 mmol/L).

2. Hypocalcemia is common in infants who are premature, small for gestational age, asphyxiated, offspring of diabetic mothers, or who have received transfusions with citrated blood or fresh-frozen plasma. Serum calcium concentration should be monitored in these patients and calcium chloride administered if the ionized calcium is less than 4.0 mg/dL (1.0 mmol/L).

H. Temperature regulation

1. Compared with adults, infants and children have a greater surface area to body weight ratio, which increases loss of body heat.

2. Infants have significantly less muscle mass and cannot compensate for cold by shivering or adjust their behavior to avoid the cold.

3. Infants respond to cold stress by increasing norepinephrine production, which enhances metabolism of brown fat. Norepinephrine also produces pulmonary and peripheral vasoconstriction, which can lead to right-to-left shunting, hypoxemia, and metabolic acidosis. Sick and preterm infants have limited stores of brown fat and therefore are more susceptible to cold. Strategies to prevent cold stress are discussed in section IV.C.

II. The preanesthetic visit. General principles of the preanesthetic visit are discussed in Chapter 1. The preoperative visit is an excellent opportunity to address the concerns of the child and parents. At least 90% of preoperative visits occur in an outpatient setting. Although some hospitals can schedule this evaluation a few weeks in advance, many preanesthetic evaluations occur on the day of surgery.

A. History should include:

1. Maternal health during gestation, including alcohol or drug use, smoking, diabetes, and viral infections.

2. Prenatal tests (e.g., ultrasound and amniocentesis).

3. Gestational age and weight.

4. Events during labor and delivery, including Apgar scores, and length of hospital stay.

5. Hospitalizations/emergency room visits.

6. Congenital chromosomal metabolic anomalies or syndromes.

7. Recent upper respiratory infections, tracheobronchitis, "croup," reactive airway disease (asthma), exposure to communicable diseases, cyanotic episodes, or history of snoring.

8. Sleeping position (prone, side, or supine).

9. Growth history.

10. Vomiting, gastroesophageal reflux.

11. Siblings' health.

12. Parents who smoke.

13. Past surgical and anesthetic history.

14. Allergies (environmental, drugs, food, and latex).

15. Bleeding tendencies.

B. **Physical examination** should include:

1. General appearance, including alertness, color, tone, congenital anomalies, head size and shape, activity level, and social interaction.

2. Vital signs, height, and weight.

3. Loose teeth, craniofacial anomalies, or large tonsils that could complicate airway management.

4. Signs of upper respiratory infection and/or reactive airways disease. Excessive secretions may predispose patients to laryngospasm and bronchospasm during induction and emergence of anesthesia.

5. Heart murmurs, which may indicate flow through anatomic shunts.

6. Potential vascular access sites.

7. Strength, developmental milestones, activity level, and motor and verbal skills.

C. **Laboratory data** appropriate for the child's illness and proposed surgery should be obtained. Most centers agree that a "routine hematocrit" is unnecessary for healthy children. If indicated, laboratory tests can often be obtained after induction of general anesthesia (e.g., blood bank sample).

III. **Premedication and fasting guidelines**

A. **Premedication**

1. Children have a range of social development. Their behavior may be influenced by experiences they have had at home, in day care or school, and during previous hospitalizations. Honesty about procedures and associated pain is essential to maintaining the trust of children regardless of their level of development. Reassuring the parents is often helpful in relieving a child's anxiety, but it is not a substitute for gentle interaction with the child.

2. Infants less than 10 months old generally tolerate short periods of separation from parents and usually do not require premedication.

3. Children 10 months to 5 years of age cling to their parents and may require sedation before the induction of anesthesia (see section V.B).

4. Older children generally respond well to information and reassurance. Parental and patient anxiety may be reduced by having parents accompany children to the operating room or to an adjacent holding area. An especially anxious child may benefit from premedication before entering the operating room. **Midazolam**, 0.5 mg/kg orally (PO), or **diazepam**, 0.2 to 0.3 mg/kg PO, given 15 to 20 minutes before surgery, is frequently used; it causes sedation with minimal respiratory depression. Opioids may produce respiratory depression. As preoperative medications, they are appropriate for the child in pain (e.g., trauma) or in the child undergoing a potentially stressful procedure (e.g., for children with congenital heart disease). **Chloral hydrate** (25 to 50 mg/kg PO or rectally) is a drug used by pediatricians and radiologists for sedation during procedures. It causes minimal respiratory depression, but may need to be repeated.

5. Premedication with intramuscular (IM) **anticholinergics** is not recommended. If vagolytic drugs are indicated, they are usually administered intravenously at the time of induction of anesthesia.

6. In the presence of **gastroesophageal reflux**, **ranitidine** (2 to 4 mg/kg PO, 2 mg/kg IV) or **cimetidine** (7.5 mg/kg PO), along with **metoclopramide** (0.1 mg/kg) can be administered 2 hours before surgery to increase gastric pH and reduce gastric volume.

7. Children receiving medications for medical problems such as reactive airways disease, seizures, or hypertension should continue to take these medications preoperatively.

8. Children with chronic diseases (e.g., seizures or sickle cell anemia) are familiar with frequent phlebotomy and may be very cooperative with intravenous placement, even without sedation.

B. Premedication and fasting guidelines

1. Milk, breast milk, formula, and solid foods should be restricted as outlined in Table 28-3.

2. The **last feeding** should consist of clear fluids or sugar water. Recent studies suggest that there may be no increased risk of aspiration if clear fluids are offered up to 2 hours preoperatively. Offering clear fluids closer to the time of surgery may decrease the chance of preoperative dehydration and hypoglycemia and contribute to a smoother induction and more stable operative course. We currently suggest that patients receive clear fluids until 2 hours before surgery is scheduled. Oral intake is then restricted (see Table 28-3).

3. If schedule delays occur, clear fluids may be given. Some patients may need to have an IV started for hydration.

IV. Preparation of the operating room

A. Anesthetic circuit

1. The **semiclosed circuit** normally used in adults has some disadvantages if used in very small infants:

Table 28-3. Fasting guidelines (hours)

Age (months)	Milk/solids	Clear Liquid
≤36	6	2
>36	8	2

Note: Water and apple juice are examples of clear liquids. Breast milk is considered a solid.

   a. The inspiratory and expiratory valves increase resistance during spontaneous ventilation.
   b. The large volume of the absorber system acts as a reservoir for anesthetic agents.
   c. The tubing has a large compression volume.
   2. The **nonrebreathing, open circuit (Mapleson D)** solves these problems (see Chapter 9). **Rebreathing** is prevented by using fresh gas flows 2.0 to 2.5 times the minute ventilation to wash out carbon dioxide. Capnography is essential in recognizing rebreathing (fraction of inspired CO_2 [F_{ICO_2}] greater than 0) and avoiding excessive hyperventilation. This circuit is useful for small infants who are allowed to breathe spontaneously.
   3. A passive heat and moisture exchanger may be used with either circuit.
   4. The **reservoir bag volume** should be at least as large as the child's vital capacity but small enough so that a comfortable squeeze does not overinflate the chest. General guidelines for bag volumes are: newborns, 500-mL bag; 1 to 3 years, 1,000-mL bag; and over 3 years, 2,000 mL bag.
   5. In children weighing 10 to 12 kg or more, the semi-closed circuit-absorber system can be utilized with a smaller reservoir bag and a circuit with small-caliber tubing. Semi-closed systems, particularly with controlled ventilation and routine end-tidal CO_2 (EtCO_2) monitoring, can also be used for children less than 10 kg.
B. Airway equipment
   1. A **mask** with minimal dead space should be chosen. A clear plastic type is preferred since the lips (for color) and mouth (for secretions and vomitus) can be visualized.
   2. The appropriate size of **oral airway** can be estimated by holding the airway in position next to the child's face. The tip of the oral airway should reach to the angle of the mandible.
   3. **Laryngoscopy**
      a. A **narrow handle** is preferred (since it has a more natural feel when using a smaller blade).
      b. A **straight blade** (Miller or Wis-Hipple) is recommended for children less than 2 years old. The smaller flange and long tapered tip of the straight blade provide better visualization of the larynx and manipulation of the epiglottis in the confined spaces of a small oral cavity.
      c. **Curved blades** are generally used for patients over 5 years old.
      d. **Guidelines for laryngoscope blade sizes** (see Table 28-4):
   4. **Endotracheal tubes.** Traditionally, uncuffed tubes were used for children under 6 to 7 years of age (5.5-mm inner diameter endotracheal tube or smaller). The ideal size will have a leak at 15- to 20-cm H_2O airway pressure. If the leak is present at less than 10 cm H_2O pressure, the endotracheal tube should be changed to the next larger size. Today, the risk of tracheal stenosis is minimal with modern low-pressure cuffs, and cuffed tubes may be used when indicated (e.g., tonsillectomy or proximal bowel obstruction). Care must be taken not to overinflate the cuff and to realize that N_2O can diffuse into the cuff. At the time of intubation, endotracheal tubes that are one size larger and

Table 28-4. Guidelines for choice of laryngoscope blades

Age	Blade
Premature and neonate	Miller 0
Infant up to 6–8 mo	Miller 0–1
9 months to 2 yr	Miller 1
	Wis-Hipple 1.5
2 to 5 yr	Macintosh 1
	Miller 1–1.5
Child over 5 yr	Macintosh 2
	Miller 2
Adolescent to adult	Macintosh 3
	Miller 2

smaller than the estimated size should be available. Special techniques of endotracheal intubation are discussed in section VI. See Table 28-5 for guidelines for endotracheal tube sizes.

C. Temperature control

1. The **operating room should be warmed** to between 80°F and 90°F before the child's arrival, and a heating blanket placed on the operating room table. Infants should be kept covered with a blanket and a hat.

2. A **servo-controlled radiant warmer** will keep infants warm during the induction of anesthesia and positioning. Skin temperature should be measured and should not exceed 39°C.

3. **Passive heat and moisture exchangers** can be used for most routine cases. Some practitioners prefer to actively heat and humidify inspired gases during prolonged surgery.

4. Fluids, blood products, and irrigation solutions should be warmed.

Table 28-5. Guidelines for endotracheal tube sizes

Age	Size (mm Internal Diameter)
Premature newborn	2.5–3.0
Full-term newborn	3.0
6–12 mo	3.5
12–20 mo	4.0
2 yr	4.5
Over 2 yr	4 + [age (years) / 4]
6 yr	5.5
10 yr	6.5

Note: Tube length at mouth (cm) = [10 + age (years)] / 2.

D. Monitoring

   1.   In addition to standard monitoring (Chapter 10), a **precordial or esophageal stethoscope** provides information about heart tones and respiratory parameters. It also helps the anesthetist to focus on the patient and not on extraneous sounds.

   2. Blood pressure

      a.   A blood pressure cuff should cover at least two-thirds of the upper arm but not encroach on the axilla or antecubital space.

      b.   The cuff can be placed on the leg if the arms are inaccessible (e.g., cast present).

   3. Pulse oximetry is important, not only because of the rapid rate of desaturation in infants and small children, but also in avoiding unnecessary hyperoxic conditions in premature infants.

   4.   Realize that observed **end-tidal carbon dioxide measurements** usually will be lower than expected when a nonrebreathing circuit is used, because exhaled gas will be diluted with high flows of fresh gases.

   5. Temperature should always be monitored. In small infants esophageal, rectal, or axillary probes are acceptable. Once the drapes are placed, the warming blanket and room temperature should be adjusted so that children (especially small infants) do not become hyperthermic.

   6. Urine output is an excellent reflection of volume status in children. In newborns, 0.5 mL/kg per hour is adequate; for infants over 1 month of age, 1.0 mL/kg per hour usually indicates adequate renal perfusion.

E. Intravenous setup and supplies

   1.   For children under 10 kg, a control chamber (burette) should be used to prevent inadvertent overhydration.

   2.   For older children, a pediatric infusion set is used where 60 drops equal 1 mL.

   3.   Extension tubing with a short T-piece connection is used so that injection ports are not draped out of reach. Drugs should be administered as close to the IV insertion site as possible to avoid excessive administration of flush solution.

   4.   Extra care should be taken to purge IV tubing of air, since, in principle, it is possible for infants to shunt right to left through a patent foramen ovale. An air filter should be used in infants and children with known intracardiac shunts.

V. Induction techniques

A. Infants less than 8 months old can be transported to the operating room without sedation; anesthesia can then be induced by an inhalation technique (see section V.C). The vessel-rich organs are proportionally larger and the muscle and fat groups smaller in neonates than in adults. This will affect uptake and distribution of inhalation agents (see Chapter 11).

B. Sedation options for children 8 months to 6 years old include:

   1.   Oral midazolam, 0.5 to 1.0 mg/kg, dissolved in sweet syrup, usually produces sedation within 20 minutes, although the time to onset of action can be quite variable. Patients often remain awake but sedated, and generally, they will have no recall of leaving their parents or of induction of anesthesia. Nasal midazolam (0.2 mg/kg) is another route, but its bitter taste often upsets children.

2. **Rectal methohexital** (Brevital), 25 to 30 mg/kg, in a 10% solution dissolved in sterile water is administered with a syringe fitted with soft plastic tubing into the distal 1 inch of the rectum. Blood flow to the proximal third of the rectum is drained into the portal circulation, where there is a significant first-pass effect for methohexital. Peak effect is after 10 to 15 minutes; if sedation does not occur after 20 minutes, the full dose is repeated. Resuscitation equipment and an anesthetist should be present after administering the drug, since it can produce respiratory depression. Parents should be advised that children frequently become excited or agitated before reaching a state of sedation.

3. **Diazepam** (0.1 to 0.5 mg/kg PO) provides sedation within approximately 30 minutes. Because this drug can be given by floor nursing personnel, its use is appropriate for inpatients.

4. **Oral transmucosal fentanyl** (Actiq, 5 to 15 μg/kg) provides both sedation and analgesia. Since respiratory depression can occur, an anesthetist must be immediately available when fentanyl is given.

5. **Pulse oximetry** is used routinely once a patient is sedated.

C. Inhalation induction

1. This is the most common approach for pediatric patients, except when a rapid sequence intravenous induction is indicated.

2. An "**excitement stage**" of anesthesia often is encountered during inhalation induction. Noise and activity in the operating room should be minimized during this time. This stage should be explained to parents if they will be present during induction since these purposeless movements can frighten parents.

3. **Techniques**

a. **Children 8 months to 5 years old** may be anesthetized after sedation with midazolam or rectal methohexital. The face mask is held near, but not touching, the child's face, and low flow rates (1 to 3 L per minute) of oxygen and nitrous oxide are begun. The concentration of volatile agent (sevoflurane or halothane) is gradually increased in 0.5% increments. When the lid reflex disappears, the mask can be applied to the child's face and the jaw gently lifted.

b. A **slow inhalation induction** may be used in cooperative toddlers and older children who have not been premedicated. Children are shown how to breathe through a clear anesthetic mask. Oxygen and N_2O are given via face mask, and then a volatile anesthetic is gradually added to the mixture. One can tell an engaging story, a fairy tale, or recount a favorite children's movie, and incorporate breathing instructions.

c. A "**single-breath induction**" may be accomplished with a few breaths of a mixture of a volatile anesthetic with nitrous oxide.

(**1**) Loss of consciousness can be achieved with a single vital capacity breath of 4% halothane or 8% sevoflurane and 70% $N_2O - O_2$. Sevoflurane has gained in popularity, because it is associated with less myocardial depression and bradycardia during induction than halothane. Desflurane, a very pungent volatile anesthetic, is not recommended for inhalation induction.

(2) The circuit is prefilled with 70% $N_2O - O_2$ and 7% to 8% sevoflurane or 4% to 5% halothane. The end of the circuit should be occluded with a plug or another reservoir bag and the pop-off valve left open to minimize nonscavenged anesthetic spillage.

(3) Painting the mask with flavor extracts may increase acceptance by children.

(4) The child is instructed to take a deep breath (vital capacity) of room air, blow it all out (forced expiration), and then hold his or her breath. At this point, the anesthetist gently places the mask on the patient's face. The child then takes a deep inspiration of the anesthetic mixture and again holds his or her breath. This sequence is repeated for four to five breaths.

(5) Most children will be anesthetized within 60 seconds; a few children will need longer.

   d. Children can become frightened, uncooperative, and even combative during an inhalation induction. Should this occur, it is imperative to have a backup plan, such as an IM injection of a sedative or hypnotic.

D. Intramuscular induction. For the extremely uncooperative or developmentally delayed child, anesthesia may be induced with ketamine (4 to 8 mg/kg IM), which takes effect in 3 to 5 minutes. Atropine (0.02 mg/kg IM) or glycopyrrolate (0.01 mg/kg IM) should be mixed with the ketamine to prevent excessive salivation. Midazolam, 0.2 to 0.5 mg/kg IM, may also be given to reduce the chance of emergence delirium that is occasionally seen with ketamine.

E. Intravenous induction

1. For children more than 8 years old, the option of IV placement should be considered. Older children may prefer an IV technique rather than a mask. Anesthesia is then induced with propofol (3 to 4 mg/kg), thiopental (4 to 6 mg/kg), or methohexital (1 to 2 mg/kg).

2. IV induction at this age is often preferable to a mask induction because many older children do not like the smell of volatile anesthetics. Local anesthesia before IV placement can be achieved with subcutaneous injection of lidocaine 1%. Alternatively (or additionally), **EMLA cream** (a eutectic mixture of 2.5% lidocaine and 2.5% prilocaine) can be applied to the skin, approximately 45 minutes before IV placement. EMLA cream is also useful to reduce the pain of accessing a Portacath.

F. Children with "full stomachs"

1. For **rapid sequence induction**, in general, the same principles apply to infants and children as for adults. In addition:

   a. Atropine (0.02 mg/kg) may be given IV to prevent bradycardia, especially if succinylcholine will be given.

   b. Children require larger doses of thiopental (4 to 6 mg/kg), propofol (3 to 4 mg/kg), and succinylcholine (1.5 to 2.0 mg/kg). This is because of a larger volume of distribution for these drugs.

   c. Infants with gastric distention (pyloric stenosis) should have their stomachs decompressed by an orogastric tube before induction of anesthesia. This gastric tube should again be suctioned before the trachea is extubated.

d. **Ranitidine** 2 to 4 mg/kg can be given to decrease gastric volume and increase gastric pH.

e. **Metoclopramide** should not be given if gastric outlet or bowel obstruction is suspected.

2. **An awake laryngoscopy and intubation** is an option for the moribund infant or an infant with a grossly abnormal airway (e.g., a severe craniofacial anomaly), with a "full stomach."

3. **A cuffed endotracheal tube** should be considered for a child with a full stomach. This option minimizes the need for replacing a small ETT. The cuff volume can be adjusted to ensure an appropriate air leak.

VI. **Endotracheal intubation**

A. **Oral approach**

1. Older children are placed in the "sniffing" position using a blanket. Infants and small children have large occiputs, and a small towel placed under the scapulae is more helpful.

2. During laryngoscopy, the tip of the blade is used to elevate the epiglottis. If this technique does not provide a good view of the glottis, the laryngoscope blade may be placed in the vallecula even with a straight blade.

3. The distance from the glottis to the carina is about 4 cm in a term neonate. Pediatric endotracheal tubes have a single black line located 2 cm from the tip and a double black line at 3 cm; these markings should be observed while the tube is passed beyond the vocal cords.

4. If resistance is met during intubation, a half-size smaller tube should be tried.

5. Following intubation, the chest should be examined for bilateral equal expansion and the lungs auscultated for equal breath sounds. There should be a leak around an uncuffed tube when 15- to 20-cm H_2O positive pressure is applied. Capnography should demonstrate consistently appropriate end-tidal CO_2 values.

6. The chest should be auscultated after every change in head or body position to verify equal bilateral breath sounds. Extension of the head can result in extubation, while flexion can result in tube advancement into either main-stem bronchus.

7. Endotracheal tubes should be securely taped, and the numerical marking on the tube closest to the gingiva noted; migration of the endotracheal tube will be apparent from any change in this relation.

8. The **laryngeal mask airway** (see Chapter 13, section IV) has revolutionized pediatric anesthesia. It has replaced the mask airway for simple cases (e.g., herniorrhaphy) and the endotracheal tube for many procedures (e.g., magnetic resonance imaging or computed tomography scan).

B. **Nasal approach**

1. This method is generally similar to that for adults (see Chapter 13).

2. The cephalad position of the infant larynx makes unaided intubation difficult; Magill forceps frequently are needed to guide the tip of the tube through the vocal cords.

3. Nasal intubation should be performed only when specifi-

cally indicated (e.g., oral surgery), due to the risk of epistaxis
from enlarged adenoids.

C.   **Apneic infants** will become hypoxemic within 30 to 45 seconds, even after preoxygenation. If bradycardia, cyanosis, or desaturation occurs, intubation attempts should cease immediately
and 100% oxygen administered until the oxygen saturation improves.

D.   **Muscle relaxants**

  1.   **Muscle relaxants** often are used to facilitate endotracheal
  intubation. Muscle relaxants may be contraindicated in infants
  and children with abnormal airway anatomy.

  2.   The use of **halothane and succinylcholine** together during induction is associated with an increased incidence of masseter spasm. This drug combination is rarely used in current
  practice; instead, nondepolarizing relaxants are generally selected unless rapid sequence induction is specifically indicated.

  3.   **Succinylcholine** can produce bradycardia, which may be
  exaggerated with repeated doses. If atropine has not been administered before the first dose of succinylcholine, it should be
  given before the second dose. In a few instances, succinylcholine has been associated with hyperkalemic cardiac arrest when
  given to children with an undiagnosed myopathy. It is our practice to limit the use of succinylcholine to situations requiring
  immediate control of the airway (e.g., laryngospasm or extreme
  gastric outlet obstruction associated with vomiting). Succinylcholine should not be given to children with a close family history of malignant hyperthermia (see Chapter 18, section XVII).

  4.   **Rocuronium** (0.6 to 1.2 mg/kg) and **mivacurium** (0.20 to
  0.25 mg/kg) have a quick onset of action. In most cases, these
  drugs have replaced succinylcholine when a rapid sequence induction is mandated.

  5.   Routine neuromuscular relaxation can be achieved with
  cisatracurium (0.1 to 0.2 mg/kg) for intubation.

  6.   For very long cases (e.g., craniotomy, cardiac surgery),
  pancuronium (0.1 mg/kg) is an option. Reversal of neuromuscular blockade with **neostigmine** (0.05 to 0.06 mg/kg) and an
  anticholinergic drug (e.g., atropine or glycopyrrolate) should
  occur if the twitch monitor or clinical exam suggests weakness.

VII.   **Fluid management.** The following calculations may be used
to estimate fluid requirements for infants and children. Other reflections of volume status, including blood pressure, heart rate, urine
output, central venous pressure, and osmolarity may guide further
adjustments.

A.   **Maintenance fluid requirements**

  1.   Administer 4 mL/kg per hour for the first 10 kg of body
  weight (100 mL/kg per day), 2 mL/kg per hour for the second
  10 kg (50 mL/kg per day), and then add 1 mL/kg per hour for
  more than 20 kg (25 mL/kg per day). For example, maintenance
  fluids for a 25-kg child would be ([4 × 10] + [2 × 10] + [1 ×
  5]) = 65 mL per hour.

  2.   The usual solution for replacement of fluid deficits and ongoing losses in the healthy child is **lactated Ringer's solution**.
  A second solution of 5% dextrose frequently is used in the perioperative period for premature infants, septic neonates, infants

of diabetic mothers, and those receiving total parenteral nutrition. These patients should have blood glucose levels measured periodically.

B. Estimated blood volume (EBV) and blood losses

1. **EBV** is 95 mL/kg in premature neonates, 90 mL/kg in full-term neonates, 80 mL/kg in infants up to 1 year old, and 70 mL/kg thereafter

2. **Estimated red cell mass (ERCM)**

$$ERCM = EBV \times patient\ hematocrit / 100.$$

3. **Acceptable red cell loss** (ARCL);

$$ARCL = ERCM - ERCM_{acceptable},$$

which is the ERCM at the lowest acceptable hematocrit.

4. **Acceptable blood loss (ABL)**

$$ABL = ARCL \times 3.$$

   a. If the amount of the blood loss is less than one-third of the ABL, it can be replaced with lactated Ringer's solution.
   b. If the amount of blood loss is greater than one-third of the total ABL, one should consider replacement with colloid (e.g., 5% albumin).
   c. If the amount of blood loss is greater than ABL, replace with packed red blood cells and an equal amount of colloid. Fresh-frozen plasma and platelet transfusions should be guided by results of coagulation tests, estimates of the present and anticipated blood losses, and adequacy of clot formation in the wound.
   d. For infants and young children, blood loss should be measured using small suction containers and by weighing sponges. Since it is sometimes difficult to measure small-volume blood losses precisely in young children, monitoring of hematocrit will help avoid unnecessary transfusions and also alert the anesthetist to the need for blood transfusion.
   e. The "**acceptable hematocrit**" is no longer considered to be 30%. Each patient is evaluated with respect to the need for red blood cell transfusion. A healthy child with normal cardiac function can compensate for acute anemia by increasing cardiac output. A debilitated child, confronting sepsis, chemotherapy, or massive surgery, may require a higher hematocrit.

C. Estimated fluid deficit = (maintenance fluid per hour) × hours since the last oral intake. The entire estimated fluid deficit is replaced during all major cases; the first half is administered during the first hour, and the remaining deficit is infused over the next 1 to 2 hours.

D. Third-space losses may require up to an additional 10 mL/kg per hour of lactated Ringer's solution or normal saline if there is extensive exposure of the intestine or a significant ileus.

VIII. Emergence and postanesthesia care

A. Extubation

1. **Laryngospasm** may occur during emergence, especially during the critical period of excitement.

2. In the majority of cases, the trachea is extubated after emergence from anesthesia. Coughing is not a sign that the child is ready for extubation. Instead, children should demonstrate purposeful activity (e.g., reaching for the endotracheal tube) or eye opening before extubation. In the infant, hip flexion and strong grimaces are useful indications of awakening.

3. Alternatively, the trachea may be extubated while the patient is still anesthetized deeply. This can be done in operations such as inguinal herniorrhaphy where coughing on emergence is undesirable or in patients with reactive airways disease. A "deep" extubation would not be appropriate for a child with an abnormal airway or one who has eaten recently.

B. During transport to the postanesthesia care unit (PACU), the child's color and ventilatory pattern should be continuously monitored. Supplemental oxygen is administered if indicated (e.g., the child with anemia or pulmonary disease).

C. In the PACU, early reunion of the child and parents is desirable.

IX. Specific pediatric anesthesia problems

A. The compromised airway

1. Etiologies

a. Congenital abnormalities (e.g., choanal atresia, Pierre Robin syndrome, tracheal stenosis, or laryngeal web).

b. Inflammation (e.g., tracheobronchitis or "croup," epiglottitis, pharyngeal abscess).

c. Foreign bodies in the trachea or esophagus.

d. Neoplasms (e.g., congenital hemangioma, cystic hygroma, or thoracic lymphadenopathy).

e. Trauma.

2. Initial management

a. Administer 100% oxygen by face mask.

b. Keep the child as calm as possible. Evaluation should be efficient, since it may increase agitation and cause further airway compromise. Parents are invaluable in their ability to pacify their children and should remain with them as long as feasible.

c. An anesthetist must be present during transport to the operating room. Oxygen, a resuscitation bag and mask, laryngoscope, atropine, succinylcholine, drugs suitable for sedation and hypnosis, appropriate endotracheal tubes and LMAs, oral airways, and pulse oximetry must be available.

3. Induction of anesthesia

a. Minimize manipulation of the patient. A precordial stethoscope and pulse oximeter are adequate monitors during the initial induction of anesthesia.

b. The child may remain in a **semi-sitting position**, with the parents present if indicated. A **gradual inhalation induction** with either sevoflurane or halothane is the next step (see section V.C.3). Airway obstruction and poor air exchange will prolong induction.

c. Parents are asked to leave when the child becomes unconscious, and an IV is started. If indicated, atropine may be given at this time.

d. Patients with croup may benefit from gentle application of continuous positive airway pressure, but any positive pressure can cause acute airway obstruction in patients with epiglottitis or a foreign body.

c. The **oral endotracheal tube** should have a stylet and be at least one size smaller than the predicted size. If postoperative ventilation is anticipated (e.g., epiglottitis), a cuffed ETT may be indicated.

f. At this point, patients usually are hypercarbic ($EtCO_2$ between 50 to 60 mmHg), but generally this is well tolerated provided they are not also hypoxemic. Bradycardia is an indication of hypoxemia and requires immediate establishment of a patent airway.

g. Perform laryngoscopy only when the child is deeply anesthetized. The decision to give a muscle relaxant depends on the situation. A muscle relaxant facilitates intubation and obviates the need for deep anesthesia in certain circumstances. In other cases, muscle relaxation may further compromise the airway. In general, orotracheal intubation should be accomplished before any further airway procedures are attempted. **Bronchoscopy** is indicated before intubation in cases of large upper airway foreign bodies or friable subglottic tumors (e.g., hemangiomas).

h. **A nasal tube** may be more appropriate for illnesses that require several days of intubation (e.g., epiglottitis). An orotracheal tube may be changed to nasotracheal tube at the end of the procedure, provided the oral intubation was easily accomplished. Never jeopardize a secure oral ETT for the sake of changing it to nasal ETT.

i. Children should be sedated during transport to the intensive care unit; a combination of a narcotic, a benzodiazepine or propofol infusion is effective. Propofol is not approved in the United States for prolonged sedation of pediatric intensive care patients. Breathing may be spontaneous or assisted during the immediate postoperative period.

B. **Recent upper respiratory infection.** Infants and children can have 6 to 10 upper respiratory infections each year. It is important to balance the severity of symptoms with the urgency of surgery. Wheezing, fever, and cough are signs of lower respiratory inflammation and are associated with an increased risk of perioperative airway complications. Conversely, myringotomy and ear tube placement may relieve the rhinorrhea associated with chronic otitis media.

C. **Intraabdominal malformations** include pyloric stenosis, gastroschisis, omphalocele, atresia of the small intestine, and volvulus (see Chapter 27).

1. **Gastrointestinal emergencies** frequently produce marked dehydration and electrolyte abnormalities. Repair of pyloric stenosis should be delayed until intravascular volume is restored and the hypokalemic, hypochloremic, metabolic alkalosis is corrected. The situation is more urgent with other diagnoses (e.g., duodenal athesia), and rehydration can be continued intraoperatively.

2. **Abdominal distention** in infants and young children rapidly causes respiratory compromise, so nasogastric drainage is mandatory. Even so, a few moribund infants may require endotracheal intubation before the induction of anesthesia.

3.   Children with less severe physiologic disturbances and only mild or moderate distention can undergo a rapid sequence induction of anesthesia.

4.   A severely dehydrated and septic child may require additional monitoring (e.g., arterial, central venous pressure, and urinary catheters).

5.   Volatile anesthetics are appropriate for the previously healthy infant undergoing a simple operation (such as pyloromyotomy). In the case of an extremely ill child (e.g., perforated viscous), the anesthetic management should include an O_2–air mixture and drugs causing minimal myocardial depression. Opioids (morphine 0.1 to 0.2 mg/kg IV; fentanyl 1 to 2 µg/kg IV; and meperidine, 1 to 2 mg/kg IV), benzodiazepines, and neuromuscular relaxants are usually better tolerated than volatile anesthetics. Nitrous oxide should be avoided since it may add to abdominal distention.

6.   **Fluid and heat losses**. When the bowel is exposed and manipulated, third-space losses may be excessive and remarkable fluid volumes may be necessary. Even when employing all possible warming strategies, heat loss may be unavoidable.

7.   Postoperative ventilatory support is often indicated until abdominal distention is diminished, hypothermia resolves, and fluid requirements decrease.

D.   Thoracic emergencies
  1.   **Tracheoesophageal fistula**. See Chapter 27.
  2.   **Congenital diaphragmatic hernia**. See Chapter 27.
E.   Congenital heart disease. See Chapters 2, 23, and 27.
F.   Head and neck procedures
  1.   Strabismus repair. See Chapter 25.
  2.   Tonsillectomy, adenoidectomy, and emergency surgery in the child with bleeding tonsils. See Chapter 25.

X.   Regional anesthesia for pediatric patients has gained acceptance because of a better understanding of the pharmacokinetics and pharmacodynamics of local anesthetics in infants and children and the availability of specifically designed equipment.

A.   Pharmacology of local anesthetics
  1.   **Protein binding** of local anesthetics is decreased in neonates because of decreased levels of serum albumin. Free drug concentration may be increased, especially for bupivacaine.
  2.   **Plasma cholinesterase activity** may be decreased in infants under 6 months old, which theoretically diminishes clearance of amino esters.
  3.   **Hepatic microsomal enzyme systems** are immature in the neonate and this will decrease the clearance of amino amides.
  4.   **The increased volume of distribution** in the infant and child acts to decrease free local anesthetic concentrations in the blood.
  5.   **Systemic toxicity** is the most frequent complication of regional anesthetics, and doses should be carefully calculated on a weight basis. The risk of accumulation of free drug following repeated doses of local anesthetics is increased in infants and children.

B.   Spinal anesthesia
  1.   **Indications**

a. Premature infants less than 60 weeks postconceptual age and infants with a history of apnea and bradycardia, bronchopulmonary dysplasia, or need for long-term ventilatory support are at increased risk for apnea and cardiovascular instability following general anesthesia. Spinal anesthesia may decrease the likelihood of these postoperative anesthetic complications. These infants still require a minimum of 24 hours of cardiorespiratory monitoring postoperatively, regardless of the anesthetic technique. Sedation during spinal anesthesia may negate all of these potential benefits.

b. Children at risk for malignant hyperthermia.

c. Children with chronic airways disease such as reactive airway disease or cystic fibrosis.

d. Cooperative older children and adolescents with full stomachs undergoing peripheral emergency surgery (e.g., fractured ankle).

2. **Anatomy.** See Chapter 16.

3. **Technique**

a. The procedure may be performed with the patient in the lateral decubitus or sitting position. Premature infants and neonates are positioned in the sitting position to limit rostral spread of drug. The head is supported upright to prevent upper airway obstruction. A 22-gauge, 1.5-inch spinal needle is used for infants, since cerebrospinal fluid flow is very slow. In children older than 2 years, a 25-gauge needle is preferable.

b. An IV should be started before spinal anesthesia and the patient should be monitored throughout the procedure. Maintaining normothermia is essential, especially for premature infants and neonates. The infant should remain supine after placement of the spinal anesthetic; Trendelenburg positioning should be avoided, since this may move the drug cephalad in the subarachnoid space.

4. **Drugs and dosage**

a. Hyperbaric solutions of bupivacaine or tetracaine are used most frequently.

b. The dosage requirements are increased and the duration of action is decreased in infants.

c. **Recommended dosages** (for a T-6 spinal level)

(1) Bupivacaine, 0.75% in 8.25% dextrose, 0.3 mg/kg in both infants and children.

(2) Tetracaine, 1%, combined with an equal volume of 10% dextrose, 0.8 to 1.0 mg/kg in the infant and 0.25 to 0.5 mg/kg in the child. This dose is large when compared with adult dosage, but is necessary in infants.

d. **Duration of surgical anesthesia** averages 90 minutes with tetracaine, and less with bupivacaine. The duration of the block may be prolonged by the addition of epinephrine, 10 μg/kg (up to 0.2 mg), or phenylephrine, 75 μg/kg (up to 2 mg).

5. **Complications and contraindications**

a. **The anesthetic level** recedes much more quickly in children than in adults. If the block wears off, supplemental sedation must be used cautiously, especially in premature infants and neonates. If subarachnoid anesthesia is inadequate, it is best to initiate general anesthesia before positioning.

b. Hypotension is rare in children less than 7 to 10 years old, perhaps because resting sympathetic vascular tone is lower than in adults. A high spinal anesthetic may be heralded only by mottled skin or apnea and bradycardia.

c. Contraindications are similar to those in adults, with particular attention to congenital anatomic defects of the central nervous system and a history of intraventricular hemorrhage.

C. **Caudal and lumbar epidural anesthesia**

1. **Indications**. These techniques are useful in combination with general anesthesia for minor and major procedures of the thorax, abdomen, pelvis, bladder, and lower extremities, particularly when significant postoperative pain is anticipated (e.g., orthopedic surgery).

2. **Anatomy** is outlined in Chapter 16. Note that the dural sac ends at the level of the S-3 vertebra in the neonate; care is required to avoid dural puncture during placement of the caudal needle.

3. **Technique** is outlined in Chapter 16.

a. Most caudal and lumbar epidural anesthetics are placed after induction of general anesthesia.

b. Caudal anesthesia may be administered as a single injection of local anesthetic through a 1.5-inch, short-bevel needle placed into the caudal epidural space. This technique is ideally suited for short procedures with mild to moderate postoperative pain such as inguinal herniorrhaphy, orchiopexy, and circumcision. For longer procedures or prolonged postoperative analgesia, a catheter may be advanced from the sacral epidural space. Intermittent boluses or a continuous infusion of local anesthetic with or without an opioid may be used. In infants, 22-gauge caudal catheters are placed through 20-gauge, 40- to 50-mm Tuohy needles; older children require 20-gauge catheters placed through 17- or 18-gauge, 90- to 100-mm Tuohy needles.

c. Caudal catheters can be advanced to lumbar or thoracic levels in young children because the epidural space is not yet extensively vascularized. The recommended levels are: T-6 to T-9 vertebral level for thoracic surgery (e.g., pectus excavatum repair); T-10 to T-12 vertebral level for abdominal surgery (e.g., Nissen fundoplication or bowel resections); and L-3 to L-4 vertebral level for pelvic procedures. Usually these catheters advance easily; resistance may indicate malpositioning. If necessary, confirmation of catheter placement can be done using contrast dye and fluoroscopy. While easy to place, compared with a lumbar catheter, the caudal catheter has a greater potential to become contaminated from stool. Also, the catheter may become dislodged postoperatively.

d. Epidural catheters may be placed via lumbar or thoracic approaches. The distance from the skin to the epidural space is short (1 to 2 cm) in children, and again, care must be taken to avoid dural puncture. Loss of resistance is usually accomplished with saline. In older children, 18-gauge Tuohy needles and 20-gauge catheters are used. Thoracic catheters are useful for pectus excavation repair or thoracotomy. Placement of a thoracic epidural catheter in anesthetized children depends on the practitioner's skills and experience. Some might argue that this method may cause inadvertent injury, while others believe that an awake 7-year-old cannot reliably remain still during this procedure.

4. **Drugs and doses**

a. In **single-dose caudal anesthesia**, a long duration of sensory blockade with minimal motor blockade is desirable. Bupivacaine, 0.125% to 0.25% with epinephrine, is administered according to the formula of 0.06 mL of local anesthetic per kilogram per segment, where number of segments is counted from the S-5 spinal level to the desired level of analgesia. A simple alternative dosing scheme is to administer 0.125% bupivacaine with epinephrine at a dose of 1 mL/kg. Increasing the concentration of bupivacaine above 0.25% does not appear to improve analgesia. Dosages of bupivacaine up to 3.5 mg/kg result in plasma levels in infants and children below the toxic range determined for adults. Ropivacaine 0.125% is now being evaluated for caudal anesthesia in children.

b. **Caudal or epidural catheter anesthesia**

(1) **Intermittent bolus dosing**. Initially, 1% lidocaine, 0.5 mL/kg, followed by 0.5% lidocaine, 0.5 mL/kg every hour as needed, or initially, 0.25% to 0.5% bupivacaine, 0.5 mL/kg, followed by 0.25% bupivacaine, 0.25 mL/kg every 1.5 to 2.0 hours as needed, is recommended.

(2) **Continuous infusion**. An initial loading dose of 0.04 mL/kg per segment of 0.1% bupivacaine with or without fentanyl, 3 μg/mL in infants and children younger than 7 years and 0.02 mL/kg per segment for children older than 7 years, is recommended. An infusion of 0.1% bupivacaine with or without fentanyl, 3 μg/mL at 0.1 mL/kg per hour, is started immediately following the bolus. The infusion rate may be increased to 0.3 mL/kg per hour as needed, with the total hourly dose of fentanyl not to exceed 1 μg/kg per hour. Infants younger than 1 year generally do not receive fentanyl in the epidural infusion, unless they are in a closely monitored setting (see Chapter 37, section III.E.).

c. **Postoperative analgesia** may be provided by infusion through the caudal or epidural catheter. Generally, an infusion of 0.1% bupivacaine with fentanyl, 3 μg/mL at 0.1 to 0.3 mL/kg per hour, will provide good analgesia without motor blockade. However, some patients benefit from omission of local anesthetic from the infusion, and fentanyl, 0.5 to 1.0 μg/kg per hour can be used in these patients. Infants younger than 1 year old, as noted above, usually do not receive epidural opioids because of concern about postoperative respiratory depression. These infants receive an infusion of 0.1% bupivacaine, 0.1 to 0.3 mL/kg per hour.

5. **Contraindications** are the same as for spinal anesthesia (see section X.B.5).

6. **Complications** of epidural and caudal anesthesia are discussed in Chapter 16.

D. **Brachial plexus blocks** (for upper extremity surgery), **penile blocks** (for circumcision), and **ilio-inguinal blocks** (for inguinal herniorrhaphy) are particularly useful regional techniques in the pediatric population. See Gregory's *Pediatric anesthesia,* and Dalen's *Regional anesthesia in infants, children and adolescents* for additional details (referenced in Suggested Readings section).

SUGGESTED READING

Behrman RE, Kliegman R, Jenson HB. *Nelson textbook of pediatrics*, 16th ed. Philadelphia: WB Saunders, 2000.

Cloherty J, Stark A. *Manual of neonatal care*, 4th ed. Philadelphia: Lippincott Williams & Wilkins, 1998.

Coté CJ, Ryan JF, Goudsouzian NG. *A practice of anesthesia for infants and children*, 3rd ed. Philadelphia: WB Saunders, 2000.

Dalens B. *Regional anesthesia in infants, children, and adolescents.* Baltimore: Williams & Wilkins, 1995.

Dorsch J, Dorsch S. The Mapleson breathing systems. In: *Understanding anesthesia equipment*, 4th ed. Baltimore: Williams & Wilkins, 1999: 207–227.

Greeley WJ. *Pediatric anesthesia.* New York: Churchill Livingstone, 1999.

Gregory GA. *Pediatric anesthesia*, 4th ed. New York: Churchill Livingstone, 2001.

Miller RD, Miller ED Jr, Reves, JG, eds. *Anesthesia*, 5th ed. New York: Churchill Livingstone, 2000.

Motoyama EK, Davis PJ. *Smith's anesthesia for infants and children*, 6th ed. St. Louis: Mosby–Year Book, 1996.

O'Neill JA, Rowe MI, Grosfeld J. *Pediatric surgery*, 5th ed. St. Louis: Mosby–Year Book, 1998.

Siberry GK, Iannone R, Childs B. *The Harriet Lane handbook: a manual for pediatric house officers*, 15th ed. St. Louis: Mosby–Year Book, 2000.

Anesthesia for Obstetrics and Gynecology

Jeannie Min and Tania Haddad

I. **Maternal physiology in pregnancy** (Table 29-1)
A. **Respiratory system**
   1. **Capillary engorgement of the mucosa** takes place throughout the respiratory tract. This swelling decreases the size of the glottic opening such that a 6.0- to 6.5-mm (inner diameter) endotracheal tube is recommended for intubation to decrease the possibility of airway trauma. **Airway edema** may also make intubation more difficult in the pregnant patient, especially during labor.
B. **Cardiovascular system**
   1. **Blood volume** increases markedly throughout the course of pregnancy. Since the plasma volume increases more than the red cell volume increases, a relative dilutional anemia occurs.
   2. **Cardiac output increases 50%** with pregnancy. During labor, contractions of the engorged uterus provides a 300- to 500-mL autotransfusion into the maternal circulation, leading to a further increase in cardiac output. **Cardiac output becomes highest immediately postpartum** and can reach 80% to 100% above the prelabor value. Blood pressure is not increased in normal pregnancy, indicative of decreased peripheral vascular resistance.
   3. After 20 weeks gestation, the gravid uterus may **obstruct the aorta and inferior vena cava** of the patient, especially when the patient is supine. This may result in decreased venous return, decreased cardiac output, hypotension, and decreased uteroplacental blood flow. Following compression of the vena cava, the parturient may become symptomatic, exhibiting hypotension, increased pallor, sweating, nausea, vomiting, and neurologic changes. Fetal distress is associated with aortic compression secondary to decreased uterine blood flow. Compression of the aorta is not associated with maternal symptoms. Left uterine displacement is used to prevent aortocaval compression when supine.
   4. The pregnant patient is **hypercoagulable** throughout gestation. This hypercoagulable state leads to decreased blood loss at delivery. Normal blood loss is about 500 mL for vaginal delivery and 1,000 mL for cesarean section.
C. **Nervous system**
   1. The **minimum alveolar concentration** for inhalational anesthetics is decreased up to 40% during pregnancy. The etiology for this is unclear but may be related to alterations of hormone and endorphin concentrations during pregnancy, which may lead to an increased pain threshold or pregnancy-induced analgesia.

Table 29-1.   Physiologic changes associated with pregnancy

System	Parameters	Changes
Respiratory	*Capacities/volume*	
	Total lung capacity	−5%
	Vital capacity	No change
	Functional residual capacity	−20%
	Inspiratory reserve volume	+5%
	Expiratory reserve volume	−20%
	Residual volume	−15
	Closing capacity	No change
	Tidal volume	+45%
	Mechanics	
	FEV_1	No change
	FEV_1/FVC	No change
	Minute ventilation	+45%
	Alveolar ventilation	+45%
	Blood gases	
	$PaCO_2$	−10%
	PaO_2	+5–10%
	pH	No change
	HCO_3^-	Decrease
	Oxygen consumption	+20%
	P50 at term	30 mm Hg
Cardiovascular	Cardiac output	+50%
	Stroke volume	+25%

Hematology	Heart rate	+20–25%
	Systematic vascular resistance	–20%
	Blood volume	+45%
	Plasma volume	+55%
	Red blood cell volume	+25%
	Coagulation factors	
	Factors VII, VIII, IX, X, XII, fibrinogen	Increase
	Prothrombin	No change
	Factors XI, XIII	Decrease
	Platelet count	No change or decrease
	Total protein (albumin, globulin)	Decrease
Central nervous system	MAC	Decrease
	Local anesthetic requirement	Decrease
Gastrointestinal	*Gastric emptying*	
	First trimester	No change
	Second trimester	No change
	Third trimester	No change
	Labor	Decrease
	Postpartum (18 h)	No change
	Barrier pressure	
	First, second, third, trimester, labor	Decrease
Hepatic	AST, ALT, LDH, bilirubin	Increase
	Alkaline phosphatase	Increase
Renal	Glomerular filtration rate	+50%
	Renal plasma flow	+75%

   2.   The pregnant patient requires **less local anesthetic** to produce the same degree of epidural anesthesia than a nonpregnant
patient. Reasons for this include:
   a.   Distended epidural veins, which decrease the effective
   size of the epidural space and prevent loss of drug through
   the intervertebral foramina.
   b.   Low cerebrospinal fluid protein, which increases the
   unbound fraction of the local anesthetic, resulting in a greater
   proportion of free active drug.
   c.   Elevated cerebrospinal fluid (CSF) pH, which increases the unionized fraction of the local anesthetic.
   d.   There may also be **hormonally induced changes** in sensitivity to local anesthetics from increased progesterone levels. The need for 30% less local anesthetic for subarachnoid
   anesthesia has also been noted.
   3.   Because of increased intraabdominal pressure, **the epidural veins become distended**, making a bloody tap during
placement of an epidural catheter more common.
   4.   During pregnancy the role of **the sympathetic nervous
system (SNS) increases**. The parturient is highly dependent
on the SNS for hemodynamic control, which reflects the significant decrease in blood pressure seen after regional anesthesia.
The role of the SNS returns to normal by approximately 48 hours
postpartum.
D.   Gastrointestinal system. The gravid uterus causes a shift
in the position of the stomach, resulting in gastric reflux and heart-
burn in most pregnant patients. Though gastric emptying is not
delayed during most of pregnancy, it is delayed during labor. Thus,
the pregnant patient should be considered at increased risk for
aspiration. If general anesthesia is planned, a nonparticulate antacid should be given routinely; a histamine (H_2) blocker and metoclopramide should be considered, and rapid sequence induction
used. Exactly when during pregnancy a woman becomes at risk
for regurgitation is controversial. Barrier pressure, which is the
difference between intragastric pressure and the tone of the lower
esophageal high-pressure zone, is decreased as early as the first
trimester. In general, any patient in her third trimester or with
symptoms of esophagitis during pregnancy should have a rapid
sequence induction.
E.   Renal system. Renal plasma flow and glomerular filtration
may increase up to 50%, leading to increased creatinine clearance
and a decrease in normal blood urea nitrogen and creatinine levels.
F.   Musculoskeletal. Exaggeration of the normal lumbar lordosis secondary to the enlarging uterus can produce a sensory loss
over the anterolateral thigh or meralgia parasthetica. This is due
to a stretching of the lateral femoral cutaneous nerve by the increased lumbar lordosis. Carpal tunnel syndrome and a widening
of the pubic symphysis is thought to be secondary to an increase
in the hormone relaxin during pregnancy.
II.   Labor and delivery
A.   Labor can be divided into three stages.
   1.   The **first stage** begins with the onset of regular contractions and ends with full cervical dilation. It is divided into a
slow latent phase and a rapidly progressive active phase.

2. The **second stage** extends from full cervical dilation to delivery of the infant.

3. The **third stage** begins with delivery of the infant and ends with delivery of the placenta.

B. **Pain** during the first part of labor is primarily caused by uterine contractions and cervical dilation. Nerve fibers that transmit pain during the first part of labor enter the spinal cord from T-10 to L-1. In late first-stage and early second-stage labor, pain is due to perineal stretching and travels through the S-2 to S-4 segments via the pudendal nerve.

C. **Physiologic changes during labor** tend to accentuate many of the changes already present during pregnancy. Oxygen uptake, which may increase 20% in a normal pregnancy, may increase an additional 60% during painful uterine contractions.

D. **Fetal monitoring** can provide a fairly accurate assessment of fetal well-being. Normal fetal heart rate (FHR) ranges from 120 to 160 beats per minute. Monitoring the response of the fetal heart rate to uterine contractions can alert physicians to possible distress. An increase in FHR may signify fetal asphyxia, maternal fever, chorioamnionitis, or maternally administered drugs. Decreased FHR is generally secondary to hypoxia; however, central nervous system depressants can also cause a decrease in FHR (Fig. 29-1).

1. **Early decelerations** occur concomitantly with uterine contraction and provide a mirror image of the contraction on the monitor printout. They are thought to be caused by an increase in vagal tone, perhaps from compression of the fetal head, and do not require intervention.

2. **Late decelerations** have their beginning and resolution delayed after the onset of uterine contraction by 10 to 30 seconds. These are caused by a decrease in uterine blood flow during the contraction, leading to fetal hypoxia. Late decelerations are cause for alarm. When associated with loss of normal baseline "beat-to-beat" variability, they may be indicative of direct neonatal myocardial hypoxia. Vigorous efforts should be made to eliminate late decelerations by correcting maternal hypotension, ensuring the adequacy of left uterine displacement, and administering oxygen by face mask to the mother.

3. **Variable decelerations** are variable in duration and appearance from one contraction to the next and are usually associated with umbilical cord compression. They may be associated with fetal compromise when severe (heart rate below 70 for more than 60 seconds), but generally only when they have occurred for periods greater than 30 minutes. Vigorous efforts should be made to correct these as well.

4. **Fetal scalp blood sampling** is used to determine the degree of fetal acidosis from asphyxia when abnormal fetal heart rate patterns cannot be corrected or their significance is unclear. In general, if the pH is above 7.25, the fetus will be vigorous at birth, while a pH below 7.20 suggests that the fetus is acidotic and asphyxiated and requires immediate delivery. If the pH is in the range of 7.20 to 7.25, close monitoring is recommended as well as repeat scalp sampling to monitor for acidosis.

III. **Medications commonly used for labor and delivery**

A. **Vasopressors.** Hypotension can result from regional anes-

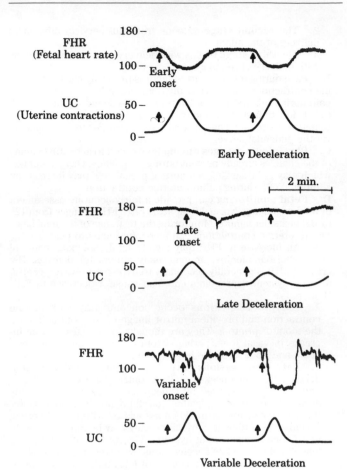

Fig. 29-1.   Patterns of periodic fetal heart rate (FHR) decelerations in relation to uterine contractions (UC).

thesia, aortocaval compression, or peripartum hemorrhage. Warning symptoms of maternal hypotension include lightheadedness, nausea, difficulty with breathing, and diaphoresis. Regional anesthesia that produces a sympathetic blockade decreases systemic vascular resistance. The uteroplacental circulation is regulated by alpha-adrenergic receptors which, when stimulated, reduce uteroplacental blood flow despite an increase in systemic blood pressure. The ideal vasopressor for obstetric anesthesia should increase maternal blood pressure without decreasing uteroplacental blood flow. Such a drug should have predominant beta-adrenergic effects and limited alpha effects.

1.   Ephedrine stimulates both alpha and beta adrenergic receptors and thus provides cardiac stimulation with a subsequent increase in peripheral and uterine blood flow. Ephedrine is the drug of choice for treatment of maternal hypotension.

2. **Pure alpha-adrenergic agents** such as phenylephrine and mixed alpha agonists such as epinephrine and norepinephrine are vasoconstrictors that will increase maternal blood pressure at the expense of uteroplacental blood flow. However, phenylephrine in small doses to treat maternal hypotension has been shown to produce no effect on uteroplacental flow. It is used only when ephedrine is ineffective or contraindicated.

B. **Oxytocics** are agents that stimulate uterine contractions.
   1. **Indications**
       a. To induce or augment labor.
       b. To control postpartum bleeding and uterine atony.
       c. To induce therapeutic abortion.
   2. The most frequently used drugs include the synthetic posterior pituitary hormone, **oxytocin** (Pitocin); and the ergot alkaloids, **ergonovine** (Ergotrate) and **methylergonovine** (Methergine).
       a. **Oxytocin** acts on the uterine smooth muscle to stimulate both the frequency and force of contractions. It also has effects on the cardiovascular system, producing vasodilation and hypotension (especially decreasing diastolic blood pressure) and also tachycardia and arrhythmias. In high doses, oxytocin may have an antidiuretic effect and produce water intoxication, cerebral edema, and convulsions in the presence of overzealous intravenous (IV) hydration. Pitocin routinely is given by continuous IV infusion.
       b. **Ergot alkaloids** in small doses increase the force and frequency of uterine contractions, which are followed by normal uterine relaxation. At higher doses, contractions become more intense and prolonged, resting tonus is increased, and tetanic contractions occur. For these reasons, the use of ergot alkaloids is restricted to control postpartum bleeding in the third stage of labor. These drugs also have effects on the cardiovascular system, including vasoconstriction and hypertension, especially in the presence of vasopressors. Intramuscular (IM) administration is recommended, since IV injection has been associated with severe hypertension, convulsions, stroke, retinal detachment, and pulmonary edema.
       c. **Prostaglandin 15-methyl $F_{2\alpha}$** has become the third line of therapy, following oxytocin and ergot alkaloids, to achieve tetanic uterine contraction as treatment for uterine atony. Transient hypertension, severe bronchoconstriction, and increased pulmonary vascular resistance have been reported following its use. Caution must be used in patients with a history of asthma. The usual dose is 250 μg IM or intramyometrially, not more frequently than every 15 minutes.

C. **Tocolytics** are used to delay or stop premature labor. They are used for fetuses with gestational ages between 20 and 34 to 36 weeks. Cervical dilation of less than 4 cm and cervical effacement of less than 80% are associated with a greater likelihood of terminating premature labor.
   1. **Indications**
       a. To delay or prevent premature labor.

    b. To slow or arrest labor while initiating other therapeutic measures (e.g., betamethasone to mature fetal lungs).

    c. Allow transfer from a community hospital to a tertiary care center with a neonatal intensive care unit.

  2. Contraindications

    a. Chorioamnionitis.

    b. Fetal distress.

    c. Preeclampsia or eclampsia.

    d. Severe hemorrhage.

  3. Specific drugs

    a. Terbutaline and **ritodrine** are selective beta-2–adrenergic agonists used to inhibit preterm labor and produce myometrial inhibition. Beta-2 stimulation will also produce bronchodilation, vasodilation, and tachycardia. Metabolic effects include hyperglycemia, hypokalemia, hyperinsulinemia, and metabolic (lactic) acidosis. Pulmonary edema (secondary to increased antidiuretic activity) and chest pain may develop but usually only after 24 hours of therapy. Before beginning treatment with a beta-2–adrenergic agonist, a baseline electrocardiogram should be obtained and preexisting hyperglycemia should be corrected.

    b. Magnesium sulfate is used for the treatment of preeclampsia (see section VII.C.4) and is also a common first-line tocolytic agent, because of the infrequency of cardiovascular side effects. Its exact mechanism of action remains uncertain, although competition with Ca^{2+} appears to play a role. Patients receiving both magnesium and terbutaline should be watched particularly closely for development of pulmonary edema.

    c. Indomethacin and **calcium channel blockers** are occasionally used for their tocolytic properties.

IV.   Placental transfer of drugs

A.   Placental transport of anesthetics occurs primarily by passive diffusion. Drugs with a high-diffusion constant more readily cross placental membranes. Factors that promote rapid diffusion include:

  1. Low molecular weight (less than 600 daltons).

  2. High lipid solubility.

  3. Low degree of ionization (the more drug in the "free" nonionized form at physiologic pH, the more available to diffuse).

  4. Low protein binding.

B. Most of the agents used to produce sedation, analgesia, or anesthesia are of low molecular weight, high lipid solubility, relatively nonionized, and minimally protein bound, accounting for their early passage across the placenta.

C. Muscle relaxants are water soluble, ionized, have high molecular weights, and therefore tend not to cross the placenta.

D. Damage to the placenta, as occurs with hypertension, diabetes, and toxemia, may lead to loss of placental capillary integrity, resulting in nonselective transfer of materials across the placenta. Once across the placenta, fetal acidosis and low pH can produce trapping of ionized drugs.

V.   Anesthesia for labor and vaginal delivery

A.   Natural childbirth. Many women opt to have no medication at all during labor and delivery. It remains prudent to know of any significant medical problems of such patients well in advance should the need for an emergency anesthetic arise.

B. Supplemental medication. Systemic medications are used to relieve pain and anxiety during labor and delivery. There is no ideal medication since they all cross the placenta and may depress the fetus. The most commonly used drugs are opioids such as **meperidine** and **oxymorphone** and agonist–antagonist agents such as **butorphanol** and **nalbuphine. Sedatives** such as diazepam, hydroxyzine, or promethazine may be used in low doses if needed. Larger doses have been associated with newborn hypotonia and impaired thermal regulation.

C. Epidural blockade can provide analgesia through labor and delivery, as well as provide anesthesia for cesarean section. Epidural analgesia usually is initiated when active labor has been achieved (cervix dilated 5 to 6 cm in a primipara, and 3 to 4 cm in a multipara). Institution of epidural analgesia may minimally slow the progress of labor such that oxytocics may be necessary.

  1. Advantages

   a. The need for systemic pain medications that may produce neonatal depression is decreased.

   b. Reducing pain will decrease endogenous catecholamine secretion and thereby improve uteroplacental perfusion.

   c. Reducing pain may reduce hyperventilation during contractions and minimize the decrease of uteroplacental perfusion that results from alkalosis.

   d. The mother is awake and able to participate in labor and delivery.

   e. The epidural can be used to provide anesthesia for cesarean section.

   f. Compared with general anesthesia, there is a lower risk of pulmonary aspiration.

  2. Disadvantages

   a. Hypotension is common and can produce uteroplacental insufficiency.

   b. The progress of labor may be delayed.

   c. Toxic reactions to local anesthetic agents are possible.

   d. Postdural puncture headache is possible.

  3. Contraindications

   a. Patient refusal.

   b. Coagulation disorder (e.g., in abruption or preeclampsia).

   c. Infection at the site of catheter placement.

   d. Hypovolemia.

  4. Technique (see Chapter 16).

   a. A large-bore IV catheter should be placed, and at least 500 to 1,000 mL of crystalloid (preferably warmed) should be infused before placement of the epidural. This will help prevent hypotension as the epidural takes effect.

   b. A 30-mL dose of a nonparticulate antacid should be administered prior to beginning epidural placement.

   c. Baseline vital signs and fetal heart rate should be recorded.

   d. Patients may be in the lateral decubitus or sitting position for lumbar catheter placement. Avoidance of the sitting position in patients being treated with magnesium for preeclampsia may be beneficial.

5. **Anesthetics**

   a. **A test dose** of 3 mL of 1.5% lidocaine with 1:200,000 epinephrine should be given to test for subarachnoid or intravascular placement. If the patient has preeclampsia, a test dose without epinephrine may be chosen because of the potential for severe hypertension if the drug is injected intravascularly.

   b. **For analgesia during labor**, the goal is to provide relief from pain without producing significant motor blockade. For labor analgesia, theoretically any local anesthetic can be used (1% to 2% lidocaine, 2% to 3% chloroprocaine, or 0.25% to 0.5% bupivacaine), although the more concentrated local anesthetics will tend to produce a motor blockade and should be reserved for cesarean sections. Epidural 0.75% bupivacaine is no longer approved for use in obstetric anesthesia because of its association with cardiac arrest in these patients. A mixture of a dilute, long-acting local anesthetic with a narcotic is most commonly used. While a variety of combinations are reasonable, our current practice is to use 0.04% bupivacaine with 1.66 µg fentanyl per milliliter. After the test dose, a bolus of 15 mL of this mixture is administered in divided doses, and followed by a continuous infusion of the same mixture, starting at a rate of 15 mL per hour. Onset of analgesia is usually within 5 minutes, and maximal in 15 to 20 minutes. As labor progresses, it is common to adjust the rate of infusion, or to bolus with more concentrated local anesthetic or opioid. In particular, as the fetal head descends, the patient may complain of aggravating rectal pressure; epidural fentanyl, 50 to 100 µg, often is effective.

   c. Whenever a bolus dose is administered via epidural, blood pressure should be monitored every few minutes for 20 to 30 minutes, and every 15 minutes thereafter. Hypotension may be treated with ephedrine, 5 to 10 mg IV, repeated as necessary. Cautious administration is recommended for patients with preeclampsia.

   d. **Patient-controlled epidural analgesia** (PCEA) is a new modality available for labor analgesia. Studies comparing PCEA with continuous epidural infusions have reported reduced drug use in the PCEA group, and no difference in pain and sedation scores between the two groups.

6. **Complications**

   a. **Neurologic complications.** The most common neurologic complication is **postdural puncture headache**. A dural puncture with an epidural needle is likely to produce headache because of the large (17-gauge) needle size. The incidence of headache in parturients with "wet-tap" is 70% to 80%. Bed rest, hydration, and analgesics are the initial treatments of choice. Caffeine preparations have proved to be of some help, although nursing mothers may prefer to avoid this. If 24 to 48 hours of conservative measures fail, the headache is best treated with an epidural blood patch. The initial blood patch produces persistent symptomatic relief in 61% to 75% of patients. This value increases to 95% with subsequent patching.

   b. **Intravascular injection** most often is heralded by agitation, visual disturbances, tinnitus, and convulsions, and may lead to loss of consciousness. If any of these symptoms is noted, the injection should be stopped and immediate attention given to the airway. The patient should be given 100% oxygen by mask. **Seizures** may be terminated with thiopental, 50 to 150 mg IV. Endotracheal intubation and hyperventilate may be necessary to ensure fetal oxygenation and to offset metabolic acidosis. If cardiovascular collapse occurs, immediate cardiopulmonary resuscitation and cesarean delivery are undertaken. Maintenance of left uterine displacement is absolutely vital during this time.

  c. Total spinal anesthesia. Subdural injection of local anesthetic intended for the epidural space may produce total spinal anesthesia. Nausea, hypotension, and unconsciousness may be followed by respiratory and cardiac arrest if appropriate interventions are not undertaken. Should a total spinal occur, the patient should be placed in supine position (with left uterine displacement), the lungs ventilated by mask with 100% oxygen while cricoid pressure is applied, and the trachea then intubated. Hypotension should be treated with fluids and ephedrine.

D. Spinal analgesia or anesthesia may be used for labor. "Saddle block" produces a motor blockade that will interfere with delivery. It can be useful as a last-minute anesthetic if a forceps delivery is required, for postpartum repair of traumatic lacerations of the vagina or rectum, or for removal of retained placenta if hypovolemia is not present. It has become popular to use a subarachnoid injection of a small dose of short acting, lipophilic opioid, with or without a small dose of local anesthetic, for labor analgesia. Sufentanil, 10 μg, or fentanyl, 25 μg, with bupivacaine, 1.25 to 2.5 mg, may be used. Analgesia, especially early in labor, is usually achieved within 5 minutes, and lasts for 1.5 to 2 hours. After subarachnoid injection of an opioid, the patient must be watched closely for signs of respiratory depression, although it is extremely rare.

E. Combined spinal-epidural analgesia has become more common as the use of intrathecal injections for labor has increased. With this technique, the epidural space is located using the standard 3.5-inch needle, and a 4-inch spinal needle is passed through the epidural needle and into the subarachnoid space. After intrathecal drug injection, the spinal needle is removed, and the epidural catheter is passed as usual. When additional analgesia becomes necessary, the epidural catheter is tested and epidural analgesia is achieved in the standard fashion. The combined spinal-epidural is used either very early in labor, before epidural analgesia would routinely be initiated, or very close to delivery, for its rapid onset. This technique has been associated with fetal bradycardia, which is possibly secondary to an effect on maternal plasma catecholamine levels caused by the rapid onset of analgesia.

VI. Anesthesia for cesarean section. The most frequent indications for cesarean section are failure to progress, fetal distress, cephalopelvic disproportion, and prior uterine surgery or cesarean section. Anesthetic choice will depend on the urgency of the procedure and the condition of mother and fetus.

A. Regional anesthesia

1. **Spinal anesthesia** is a simple, rapid, and reliable technique to provide anesthesia for cesarean delivery if no contraindications exist. The patient is hydrated and given metoclopramide and a nonparticulate antacid. The patient may be sitting or in a lateral decubitus position. Bupivacaine 0.75% in 8.25% dextrose is a commonly used local anesthetic. For surgical procedures lasting less than 45 minutes, 5% lidocaine had been used, but an increased incidence of neurotoxicity associated with the subarachnoid administration of lidocaine has been reported (see Chapter 16, section IV.F.11). It currently appears prudent to avoid the use of lidocaine for spinal anesthesia. A T-4 spinal level is sought, although the patient may still experience visceral discomfort and vagal symptoms with exteriorization of the uterus. Addition of small amounts of opioids such as fentanyl, 10 to 25 μg, to the local anesthetic or ephedrine, 5 mg IV, may decrease the incidence of symptoms during the surgery. Subarachnoid morphine, 0.1 to 0.25 mg, may be mixed with the local anesthetic for postoperative analgesia. If it is used, a protocol should be established for monitoring for delayed respiratory depression, and for the treatment of aggravating minor side effects such as pruritis.

2. **Epidural anesthesia** is an alternative for patients who are having elective cesarean sections. The dose of anesthetic can be titrated and repeated as necessary. For elective cesarean section, 2% lidocaine or 0.5% bupivacaine may be used. The addition of fentanyl, 50 to 100 μg, is helpful in reducing discomfort of uterine manipulation. An epidural can be used effectively for an emergency cesarean section in a patient who already has a catheter in place for labor analgesia. A dose of 3% 2-chloroprocaine or 2% lidocaine may be used. For rapid onset, sodium bicarbonate, 1 mL for each 10 mL of 2-chloroprocaine or lidocaine, can be added. Morphine, 3 mg, may be added after the cord is clamped to provide postoperative analgesia. If morphine is used, a protocol should be established for monitoring for delayed respiratory depression and for the treatment of aggravating minor side effects.

B.   General anesthesia is the technique of choice for emergency cesarean sections when regional anesthesia is refused or contraindicated, when substantial hemorrhage is anticipated, or when uterine relaxation is required.

1. **Advantages**
   a.   Rapid induction allows surgery to be started immediately.
   b.   Optimal control of the airway and ventilation is ensured.
   c.   Decreased incidence of hypotension in the hypovolemic patient.

2. **Disadvantages**
   a.   **The inability to intubate the trachea remains a major cause of maternal morbidity and mortality. The incidence of failed intubation in obstetric patients may be as much as eight times greater than it is in nonpregnant patients.**
   b.   The risk of aspiration is increased.
   c.   General anesthetics may cause fetal depression.
   d.   Awareness under anesthesia is possible with anesthesia

for cesarean section, because light anesthesia is used and the incision is made immediately following induction.

3. Technique

a. Thirty milliliters of a nonparticulate antacid is administered before induction. If time permits, metoclopramide, 10 mg, and cimetidine, 300 mg, or ranitidine, 50 mg, may be given IV. A large-bore (16-gauge) IV catheter and standard monitoring are used. The patient is positioned supine with left uterine displacement.

b. The patient breathes 100% oxygen for 3 minutes if time allows or takes five to six deep breaths if time is of the essence. The obstetricians should prepare and drape the abdomen at this time.

c. A rapid sequence intubation with cricoid pressure is performed with 4 to 5 mg/kg of thiopental IV (reduce dose for hypovolemic or bleeding patients) and 1.5 mg/kg of succinylcholine IV. Etomidate or ketamine may be used in cases of maternal hypovolemia. Etomidate demonstrates the same neonatal outcome as thiopental. Ketamine has been reported to cause neonatal depression at doses greater than 2 mg/kg.

d. Until delivery, a 50% mixture of nitrous oxide and oxygen is used with either enflurane or 0.75% to 1.0% isoflurane. A succinylcholine infusion or short-acting, nondepolarizing muscle relaxant is administered. Hyperventilation should be avoided because of its adverse effects on uterine blood flow.

e. Oxytocin (Pitocin) (10 to 20 units per liter) is added to the IV infusion and administered after delivery of the placenta to stimulate uterine contraction.

f. Volatile anesthetics may be used in low doses for maintenance of anesthesia after the Pitocin infusion is begun, recognizing that they may decrease uterine tone. Alternatively, once the cord is clamped, a balanced technique with nitrous oxide, opioid, and relaxant may be chosen.

g. An orogastric tube is passed to empty the stomach. Extubation is performed when the patient is fully awake.

VII. Preeclampsia and eclampsia

A. Preeclampsia is a syndrome of hypertension, proteinuria, and generalized edema. It occurs in about 7% of all pregnancies. If seizures occur, the condition is known as **eclampsia**, which has an incidence of about 0.3%. These disorders do not manifest themselves before the twentieth week of pregnancy and usually abate within 48 hours of delivery. **Hypertension** in these disorders is defined as a systolic blood pressure greater than 140 mm Hg (or an increase of more than 30 mm Hg above baseline blood pressure) or a diastolic blood pressure greater than 90 (or an increase of more than 15 mm Hg above baseline). The condition is most often seen in young nulliparous women, but also is associated with hydatidiform mole, multiple pregnancy, diabetes, and Rh incompatibility. Genetic contributions from both parents are important determinants of the predisposition and development of preeclampsia.

B. The pathophysiology of preeclampsia is thought to be related to immunologic rejection of fetal tissues, which results in incomplete invasion of the trophoblast, placental vasculitis, and ischemia. Decreased placental perfusion increases circulating levels of renin, angiotensin, aldosterone, and catecholamines, which can produce generalized vasoconstriction and endothelial damage. Fluids shift from the intravascular fluid into the extravascular space with resultant edema, hypoxemia, and hemoconcentration. Disseminated intravascular coagulation (DIC) is rare, but coagulation abnormalities such as thrombocytopenia, increased fibrin split products, and a slightly prolonged partial thromboplastin time may occur. Renal blood flow, glomerular filtration rate, and urine output are reduced. Hyperreflexia occurs, and central nervous system irritability often increases.

C. Management. Definitive treatment involves prompt delivery of the fetus. Symptoms usually abate within 48 hours of delivery. Until then, treatment of hypertension, intravascular volume, coagulation abnormalities, and prevention or termination of seizures are high priorities.

    1. Hypertension

        a. Hydralazine is a commonly used vasodilator because it increases both uteroplacental and renal blood flow.

        b. Labetalol is a very useful alternative, because of its alpha- and beta-adrenergic blocking effects.

        c. Sodium nitroprusside may be useful for treating a hypertensive crisis or the acute increases of blood pressure that may accompany laryngoscopy.

    2. Fluid management. Intravascular depletion should be corrected with crystalloid and may be guided by central venous pressure and rarely pulmonary artery occlusion pressure measurements.

    3. Coagulation abnormalities. The patient's coagulation status should be assessed, especially in severe preeclampsia. Administration of platelets, fresh-frozen plasma, and red cells may be necessary.

    4. Magnesium sulfate is a mild vasodilator and central nervous system depressant. By relaxing the myometrium, it also causes an increase in uteroplacental blood flow. Magnesium increases the sensitivity to both depolarizing and nondepolarizing muscle relaxants. It may also cause postpartum uterine atony, especially when Oxytocin has been used to augment a long labor. Magnesium may cross the placenta, resulting in muscle weakness or apnea in the neonate. Intravenous calcium may counteract this weakness in both mother and newborn, but calcium may also antagonize the anticonvulsant effect of magnesium in the mother. After an initial IV-loading dose of 2 to 4 g over 15 minutes, a continuous infusion of 1 to 3 g per hour is used to maintain therapeutic blood levels of 4 to 8 meq/L. Systemic effects of magnesium are presented in Table 29-2.

D. Anesthesia

    1. Epidural anesthesia is recommended for cesarean delivery in the preeclamptic patient with hypovolemia. Epidural analgesia early in labor may help to reduce circulating levels of maternal epinephrine and norepinephrine, thus improving uteroplacental perfusion.

    2. Spinal anesthesia generally has not been recommended because of the rapid onset of sympathectomy causing hypotension in a hypovolemic patient. However, neonatal assessment and maternal morbidity outcomes have not been found to be

Table 29-2.   Systemic effects of magnesium

Plasma Level of Magnesium (mEq/L)	Systemic Effect
4–8	Therapeutic range
5–10	Electrocardiographic changes ↑ PR interval, ↑ QRS
10–15	↓ DTRs Respiratory depression
15–20	Respiratory arrest SA and AV conduction defects
>20	Cardiac arrest

AV, atrioventricular; DTR, deep tendon reflex; PR, pulse rate; QRS, principal deflection in electrocardiogram; SA, sinoatrial.

different among spinal, epidural or general anesthetic techniques.

3.   General anesthesia is employed for emergency cesarean deliveries if the patient has a coagulopathy or other contraindication to regional anesthesia. These patients are particularly prone to periglottic edema, making rapid-sequence induction particularly difficult. The hemodynamic response to intubation may be blunted by administration of labetalol, 10 mg IV. Systemic and pulmonary hypertension increases the incidence of stroke and pulmonary edema. The sensitizing effects of magnesium on muscle relaxants must be considered.

VIII.   Peripartum hemorrhage is the major cause of maternal mortality.

A.   Antepartum hemorrhage most commonly is due to placenta previa or placental abruption.

1.   Placenta previa occurs when the placenta is implanted at or very near the cervical opening. This can result in bleeding that is usually painless and can vary from minimal spotting to massive hemorrhage. Placenta previa in a patient with a previous cesarean section has a higher incidence of abnormal placental attachment (**placenta accreta**). The incidence of gravid hysterectomy is higher in this population. If the patient is not actively bleeding and is euvolemic, subarachnoid or epidural anesthesia may be performed. Pelvic examination in patients with placenta previa may also precipitate hemorrhage and should only be done in an operating room that is prepared for emergency cesarean section. This is called a "**double setup**" and generally consists of the following:

a.   Administration of 30 mL of a nonparticulate antacid.

b.   Placement of a large-bore (14- or 16-gauge) IV with a pump set.

c.   Blood (two to four units) in the room.

d.   Abdomen prepared and draped by the obstetricians.

e.   All preparations for general anesthesia available.

f.   Assistance available.

2. Placental abruption is the premature separation of the normally implanted placenta before birth. The bleeding is usually painful and may be either external (obvious bleeding from the vagina) or concealed (blood is trapped behind the placenta and remains inside the uterus). Abruption is the most common cause of DIC in pregnancy. Anesthetic management is essentially the same as for placenta previa except that coagulation studies are checked before initiating regional anesthesia. Regional anesthesia should only be used in cases of mild abruption when there is no fetal distress, hypovolemia, or coagulopathy. Consumption of coagulation factors and activation of the fibrinolytic system occur frequently and should be treated with blood products as needed.

B. Intrapartum hemorrhage

1. Uterine rupture can occur at any point during labor and delivery and is associated with:

    a. Separation of a prior uterine scar or traumatic rupture such as during a difficult forceps application.

    b. History of previous difficult deliveries.

    c. Rapid, spontaneous, tumultuous labor.

    d. Prolonged labor in association with excessive oxytocin stimulation.

2. Vaginal birth after cesarean section (VBAC). Certain patients who have had prior cesarean section may have a trial of labor, attempting to have a vaginal birth after cesarean section. The concern is for possible uterine rupture at the site of a prior incision. In general, patients with a singleton fetus in vertex presentation, whose prior uterine incision was low transverse and with no other maternal risk factors, are the best candidates for VBAC. Dehiscence of a low transverse scar has been shown to be less catastrophic, both to the mother and fetus, than rupture of a classic vertical incision scar. It is safe and probably desirable to use regional techniques in these patients. The most reliable signs of rupture are a change in uterine tone, contraction pattern, and fetal heart rate, which should be unaffected by epidural analgesia. In a patient with a functioning epidural, the onset of pain that is constant during and between contractions may be an indication of uterine rupture, although most patients with uterine rupture will have no pain. If uterine rupture occurs, a functioning epidural provides a means for establishment of a quick, safe anesthetic for surgical intervention.

    If uterine rupture causes massive hemorrhage, anesthetic management is the same as it would be for any actively bleeding, acutely hypovolemic patient. General anesthesia usually is indicated in this situation.

3. Vasa previa is a condition in which the fetal umbilical cord passes in front of the presenting part. The vessels of the umbilical cord are vulnerable to trauma during vaginal examination or during artificial rupture of membranes. Bleeding is only from the fetal circulation in this circumstance. This obviously puts the fetus at great risk and is a reason for immediate delivery.

C. Postpartum hemorrhage

1. Retained placenta occurs in up to 1% of all vaginal deliveries, and it usually requires manual exploration of the uterus. Removal of the placenta is facilitated if the patient still has an epidural or spinal block. If uterine relaxation is necessary, and bleeding has not been excessive, nitroglycerin in 50- to 100-μg boluses will effectively relax the uterus. Small doses of ketamine may be used if a regional anesthetic is not in place.

If bleeding has been brisk and the patient shows signs of hypovolemia, a regional block may be contraindicated and may produce severe hypotension. Rapid sequence induction and general anesthesia with a potent volatile inhalation agent may be necessary. As soon as the uterus is relaxed sufficiently to allow extraction, the volatile anesthetic should be discontinued to prevent uterine atony and further bleeding.

2. Uterine atony occurs in up to 2% to 5% of patients. Infusion of crystalloid, colloid, and blood products, as needed, should begin when the diagnosis is made. Pharmacologic therapy involves IV oxytocin to cause uterine contracture. If this fails, the ergot preparation methergine, 0.2 mg IM, should be administered. If this fails to produce uterine contraction, then 15-methyl prostaglandin $F_{2\alpha}$ should be given IM or injected directly into the uterus by the obstetrician. If these measures fail, then emergency hysterectomy or internal iliac artery ligation may be necessary.

3. Laceration of the vagina, cervix, or perineum is a common cause of postpartum hemorrhage. Bleeding may be insidious, and can be difficult to estimate. If epidural analgesia must be intensified for repair, care must be taken to ensure adequate volume resuscitation and avoid significant hypotension.

4. Uterine inversion is a very rare cause of postpartum hemorrhage. This represents a true obstetric emergency, since the patient can exsanguinate rapidly. General anesthesia is often required to produce immediate uterine relaxation in the face of rapidly developing hypovolemia. Help should be summoned immediately.

IX. Amniotic fluid embolism

A. Pathophysiology. Amniotic fluid embolism occurs in 1:20,000 to 30,000 deliveries, and most cases are fatal. As many as 10% of the maternal deaths from all causes result from amniotic fluid embolism. The pathogenesis of this disorder involves a tear through the amnion or chorion (opening uterine or endocervical veins) and pressure sufficient to force the fluid into the venous circulation.

B. Clinical features include respiratory distress with pulmonary edema and cyanosis; shock; coagulopathy and hemorrhage (from DIC); and altered mental status, which may be characterized by seizures and coma.

C. Predisposing factors include a tumultuous or oxytocin-augmented labor, meconium in the amniotic fluid, intrauterine fetal demise, abruptio placentae, advanced maternal age, multiparity, and vaginal manipulation or cesarean section.

D. Laboratory studies. The diagnosis may be supported by the presence of fetal squamous cells, lanugo hair, vernix, or mucin in the buffy coat of heparinized maternal blood sampled from a pulmonary artery catheter, but these signs are not always present and are not pathognomonic. Diagnostic workup includes arterial blood gas tensions and pH, coagulation studies, chest radiograph, and electrocardiogram. Pulmonary hypertension may be present.

E.   Treatment is supportive and consists of cardiopulmonary resuscitation, if necessary, and immediate delivery of the fetus. Endotracheal intubation and respiratory support using increased oxygen concentrations and positive end-expiratory pressure may be necessary. Diuretics are used to correct the pulmonary edema and transfusions of blood products may be necessary because of hematologic derangements.

XI.   Anesthesia for nonobstetric surgery during pregnancy
A.   Approximately 1.5% of women undergo nonobstetric surgery during pregnancy. The objectives in the anesthetic management of these procedures include:

   1.   Maternal safety. The anesthetic plan must take into consideration that physiologic changes of pregnancy begin in the first trimester.

   2.   Fetal safety. Efforts should be made to prevent preterm labor, maintain uteroplacental blood flow, and avoid teratogenic substances. No anesthetic agent has been proven to be teratogenic in humans, although nitrous oxide has been shown to be teratogenic in certain situations in animals.

B.   Procedures directly related to pregnancy

   1.   Ectopic pregnancy results when the fertilized ovum implants abnormally outside the endometrial lining of the uterus. Ruptured ectopic pregnancy is the leading cause of first trimester death and usually requires emergent laparoscopy or laparotomy. It is prudent to volume resuscitate these patients and to have blood products available before the induction of anesthesia.

   2.   Abortion or miscarriage refers to the loss of pregnancy before 20 weeks gestation or fetal weight less than 500 g. A **complete abortion** refers to spontaneous expulsion of products of conception; an **incomplete abortion** refers to a partial expulsion of products of conception; and a **missed abortion** refers to unrecognized fetal demise. A dilation and evacuation are indicated in incomplete abortions and in missed abortions without spontaneous expulsion. Monitored anesthesia care, spinal, epidural, or general anesthesia can be used after careful assessment of the patient to evaluate volume status, presence of disseminated intravascular coagulopathy and sepsis, and fasting (NPO) status.

   3.   Surgeries for incompetent cervix include the Shirodkar cerclage and the McDonald cerclage. They are both performed transvaginally during the first or the second trimester, either prophylactically or emergently with the onset of cervical change. Either spinal or epidural anesthesia usually is the anesthetic of choice. General anesthesia may be preferable, however, to decrease intrauterine pressure in patients with a dilated cervix and bulging fetal membranes.

   4.   Anesthesia for postpartum sterilization. Many patients and obstetricians prefer to schedule tubal ligation for the immediate postpartum period. Timing of tubal ligation and choice of anesthesia are controversial areas in obstetric anesthesia.

      a.   Advantages
         (1)   The enlarged uterus brings the fallopian tubes up out of the pelvis, so that the surgery can be done through a minilaparotomy incision under direct vision.

(2) A second hospital visit is avoided, which is an advantage with respect to cost, convenience, and childcare, compared with laparoscopic tubal ligation done at 6 weeks postpartum.

(3) There is essentially no chance that the patient will experience an undesired pregnancy while waiting for sterilization.

b. Disadvantages

(1) Physiologic changes of pregnancy do not fully return to prepregnant status until 6 weeks postpartum. In particular, gastric emptying slows during labor and after administration of opioids. It is not clear how soon after delivery that emptying returns to baseline. Also, failed intubation is significantly more likely at term than in the nonpregnant state.

(2) Tubal ligation is an elective procedure, with effective alternatives available. Therefore, the procedure should not be performed when the patient has a full stomach.

c. Recommendations. Patients who refuse regional anesthesia are scheduled for laparoscopic tubal ligation at least 6 weeks postpartum. If the patient has a labor epidural anesthetic that is functioning well, if the patient is stable postpartum, and if her infant is stable, she will be kept NPO after delivery, and the procedure performed as soon as personnel and labor floor resources allow. In some cases, the epidural catheter will be nonfunctional. If no effect is seen after a test dose of 3 to 5 mL of bicarbonated 2% lidocaine, the catheter is removed, and either another one placed or a spinal anesthetic performed. If the patient does not have an epidural for labor, she is generally kept NPO for 8 hours, and her procedure then performed under spinal anesthesia. Under regional anesthesia, a T-6 sensory level, comparable to that for cesarean section, is required for patient comfort.

C. Procedures incidental to pregnancy

1. Postpone elective surgery until 6 weeks postpartum (when the physiologic changes of pregnancy have returned to normal). Postpone semielective procedures until the second or third trimester.

2. Consult with an obstetrician preoperatively for all but the most minor surgical procedures.

3. Use regional techniques when possible, especially spinal anesthesia, to minimize fetal exposure to local anesthetic and the risk of aspiration or loss of airway.

4. Depending on the operative site, after the sixteenth week of gestation **continuous fetal monitoring** may be employed perioperatively (although fetal viability is not until after the twenty-sixth week of gestation). Communication with the obstetrician is important for interpretation of fetal heart rate tracings.

5. A uterine tocodynamometer should be used to detect preterm labor, especially in the postoperative period.

XII. Cardiopulmonary resuscitation during pregnancy

A. Cardiac arrest during pregnancy is rare. When it occurs, resuscitation is more difficult and less successful than in nonpregnant individuals for several reasons.

1. After approximately 24 weeks gestation, **aortocaval compression** by the gravid uterus hampers venous return such that closed chest compressions may be ineffective.

2. The increased oxygen demands of pregnancy makes hypoxia more likely even with adequate perfusion.

3. Enlarged breasts and upward displacement of abdominal contents makes effective closed chest compressions more difficult.

B. **Recommendations** when cardiac arrest occurs:

1. **Immediately intubate** the trachea and secure the airway.

2. **Maintain left uterine displacement** in the case of cardiac arrest after 24 weeks gestation and in the immediate postpartum period.

3. **Immediately page a neonatologist** for likely imminent delivery of a depressed, possibly preterm infant.

4. **Consider cesarean section** to alleviate aortocaval compression and increase the chance of survival of both mother and fetus, if efforts at resuscitation are unsuccessful by 4 minutes.

5. **Utilize standard advanced cardiac life support protocols** (see Chapter 36), using the usual recommended drugs, doses, and countershocks.

6. **Consider open-chest cardiac massage** if perfusion is inadequate.

7. **Consider institution of cardiopulmonary bypass** in cases of bupivacaine toxicity or massive pulmonary embolus.

XIII. **Anesthesia for gynecologic surgery**

A. **Laparoscopy** (see also Chapter 20, section IV.A).

1. Laparoscopy requires **pneumoperitoneum**, occasionally extreme Trendelenburg positioning, and the use of electrocoagulation during sterilization procedures.

2. **Insufflation** of the peritoneal cavity with carbon dioxide often causes an elevation of the partial pressure of arterial CO_2. Hypercarbia results from decreased pulmonary compliance, decreased functional residual capacity, and absorption of the carbon dioxide used for pneumoperitoneum. Excess carbon dioxide may be eliminated with controlled ventilation 1.5 times the basal requirements. Increased intraabdominal pressure secondary to gas insufflation at pressures of 20- to 25-cm H_2O produces increases in central venous pressure and cardiac output, secondary to central redistribution of blood volume. Pressures greater than 30- to 40-cm H_2O produce a decrease in central venous pressure and cardiac output by decreasing right heart filling.

3. **Techniques.** General anesthesia is most commonly used for laparoscopic procedures. Spinal or epidural techniques generally are not well tolerated because of the increased ventilatory load associated with pneumoperitoneum, unless insufflation is less than 2 L.

B. **Abdominal procedures** (also see Chapter 20). Most of these procedures are performed through a low abdominal incision, and a regional or general anesthetic is appropriate. The patient may experience discomfort from peritoneal tugging, though the addition of epidural or intrathecal fentanyl may help. General anesthesia usually is chosen for extensive pelvic and abdominal procedures with large blood loss and fluid shifts. In addition, steep Trendelenburg position, commonly used for pelvic surgery, may not be well tolerated for very long in an awake patient.

C. Vaginal procedures. Both regional and general anesthetics may be used, although regional techniques are more common. When placing the regional anesthetic, having the patient sitting will help ensure adequate sacral anesthesia. Some procedures require extreme Trendelenburg with lithotomy position. This may impair ventilation, necessitating general anesthesia. Major transvaginal procedures may be associated with large occult blood losses.

XIV. Anesthesia for assisted reproductive techniques

A. *In vitro* **fertilization and embryo transfer** have become increasingly popular for the treatment of infertility. Hormone manipulation is used to stimulate the maturation of multiple ovarian follicles. Preovulatory oocytes are then harvested, combined with semen, and the resulting embryos are transferred into the uterine cavity. Ultrasonically guided follicle aspiration is the most commonly used method for oocyte retrieval. The procedure involves puncture and aspiration of follicles using real-time ultrasound through a transvaginal approach.

1. Local infiltration of the posteriolateral vaginal fornix, combined with small doses of sedatives and narcotics, have been used successfully. The surgeons, however, may desire an immobile patient to maximize oocyte retrieval. If so, this technique may be inadequate.

2. Spinal anesthesia will provide excellent operating conditions. Some centers avoid spinal anesthesia because of the risk of postdural puncture headache and to avoid prolonged recovery. With a 24-gauge Sprotte needle, or 25-gauge Whittacre needle, however, the incidence of postdural puncture headache should be under 1%, and the need for epidural blood patch very low. Hyperbaric 5%, 2%, or 1.5% lidocaine may be used depending on the expected length of surgery; however, there are concerns over neurotoxicity with lidocaine, especially in the 5% concentration. Alternatively, hyperbaric 0.75% bupivacaine may be used. Fentanyl, 10 to 25 μg, may be added to any of the local anesthetics to decrease the pain of peritoneal stimulation.

3. General anesthesia may be used for oocyte retrieval. The effects of inhalation anesthetics on cell division and implantation are incompletely understood. All inhalational anesthetics can interfere with some stages of reproductive physiology *in vitro*. In particular, nitrous oxide inhibits methionine synthetase activity, and could affect DNA synthesis. There is no convincing evidence, however, that any of the commonly used inhalational anesthetics adversely affect pregnancy and live-birth rates for *in vitro* fertilization procedures. General anesthesia with a benzodiazepine, opioid, and propofol appears to be a safe alternative to inhalational anesthesia for oocyte retrieval.

B. Gamete intrafallopian transfer begins with transvaginal oocyte retrieval. If oocytes are confirmed in the laboratory, laparoscopy is performed immediately; the oocytes along with washed sperm are injected into the fallopian tube. Thus, fertilization is *in vivo*, and requires a normal fallopian tube for success. Regional anesthesia is possible. Since this is a laparoscopic procedure and immobility is extremely important, however, general anesthesia is usually chosen.

SUGGESTED READING

Birnbach DJ, Ostheimer GW. *Ostheimer's manual of obstetric anesthesia*, 3rd ed. New York: Churchill Livingstone, 2000.

Briggs GG, Freeman RK, Yaffe SJ. *Drugs in pregnancy and lactation: a reference guide to fetal and neonatal risk*, 6th ed. Philadelphia: Lippincott Williams & Wilkins, 2001.

Chestnut DH. *Obstetric anesthesia: principles and practice*, 2nd ed. St. Louis: Mosby–Year Book, 1999.

Cunningham FG, Gant NF, Leveno LJ, et al. *Williams obstetrics*, 21st ed. New York: McGraw-Hill, 2001.

Datta S. *Anesthetic and obstetric management of high risk pregnancy*, 2nd ed. St. Louis: Mosby–Year Book, 1996.

Datta S. *The obstetric anesthesia handbook*, 3rd ed. Philadelphia: Hanley & Belfus, 2000.

Duffy PJ, Crosby ET. The epidural blood patch: resolving the controversies. *Can J Anesth* 1999;46: 878–886.

Hughes SC, Levinson G, Rosen MA. *Shnider and Levinson's anesthesia for obstetrics*, 4th ed. Philadelphia: Lippincott Williams & Wilkins, 2002.

Martin RW. Amniotic fluid embolism. *Clin Obstet Gynecol* 1996;39: 101–106.

Ngan Kee WD, Khaw KS, Ma ML. Patient-controlled epidural analgesia after caesarean section using meperidine. *Can J Anaesth* 1997;44: 702–706.

Santos AC, O'Gorman DA, Finster M. Obstetric anesthesia. In Barash PG, Cullen BF, Stoelting RK, eds. *Clinical anesthesia*, 4th ed. Philadelphia: Lippincott Williams & Wilkins, 2001:1141–1170.

Ambulatory Anesthesia

James B. Mayfield

I. Patient selection

A. The **volume of patients** receiving ambulatory anesthesia and surgical care now far exceeds the number of inpatient procedures. There is a continual shift of formerly inpatient procedures to the outpatient surgicenter, and surgeon's office. Outpatient surgery is now routinely performed on many American Society of Anesthesiologists (ASA) class III and IV patients who are stable medically as well as on ASA I and II patients. Recent studies have documented the safety of this practice. Admissions and complications correlate with type of procedure, duration of surgery, use of general anesthesia, and patient age, rather than ASA classification.

B. Patients inappropriate for outpatient surgery

   1. Pediatric

   a. Formerly premature infants of less than 46 weeks postconceptual age, even if healthy, have an increased risk of postanesthetic apnea. Regardless of type of anesthesia, these infants should be admitted for a day of postoperative apnea monitoring.

   b. Infants with respiratory disease such as severe bronchopulmonary dysplasia, apnea, or bronchospasm.

   c. Infants with cardiovascular disease such as congestive heart failure or hemodynamically significant congenital heart anomalies.

   d. Children with fever, cough, sore throat, coryza, or other signs of recent onset or worsening upper respiratory infection.

   2. Adult

   a. Patients expected to have **major blood loss** or undergoing major surgery.

   b. ASA III and IV patients who require complex or extended monitoring or postoperative treatment.

   c. Morbidly obese patients with significant respiratory disease.

   d. Patients with a need for **complex pain management**.

   e. Patients with significant fever, wheezing, nasal congestion, cough, or other symptoms of a recent upper respiratory infection.

II. Patient preparation

A. Preoperative testing. The need for preoperative testing is minimal in healthy patients. Current guidelines are for a complete blood count starting at age 50 years in women and 65 years in men, an electrocardiogram for men at 40 and women at 50 years of age, and creatinine and blood urea nitrogen levels at age 65 years. All other testing is performed as indicated by patient disease.

B. Prehospital instructions

1. Patients are instructed (by either the physician's office or the preadmission area) as to the time of expected arrival, appropriate clothing, diet restrictions, duration of surgery, and the need for escort home.

2. Current diet guidelines. Current recommendations are taken from the recent ASA Task Force on preoperative fasting. Intake of clear liquids until 2 hours and solids until 8 hours preoperatively has been accepted and found to be safe.

3. Medications. Patients should be instructed to continue their cardiovascular, asthma, pain, anxiety, anticonvulsant, and antihypertensive medications until the time of surgery. Warfarin (Coumadin) should be stopped several days prior to surgery to allow the prothrombin time to return to normal. Diuretics are usually withheld on the morning of surgery. An accepted regimen for diabetic patients is to withhold regular insulin the morning of surgery and give half the usual dose of long-acting insulin such as neutral-protamine-Hagedorn (NPH) insulin. If the patient is traveling alone or over a long distance, the insulin may be given on arrival coincident with an intravenous (IV) infusion of glucose.

4. Preanesthetic visit. For healthy ambulatory patients, an evaluation by an anesthesiologist is usually performed immediately prior to the planned procedure. When a patient has a potentially serious problem or a complex medical condition, a consultation with an anesthesiologist should be arranged in advance. The consultation occurs in a preadmission testing clinic where patients are seen prior to their inpatient procedures. A standard history and physical examination are performed with special attention to the heart, lungs, and airway, and any significant new problems are explored (e.g., symptoms of an upper respiratory infection or unexplained chest pain). Time of last oral intake is confirmed and compliance with preoperative medications determined. Any required preoperative laboratory tests are also performed at this time. The anesthetic plan is discussed, and informed consent is obtained.

III. Anesthetic management

A. Premedication

1. Anxiolytics. Reassurance and rapport with the patient usually are all that are required. If necessary, **midazolam** (Versed), 1 to 2 mg intravenously may be administered.

2. Aspiration prophylaxis. Patients with extreme anxiety, morbid obesity, diabetic gastroparesis, symptomatic hiatal hernias, or other conditions causing esophageal reflux are at higher risk of pulmonary aspiration of gastric contents. They should be premedicated with one or more of the following:

a. Nonparticulate antacids (Bicitra), 30 mL by mouth (PO), just before the procedure.

b. Histamine (H_2)-receptor antagonist such as ranitidine, 150 mg PO, preferably the night before surgery and the morning of, or 50 mg IV before surgery.

c. Metoclopramide, 10 mg PO or IV before surgery. Metoclopramide may be most useful to increase gastric emptying in patients with diabetic gastroparesis.

3. Opioids. Fentanyl, 50 to 100 µg IV, may be given, especially if preoperative pain is present. Nurse supervision and oxygen saturation monitoring should be employed after administration of IV sedatives or opioids in the preinduction area.

B. **Intravenous access.** A small IV catheter (20 gauge) is started, frequently in an antecubital vein to diminish the pain associated with injection of propofol.

C. **Standard monitoring** is used (see Chapter 10). In addition, a bispectral index monitor (Aspect Medical Systems, Newton, MA) often is used during general anesthesia to allow more accurate titration of hypnotic agents, and speed recovery in the ambulatory patient.

D. **General anesthesia**

  1. **Induction. Propofol** is used most commonly for induction in adults because of its short duration, depression of pharyngeal reflexes, and reduced incidence of postoperative emesis compared with barbiturates. **Lidocaine,** 20 mg, may be added to each 200 mg of propofol to decrease the pain associated with injection into small veins. Small doses of alfentanil or fentanyl may be added, or given prior to the propofol to reduce the induction dose. **Sevoflurane** adds the option of a mask induction for adults and is an alternative to halothane for mask induction in children.

  2. **Airway management.** The choice of employing a face mask, a laryngeal mask, or tracheal intubation is discussed in Chapters 13 and 14. Succinylcholine or mivacurium is used to facilitate intubation for short procedures. Pretreatment with small doses of a nondepolarizing muscle relaxant may minimize the myalgias that follow succinylcholine administration. For longer procedures, an intubating dose of a short-acting nondepolarizing agent (cisatracurium) is used.

  3. **Maintenance.** Volatile anesthetics (e.g., isoflurane, desflurane, or sevoflurane), with or without nitrous oxide, are commonly employed with total gas flow rates of less than 1 L per minute (2 L per minute for sevoflurane) after the first 10 to 15 minutes to reduce wastage. Propofol and alfentanil or remifentanil infusions are also used in conjunction with nitrous oxide. Supplemental local anesthesia provided by the surgeon early in the procedure reduces general anesthetic requirements and provides early postoperative analgesia, and greater efficiency for recovery services.

E. **Regional anesthesia**

  1. The ideal outpatient technique involves the use of agents with rapid onset to minimize case delay and short duration to facilitate quick recovery and discharge. Patient selection is important, since the benefits of regional anesthesia will be negated if heavy sedation is required. Performing peripheral nerve blocks in a separate designated area well in advance of the scheduled surgery time will decrease time in the operating room (OR) waiting for onset of anesthesia. Separate areas for regional blocks should be fully equipped with the usual monitoring and resuscitative devices in the event that complications occur.

  2. **Specific blocks**

   a. **Spinal anesthesia**

    (1) **Subarachnoid anesthesia** is a fast, reliable technique providing adequate conditions for lower abdominal, groin, pelvic, perineal, and lower extremity surgery. The duration can be adjusted by appropriate selection of local anesthetic.

(2) Mepivacaine, lidocaine, and bupivacaine are used most commonly in ambulatory surgery (see Chapter 15).

(3) Complications

(a) Postdural puncture headache (PDPH) occurs in 5% to 10% of outpatients. Patients under 40 years of age and women are at greater risk. Informed consent should include the discussion of the risk of PDPH and treatment options. Routine use of a 24- to 27-gauge Sprotte needle has reduced the incidence of spinal headaches.

(b) Urinary retention. Men are at greater risk of delayed return of bladder tone and subsequent urinary retention. Catheterization may be required, and persistent inability to void may be an indication for admission. Reducing intraoperative IV fluids to a minimum may help avoid the problem.

(c) Transient radicular irritation and neurologic symptoms occurring with the use of lidocaine preparations have led some anesthetists to use exclusively low-dose bupivacaine or mepivacaine for spinal anesthesia.

b. Epidural anesthesia can be used to reduce the risk of PDPH. Common use is predicated on the ability to initiate the block in a separate area to reduce the time between operations. When used with a catheter, it provides regional anesthesia for appropriate procedures of uncertain duration.

c. Peripheral nerve blocks (see Chapter 17).

(1) Intravenous regional for hand or forearm surgery. The advantages include simplicity, rapid onset, high reliability, and early recovery and discharge. In the average patient, 50 mL of 0.5% lidocaine without epinephrine is used. The addition of **clonidine** (1 μg/kg) to the lidocaine has been shown to significantly enhance the duration of analgesia in the postoperative period. Disadvantages include a maximum case time of approximately 1.5 hours due to the need for an inflated tourniquet, lack of postoperative analgesia, and risk of local anesthetic toxicity if the tourniquets fail within the first few minutes after injection.

(2) Brachial plexus blockade for upper extremity surgery usually is indicated when patients prefer regional anesthesia as an alternative to general anesthesia, and when their medical condition increases the risks associated with general anesthesia. For shoulder surgery, the **parascalene** or **interscalene block** is utilized to provide anesthesia to the upper extremity above the midhumeral line. For elbow or hand surgery, an **axillary** or **infraclavicular block** is most effective.

(3) Lower extremity anesthesia using femoral or sciatic nerve blocks is not performed as frequently due to the requirement for early ambulation and discharge. **Popliteal** and **ankle blocks**, however, can provide an excellent alternative for the ambulatory patient wishing to avoid general anesthesia.

F.   Monitored anesthesia care. For some patients with complex medical problems whose operations would ordinarily be done under local anesthesia, an anesthetist may be asked to monitor the patient and provide medications, usually sedatives or opioids, supplemental to the local anesthesia provided by the surgeon. Standard monitoring should be used, and the anesthetist should be prepared to administer general anesthesia if the local anesthesia plus sedation is not sufficient.

IV.   Postoperative care

A.   Postanesthesia care unit (PACU) admission. Patients usually are admitted from the OR to a phase-I PACU. Some patients who are awake after minor procedures may be ready for a phase-II recovery area directly from the OR. Indications for this accelerated recovery process are being developed. Currently, the usual recovery protocol for outpatients receiving general anesthesia is a criteria-driven progression from the OR to the PACU and then to the phase-2 PACU, followed by discharge to home when they have met the discharge criteria. If the criteria used to discharge patients from the PACU are met in the OR, it is usually appropriate to "fast track" the patient, bypassing the PACU and transferring the patient directly to the phase-2 PACU. For patients to bypass the phase-1 PACU, they must be awake and oriented, have stable vital signs, have no nausea or vomiting, have minimal pain or discomfort, and be able to sit up without assistance. If these criteria are met, the anesthetist assists the patient into a reclining lounge chair, and transfers the patient to the phase-2 PACU.

B.   Pain. If the patient has pain on admission to the PACU, intravenous supplementation with an opioid, usually fentanyl or meperidine, is administered. When awake, the patient is usually given oral acetaminophen (Tylenol, 975 mg), oxycodone (Percocet, 1 to 2 tablets), or ibuprofen (Motrin, 600 mg).

C.   Nausea and vomiting. Predisposing factors include a previous history of vomiting after anesthesia, a history of severe motion sickness, use of large doses of opioids as part of the anesthetic technique, pelvic procedures in young females, gastric distension, and severe postoperative pain. **Ondansetron**, 4 mg IV, may be given if a history of severe nausea and vomiting is elicited preoperatively. Scopolamine (100 µg SC) has been shown in our institution to be very effective for rescue treatment after other medications have failed.

D.   Discharge criteria. Criteria for final discharge from the recovery areas include an operative site without hematoma or excessive bleeding, stable vital signs, ambulation, ability to urinate after spinal anesthesia, and adequate pain control. Discharge instructions are reviewed with the patient by the surgeon or nurse in the recovery areas.

V.   Unanticipated admission. The unanticipated admission rate after outpatient surgery is about 1%. Nausea, vomiting, pain, and operative site bleeding are the most common causes. Extended stay or inpatient facilities should be available for those patients who cannot be discharged after a reasonable stay in the PACU areas.

SUGGESTED READING

American Society of Anesthesiologists. *ASA guidelines for ambulatory anesthesia and surgery*. Park Ridge, IL: ASA. Amended by ASA House of Delegates, October 21, 1998.

American Society of Anesthesiologists Task Force on Preoperative Fasting. Report by the American Society of Anesthesiologists Task Force on Preoperative Fasting. Practice guidelines for preoperative fasting and the use of pharmacologic agents to reduce the risk of pulmonary aspiration: application to healthy patients undergoing elective procedures. *Anesthesiology* 1999;90:896–905.

Apfelbaum JL. Bypassing PACU: a cost-saving measure. *Can J Anaesth* 1998;45:R91–R94.

Auroy Y, Narchi P, Messiah A, et al. Serious complications related to regional anesthesia results of a prospective survey in France. *Anesthesiology* 1997;87:479–486.

Gan TJ, Glass PS, Windsor A, et al. Bispectral index monitoring allows faster emergence and improved recovery from propofol, alfentanil, and nitrous oxide anesthesia. *Anesthesiology* 1997;87:808–815.

Hampl KF, Heinzmann-Wiedmer S, Luginbuehl I, et al. Transient neurological symptoms after spinal anesthesia: a lower incidence with prilocaine and bupivacaine than with lidocaine. *Anesthesiology* 1998;88: 629–633.

Joshi GP, Inagaki Y, White PF, et al. Use of the laryngeal mask airway as an alternative to the tracheal tube during ambulatory anesthesia. *Anesth Analg* 1997;85:573–577.

Mayfield, J. BIS Monitoring reduces phase 1 PACU admissions in an ambulatory surgical unit. *Anesthesiology* 1999;91:3A:A28.

Meridy HW. Criteria for selection of ambulatory surgical patients and guidelines for anesthetic management: a retrospective study of 1553 cases. *Anesth Analg* 1982;61:921–926.

Song D, Joshi GP, White PF. Fast-track eligibility after ambulatory anesthesia: a comparison of desflurane, sevoflurane, and propofol. *Anesth Analg* 1998;86:267–273.

Tang J, Watcha MF, White PF. A comparison of costs and efficacy of ondansetron and droperidol as prophylactic antiemetic therapy for elective outpatient surgery. *Anesth Analg* 1996;83:304–313.

Tong D, Chung F, Wong D. Predictive factors in global and anesthesia satisfaction in ambulatory surgical patients. *Anesthesiology* 1997:87: 856–864.

Vaghadia H. Spinal anesthesia for outpatients: controversies and new techniques. *Can J Anaesth* 1998;45[Suppl 5 Part 2]:R64–R70.

Watcha MF, White PF. Economics of anesthesia practice. *Anesthesiology* 1997;86:1170–1196.

White PF. Ambulatory anesthesia—past, present and future. In: White PF, ed. *Ambulatory anesthesia and surgery.* London: WB Saunders: 1997:1–34.

Wilson JL, Brown DL, Wong GY, et al. Infraclavicular brachial plexus block: parasagittal anatomy important to the coracoid technique. *Anesth Analg* 1998;87:870–873.

Anesthesia Outside the Operating Room

William E. Hurford and Susan A. Vassallo

I. **General considerations**. The anesthetist may be called on to provide sedation or general anesthesia in locations remote from the familiar surroundings and backup capabilities of the operating room. The same principles and requirements for anesthesia equipment and monitoring standards outlined in Chapters 9 and 10 should be met.

A. **Equipment.**

1. Outlets for electrical power, oxygen, nitrous oxide, suction, and scavenging must be available and function properly. **A central supply of oxygen** is a minimum requirement, although some locations may not have a central supply of nitrous oxide. The presence of full reserve tanks for oxygen and nitrous oxide must be checked. A source of compressed air is desirable in cases (such as embolization) where nitrous oxide is not used.

2. A complete anesthesia cart, similar to the one used in the operating room, should be available.

3. **Resuscitation equipment** (e.g., defibrillator and medications) must be available.

B. **Workspace area and patient access** often are limited.

1. Adequate monitoring during the procedure may need to be modified if the anesthetist cannot stay in the room (e.g., during irradiation). Alternative methods of monitoring (e.g., through a window or by closed-circuit television) must then be used. Monitoring needs during transport of the patient must be anticipated.

2. It is important to establish direct communication channels, particularly in case of emergency.

3. Areas outside the operating room where anesthesia will be performed should be designated as "approved anesthesia locations."

4. Anesthetists should take appropriate precautions and employ appropriate techniques to minimize their risk of radiation exposure during procedures.

II. **Anesthesia for computed tomography**

A. **Computed tomography scans** are usually performed without general anesthesia, but children and uncooperative adults (e.g., head-injured patients) may need sedation or general anesthesia to avoid motion artifacts during the scan. Standard monitors (electrocardiogram [ECG], pulse oximetry, and blood pressure) should be used; capnography is useful to provide evidence of ventilation. A side-stream capnography sampling tube may be fitted to a nasal cannula or oxygen face mask to provide a qualitative assessment of ventilation.

B.   In adults, small intravenous (IV) doses of a benzodiazepine or short-acting hypnotic (e.g., propofol) can be used for sedation.

C.   Infants and children

   1.   In some children less than 3 months of age, scans can be done without sedation. However, most children require either sedation or general anesthesia. If deep sedation or general anesthesia is required, a patent airway is maintained with a laryngeal mask airway (LMA) or an endotracheal tube.

   2.   Chloral hydrate (30 to 50 mg/kg orally or per rectum [PR] administered 30 to 60 minutes before the procedure) is often chosen as a mild sedative for children. In sedating doses, choral hydrate is safe to use, and is not associated with respiratory depression or loss of airway. This drug can be safely administered by nonanesthesia personnel. However, there is a "failure" rate (defined as movement during the scan) of 15%.

   3.   Rectal methohexital (25 to 30 mg/kg) has a more rapid onset (5 to 10 minutes) than chloral hydrate and a reasonably long duration (approximately 30 minutes). It is useful for the induction of general anesthesia. Its absorption, and consequently its effects, however, are somewhat unpredictable. A state of deep sedation or general anesthesia may be produced; therefore, the drug should only be administered by an anesthetist under monitored conditions, provisions for securing the airway should be present, and patients should not be at risk of reflux of gastric contents.

   4.   General anesthesia using either intravenous or inhalational agents may be required.

III.   Anesthesia for magnetic resonance imaging

A.   Anesthetizing a patient in the magnetic resonance imaging (MRI) suite presents several challenging problems related to the physical environment.

   1.   The "tunnel" in which the patient is placed is long and narrow (2x0.5m) and does not allow access to the patient during the procedure.

   2.   There is a **constant magnetic field** present, which will exert a strong pull on any equipment containing ferromagnetic materials (e.g., steel gas tanks and batteries) and will also interfere with mechanical components (solenoids) in automated, noninvasive, blood pressure monitors, ventilators, and infusion pumps. Personnel working around an MRI scanner should be extremely careful not to have ferromagnetic materials with them. **Ferromagnetic objects can be forcibly pulled toward the magnet, possibly injuring people or equipment in their path**. Equipment that cannot be used includes standard stethoscopes and laryngoscopes. Aluminium laryngoscopes and plastic stethoscopes must be available in case an emergency occurs within the MRI. Credit cards, watches, and pagers should also be left outside the scanning area since they may be damaged by the magnetic field.

   3.   Metallic implants or devices in patients may be at risk of dislodgment when MRI procedures are performed. Patients with implanted pacemakers or cerebrovascular clips should not have MRI scans. Other devices may or may not be affected by MRI. Each MRI site carries a list of medical devices and whether they have been deemed MRI "safe" by the U.S. Food and Drug

Administration (FDA). Since medical devices may be upgraded or altered by a manufacturer without notifying the FDA, MRI centers should, in addition, contact the manufacturer if questions arise about certain devices.

4. Radio-frequency signals are present during scans and disturb electronic monitoring devices and produce loud rhythmic noises, making it difficult to hear breath and heart sounds.

B. The duration of the MRI procedure varies, and immobility is required during the actual scans, which take 5 to 8 minutes each. General anesthesia with an LMA for airway patency will be necessary for most infants and children. For reasons of safety and convenience, general anesthesia is induced in an area away from the magnetic field. When stable, the patient is moved into the scanner. A specially modified anesthesia machine that contains only nonferrous metal is used during maintenance of anesthesia. The patient should be removed from the area of the magnetic field if airway manipulations or cardiopulmonary resuscitation is required.

C. Monitors must be safe for the patient, function within the magnetic field, and have no effect on the images obtained by the scan. Existing equipment may be used as long as it is distanced from the magnetic field by using long cables. Electrical currents can be induced in coiled cables; cables should be kept as straight as possible to minimize the risk of burns and interference. Specialized "MRI-compatible" equipment (e.g., anesthesia machines, ventilators, and monitors) composed of nonferromagnetic materials such as aluminium and plastic are available.

1. The standard ECG suffers interference during the actual scans. A specialized, gated ECG monitor that will function even during scanning is available.

2. Standard, unmodified **pulse oximeters** also suffer interference during scans and may themselves interfere with imaging. Specialized "MRI-compatible" pulse oximeters are available that can function safely during MRI. Their sensors should be placed away from the center of the magnetic field.

3. Temperature probes are not used because of the potential for causing cutaneous burns.

4. Closed-circuit television can be used to visualize the patient and monitors during the scan.

IV. Anesthesia for neuroradiology. Neuroradiologic procedures include diagnostic arteriography, embolization of arteriovenous malformations and aneurysms, treatment of vasospasm with localized injections of vasodilating drugs, and diagnosis and ablation of trigeminal neuralgia.

A. Intracranial vascular procedures

1. Anesthetic goals include maintaining patient consciousness to facilitate neurologic evaluation (unless general anesthesia is indicated), providing sedation to allow patients to be immobile during dye injection, and maintaining stable hemodynamics. Children and patients with neurologic defects may require a general anesthetic. General anesthesia may also be indicated for lengthy or difficult procedures, even for cooperative adults. Anesthesia can be accomplished with intravenous techniques (propofol, muscle relaxant, and opioid) and supplemented with low doses of volatile anesthetics. Nitrous oxide is avoided to reduce the consequences of air embolization. High doses of volatile anesthetics and hypercarbia can cause cerebral vasodilation and should be avoided.

2. Sedation is used to minimize the discomfort associated with arterial puncture and dye injection. Small doses of an opiate along with a benzodiazepine or propofol usually are adequate.

3. Hyperosmolar contrast dyes produce a brisk diuresis requiring urinary catheterization and IV fluid administration.

4. An arterial catheter is frequently placed in the radial artery, or alternatively, blood pressure may be transduced from the femoral artery catheter sheath used during the procedure. Intravenous phenylephrine and nitroglycerin must be immediately available.

5. Hypertension should be avoided, since it may increase the risk of hemorrhage or aneurysm rupture.

6. Embolization procedures may be lengthy and can place the patient at risk for untoward embolic events. Emergency airway management and endotracheal intubation may be required if sudden neurologic deterioration occurs.

7. A cooling blanket can be used to induce moderate hypothermia (33.5°C) during aneurysm procedures. A warming blanket is used to return body temperature to normal once the embolization is complete.

B. Embolization for control of extracranial vascular lesions presents potential problems of hemorrhage, hemodynamic instability, and aspiration. Typed and cross-matched blood should be available, large-bore IV access must be obtained, and endotracheal intubation may be required for airway control.

C. Trigeminal neuralgia. Neurolytic block of the trigeminal nerve and its branches has been used effectively in the management of chronic pain. In general, a local anesthetic block is performed to reproduce the anesthesia that will accompany permanent gangliolysis.

1. Diagnostic local anesthetic block of the trigeminal ganglion. Standard monitoring is used, and a brief period of unconsciousness, produced by either methohexital 1% (0.5 to 1.0 mg/kg IV) or propofol (1 to 2 mg/kg IV), is induced to allow needle placement in the trigeminal ganglion by way of the foramen ovale. Proper position of the needle is confirmed using fluoroscopy, a test dose of local anesthetic is injected, and the patient's neurologic examination is evaluated when the patient is awake and fully cooperative.

2. Neurolytic lesion of the trigeminal ganglion. Once the degree of anesthesia induced by the temporary trigeminal block is deemed to be satisfactory, permanent neurolytic block may be performed. Neurolytic techniques include alcohol or glycerol injection, surgical rhizotomy, and thermogangliolysis. The anesthetic technique is identical to that used for diagnostic local anesthetic block of the trigeminal ganglion. Hypertension is common during gangliolysis, may require continuous arterial monitors and control with esmolol, labetalol, or nitroprusside. Airway support may be difficult in these patients when the block needles are in place.

V. Anesthesia for cyclotron therapy

A. Proton-beam radiation therapy is used in the treatment of arteriovenous malformations, pituitary tumors, and retinoblastomas. The irradiation is painless, but targeting and exact positioning may take several hours, during which the patient's head must remain in a fixed position. To achieve this, the head is usually placed in a stereotactic frame locked to the positioning device.

B. **In adults**, placement of small pins or screws in the skull can be performed under local anesthesia with 2% lidocaine with epinephrine. If "ear bars" are used, a satisfactory ear block can be performed by subcutaneous injection of 3 mL of 2% lidocaine with epinephrine in the outer ear canal. Sedation is usually not recommended, since patient cooperation is required.

C. **For children**, a general anesthetic is usually administered.. The procedure typically is performed daily for about 4 weeks; a propofol induction (3 mg/kg IV) and maintenance infusion (approximately 75 µg/kg per minute) through an implanted Broviac or Hickman catheter is a suitable technique. Whenever possible, spontaneous ventilation should be permitted. The patient's head is placed in a sniffing position, and a plaster mold is made that holds in head in the correct position for treatment. Supplemental oxygen can be provided by nasal prongs or a face mask. A LMA can be considered if an adequate natural airway cannot be maintained. Standard monitoring is employed and the patient is monitored viewed via closed-circuit television, since the anesthetist must leave the room during the brief period of radiation.

VI. **Anesthesia for radiation therapy**. Children receiving radiation therapy often require general anesthesia.

A. A typical treatment course is 3 to 4 times a week for a 4-week period. It is desirable to choose an anesthetic that allows rapid recovery with minimal risk of nausea and vomiting.

B. The first radiation procedure may be quite time consuming (1 to several hours) since measurements must be performed and molds of the patient made. Subsequent treatments are usually much shorter (less than 30 minutes).

C. Many patients will have indwelling venous access in place for chemotherapy. An IV induction and maintenance with a propofol infusion (see section V.C) is a suitable technique. A combination of midazolam, glycopyrrolate, and ketamine administered intramuscularly may be used in children with difficult venous access.

VII. **Conscious sedation and monitored anesthesia care**

A. Most invasive procedures outside the operating room requiring sedation are accomplished with the administration of conscious sedation by a nonanesthetist. **Conscious sedation** is defined as a medically controlled state of depressed consciousness that allows protective reflexes to be maintained, and retains the patient's ability to maintain a patent airway and the ability to respond appropriately to physical and verbal stimulation. Standards for the roles of nonanesthesiologists and nonphysicians in conscious sedation have been set by the Joint Commission on Accreditation of Healthcare Organizations and various state agencies such as licensing boards. All guidelines and standards require the same level of vigilance and patient monitoring in all settings.

B. As with any anesthetic, **a thorough preprocedure evaluation**, anesthetic plan, and informed consent are necessary (see Chapter 1). Formal consultation with an anesthesiologist and the presence of an anesthesiologist (**monitored anesthesia care**) during the procedure may be desirable for high-risk patients.

C. **Drug choices for conscious sedation**

   1. **Benzodiazepines** (see Chapter 11, section I.C) provide anxiolysis, anterograde amnesia, and drowsiness. Common choices are midazolam, diazepam, and lorazepam. Their effects can be reversed by a specific antagonist, flumazenil.

   2. **Opioids** (see Chapter 11, section I.F) provide analgesia and sedation. Commonly used opioids for IV conscious sedation include morphine, fentanyl, and meperidine. Continuous infusions of short-acting opioids, such as remifentanil, are difficult to titrate safely and are not commonly used by nonanesthetists. Naloxone can be used to reverse unintended respiratory depression resulting from opioid administration.

   3. **Propofol** (see Chapter 11, section I.A) has the advantage of rapid awakening after its administration. Careful attention to its administration during conscious sedation is necessary, because unintended unconsciousness, loss of airway reflexes, and apnea may occur.

   4. **Droperidol** is a butyrophenone that is used for conscious sedation in many centers. It is often combined with an opioid such as fentanyl to produce neuroleptanalgesia. While it does not produce respiratory depression, extrapyramidal effects and hypotension may occur. Recent concerns over QT-interval prolongation and induction of ventricular arrhythmias may limit its use (see *Droperidol* in Appendix I).

   5. **Diphenhydramine** is a histamine-1 receptor antagonist that has weak sedative properties and lacks significant respiratory depression. Prolonged drowsiness after diphenhydramine may delay recovery in elderly patients.

   6. **Barbiturates** and **ketamine** (see Chapter 11, sections I.B and I.D, respectively) are occasionally used for conscious sedation, but recovery from these agents tends to be prolonged.

   7. **Considerations for pediatric patients** are as outlined in section II.C.

VIII. Electroconvulsive therapy (ECT) is used for treatment of major depression for patients who have not responded to medications, are debilitated by serious side effects, or are acutely suicidal. Patients who suffer from delusions, hallucinations, or profound psychomotor retardation are less responsive to medication, and thus early ECT is preferred for them as well. Of those receiving ECT, 75% to 85% have a favorable response. Usually a series of 6 to 12 treatments over 2 to 4 weeks is required for a clinical response.

A. **Physiologic effects of ECT**

   1. The electrical stimulus produces a grand mal seizure consisting of a tonic phase lasting 10 to 15 seconds, followed by a 30- to 50-second clonic phase.

   2. An increase in cerebral blood flow and cerebral metabolic rate leads to an increase in intracranial pressure (ICP).

   3. An initial vagal discharge is manifested as bradycardia and mild hypotension.

   4. Sympathetic nervous system activation subsequently produces hypertension and tachycardia, which can persist for 5 to 10 minutes. ECG changes are common and may include pulse-rate interval prolongation, increased QT interval, T-wave inversions, and atrial or ventricular arrhythmias.

5. Increased intraocular and intragastric pressure may occur.

B. Anesthetic goals

1. Provide amnesia and a rapid return to consciousness.

2. Prevent damage from the tonic-clonic contracture (e.g., long-bone fracture).

3. Control the hemodynamic response.

4. Avoid interference with the initiation and duration of the induced seizure.

C. The one absolute contraindication to ECT is **intracranial hypertension** (elevated ICP). **Relative contraindications** include presence of an intracranial mass lesion (with normal ICP), intracranial aneurysm, recent myocardial infarction, angina, congestive heart failure, untreated glaucoma, major bone fractures, thrombophlebitis, pregnancy, and retinal detachment. Patients on maintenance treatment with either benzodiazepines or lithium should discontinue these treatments before undergoing ECT. Benzodiazepines are anticonvulsant and abolish or attenuate the induced seizure. Lithium treatment is associated with post-ECT confusion and delirium.

D. Anesthetic management

1. Sedative premedication generally is not indicated and may prolong emergence. Anticholinergic drugs are administered only to patients who are prone to bradycardia.

2. A capped (saline-lock), small-gauge IV cannula is placed for drug administration, standard monitors (ECG, pulse oximetry, and blood pressure) are applied, and the patient is preoxgenated with 100% oxygen.

3. Anesthesia is induced, usually with methohexital (0.5 to 1.0 mg/kg IV) and succinylcholine (0.5 to 1.0 mg/kg IV), and the patient's lungs are ventilated with 100% oxygen with an Ambu bag and mask. Mivacurium can be used in those patients with contraindications to succinylcholine use. Patients with hypertension or coronary artery disease are pretreated with labetalol (10 to 50 mg IV) or esmolol (40 to 80 mg IV) to blunt the hypertensive response to the stimulus.

4. Other anesthetic induction agents may be used; however, thiopental prolongs emergence, midazolam raises the seizure threshold, and propofol reduces seizure duration. Pretreatment with ondansetron may be considered for those with a history of nausea and vomiting after ECT, and ketorolac may be useful for patients with muscle pains after the procedure.

5. Rolled gauze pads are placed between the maxilla and jaw on each side of the mouth, which will protect the gums and lips from biting, and a unilateral or bilateral electrical stimulus is applied.

6. The nature and duration of the induced seizure can be monitored with either an electroencephalogram or the "isolated arm" technique. With the latter, the blood supply to one arm is interrupted by an inflated blood pressure cuff before injecting the muscle relaxant so that unopposed seizure activity can be seen in the isolated arm.

7. Patients are ventilated with oxygen by face mask until spontaneous ventilation has resumed. They are then turned to the lateral decubitus position and monitored in a recovery area until awake and alert. An agitated delirium, which may be caused by tardive seizures, may occur after an ECT treatment and can be treated with small doses of propofol or a benzodiazepine.

8.   Patients with underlying medical conditions may require special attention before ECT.

    a.   Patients with gastroesophageal reflux may require aspiration prophylaxis and rapid sequence intubation.

    b.   Patients with severe cardiac dysfunction may require invasive monitoring.

    c.   Patients with intracranial lesions should be monitored with an arterial line, require tight hemodynamic control, and should be hyperventilated before the stimulus is applied.

    d.   Pregnant patients may require endotracheal intubation, fetal monitoring, and left uterine displacement.

9.   Rarely an induced seizure will not terminate spontaneously. Ventilation with 100% oxygen is continued, and the seizure terminated within 3 minutes with propofol (20 to 50 mg IV).

E.   Psychiatric drug interactions. The patient for ECT may be treated with psychotropic drugs that have potent side effects and interactions with anesthetic drugs.

1.   Tricyclic antidepressants (e.g., amitriptyline, nortriptyline, desipramine, imipramine, and doxepin) potentiate the effects of norepinephrine and serotonin by preventing their reuptake. Adverse effects may limit the usefulness of tricyclics for chronic treatment of depression, and include postural hypotension, sedation, dry mouth, urinary retention, and tachycardia. Anesthesia and ECT-induced ECG changes (including prolonged PR interval, widened QRS complex, and T-wave changes) are relatively common in patients receiving tricyclic antidepressants.

2.   The use of **monoamine oxidase inhibitors (MAOIs)** (e.g., phenelzine and isocarboxazid) for long-term treatment of depression may also be limited by adverse effects. By inhibiting monoamine oxidase, these drugs increase the intracellular concentrations of the amine neurotransmitters dopamine, epinephrine, norepinephrine, and serotonin, and increase the availability of norepinephrine at postsynaptic receptors. The drugs have complex adverse effects and drug interactions that include orthostatic hypotension and severe hypertension. Patients taking MAOIs have dietary restrictions since the tyramine in certain foods produce hypertensive crisis. Although it has been recommended that MAOI therapy be discontinued at least 10 days before elective surgery, usually the risk of severe depression outweighs the risks of continuing the drug. **Important interactions** between MAOIs and anesthetics include exaggerated hypotension during spinal anesthesia and severe hypertension with indirectly acting vasopressors such as ephedrine. Administration of even a single dose of **meperidine** (and meperidine derivatives) to patients receiving MAOIs has been associated with a syndrome of serotonin excess, which can produce severe hemodynamic instability, respiratory depression, malignant hyperpyrexia, seizures, coma, and death.

3.   Selective serotonin reuptake inhibitors (e.g., fluoxetine, sertraline, fluvoxamine, and paroxetine) are used often in the treatment of chronic depression because they are safe and associated with only a few, mild adverse effects (most commonly gastrointestinal disturbance, insomnia, agitation, and loss of libido). There are no significant interactions with anesthetic drugs.

SUGGESTED READING

Coté CJ. Anesthesia outside the operating room. In: Coté CJ, Todres ID, Goudsouzian NG, Ryan JF, eds. *A practice of anesthesia for infants and children*, 3rd ed. Philadelphia: WB Saunders, 2001:571–583.

El-Ganzouri AS, Ivanovich AD, Braverman B, et al. Monoamine oxidase inhibitors: should they be discontinued preoperatively? *Anesth Analg* 1985;64:592–596.

Gaines GY III, Rees DI. Anesthetic considerations for electroconvulsive therapy. *South Med J* 1992;85:469–482.

Gilbertson LI, cd. Conscious sedation. *Int Anesthesiol Clin* 1999;37: 1–129.

Jorgensen NH, Messeck JM Jr, Gray J, et al. ASA monitoring standards and magnetic resonance imaging. *Anesth Analg* 1994;79:1141–1147.

Mackenzie RA, Southorn PA, Stensrud PE. Anesthesia at remote locations. In: Miller RD, ed. *Anesthesia*, 5th ed. New York: Churchill Livingstone, 2000:2241–2270.

Martin LD, Pasternak LR, Pudimat MA. Total intravenous anesthesia with propofol in pediatric patients outside the operating room. *Anesth Analg* 1992;74:609–612.

Patteson SK, Chesney JT. Anesthetic management for magnetic resonance imaging: problems and solutions. *Anesth Analg* 1992;74: 121–128.

Stoelting RK, Dierdorf SF. *Psychiatric illness and substance abuse: anesthesia and co-existing disease*, 3rd ed. New York: Churchill Livingstone, 1993:517–538.

Welch CA. Electroconvulsive therapy in the general hospital. In: Cassem NH, ed. *Massachusetts General Hospital handbook of general psychiatry*. St. Louis: Mosby–Year Book, 1997:89–99.

Young WL, Pile-Spellman J. Anesthetic considerations for interventional neuroradiology. *Anesthesiology* 1994;80:427–456.

Anesthesia for Trauma and Burns

Christopher Carter and Keith H. Baker

I. Initial evaluation of the trauma patient
A. Airway and breathing

1. Since hypoxemia poses an immediate threat to the trauma patient, the anesthetist initially should focus on the airway. **Assume all multiple-trauma patients have a cervical spine injury, a full stomach, and are hypovolemic.**

2. All patients should have **initial stabilization of the cervical spine** before any airway manipulation. No method is foolproof. Manual immobilization or sandbags on either side of the head, and joined by tape across the forehead, can keep the head in a neutral position. Stabilization can also be accomplished with a rigid cervical (Philadelphia) collar. Soft collars are ineffective for immobilizing the neck.

3. Remove all secretions, blood, vomitus, and any existing foreign bodies (e.g., dentures or teeth). If the airway is patent and ventilation is adequate, provide supplemental oxygen and closely monitor the patient while initiating other resuscitative measures. The anesthetist always should be prepared to immediately secure the airway.

4. Patients with a variety of clinical presentations may require endotracheal intubation:

    a. **The awake patient.** Depending on the nature of the injuries, the ability of the patient to cooperate, and the general stability of the patient, several options are available (see Chapter 13):

        (1) Awake nasal or orotracheal intubation with or without the use of a laryngoscope or fiber-optic bronchoscope.

        (2) Blind nasal intubation.

        (3) Rapid sequence intubation.

        (4) Awake tracheostomy.

    b. **The combative patient.** A rapid-sequence induction and orotracheal intubation is often the most expedient approach, provided there are no problems precluding neuromuscular blockade. Hypoxemia must always be excluded in an agitated patient. Blind nasal intubation may be attempted; however, sedating these patients to control their agitation may lead to further airway compromise.

    c. **The unconscious patient.** Generally an orotracheal intubation is the safest and most expeditious approach.

    d. If the patient arrives with an esophageal obturator airway or esophageal gastric tube airway, perform **endotracheal intubation before removing these devices**, since vomiting frequently occurs with removal.

5. The intubated patient. Verify the position of an endotracheal tube by auscultating for breath sounds bilaterally and by detecting exhaled or end-tidal CO_2. Secure the endotracheal tube and ensure adequate ventilation and oxygenation.

B. Circulation

1. Hemodynamics are initially assessed by palpating pulses and measuring the blood pressure.

2. Intravenous access. Check intravenous (IV) lines already in place to ensure that they function well. At least two large (minimum 16-gauge) catheters are required. These lines should be placed above the level of the diaphragm in patients with injuries of the abdomen (and with the potential for major venous disruption). Intravenous access below the level of the diaphragm is helpful if obstruction or disruption of the superior vena cava is suspected.

3. Peripheral venous cannulation failure. In this event, percutaneous subclavian or femoral vein cannulation should be carried out. Although the internal and external jugular veins remain options, access to these structures is frequently hindered by immobilization of the head and neck for a suspected cervical spine injury. If these approaches prove unsuccessful, **surgical cutdowns** should be performed. The saphenous vein at the ankle or the thigh and the antecubital venous system are acceptable options. Intraosseous infusion is also an option but is better suited for the pediatric patient.

4. Volume resuscitation begins immediately with the establishment of venous access.

    a. Most trauma patients experience hypovolemia and their hemodynamics will improve with the rapid administration of warmed crystalloid. If possible, defer blood replacement until cross-matched units are available.

    b. Patients who do not respond to rapid infusion of crystalloid are candidates for transfusion of type-specific, non–cross-matched blood as soon as it is available (This should be available within 15 minutes of the patient's arrival.)

    c. Rarely, a patient remains moribund despite rapid infusion of crystalloid. Low-titer, type O-negative, non–cross-matched blood may be lifesaving.

    d. Controversy still exists regarding the use of colloid (e.g., albumin and hetastarch) in resuscitation. Albumin offers no advantage as a therapy for the management of hypovolemia. Currently available dextrans are not used in the management of hemorrhagic shock because of potential coagulopathy.

5. Vasopressor infusions should not substitute for adequate volume replacement during initial resuscitation. They may be necessary as a temporizing measure if perfusion pressure is clearly inadequate during ongoing volume resuscitation.

C. History

1. Interview the patient, family members, and prehospital care personnel about the events surrounding an accident.

2. Obtain an **abbreviated history** including allergies, medications, and medical and surgical histories.

3. Mechanisms of injury. Determine the pattern of injury and allow the clinician to focus the treatment priorities for each patient.

a. Because **blunt trauma** (e.g., motor vehicle accidents or falls) results in widespread energy transfer to the body, multiple injuries can occur in various anatomic locations.

b. **Penetrating trauma** (e.g., knives and bullets) produces injuries that are generally confined to the penetration track. High-velocity gunshot wounds may cause tissue disruption in areas adjacent to the penetration track.

D. Physical examination

1. Frequent monitoring of vital signs is mandatory and provides an ongoing assessment of airway, neurologic, cardiovascular, and pulmonary stability.

2. Assess obvious **sites of hemorrhage**, as well as less obvious sites (e.g., chest, abdomen, pelvis, thighs, and retroperitoneum) for evidence of blood loss.

3. Investigate **neurologic deficits and vascular compromise** without delay.

E. Diagnostic studies

1. Laboratory studies include blood type and cross-matching, complete blood count, platelet count, prothrombin time, activated partial thromboplastin time, electrolytes, glucose, blood urea nitrogen, creatinine, urinalysis, and, if indicated, toxicologic screening.

2. Radiographic studies should include a lateral cervical spine film, a chest radiograph (CXR), and an anteroposterior view of the pelvis on all patients with blunt trauma. At the minimum, obtain a CXR in all patients with penetrating injuries of the trunk. Additional studies include thoracic, lumbar, and sacral spine films, and chest and abdominal computed tomography (CT) studies.

a. Lateral radiographs of the cervical spine must include the C-7–T-1 interface and be of sufficient quality to delineate the structures of interest (i.e., soft tissues and bones).

b. If the patient's clinical condition allows time for additional studies, obtain **open-mouth odontoid and anteroposterior views of the neck** (standard trauma cervical-spine series).

c. If the clinical evaluation demonstrates a patient with significant neck pain and tenderness but no evidence of fracture or dislocation on the plain radiographs, CT and magnetic resonance imaging may help delineate an occult injury.

3. Obtain a **12-lead electrocardiogram (ECG)** on all major trauma patients to help evaluate the presence of myocardial injury (e.g., contusion, tamponade, ischemia, and arrhythmia).

F. Monitoring is dictated by the severity of the patient's injuries and preexisting medical problems.

1. An arterial line may prove useful in patients with hemodynamic instability or respiratory failure.

2. A central venous pressure line may be required to assess volume status and administer vasoactive drugs.

3. A **pulmonary artery catheter** may be helpful in patients with ventricular dysfunction, severe coronary artery disease, valvular heart disease, or multiple organ system involvement. Placement is planned according to the time available and the clinical status of the patient.

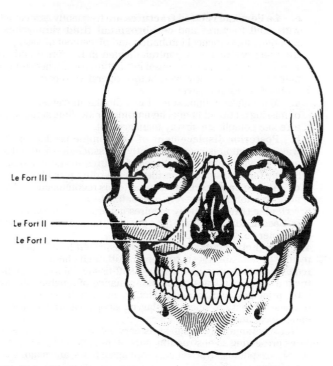

Fig. 32-1. The LeFort classification. (From Rosen P, et al., eds. *Emergency medicine: concepts and clinical practice*, 2nd ed. St. Louis: Mosby, 1988:407.)

II. Specific injuries

A. Intracranial and spinal cord trauma (see Chapter 24).

B. Facial trauma. Brisk oral or nasal bleeding, broken teeth, vomitus, or tongue or pharyngeal injury may occlude the airway and complicate airway management. Emergency cricothyroidotomy or tracheostomy may be lifesaving.

    1. Maxillary fractures are grouped by the **LeFort classification** (Fig. 32-1).

        a. Type I (transverse or horizontal). The body of the maxilla is separated from the base of the skull above the level of the palate and below the level of the zygomatic process.

        b. Type II (pyramidal). Vertical fractures through the facial aspects of the maxilla extend upward to the nasal and ethmoid bones.

        c. Type III (craniofacial dysjunction). Fractures extend through the frontozygomatic suture lines bilaterally, across the orbits, and through the base of the nose and the ethmoid region.

        d. Common coexisting injuries include intracranial hemorrhage, cerebral contusions, and cervical spine trauma.

e.   Le Fort and related fractures are frequently associated with skull fractures and **cerebrospinal fluid rhinorrhea**. Emergent nasotracheal intubation and placement of nasogastric tubes are relatively contraindicated in Le Fort II and Le Fort III fractures. Elective nasal intubation (or tracheostomy) may be necessary, however, before operative repair.

2.   Mandibular fractures

a.   Malocclusion, limitation of mandibular movement, loose or missing teeth, sublingual hematoma, or swelling at the fracture site complicate airway management.

b.   Posterior displacement of the tongue producing airway obstruction is seen frequently in association with bilateral condylar or parasymphyseal fractures of the mandible. Simple forward traction on the tongue often provides relief.

c.   Awake nasotracheal intubation is recommended if the nose has not been severely traumatized.

3.   Ocular trauma usually requires general anesthesia for repair. Special considerations for open-eye injuries are discussed in Chapter 25, section I.C.1.

4.   Anesthetic management. Most displaced facial fractures require general anesthesia for repair. Although children usually require general anesthesia, many soft-tissue injuries can be treated using local anesthesia. Maintenance of a patent airway is the principal concern, and induction may require awake nasotracheal intubation, fiberoptic laryngoscopy, or tracheostomy under local anesthesia.

C.   Neck trauma may manifest as cervical spine injury, airway injuries presenting as obstruction, subcutaneous emphysema, hemoptysis, dysphonia, hypoxemia, esophageal tears, and major vascular injuries.

1.   "Clothesline" injuries occurring from direct trauma to the upper airway do not always present with an open neck wound. Additional injuries include laryngotracheal transection, laryngeal fractures, and vascular injury.

2.   Initial management of **penetrating trauma** includes direct compression of involved vessels to control hemorrhage and prevent air embolism.

3.   Associated **thoracic injuries**, such as pneumothorax and hemorrhage from injury to the great vessels, may occur with lower neck injuries.

4.   Anesthetic management

a.   Securing the airway is the most important issue in these patients. A coordinated approach among members of the trauma team is necessary. A surgical airway or direct intubation of an open airway defect can be lifesaving.

b.   Great vessel injuries in the neck may necessitate lower extremity IV access.

D.   Chest trauma can involve injuries to the trachea or larynx, heart, great vessels, thoracic duct, esophagus, lung, or diaphragm.

1.   Rib fractures are a common feature of major thoracic trauma and mandate assessment for pneumothorax by CXR. First-rib fractures should alert the clinician to the potential for associated internal injuries. Multiple rib fractures most commonly involve ribs 7 to 10 and often accompany lacerations of the spleen or liver.

2. A "**flail chest**" refers to the paradoxical inspiratory retraction and expiratory expansion of an unstable chest wall segment that results from sequential segmental rib fractures. The hypoxemia and respiratory failure that accompany flail chest and other major chest injuries are indicative of underlying pulmonary contusion.

3. The presence of **subcutaneous emphysema** may indicate the presence of a pneumothorax or laryngeal, tracheobronchial, or esophageal trauma. Pneumothorax and hemothorax may lead to respiratory and cardiovascular collapse. If these conditions are present or highly suspected, chest tubes should be placed under local anesthesia before induction of general anesthesia. Avoid central line insertion (particularly by the subclavian route) on the side opposite an injury, because of the consequences of bilateral pneumothorax. Also, avoid the ipsilateral side if a concomitant major venous injury is suspected.

4. Anesthetic management

a. Patients with significant chest injuries almost always require general anesthesia.

b. The necessity for mechanical ventilation may extend into the postoperative period.

c. Avoid nitrous oxide when a pneumothorax is suspected and a chest tube has not yet been placed. Airway pressures must be closely monitored during positive-pressure ventilation.

d. Isolate a hemorrhaging lung before blood floods the uninjured side. Double-lumen endotracheal tube placement, mainstem intubation or endobronchial blockade may be lifesaving under these circumstances (see Chapter 21).

e. Regional anesthesia (i.e., intercostal nerve blockade or thoracic epidural anesthesia) frequently is useful for multiple painful rib fractures, which can cause chest wall splinting, regional hypoventilation, and progressive hypoxemia.

E. Cardiac and major vascular trauma

1. Signs of cardiac trauma include a fractured sternum, hemothorax, pericardial tamponade, and ECG changes (persistent sinus tachycardia and other arrhythmias, nonspecific ST-segment and T-wave changes, and overt ischemia).

2. A widened mediastinal profile and lack of clarity of the aortic knob on the CXR mandate **emergency angiography** to rule out traumatic aortic rupture. High-resolution CT and transesophageal echocardiography also are used to diagnose aortic dissection.

3. Cardiac abnormalities resulting from nonpenetrating cardiac trauma include arrhythmias, ventricular dysfunction, myocardial ischemia, and tamponade. An abnormal ECG should alert the anesthetist to the possibility of accompanying cardiac trauma.

4. The subclavian artery is subject to injury with hyperextension of the neck and shoulder.

5. Anesthetic management

a. These patients are often **severely hypovolemic** and may have compromised cardiac function. Cardiopulmonary bypass may be required.

b. Etomidate and ketamine are good choices for induction, but use of the latter must be weighed against its risk in patients with concomitant head injury.

F.   Abdominal trauma

1.   Penetrating abdominal wounds (with the exception of gunshot wounds) are initially evaluated in stable patients by local wound exploration to determine whether the peritoneal cavity has been violated. If the exploration is equivocal, diagnostic peritoneal lavage, abdominal ultrasound, or an abdominal CT scan may be performed.

2.   All patients with gunshot wounds of the abdomen are surgically explored.

3.   With impalement injuries (e.g., stab wounds or falls onto sharp objects), the penetrating object, if still present in the wound, will usually be removed in the operating room after anesthesia has been induced and the patient stabilized. Removal in an uncontrolled environment may result in exsanguination.

4.   Blunt trauma may result in intraabdominal or retroperitoneal bleeding.

   a.   The **spleen** is the most frequently injured abdominal organ in blunt trauma. Symptoms include abdominal or referred shoulder pain, abdominal rigidity, and a falling hematocrit or hypotension.

   b.   The **liver** frequently fractures with blunt abdominal trauma, which can produce massive blood loss.

G.   Genitourinary trauma

1.   All multiple trauma patients should have a **Foley catheter** placed. If pelvic or perineal injury has occurred, as evidenced by blood at the urethral meatus, a perineal hematoma, or a high-riding prostate, retrograde urethrography should be performed before urethral catheterization.

2.   All patients with penetrating abdominal or back injuries and those with significant hematuria following blunt trauma should have a radiographic **kidney-ureter-bladder** examination and undergo **intravenous pyelography**.

3.   Eighty-five percent of renal injuries can be managed nonoperatively, but patients with refractory hypotension should go directly to the operating room for exploration.

   a.   **Ureteral laceration** is managed by surgical intervention after locating the disruption by retrograde urography.

   b.   **Bladder** contusions may be treated nonoperatively, but rupture usually requires exploration.

   c.   The inability of the patient to void and clinical signs of injury indicate **injury to the urethra** (see section II.G.1). Diagnostic urethrography should precede treatment with suprapubic cystostomy for urinary diversion and control of hemorrhage. Most disruptions can undergo delayed repair.

H.   Peripheral vascular trauma

1.   Check peripheral pulses in all extremities during the evaluation of trauma patients. Arteriography is advisable when doubt exists.

2.   Anesthetic management should focus on the recognition of hypovolemia secondary to uncontrolled hemorrhage. Repair of injuries in stable patients may be amenable to regional anesthetic techniques.

I.   Orthopedic trauma

1. All **fractures or dislocations** that compromise nerve or vascular function may constitute surgical emergencies (e.g., radial nerve injury with humeral shaft fractures and aseptic necrosis of the femoral head with hip dislocation), and must be reduced immediately.

2. **Upper extremity**

   a. Severe **depression or hyperabduction of the shoulder girdle** can stretch or tear the brachial plexus. Horner's syndrome may present with damage to the cervical sympathetic chain.

   b. When the shoulder is struck hard from the side, the medial end of the clavicle may be dislocated upward or retrosternally. Pressure on the trachea in a retrosternal dislocation may cause life-threatening airway compromise.

   c. Dislocation of the glenohumeral joint can cause axillary nerve injury.

   d. **Fractures of the humeral shaft**, especially the middle or distal part, are frequently associated with radial nerve injury.

   e. Neurovascular compromise of the forearm can occur with fracture or dislocation of the elbow.

   f. Median nerve compression is possible with **fractures at the wrist**.

   g. **Fractures of the elbow** or direct trauma to the forearm may cause edema of the anterior compartment of the forearm. Increased pressure on the blood vessels of the anterior compartment may result in ischemic necrosis. Fasciotomy may be indicated.

3. **Pelvis**

   a. Patients who have sustained pelvic injuries can be divided into one of three major categories:

      (1) **Exsanguinating hemorrhage** from external bleeding in open fractures or from retroperitoneal hematoma in closed fractures (0.5% to 1.0%). These patients almost always present with either severe hypotension or cardiac arrest and rarely respond to resuscitative measures.

      (2) **Hemodynamically stable** with a relatively uncomplicated course (75%). Urgent or elective surgery for repair of bony and ligamentous pelvic disruptions may be required.

      (3) An **intermediate group** in critical condition with varying degrees of overall injury, hemorrhage, and hemodynamic instability (25%).

   b. **Initial management** for these injuries may include the application of a compressive binder for "open book" fractures, pelvic angiography (with or without therapeutic embolization to control hemorrhage), and external pelvic fixation.

   c. **Fat embolism** can occur with pelvic and major long-bone fractures (see Chapter 18, section XV.C).

   d. **Crush injuries** may be associated with **hyperkalemia and myoglobinuria**. Early reversal of hypovolemia and alkalinization of the urine may help prevent acute renal failure.

4. **Lower extremity**

   a. Fractures of the **tibia and fibula,** the most common

major skeletal injuries, can be associated with neurovascular trauma.

b. With a fracture of the **femur or pelvis**, blood loss can be much greater than evident from superficial inspection.

c. **Hip fractures** are common in the elderly whose clinical picture is often dominated by other complicating medical illnesses. Traction is used initially for pain relief, but most fractures require open reduction and internal fixation to ensure adequate healing and function and to avoid the complications of prolonged immobilization.

d. Regional, general anesthesia, and combined techniques all are excellent choices for patients with isolated hip fractures.

5. Extremity reimplantation

a. Indications. In general, these procedures are performed only on the upper extremities and only in patients who are otherwise stable. An amputated arm, hand, or digit will not be reimplanted if it has sustained a severe crush injury or has been raggedly torn from attachments to major nerves and blood vessels. Reimplantations may be extremely lengthy procedures, occasionally in excess of 24 hours.

b. Anesthetic management

(1) General anesthesia is usually chosen because of the long duration of these procedures. A combined technique will reduce anesthetic requirements, provide for postoperative analgesia (especially with catheter placements, rather than single-dose brachial plexus blocks), and the resulting sympathectomy may improve blood flow.

(2) During general anesthetics, the head and pressure points must be evaluated at every 1 to 2 hours to avoid pressure-induced injury (e.g., scalp ulceration and hair loss). Low-pressure mattresses and padded sponge blocks should be used to minimize pressure on susceptible peripheral nerves (e.g., ulnar, sciatic, peroneal, or sural). The endotracheal tube cuff pressure should be periodically assessed, since nitrous oxide will diffuse into the cuff and increase the pressure on the tracheal mucosa.

III. The pediatric trauma patient

A. General considerations

1. A clear understanding of the salient anatomic and physiologic differences among adults, children, and infants as well as a working knowledge of the specific anesthetic considerations for this patient population is required (see Chapters 27 and 28).

2. Blunt trauma, usually from falls or motor vehicle accidents, predominates in children. Multiple injuries are the rule rather than the exception, but diagnosis is often more difficult because of the child's inability to provide an accurate history.

B. Specific considerations

1. Although the pediatric trauma patient frequently presents with significant blood loss, initially the **vital signs** may be minimally altered. **Reliance on vital signs alone may seriously underestimate the severity of injury.**

2. Surgical cricothyroidotomy is rarely performed in the infant or small child because of technical difficulties.

3. Intraosseous infusion is an acceptable procedure for critically injured pediatric patients in whom venous access cannot be established (see Chapter 28).

4. The small child who is **hypothermic** may be refractory to therapy for shock. While the child is exposed during initial evaluation and management, overhead heaters or thermal blankets will be needed to maintain body temperature.

IV. The pregnant trauma patient

A. General considerations

1. Pregnancy must always be suspected in any female trauma patient of childbearing age (see Chapter 29 for management of the pregnant patient).

2. Because the fetus is dependent on its mother for its oxygen requirements, an **uninterrupted supply of oxygenated blood** must be provided to the fetus at all times.

    a. Compression of the vena cava by the gravid uterus (after 20 weeks gestation) reduces venous return to the heart, thereby decreasing cardiac output and exacerbating shock. Unless a spinal injury is suspected, the pregnant patient should be transported and evaluated with left uterine displacement.

3. Although diagnostic irradiation poses a risk to the fetus, necessary radiographic studies should be obtained.

B. Treatment

1. If the mother's condition is stable, the status of the fetus and the extent of uterine injury will determine further management.

2. A potentially viable fetus that shows no signs of distress should be monitored by external ultrasound. Since premature labor is always a possibility in these patients, an external tocotransducer must be used to detect the onset of contractions. Initiate tocolytic therapy if premature labor develops.

3. When a viable fetus shows signs of distress despite successful resuscitative measures, a cesarean delivery must be performed expeditiously. A nonviable fetus may be managed conservatively in utero in order to optimize maternal oxygenation and circulation.

4. Primary repair of all maternal wounds should be attempted in a critically injured mother carrying a viable gestation, even at the expense of fetal distress.

V. Burns

A. Deep thermal injury destroys skin, the body's barrier to the external environment. Skin plays a vital role in thermal regulation, fluid and electrolyte homeostasis, and protection against bacterial infection. Significant heat loss, massive fluid shifts and protein losses, and infections commonly occur in patients with severe thermal injuries. There is also a diffuse alteration in the permeability of cell membranes to sodium, resulting in generalized cellular swelling. Microvascular injury results from local damage by heat and from the release of vasoactive substances from the burned tissue. Therefore, edema occurs in both burned and unburned tissues.

B. In **electrical burns**, current passage creates thermal energy that actually destroys tissue, particularly those tissues with high resistance such as skin and bone. The course of the electrical current is often occult. The precise location and extent of tissue damage may not be revealed by physical examination.

C. In **chemical burns**, the degree of injury depends on the particular chemical, its concentration, duration of contact, and the penetrability and resistance of the tissues involved. Some substances producing chemical burns, such as phosphorus, are absorbed systemically, producing significant and often life-threatening injury.

D. **Infections and drug reactions** may also cause extensive and life-threatening dermal injury.

VI. **Preoperative evaluation of burn patients**

A. **Burns are a form of trauma**; thus, the airway, breathing, and circulation should be initially assessed (see section I).

B. **The size of the burn** should be estimated as a percentage of the total body surface area (percent TBSA).

   1. The **rule of nines** guides estimations (Fig. 32-2).

     a. **Adults**

       (1) The head and both of the upper extremities represent 9% TBSA each.

       (2) The anterior trunk, posterior trunk, and both of the lower extremities represent 18% each.

     b. **Infants and children.** Because of the different proportions of body surface area relative to patient age, reference must be made to the proper burn chart when calculating percent TBSA to avoid significant errors (Fig. 32-2).

   2. Another practical method to estimate percent TBSA is that the area of the patient's hand will cover about 1% TBSA.

C. The **depth of the burn** determines therapy (i.e., conservative management versus excision and grafting). Burn depth is difficult to determine visually; however, there are some useful guidelines.

   1. The area under a **partial-thickness burn** should have normal or increased sensitivity to pain and temperature and should blanch with pressure.

   2. A **full-thickness burn** will be anesthetic and will not blanch with pressure.

VII. **Perioperative management of burns**

A. **Cardiovascular system**

   1. **Fluid loss**

     a. During the first 24 to 48 hours, massive evaporative losses and sequestration of fluid in the extracellular compartment (third spacing) are to be expected. Aggressive fluid repletion will be necessary to prevent hypotension, hypoperfusion, and shock.

     b. The composition of lost or sequestered fluid is very similar to that of plasma (i.e., the fluid has a high protein content).

     c. **Fluid replacement** consists of crystalloid, usually Ringer's lactate, with or without the addition of colloid.

     d. **Standard protocols** for fluid replacement use body weight in kilograms and percent TBSA burned.

       (1) **Parkland formula** (most commonly used at the Massachusetts General Hospital): 4.0 mL of Ringer's lactate per kilogram per %TBSA burn per 24 hours.

       (2) **Brooke formula:** 1.5 mL of crystalloid per kilogram per %TBSA burn per 24 hours plus 0.5 mL of colloid per kilogram per %TBSA burn per 24 hours plus 2000 mL of 5% dextrose in water per 24 hours.

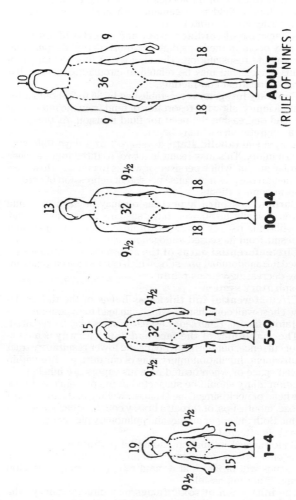

Fig. 32-2. Rule of nines (Lung and Browder chart). (Modified from Ryan JF, et al. (eds.). *A practice of anesthesia for infants and children.* Philadelphia: WB Saunders, 1986:230.)

e. Generally, half the calculated fluid deficit is administered during the first 8 hours postburn and the remainder over the next 16 hours. The patient's daily maintenance fluid requirements are given concurrently.

f. The endpoints of fluid therapy are hemodynamic stability and maintenance of an adequate urine output. In extensive burns, follow fluid management with appropriate invasive monitoring and laboratory studies.

2. A decrease of cardiac output and arterial blood pressure may occur in the immediate postburn period despite adequate volume resuscitation. The etiology of this phenomenon remains unclear but may be related to circulating factors that depress myocardial contractility.

3. Capillary integrity is reestablished by 36 to 72 hours after the initial injury, allowing resorption of fluid from the interstitial space and decreasing the need for fluid infusion. At this juncture, a "diuretic phase" may begin.

4. A hypermetabolic state develops 3 to 5 days following the burn injury. This may result in a two- to three-fold increase in cardiac output, which persists for weeks to months. However, gram-negative sepsis may cause persistent depression of cardiac output in some patients.

5. Chronic postburn hypertension may be seen in young children (usually boys) who have sustained extensive burns. The syndrome usually develops within 2 weeks of injury and may result from increased endogenous catecholamine levels.

6. Circumferential burns of the abdomen may produce increased intraabdominal pressure, which can reduce cardiac output by decreasing venous return.

B. Respiratory system

1. Circumferential full-thickness burns of the thorax decrease chest-wall compliance, which can lead to hypoxemia and respiratory failure. Emergency escharotomies may be required.

2. Thermal injury of the face and upper airway is a common occurrence, but burns involving the lower respiratory tract are infrequent. Inhalation injury may occur during a fire within a closed space or when heated noxious vapors are inhaled. An inhalation injury should be suspected in the presence of burns of the head or neck; singed nasal hairs; swelling of the mucosa of the nose, mouth, lips, or throat; a brassy cough; or carbonaceous sputum. Both the upper airway and pulmonary parenchyma may be severely affected.

3. Endotracheal intubation should be performed before airway edema occurs. Continued swelling and distortion of the soft tissues will progress at a rapid rate, rendering intubation difficult, if not impossible.

4. The **inhalation of toxic fumes** may directly damage the tracheobronchial tree and produce additional systemic effects.

a. Combustion of polyurethane-containing products (e.g., insulation and wall paneling) releases hydrogen cyanide, a cellular poison that can produce tissue hypoxia and cause death.

b. Carbon monoxide poisoning occurs when carbon monoxide combines with hemoglobin, displacing oxygen (carbon monoxide is bound more than 200 times as firmly as oxygen) and shifting the oxyhemoglobin curve to the left. Tissue hypoxia ensues.

(1) The ambient oxygen concentration is reduced and the carbon monoxide concentration is increased during a fire. All burned patients, especially those burned while within a closed space, may have sustained some degree of tissue hypoxia with their thermal injury. Oxygen administration should begin at the scene.

(2) Carbon monoxide toxicity may be difficult to diagnose because carboxyhemoglobin is visually the same as oxyhemoglobin, and PaO_2 measurements may be in the normal range (unless there is underlying pulmonary parenchymal injury). Conventional pulse oximetry is unable to differentiate between oxyhemoglobin and carboxyhemoglobin. Diagnosis is made by the direct measurement of carboxyhemoglobin levels.

(3) The half-life of carboxyhemoglobin is directly related to the inspired oxygen concentration (FIO_2); it is 5 to 6 hours when breathing room air, but 30 to 60 minutes when breathing 100% oxygen. Hyperbaric oxygen at 3 atmospheres further reduces carboxyhemoglobin half-life to 20 to 30 minutes. Thus, treatment consists of supplemental oxygen (hyperbaric oxygen in severe cases) and supportive care until the carbon monoxide is eliminated.

   5. The **inhalation of particulate matter** (i.e., smoke and soot) may result in mechanical obstruction of the airways.
C. **Central nervous system.** A high incidence of encephalopathy occurs in burned patients.
D. **Renal blood flow** may be decreased from:
   1. **Prerenal factors** (see Chapter 4).
   2. **Intrinsic renal factors** specific to burn trauma, including tubular obstruction secondary to rhabdomyolysis and hemoglobinuria from hemolysis. The former is more common in electrical injury, while the latter is seen following severe cutaneous burns (see Chapter 4 for appropriate therapy).
E. **Gastrointestinal system**
   1. **Gastrointestinal function** is diminished immediately following burn injury, secondary to the development of gastric and intestinal ileus. Because of the danger of pulmonary aspiration of gastric contents, the stomach should be adequately vented with a nasogastric tube, particularly in patients unable to protect their airway.
   2. **Serum enzyme changes** indicative of liver damage are sometimes evident in the early postburn period.
   3. **Curling's ulcers (mucosal erosion)** will occur at variable times after major burns, leading to gastric hemorrhage or perforation. These seem to be more common in children than in adults. Therapy consists of antacids and histamine (H_2) receptor antagonists.
   4. **Other gastrointestinal complications of burns** include esophagitis, tracheoesophageal fistula (from prolonged intubation and the presence of a nasogastric tube), acalculous cholecystitis, and mesenteric artery thrombosis.
F. **Endocrine system.** The stress of a burn injury causes marked changes in catecholamine, corticosteroid, and glucagon levels. In-

creases in these catabolic hormones result in loss of muscle mass and accelerated nitrogen breakdown.

G.   Musculoskeletal system. Circumferential burns of the extremities can lead to vascular compromise from increased interstitial pressure. Escharotomy may be required to prevent ischemic necrosis of distal structures, particularly the digits.

H.   Hematologic system

1.   Microangiopathic hemolytic anemia can occur.

2.   Thrombocytopenia, secondary to increased platelet aggregation and trapping of platelets in the lungs, is seen early in the postburn period and is followed by an increase in the platelet count 10 to 14 days following the injury. This elevation will persist for several months.

3. Sepsis can lead to **disseminated intravascular coagulation** as well as bone marrow suppression.

I.   Bacterial infection

1.   Infection of burned areas delays healing and prevents successful skin grafting. Bacterial invasion of underlying tissues may result in septicemia.

2. The **most common organisms** involved are staphylococci, beta-hemolytic streptococci, and the gram-negative rods such as *Pseudomonas* and *Klebsiella* species.

3.   Local treatment consists of topical antimicrobials.

a.   Silver nitrate. Methemoglobinemia is a rare complication.

b.   Mafenide cream may cause metabolic acidosis if absorbed, since it is a carbonic anhydrase inhibitor.

c.   Silver sulfadiazine. Leukopenia is the main disadvantage but reverses with discontinuation.

d.   Povidone-iodine elevates serum iodide levels and is contraindicated in any patient with renal dysfunction.

4. The incidence of **sepsis** may be reduced by using temporary biologic dressings, which may be allografts (cadaver skin or amnion) or xenografts (porcine). "Artificial skin," which is bioengineered from collagen and cultured epidermis, can be used when conventional autograft is not available.

5. The use of **systemic antibiotics** is limited to treatment of documented systemic infection (as opposed to colonization) and as prophylaxis before surgical procedures.

VIII.   Anesthetic considerations for burn patients

A.   General considerations

1.   Early excision and grafting of burned areas is a widely accepted procedure. Patients may be brought to the operating room in the acute phase of injury, with hemodynamic instability and respiratory dysfunction. Special emphasis should be placed on correcting acid-base and electrolyte disturbances and coagulopathy. Adequate colloid and blood products should be ordered in advance.

2. During the **chronic phase of burns,** when reconstructive procedures are performed, altered pharmacokinetics, drug tolerance, difficult IV access, and anatomic derangements of the airway (neck scar or mouth contracture) are the main considerations.

B.   Monitoring and intravenous access

1. Often IV access will still be in place from the initial resuscitation. Large-bore IVs are mandatory to allow for massive fluid replacement.

2. In massive burns, ECG electrodes may be placed directly on debrided tissue. Alternatively, needle electrodes can be used.

3. Arterial lines are indispensable for continuous blood-pressure monitoring and to facilitate frequent blood sampling. The cannulation site will depend on the availability of unburned areas. If all appropriate sites are burned, the line may have to be placed through the burn wound after the area has been prepared in a sterile fashion.

4. Central venous pressure lines are useful, both for monitoring central volume and as central access for drug infusions.

5. A **pulmonary artery catheter** may be required for management of patients with myocardial dysfunction, persistent oliguria or hypotension, or sepsis.

C. Airway. Obtaining an adequate mask fit may be difficult because of edema in the early phases of burn injury or because of scars and contractures later on. These same processes can render endotracheal intubation extremely difficult in burn patients.

D. Muscle relaxants

1. Succinylcholine is absolutely contraindicated 24 hours to 2 years following major burns, since it can produce profound hyperkalemia and cardiac arrest.

2. Nondepolarizing relaxants are used when muscle relaxation is required. Burn patients show a "resistance" to these drugs (i.e., diminished response to conventional doses), in some cases requiring three- to five-fold greater doses than nonburn patients.

E. Anesthetics

1. There is no single preferred agent or combination of agents; however, **ketamine** and **etomidate** may have advantages in patients with uncertain volume status.

2. These patients may have **greatly increased opioid requirements** due to tolerance and increases in the apparent volume of distribution for drugs. It is important to provide adequate analgesia.

F. Temperature regulation. The most comfortable body temperature for a burn patient is about 100°F (38°C). In the burn intensive care unit, patients are cared for in warmed, humidified rooms. Every effort should be made to maintain normothermia during transport and surgery. The operating room, IV fluids, and blood products should be warmed and inspired gases heated and humidified. Pediatric patients should be placed under a radiant heat source and on a warming blanket whenever possible.

G. Immunosuppression. The immune system is suppressed for weeks to months following burn injury, and the wound itself serves as an excellent medium for bacterial growth. Every attempt should be made to practice aseptic technique when handling patients, suctioning airways, or inserting intravascular lines.

H. Postanesthetic care. It is important to maintain normothermia while transporting patients back to the intensive care unit, since shivering could contribute to graft loss. Supplemental oxygen should be given until patients are fully recovered from anesthesia.

SUGGESTED READING
Baud FJ, Barriot P, Toffis V, et al. Elevated blood cyanide concentrations in victims of smoke inhalation. *N Engl J Med* 1991;325:1761–1766.

Beushausen T, Mucke K. Anesthesia and pain management in pediatric burn patients. *Pediatr Surg Int* 1997;12:327–333.

MacLennan N, Heimbach DM, Cullen BF. Anesthesia for major thermal injury. *Anesthesiology* 1998;89:749–770.

Monafo WW. Initial management of burns. *N Engl J Med* 1996;335: 1581–1586.

Phillips TF, Soulier G, Wilson RF. Outcome of massive transfusion exceeding two blood volumes in trauma and emergency surgery. *J Trauma* 1987;27:903–910.

Szy Felbein SK, Martyn JAJ, Sheridan RL, Coté CJ. Anesthesia for children with brain injuries. In: Coté CJ, Todres ID, Goudsouzian NG, Ryan JF, eds. *A practice of anesthesia for infants and children*, 3rd ed. Philadelphia: WB Saunders, 2001:522–543.

Trunkey D. Initial treatment of patients with extensive trauma. *N Engl J Med* 1991;324:1259–1263.

Transfusion Therapy

Rae M. Allain

I. Indications for transfusion therapy. Blood component transfusion usually is performed because of decreased production; increased utilization, destruction, or loss; or dysfunction of a specific blood component (red cells, platelets, or coagulation factors).

A. Anemia

1. Hematocrit. The main reason for transfusing red cells is to maintain oxygen-carrying capacity to the tissues. Healthy individuals or individuals with a chronic anemia can usually tolerate a hematocrit (Hct) of 20% to 25%, assuming normal intravascular volume. In patients with coronary or peripheral arterial disease, it is clinical practice to maintain higher Hcts (30%), although the efficacy of this is unproved.

2. If a patient is anemic preoperatively, the etiology should be clarified. It may be secondary to decreased production (marrow suppression), increased loss (hemorrhage), or destruction (hemolysis).

3. Estimating blood volumes

a. Intraoperative blood transfusion is dependent on red cell loss. This can be roughly estimated by measuring blood in suction canisters, weighing sponges, and checking blood loss on the drapes.

b. Estimated allowable blood loss (EABL) can be calculated as follows:

$$EABL = [(Hct_{starting} - Hct_{allowable})$$
$$\times BV] / [(Hct_{starting} + Hct_{allowable}) / 2]$$

Blood volume (BV) in an adult is approximately 7% of lean body mass. This may be calculated as approximately 70 mL/kg of body weight in a normal adult man and approximately 65 mL/kg of body weight in a normal adult woman (see Chapter 28, section VII.B for pediatric considerations).

c. Estimating the volume of blood to transfuse can be calculated as follows:

Volume to transfuse

$$= [(Hct_{desired} - Hct_{present}) \times BV] / Hct_{transfused\ blood}$$

A unit of packed red blood cells has a Hct of about 70%.

B. Thrombocytopenia. Thrombocytopenia is due to either decreased bone marrow production (e.g., chemotherapy, tumor infiltration, or alcoholism) or increased utilization or destruction (e.g., hypersplenism, idiopathic thrombocytopenia purpura, or drug effects). It is also seen with massive blood transfusion (see section IX.A.1). Spontaneous bleeding is unusual with platelet counts above 20,000/mm^3. Platelet counts above 50,000/mm^3 are preferable for surgical hemostasis.

C.   Coagulopathy. Bleeding associated with documented factor deficiencies or prolonged clotting studies (prothrombin time and partial thromboplastin time) mandates replacement therapy to maintain normal coagulation function. See sections II and IX for a discussion of coagulopathy.

II.   Coagulation studies. The most important clue to a clinically significant bleeding disorder in an otherwise healthy patient remains the history. Prior surgical bleeding, gingival bleeding, easy bruising, epistaxis, or menorrhagia should raise concern. There are many tests available to assess the coagulation system. However, the clinician must remember that the coagulation system is a complex interplay of platelets and coagulation factors. There is no single test that measures the integrity of the entire coagulation system.

A.   Partial thromboplastin time (PTT) is performed by adding particulate matter to a blood sample to activate the intrinsic coagulation system. Normal values for the PTT are between 25 and 37 seconds and depend on normal levels of clotting factors in the intrinsic coagulation system. The test is sensitive to decreased amounts of coagulation factors and is elevated in patients on heparin therapy. The PTT will also be abnormal if there is a circulating anticoagulant present (e.g., lupus anticoagulant or antibodies to factor VIII). The clinician should remember that an abnormal PTT does not necessarily correlate with clinical bleeding. Aggressive correction of an abnormal PTT in surgical patients is not always indicated, unless the patient is actively bleeding.

B.   Prothrombin time (PT) is a measure of the extrinsic coagulation system and is measured by adding tissue factor to a blood sample. While both PT and PTT are affected by levels of factors V and X, prothrombin, and fibrinogen, the PT is specifically sensitive to deficiencies of factor VII. The PT is normal in deficiencies of factors VIII, IX, XI, XII, prekallikrein, and high-molecular-weight kininogen.

C.   The INR (International Normalized Ratio) is a means of standardizing PT values to allow comparisons among different laboratories or at different times. It is the ratio of patient's PT to the control PT value that would be obtained if international reference reagents had been used to perform the test. Before development of the INR, differences in thromboplastin reagent activity prevented meaningful comparisons of PT values. Now, oral anticoagulation therapy may be guided by a target INR value that is independent of laboratory variability of the PT. For example, an INR of 2.0 to 3.0 is recommended for prophylaxis against thromboembolism in atrial fibrillation.

D.   Bleeding time reflects the interaction of platelets with the vessel endothelium, which leads to formation of an initial clot. An abnormal bleeding time may reflect dysfunctional or diminished platelets, but may also be seen with decreased von Willebrand factor or fibrinogen. Performance of the test requires adherence to a standardized protocol; nevertheless, results are technician dependent and poorly reproducible. Results do not correlate with clinical observations of hemostasis in the perioperative period.

Thus, the bleeding time is not recommended for assessment of perioperative coagulation status and the test is no longer used or available in many institutions.

E. Activated clotting time (ACT) is a modified whole-blood clotting time in which diatomaceous earth is added to a blood sample to activate the intrinsic clotting system. The ACT is the time until clot formation. A normal ACT is between 90 and 130 seconds. The ACT is a relatively easy and expedient test to perform and is useful in monitoring heparin therapy in the operating room.

F. D-dimer and fibrin split products. When fibrinolysis occurs, plasmin degrades both fibrin and fibrinogen. Fibrin-split products reflect degradation of both fibrinogen and fibrin. D-dimer measurements, which reflect degradation of cross-linked fibrin, are more specific for primary fibrinolysis and **disseminated intravascular coagulation** (DIC). The test is performed by mixing antibody-coated latex beads with patient plasma in serial dilutions. An elevated titer of D-dimer is common in patients with DIC but may also be seen with deep venous thrombosis, liver disease, or after recent surgery (within 48 hours). Fibrin fragments can interfere with normal coagulation by impairing platelet function and the normal formation of fibrin clot.

III. Blood typing and cross-matching

A. Donor and recipient blood is typed in the red cell surface **ABO and Rh systems** and screened for antibodies to other cell antigens. Cross-matching involves directly mixing the patient's plasma with the donor's red cells to establish that hemolysis does not occur from any undetected antibodies. An individual's red cells have either A, B, AB, or no surface antigens. If the patient's red cells are lacking either surface antigen A or B, then antibodies will be produced against it. A person who is type B will have anti-A antibodies in the serum, and a type O individual (having neither A nor B surface antigens) will have circulating anti-A and anti-B antibodies. Consequently, a person who is type AB will not have antibodies to either A or B and can receive red blood cells from any blood type. Type O blood has neither A nor B surface antigens and can donate blood cells to any other type (universal red cell donor).

B. Rh-surface antigens are either present (Rh-positive) or absent (Rh-negative). Individuals who are Rh-negative will develop antibodies to the Rh factor when exposed to Rh-positive blood. This is not a problem with the initial exposure, but with subsequent exposures hemolysis will occur due to the circulating antibodies. This can be a particular problem during pregnancy. The anti-Rh antibodies are IgG and freely cross the placenta. In Rh-negative mothers who have developed Rh antibodies, these antibodies are transmitted to the fetus. If the fetus is Rh-positive, massive hemolysis will occur. **RHO-immune globulin,** an Rh-blocking antibody, prevents the Rh-negative patient from developing anti-Rh antibodies. It should be administered to individuals who receive Rh-positive blood and to Rh-negative mothers delivering Rh-positive babies (some fetal maternal blood mixing occurs at delivery). The recommended dose is 300 μg IM for every 15 mL of Rh-positive blood transfused.

C. If an emergency blood transfusion is needed, type-specific (ABO) red cells usually can be obtained within minutes if the patient's blood type is known. If type-specific blood is unavailable, type O Rh-negative red cells should be transfused (Type O+ blood can be used emergently in males). Type-specific blood should be substituted as soon as possible to minimize the amount of type O plasma (containing anti-A and anti-B antibodies) transfused.

IV. Blood component therapy

A. General considerations

1. One unit of **packed red blood cells** (PRBCs; Hct about 70%, volume about 250 mL) usually will increase the Hct of an euvolemic adult by 2% to 3% once equilibration has taken place. PRBCs must be ABO compatible to the recipient.

2. One unit of **platelets** increases the platelet count by 5,000 to 10,000/mm^3. A usual platelet transfusion is one unit per 10 kg of body weight. If thrombocytopenia is caused by increased destruction (due to development of antiplatelet antibodies) or if platelets are dysfunctional, platelet transfusions will be less efficacious. Transfusion of ABO-compatible platelets is not obligatory, although they may provide a better posttransfusion platelet count. Single-donor or HLA-matched platelets may be required for patients with a refractory response to platelet transfusion. A unit of single-donor platelets provides the equivalent of approximately six random-donor units of platelets.

3. Fresh-frozen plasma (FFP), in a dose of 10 to 15 mL/kg, generally will increase plasma coagulation factors to 30% of normal; fibrinogen levels increase by 1 mg per milliliter of plasma transfused. Acute reversal of warfarin requires only 5 to 8 mL/kg of FFP. FFP transfusions must be ABO compatible.

4. Cryoprecipitate is prepared from FFP and contains concentrated factor VIII, factor XIII, fibrinogen, von Willebrand factor, and fibronectin. Indications for cryoprecipitate include hypofibrinogenemia, von Willebrand disease, hemophilia A (when factor VIII is unavailable), and preparation of fibrin glue. Dosage is one unit per 7 to 10 kg, which will raise the plasma fibrinogen by about 50 mg/dL in a patient without massive bleeding. ABO compatibility is not mandatory for cryoprecipitate transfusion.

B. Technical considerations

1. Compatible infusions. Blood products should not be infused with 5% dextrose solutions, since they cause hemolysis, or with lactated Ringer's, which contains calcium and may induce clot formation. Normal saline (0.9%) solution, albumin (5%), and FFP are compatible with red blood cells.

2. Blood filters. Standard blood filters (170 to 200 μm) remove debris and should be used for all blood components. Microaggregate filters (20 to 50 μm), which should not be used for platelets, remove 70% to 90% of leukocytes. Third-generation or adhesion filters remove more than 99.9% of leukocytes and may be recommended for use in patients with a history of febrile, nonhemolytic transfusion reactions, for prevention of alloimmunization to foreign leukocyte antigens, or to prevent cytomegalovirus (CMV) transmission in organ transplant recipients. Other potential but as yet unproved benefits of leukocyte reduction include diminished immunomodulatory effect of allogeneic transfusion; reduced transmission of bacterial, viral, or prion diseases; prevention of transfusion-related acute lung injury; and decreased incidence of graft-versus-host disease. Possible future government regulations mandating use of leukocyte-reduced blood products for all patients has generated significant controversy within the transfusion community.

C. **Blood substitutes.** Despite years of research intent upon finding a blood substitute capable of oxygen transport, none provides general clinical usefulness at this time. Fluosol-DA, a synthetic perfluorocarbon capable of carrying oxygen, has been tested in humans, but offers limited applicability of oxygen transport *in vivo*. Free hemoglobin solutions also are being tested as potential alternatives or supplements to blood transfusion. Limiting problems include short plasma half-lives (about 8 hours) and hypertension with administration.

V. **Plasma substitutes.** Various colloid products are available commercially. Their main limitations are their cost and the dilution of red cells and coagulation factors that occurs with their administration.

A. **Albumin** is available as either an isotonic 5% or a hypertonic 20% or 25% solution. Albumin has an intravascular half-life of 10 to 15 days.

B. **Dextran** 70 and dextran 40 are high–molecular-weight polysaccharides. Dextran 70, having a higher molecular weight, is not filtered by the kidney. The dextrans have relatively short half-lives (2 to 8 hours) and are either excreted or metabolized. Decreased platelet adhesiveness and depressed von Willebrand factor (vWf) levels are side effects of dextrans that are commonly seen at dosages greater than 1.5 g/kg. Anaphylactoid reactions have been seen in approximately 1% of patients. These reactions can be avoided by pretreating with dextran 1 (20 mL IV), a hapten that binds the patient's dextran-binding antibodies.

C. **Hydroxyethyl starch** (hetastarch) is manufactured from amylopectin. After infusion, hydroxyethyl starch undergoes both renal excretion and tissue redistribution, including storage in the reticuloendothelial cells of the liver for many weeks. Metabolic degradation occurs by serum amylase; this process can cause an increase in serum amylase for several days, which may confuse the diagnosis of pancreatitis. Hetastarch's effects on coagulation include decreased fibrinogen, vWf, and factor VIII levels, and decreased platelet function. Nonetheless, dosages up to 1 g/kg have been used without adverse bleeding problems. Anaphylactoid reactions are rare.

VI. **Pharmacologic therapy**

A. **Erythropoietin** increases red blood cell mass by stimulating proliferation and development of the erythroid precursor cells. It can be used before elective surgery to increase red blood cell (RBC) production. A higher preoperative Hct has been shown to allow increased autologous red blood cell donation. Results about erythropoietin's ability to diminish allogeneic blood exposure perioperatively have been mixed, with baseline mildly anemic patients seeming to gain the greatest benefit. Preoperative erythropoietin treatment should be accompanied by supplemental iron administration. Several dosing regimens for preoperative erythropoietin are used, including 300 IU/kg subcutaneously (SC) daily for 15 days beginning 10 days before surgery or 600 IU/kg SC weekly for 3 weeks before surgery.

B.   Desmopressin (DDAVP) is an antidiuretic hormone that is known to be helpful in patients with mild hemophilia A and in some patients with von Willebrand disease. Desmopressin increases endothelial cell release of von Willebrand factor, factor VIII, and plasminogen activator. Desmopressin is also useful for patients with platelet defects associated with uremia. The dosage of desmopressin is 0.3 μg/kg. Tachyphylaxis may occur if dosing is greater than every 48 hours. The IV dose should be given slowly, since hypotension may result.

C.   The lysine analogues, aminocaproic acid and tranexamic acid, inhibit fibrinolysis, the endogenous process by which fibrin clot is broken down. They act by displacing plasminogen from fibrin, diminishing plasminogen conversion to plasmin, and preventing plasmin from binding to fibrinogen or fibrin monomers. The uses of aminocaproic acid include prophylaxis for dental surgery in hemophiliacs, prevention of bleeding in prostatic surgery, and reduction of hemorrhage in cases of excessive fibrinolysis. Since cardiopulmonary bypass has been shown to initiate fibrinolysis, aminocaproic acid has been used during cardiac surgery to decrease postoperative chest tube drainage. The drug's efficacy at diminishing blood transfusion has been demonstrated only when the transfusion trigger was low (Hct approximately 20%). Theoretic risks of thrombosis with aminocaproic acid have not been demonstrated clinically; nevertheless, the drug is contraindicated in DIC. Dosage in adults is 5 g IV load over 1 hour followed by 1 to 2 g per hour IV infusion.

D.   Aprotinin is a serine protease inhibitor shown to be effective in diminishing blood loss after cardiopulmonary bypass. In a dose-dependent fashion, aprotinin inhibits trypsin, plasmin, and kallikrein. In addition, aprotinin protects the glycoprotein Ib receptor on platelets during cardiopulmonary bypass, thereby preserving platelet adhesive capability. The drug also has anti-inflammatory and antioxidant effects. Of note, celite ACTs are artificially prolonged following heparinization of patients receiving aprotinin. To maintain appropriate heparin anticoagulation for cardiopulmonary bypass, kaolin-activated ACTs should be performed or heparin should be administered by a fixed dose regimen. Complications of aprotinin treatment include potential anaphylactic reaction. The incidence is approximately 0.3%, but rises with repeat exposure; an initial test dose of 1 mL administered intravenously is recommended. Aprotinin may increase serum creatinine levels, but this appears to be reversible and dose related. For cardiac surgery, "high-dose" aprotinin consists of 2 million kallikrein inactivation units (KIU) IV load after induction of anesthesia and 500,000 KIU per hour IV infusion through completion of surgery; another 2 million KIU is added to the cardiopulmonary bypass pump prime. "Low-dose" aprotinin is one-half this regimen. Advantages of low-dose therapy may be preserved blood conservation with potentially less renal toxicity, but this remains controversial. The precise role for intraoperative aprotinin therapy continues to be defined. It has an established role in patients undergoing cardiac procedures at high risk for hemorrhagic complications. It has also been used to decrease bleeding and transfusion requirements in patients undergoing prostatectomy, total hip replacement, and liver resection or transplantation. Risks of thrombosis with aprotinin remain unclear. One large study on cardiac patients showed no increased risk of myocardial infarction, but a higher early graft occlusion rate when aprotinin was used.

VII. Conservation and salvage techniques

A. Autologous donation usually begins 6 weeks before surgery and can greatly reduce the amount of homologous blood transfused. The length of the predonation period is limited by the length of time that blood can be stored, currently 42 days unless the blood is frozen. Current blood bank guidelines require a predonation hemoglobin of at least 11 g/dL, donations no more frequently than every 3 days, and no donations in the 72 hours before surgery. Most patients tolerate autologous donation without complication. Patients with severe aortic stenosis or unstable angina are not candidates for autologous donation. Patients donating autologous blood should receive supplemental iron since depleted iron stores frequently limit RBC recovery. Recombinant erythropoietin treatment (see section VI.A) also may be considered. Since a risk of transfusion reaction exists due to clerical error, autologous blood should not be transfused unless indicated.

B. Normovolemic hemodilution. Preoperative or intraoperative hemodilution entails phlebotomizing a patient of one or more units of fresh whole blood while replacing the lost volume with either colloid or crystalloid. By using normovolemic hemodilution before intraoperative blood loss, fresh autologous blood is available for later reinfusion after surgical blood loss is complete. Also, by hemodiluting a patient to a Hct of 30% or less, any blood loss intraoperatively will constitute more plasma loss and less red cell loss. Hemodilution may also be helpful in situations where platelet function is altered intraoperatively (e.g., cardiopulmonary bypass), since the phlebotomized blood has normal platelets and clotting factors when reinfused. Obviously, if surgical blood loss is extreme, the fresh autologous blood should be transfused before any homologous blood. It should also be remembered that the autologous blood has a Hct similar to the patient's preoperative Hct, as opposed to a unit of packed red blood cells, which has a Hct of approximately 70%. While hemodilution alone may not eliminate the need for homologous transfusion, when used in combination with preoperative autologous donation, it may decrease the need for homologous units.

C. Intraoperative autotransfusion (cell saver) utilizes blood collected from the surgical field by a double-lumen suction device. Heparinized normal saline is infused through one lumen so that the blood is anticoagulated as it is suctioned from the surgical field. The scavenged, heparinized blood is filtered and collected in a reservoir. The blood is then centrifuged to remove plasma and any debris. The red blood cells are suspended in normal saline and then recentrifuged to further remove debris, plasma, free hemoglobin, and anticoagulant. The washed red cells are then ready for reinfusion. The Hct of these processed units is approximately 50%. Processing time is about 3 minutes. These units are washed, packed, red blood cells deficient in plasma, clotting factors, and platelets. Intraoperative autotransfusion is generally restricted to clean surgical fields and nononcologic procedures because of risks of reinfusing bacteria or tumor cells into patients.

VIII. **Complications of blood transfusion therapy**

A. **Transfusion reactions**

   1. **Acute hemolytic transfusion reactions** occur when ABO-incompatible blood is transfused, resulting in recipient antibodies attaching to donor RBC antigens and forming an antigen–antibody complex. This antigen–antibody complex activates complement, resulting in intravascular RBC lysis with release of RBC stroma and free hemoglobin. Immune system activation also results in bradykinin release (leading to hypotension) and mast cell activation (causing serotonin and histamine release). The net result may be shock, renal failure due to hemoglobin precipitation in renal tubules, and DIC (see section IX.B). Symptoms of an acute hemolytic transfusion reaction appear immediately and include fever, chest pain, anxiety, back pain, and dyspnea. Many are masked by general anesthesia, but clues to the diagnosis include fever, hypotension, hemoglobinuria, unexplained bleeding, or failure of Hct to increase following transfusion. Table 33-1 indicates steps to take if a transfusion reaction is suspected. The incidence of fatal hemolytic transfusion reaction in the United States is approximately 1 out of every 250,000 to 1,000,000 units transfused. Most reactions occur because of administrative errors, with the majority due to improper identification of the blood unit or patient. The importance of adhering to strict policies of checking blood and matching to the correct patient in the operating room cannot be overemphasized.

   2. **Delayed hemolytic transfusion reactions** occur because of incompatibility of minor antigens (e.g., Kidd) and are characterized by extravascular hemolysis. They present 2 days to

Table 33-1.   Approach to suspected acute hemolytic transfusion reaction

1. *Stop the transfusion.*

2. Quickly check for error in patient identity or donor unit.

3. Send donor unit and newly obtained blood sample to blood bank for recross match.

4. Treat hypotension with fluids and vasopressors as necessary.

5. If transfusion is required, use type O-negative PRBC and type AB FFP as necessary.

6. Support renal function: first, administer fluids to correct hypovolemia and second, administer diuretics (furosemide ± mannitol) to maintain brisk urine output.

7. Monitor for signs of DIC clinically and with appropriate laboratory studies; treat supportively (see section IX.B.).

8. Send patient blood sample for direct antiglobulin (Coombs) test, free hemoglobin, haptoglobin; send urine for hemoglobin.

DIC, disseminated intravascular coagulation; FFP, fresh-frozen plasma; PRBC, packed red blood cells.

months following transfusion. Patients complain of no or minimal symptoms, but may display signs of anemia and jaundice. Laboratory studies reveal a positive direct antiglobulin test, hyperbilirubinemia, decreased haptoglobin levels, and hemosiderin in the urine. Treatment is aimed at correcting the anemia.

3. Febrile nonhemolytic transfusion reactions (FNHTR) are the most common transfusion reactions, occurring in approximately 1% of RBC transfusions and up to 30% of platelet transfusions. They occur when antileukocyte antibodies in a recipient react with white blood cells in a transfused blood product. Signs and symptoms include fever, chills, tachycardia, discomfort, nausea, and vomiting. Approach to treatment involves first stopping the transfusion and excluding an acute, hemolytic transfusion reaction or bacterial contamination of the donor unit. Acetaminophen and meperidine may diminish fever and rigors. Once the diagnosis of FNHTR has been made, future reactions may be avoided or diminished by administering leukocyte reduced blood products (see section IV.B.2), premedicating at-risk patients with acetaminophen and hydrocortisone (50 to 100 mg IV), and administering the transfusion slowly.

4. Allergic transfusion reactions are common, occurring in 1% to 3% of transfusions. They arise from recipient antibody response to donor plasma proteins. Urticaria with pruritus and erythema is the most common manifestation, but rarely bronchospasm or anaphylaxis presents. Many patients also have fever. Patients with IgA deficiency may be at increased risk of allergic transfusion reaction because of the presence of anti-IgA antibodies that react with transfused IgA. Treatment involves stopping the transfusion, excluding a more severe reaction (see above), and administering antihistamines (diphenhydramine 50 mg IV and ranitidine 50 mg IV). A significant reaction may warrant treating with a corticosteroid (methylprednisolone 80 mg IV). Bronchospasm and anaphylaxis should be treated as described in Chapter 18.

5. Transfusion-related acute lung injury is a condition of severe pulmonary insufficiency occurring as a result of blood transfusion. Signs and symptoms include fever, dyspnea, hypoxemia, hypotension, and pulmonary edema developing within 4 hours of transfusion. The pathophysiology likely involves a reaction between recipient white blood cells and leukocyte antibodies present in donor plasma. The incidence, likely underestimated, is 1 out of 5,000 units transfused. Therapy is supportive, mimicking the treatment of acute respiratory distress syndrome, from which the diagnosis may be clinically indistinguishable. Mechanical ventilation usually is required during the acute phase, but resolution often occurs within 4 days. Preventive measures have not yet been identified.

B. Metabolic complications of blood transfusions

1. Potassium (K^+) concentration changes are common with rapid blood transfusion, but usually are clinically important only in massive transfusion or renal failure. With storage, red cells leak K^+ into the extracellular storage fluid. However, with transfusion and replenishment of cellular energy stores, this is rapidly corrected.

2. Calcium. Citrate, which binds calcium, is used as an anticoagulant in stored blood products. Consequently, rapid transfusion may cause a decreased ionized calcium level. Hypocalcemia is usually not significant because the liver rapidly metabolizes the infused citrate, but may become an important problem in patients with impaired liver function, during the anhepatic phase of liver transplantation, in hypothermic patients, or in patients with decreased hepatic blood flow. Ionized calcium levels should be followed, since total serum calcium measures the citrate-bound calcium and may not accurately reflect free serum calcium.

3. Acid-base status. Banked blood is acidic because of accumulated red cell metabolites. However, the actual acid load to the patient is minimal. Acidosis in the face of severe blood loss is more likely due to hypoperfusion and will improve with volume resuscitation. Alkalosis is frequent following massive blood transfusion because citrate is metabolized in the liver to bicarbonate.

C. Infectious complications of blood transfusions have decreased with improved laboratory testing for transmissible diseases. Exposure to pooled products (e.g., cryoprecipitate) increases the risk proportional to the number of donors.

   1. Hepatitis

      a. Hepatitis B (see Chapter 7, section III.A.2). The risk of hepatitis B infection from a blood transfusion has decreased since testing donated blood for hepatitis B antigen became routine in 1971. The current risk is estimated to be 1:60,000 units transfused.

      b. Hepatitis C (see Chapter 7, section III.A.3). Institution of routine testing for antibody to HCV in 1990 has reduced the risk of transfusion-related HCV to approximately 1:100,000 units.

   2. Human immunodeficiency virus (HIV; see Chapter 7, section III.A.1). Because of improved screening and testing, the risk of transfusion-associated HIV has been estimated to be about 1:450,000 per unit transfused in the United States.

   3. Cytomegalovirus (see Chapter 7, section II.A.5). The prevalence of antibodies to CMV in the general population is approximately 70% by adulthood. The incidence of transfusion-associated CMV infection in previously noninfected patients is quite high. Usually the infection is asymptomatic, but because immunosuppressed patients and neonates can have severe reactions, CMV-negative blood or leukocyte-reduced blood may be recommended.

   4. Lymphotrophic viruses. Retroviruses have been implicated as causative agents of some leukemias and lymphomas. Human T-cell lymphotrophic virus-I (HTLV-I), known to cause a T-cell malignancy, and HTLV-II, associated with hairy-cell leukemia, may be transmitted by blood at a rate of less than 1:640,000 units transfused.

   5. Prion diseases (see Chapter 7, section III.A.8). Transmissible spongiform encephalopathies are very rare, infectious neurodegenerative diseases with very long latencies. They affect humans and animals and are fatal. The recent emergence of the new variant, Creutzfeldt-Jakob disease, in Britain and its association with a similar disease in cattle, bovine spongiform encephalopathy, has raised fears of possible blood-borne transmission of prions, the proteins implicated as causative agents in these diseases. To date, there exists no scientific evidence to support these fears. However, current U.S. Food and Drug Administration policy is to exclude blood donation from individuals who have spent more than 6 months in the United Kingdom between 1980 and 1996.

   6. Bacterial sepsis caused by transfused blood products is rare. Donors with evidence of infectious disease are excluded and the storage of RBCs at 4°C minimizes infectious risk. Nonetheless, RBCs may become infected, most commonly with *Yersinia enterocolitica*. Platelets, which are stored at room temperature, are more problematic, with an estimated sepsis incidence of 1:12,000 transfused units. Organisms associated with platelet contamination are usually *Staphylococcus* (*aureus* and *epidermidis*) and diphtheroids. The risk of infection is directly related to the storage time of the product. Signs of sepsis usually are apparent during transfusion and should trigger immediate halt of the transfusion and testing of the unit for contamination. The impact on the individual patient depends on the size of the bacterial inoculum and the immunocompetence of the recipient.

D. Immunomodulation of blood transfusion. Transfusion of allogeneic blood is known to suppress the immune system. Although the exact mechanism is unknown, theories suggest that transfusion of donor leukocytes may induce an immune-"tolerant" state in the recipient. Thus, allogeneic blood transfusion has been used pre- and intra-operatively in renal transplant recipients to improve graft viability. Less clear and more controversial are the potential detrimental effects of intraoperative allogeneic blood transfusion on cancer recurrence rates and postoperative infection. If new government guidelines recommending leukocyte-reduced blood transfusion for all patients are implemented (see section IV.B.2), immunomodulation associated with blood transfusion may be decreased.

IX. Perioperative coagulopathy

A. Coagulopathy of massive transfusion is unusual before the transfusion of greater than 1.0 to 1.5 blood volumes, assuming the patient had a normal coagulation profile, platelet count, and platelet function to start.

   1. Thrombocytopenia. Diffuse oozing and failure to form clot after massive transfusion are often at least in part due to thrombocytopenia. The decreased platelet count is due to the transfusion of platelet-poor blood products. Clinical bleeding is unlikely with platelet counts above 50,000 cells/mm^3. If loss of one blood volume or more is expected, platelets should be available and transfused to maintain a count of more than 50,000 cells/mm^3 or greater if ongoing blood loss is expected.

   2. Clotting factors. The normal human body has tremendous reserves of clotting factors. In addition, the patient receives small amounts of the stable clotting factors in the plasma of each unit of red cells. Bleeding from factor deficiency in the face of massive transfusion is usually due to decreased levels of fibrinogen and labile factors (V, VIII, or IX). Bleeding from hypofibrinogenemia is unusual unless the fibrinogen level is below 75 mg/dL. In some patients, factor-VIII levels increase with massive transfusion because of increased release from endothelial cells. Labile clotting factors are administered in the form of FFP. Six units of platelets contain the equivalent of one unit of FFP. Cryoprecipitate provides a source of concentrated fibrinogen for the patient who cannot tolerate FFP due to volume overload.

B. Disseminated intravascular coagulation refers to the abnormal, diffuse systemic activation of the clotting system. The pathophysiology involves excessive formation of thrombin, resulting in fibrin formation throughout the vasculature, and accompanied by platelet activation, fibrinolysis, and consumption of coagulation factors.

   1. Causes of DIC include infection, shock, trauma, complications of pregnancy (e.g., amniotic fluid embolism, placental abruption, or septic abortion), burns, and fat or cholesterol embolism. DIC is common in extensive head injury because of the high content of thromboplastin in brain tissue. A chronic form of DIC may accompany cirrhotic liver disease, aortic dissection, and malignancy.

   2. Clinical features include petechiae, ecchymoses, bleeding from venipuncture sites, or frank hemorrhage from operative incisions. The bleeding manifestations of DIC are most obvious, but the diffuse microvascular and macrovascular thromboses are usually more common, more difficult to treat, and more frequently life-threatening because of ischemia to vital organs. Bradykinin release in DIC may also cause hypotension

   3. Laboratory features of DIC include an elevated D-dimer, indicating fibrin degradation by plasmin, in all cases. Fibrinogen degradation products (FDPs) are increased, but this is not specific to DIC since FDPs may be present from the formation of fibrin by fibrinogen or from the degradation of fibrinogen by plasmin. The PT and PTT typically are prolonged and serial measurements reveal falling fibrinogen levels and platelet counts.

   4. Treatment of DIC involves treating the precipitating cause and transfusion of appropriate blood products (e.g., FFP, platelets, and cryoprecipitate) to correct bleeding. In cases associated with inappropriate thrombosis rather than bleeding, the use of heparin to decrease fibrin formation can be considered, although this may risk life-threatening hemorrhage in the operating room. Inhibitors of fibrinolysis (e.g., aminocaproic acid and aprotinin) are not recommended for treatment of DIC because of the possibility of diffuse intravascular thrombosis.

C. Chronic liver disease. With the exception of factor VIII and von Willebrand factor, which are manufactured by the endothelium, the liver synthesizes coagulation factors. Patients with hepatic dysfunction may have decreased production of coagulation factors and decreased clearance of activated factors. Patients may have an ongoing consumptive coagulopathy, similar to DIC, if circulating activated clotting factors are increased. Since the liver is also instrumental in removing the byproducts of fibrinolysis, circulating fibrin degradation products may be elevated.

D. Vitamin K deficiency. Vitamin K is required by the liver for production of factors II, VII, IX, and X, and proteins C and S. Since vitamin K cannot be synthesized by humans, interference with vitamin K absorption will cause a coagulopathy (see Chapter 5, section IV.B.6) and a prolonged prothrombin time. These patients can be treated with vitamin K, 10 mg SC daily for 3 days. Intravenous administration of vitamin K may decrease bleeding at the injection site and may result in a slightly faster correction of the PT, but is accompanied by a rare risk of anaphylaxis. If used, intravenous vitamin K should be administered very slowly. If faster correction of PT than vitamin K is required, FFP (5 to 8 mL/kg) can be used.

E. **Pharmacologic intervention**

1. **Heparin** acts by accelerating the effect of antithrombin III. It prolongs the PTT and has a short half-life so that its anticoagulant effect is usually fully reversed approximately 2 to 4 hours following discontinuation of the infusion. If faster reversal is required, protamine, a natural antagonist, may be administered or FFP transfused.

2. **Low–molecular-weight heparins** are commercially prepared by fractionating heparin into molecules of 2,000 to 10,000 daltons. They exert their anticoagulant effect primarily by inhibiting factor X and usually do not prolong the PTT. These drugs have a longer half-life than heparin and are incompletely reversed by protamine. Fast reversal may require FFP transfusion.

3. **Warfarin (Coumadin)** inhibits vitamin-K epoxide reductase. This causes a deficiency of vitamin K, preventing the hepatic carboxylation of factors II, VII, IX, and X, and proteins C and S to the active form. The PT and the INR are prolonged in patients taking warfarin. The drug's half-life is approximately 35 hours, requiring days for reversal. If quick reversal of warfarin is required, active factors can be given in the form of FFP (5 to 15 mL/kg). Vitamin K (2.5 to 10 mg IV or SC) can also be given for warfarin reversal, but its effect requires 6 or more hours.

4. **Platelet inhibitors. Aspirin** and **nonsteroidal anti-inflammatory drugs** (NSAIDs) inhibit platelet aggregation by interfering with the cyclooxygenase pathway. Aspirin permanently inhibits the pathway for the 10-day lifespan of the platelet. The other NSAIDS reversibly inhibit the cyclooxygenase pathway; their effects are reversed within 3 days of discontinuing the drug. **Dipyridamole** is a phosphodiesterase inhibitor that increases platelet cAMP, thereby inhibiting platelet aggregation. **Ticlopidine** and **clopidogrel** are newer antiplatelet agents that inhibit ADP-mediated platelet aggregation. **Abciximab** is an intravenous monoclonal antibody against the platelet glycoprotein IIb/IIIa receptor. It causes profound platelet inhibition and produces thrombocytopenia. Although the drug's plasma half-life is short, impairment of platelet function may last for days and reversal of the effect may require multiple platelet transfusions due to absorption of the antibody to donor platelets. Immediate reversal of platelet inhibitors may require platelet transfusion.

5. **Thrombolytic agents** act by dissolving thrombi via conversion of plasminogen to plasmin, which lyses fibrin clot. They are intended to reverse thrombosis and recanalize blood vessels. Two thrombolytic agents, **tissue plasminogen activator (tPA)** and **streptokinase**, are commonly used in clinical practice, each with slightly different pharmacodynamic and side ef-

fect profiles. Each of these drugs results in a hypofibrinogenemic state and carries a substantial risk of bleeding. They are generally contraindicated perioperatively. If emergent surgery is required following thrombolytic therapy, the effect may be reversed by administration of aminocaproic or tranexamic acid. The fibrinogen level may be restored by transfusion of cryoprecipitate or FFP.

X.   Special considerations

A.   Hemophilia. Hemophilia A and B are rare, sex-linked diseases affecting males almost exclusively. **Hemophilia A** is due to an abnormality in factor VIII while **hemophilia B (Christmas disease)** is due to a factor IX abnormality. The incidence in the United States is 1:10,000 males for hemophilia A and 1:100,000 males for hemophilia B.

    1.   Clinical features. Patients usually present early in childhood with hemarthroses and soft-tissue hematomas after minor trauma. Laboratory tests demonstrate a markedly prolonged PTT with normal PT and platelet count.

    2.   Treatment with the appropriate factor (of either recombinant or lyophilized concentrate source) should be coordinated with the patient's hematologist. Hemophilia A is treated with factor VIII to achieve preoperative activity levels of 25% to 100%, depending on the extent of the procedure. Some patients with mild hemophilia A may respond to DDAVP therapy. In an emergency, if factor VIII is unavailable, cryoprecipitate transfusion can provide the deficient factor. Hemophilia B is treated with factor IX to achieve at least 30% to 50% activity before surgery.

B.   Von Willebrand disease is caused by a deficiency or abnormality in von Willebrand factor, a protein involved in anchoring platelets to injured subendothelium and stabilizing factor VIII. It is the most common inherited bleeding disorder, affecting 1% to 2% of the population. It is autosomally dominant and affects both sexes equally.

    1.   Clinical presentation. The phenotypic expression is variable so that clinical manifestations may range from very mild to severe bleeding. Usually, patients have a history of easy bruisability and bleeding from mucosal surfaces, but some patients are not diagnosed with a bleeding disorder until suffering major trauma or surgery complicated by bleeding. Laboratory tests usually reveal a prolonged bleeding time.

    2.   Treatment of von Willebrand disease depends on the subtype. Many patients respond to DDAVP treatment, but others may require cryoprecipitate. The lysine–analogue antifibrinolytics also have been used in some patients to reduce surgical bleeding. Preoperative consultation with the patient's hematologist is recommended.

C.   Sickle cell anemia affects 1:600 African Americans. The disease is caused by the substitution of valine for glutamic acid at the sixth position on the beta chain of hemoglobin. Homozygotes for this substitution (as well as double heterozygotes SC or beta-thalassemia) have clinical sickle cell disease.

    1.   Clinical features. The abnormal hemoglobin polymerizes and causes a sickling deformity of the red cell under certain conditions (e.g., hypoxia, hypothermia, acidosis, and dehydration). Sickled cells cause microvascular occlusion with tissue ischemia and infarction. A sickle cell crisis typically presents with excruciating chest or abdominal pain, fever, tachycardia, leukocytosis, and hematuria. Signs and symptoms may be masked by anesthesia. The RBCs have a shortened survival time of 12 days, leading to anemia and extramedullary hematopoiesis.

2. The anesthetic management of these patients includes avoiding conditions that promote sickling (e.g., hypoxia, hypovolemia, acidemia, and hypothermia). In addition, transfusing to a preoperative Hct of approximately 30% prevents postoperative complications as effectively as the traditional "exchange transfusions" that sought to reduce the amount of hemoglobin S to 30% of total hemoglobin.

D.   Jehovah's Witness patients generally may refuse to receive blood or blood products because of their religious beliefs, even if such refusal results in death. Special considerations may apply if the patient is a minor, is incompetent, or has responsibilities for dependents, and in certain emergency circumstances (see also Chapter 39, section II.F). However, a physician is not required to agree to treat a patient who refuses a transfusion if doing so is contrary to the physician's ethical beliefs. Blood conservation measures are crucial in these patients (see section VII). Jehovah's Witnesses may allow transfusion of intraoperatively phlebotomized blood (see section VII.B) as long as the blood remains in continuity with the body (i.e., the blood tubing must always remain connected to the patient). Erythropoietin is sometimes used to increase red cell mass perioperatively. It is incumbent on the anesthesiologist to fully discuss the patient's beliefs and decisions concerning transfusion and document these decisions clearly in the medical record as well as operative consents.

SUGGESTED READING

American Society of Anesthesiologists Task Force on Blood Component Therapy. Practice guidelines for blood component therapy. *Anesthesiology* 1996;84:732–747.

Baron JF. Haemoglobin therapy in clinical practice: use and characteristics of DCLHb. *Br J Anaesth* 1998;81[Suppl 1]:34–37.

Goodnough LT, Brecher ME, Kanter MH, et al. Transfusion medicine. I. Blood transfusion. *N Engl J Med* 1999;340:438–447.

Goodnough LT, Brecher ME, Kanter MH, et al. Transfusion medicine: II. Blood conservation. *N Engl J Med* 1999;340:525–533.

Gross JB. Estimating allowable blood loss: corrected for dilution. *Anesthesiology* 1983;58:277–280.

Kopko PM, Holland PV. Transfusion-related acute lung injury. *Br J Haematol* 1999;105:322–329.

Lake CL, Moore RA, eds. *Blood: hemostasis, transfusion, and alternatives in the perioperative period.* New York: Raven Press, 1995.

McFarland JG. Perioperative blood transfusions: indications and options. *Chest* 1999;115[5 Suppl]:113S–121S.

Peters DC, Noble S. Aprotinin: an update of its pharmacology and therapeutic use in open heart surgery and coronary artery bypass surgery. *Drugs* 1999;57:233–260.

Schreiber GB, Busch MP, Kleinman SH, et al. The risk of transfusion-transmitted viral infections. *N Engl J Med* 1996;334:1685–1690.

Sharma AD, Sreeram G, Erb T, et al. Leukocyte-reduced blood transfusions: perioperative indications, adverse effects, and cost analysis. *Anesth Analg* 2000;90:1315–1323.

Spahn DR, Casutt M. Eliminating blood transfusions: new aspects and perspectives. *Anesthesiology* 2000;93:242–255.

Steinberg MH. Management of sickle cell disease. *N Engl J Med* 1999; 340:1021–1030.

Perioperative Issues

The Postanesthesia Care Unit

Edward E. George and Luca M. Bigatello

I. General considerations. For most patients, recovery from anesthesia is uneventful. Postoperative complications, however, may be sudden and life-threatening. The **postanesthesia care unit** (PACU) is designed to provide close monitoring and care to patients recovering from anesthesia and sedation, assuring safety to the transition between anesthesia and the fully awake state, before patients are transferred to unmonitored general wards. The PACU is staffed by a dedicated team of an anesthesiologist, nurses, and aides. It is located in immediate proximity to the operating room (OR), with access to radiology and the laboratory. Drugs and equipment for routine care (O_2, suction, and monitors) and advanced support (mechanical ventilators, pressure transducers, infusion pumps, and code cart) must be readily available.

II. Admission to the PACU

A. Transport from the OR is carried out under direct supervision of the anesthetist, preferably with the head of the bed elevated or with the patient in the lateral decubitus position to maximize airway patency. Oxygen delivered by face mask is indicated in most patients to prevent hypoxemia from hypoventilation and diffusion hypoxia (see section VI.A.1).

B. Report. Upon arrival, vital signs are recorded and the anesthetist provides a complete report to the PACU team. The anesthetist remains in charge of the care of the patient until the team is ready to take over. In addition, the anesthetist may speak directly to the anesthesiologist in charge of the PACU, the surgeon, or a consultant about issues of particular importance. This report is often the only formal account of the intraoperative events between the operating team and the personnel who will carry out the immediate postoperative care.

C. Report includes:

1. Patient identification, age, surgical procedure, diagnosis, a summary of prior medical history, medications, allergies, and preoperative vital signs. Specific features such as deafness, psychiatric issues, or language barriers should be mentioned.

2. Location and size of intravascular catheters.

3. Premedication, antibiotics, anesthetic drugs for induction and maintenance, opioids, muscle relaxants, and reversal agents. Vasoactive drugs, bronchodilators, and other relevant drugs administered should be listed.

4. Exact nature of the surgical procedure. If relevant surgical issues exist (e.g., adequacy of hemostasis, care of drains, restrictions on positioning, etc.), the PACU staff should be informed.

5. Anesthetic course, with emphasis on problems that may impact on the immediate postoperative course including laboratory values, difficult intravenous (IV) access, difficult intubation, intraoperative hemodynamic instability, electrocardiographic (ECG) changes, and so on.

6. Fluid balance, including amount, type, and rationale of fluid replacement, urine output, and estimated fluid and blood loss.

III. Monitoring. Close observation of the patient's level of consciousness, breathing pattern and peripheral perfusion is most important. The nurse/patient ratio for routine cases is one nurse to two or three patients and increases to 1:1 for high acuity patients, those with a significant medical history, and those with intraoperative complications. Vital signs are monitored and charted at regular intervals according to the patient's need. Standard monitoring includes **respiratory rate** measurement by impedance plethysmography, continuous **electrocardiogram**, manual or automated oscillometric **blood pressure**, and **pulse oximetry**. When necessary, invasive monitoring can be instituted. An arterial catheter provides continuous measurement of the systemic blood pressure in patients with tenuous hemodynamics and provides access for blood sampling. Central venous and pulmonary artery catheters may be used when the etiology of hemodynamic instability is unclear (see Chapter 10). When monitoring and care requirements are increasing, plans should be made to transfer the patient to an intensive care unit (ICU).

IV. Complications. The incidence of complications in the PACU varies with the patient population. From several studies over the last 10 years, it appears that complications causing at least moderate morbidity occur in approximately 5% to 10% of PACU admissions.

V. Hemodynamic complications were the most frequently recorded adverse events in studies at the Massachusetts General Hospital and at a large Canadian university hospital. Hypotension (4% of admissions), arrhythmias (4%), hypertension (1% to 2%), and hypovolemia (1%) were the most common complications recorded.

A. Hypotension. The differential diagnosis is aided by a review of the patient's history and intraoperative management. The anesthetist who performed the case can be contacted to help in the interpretation of the current events. **Hypovolemia** is the most common cause of hypotension in the PACU and administration of a fluid bolus during the initial assessment is generally a safe maneuver to start. In any case, the following algorithm is helpful in the differential **diagnosis of hypotension**.

1. **Inadequate venous return**.

a. **True hypovolemia**. Ongoing hemorrhage, inadequate fluid replacement, osmotic polyuria, and fluid sequestration (intestinal obstruction or ascites) are among the causes of hypovolemia in the PACU. Nonspecific signs include hypotension, tachycardia, tachypnea, decreased skin turgor, dryness of mucous membranes, oliguria, and thirst. A meaningful volume challenge (250 to 1,000 mL of an electrolyte solution or a synthetic colloid, blood products, or both) should be administered. Persistent hypotension following a seemingly adequate volume replacement mandates further assessment, starting with placement of a urinary catheter and followed by invasive monitoring.

b. **Relative hypovolemia** occurs when the venous return to the heart is decreased, not by an absolute reduction of circulating volume, but by mechanical forces. Common causes include **positive pressure ventilation**, dynamic hyperinflation of the lungs with subsequent **intrinsic positive end-expiratory pressure** (see Chapter 35), **pneumothorax**, and **pericardial tamponade**. Signs of obstruction to venous return are similar to those of true hypovolemia, except for the presence of jugular venous distention, an elevated central venous pressure, and decreased breath sounds and heart tones. Volume administration is the mainstay of symptomatic therapy, but treatment of the cause is the ultimate intervention.

2.   Vasodilation. General and neuroaxial anesthesia, rewarming from hypothermia, transfusion reactions, adrenal insufficiency, anaphylaxis, systemic inflammation, sepsis, liver failure, and the administration of vasodilator drugs are causes of hypotension resulting from vasodilation. Hypovolemia accentuates the hypotension of vasodilation, but volume replacement alone cannot fully restore the blood pressure. Pharmacologic treatment includes α-adrenergic–receptor agonists such as **phenylephrine, epinephrine**, and **norepinephrine** and should be carried out under close monitoring. Diagnosis and treatment of the specific etiology should be concurrent with symptomatic treatment.

3.   Decreased inotropy. Myocardial ischemia and infarction, arrhythmias, congestive heart failure, negative inotropic drugs (anesthetics, β-adrenergic blockers, calcium-channel blockers, and antiarrhythmics), sepsis, hypothyroidism, and malignant hyperthermia are possible etiologies of perioperative myocardial dysfunction. Symptoms include dyspnea, diaphoresis, cyanosis, jugular vein distention, oliguria, rhythm disturbances, wheezes, dependent crackles, and an S_3 gallop at auscultation. A chest radiograph (CXR), 12-lead ECG, and basic laboratory values help in the diagnosis. Invasive monitoring generally is necessary to guide therapy (see Chapters 2 and 19), which may include:

a.   Positive inotropes such as dopamine, dobutamine, epinephrine, norepinephrine, and milrinone.

b.   Afterload reduction with nitrates, calcium-channel blockers, or angiotensin-converting enzyme inhibitors.

c.   Diuresis (see Chapter 4).

B.   Hypertension is most commonly observed in patients with preexisting hypertensive disease, particularly if antihypertensive medications were not administered preoperatively. Other postoperative etiologies include pain, bladder distention, fluid overload, hypoxemia, increased intracranial pressure (ICP), and administration of vasoconstrictive agents. Hypertension may present with headache, visual disturbances, dyspnea, restlessness, and chest pain, but is often asymptomatic. In the initial assessment, one should verify the accuracy of blood pressure measurement, review the patient's history and operative course, and rule out correctable etiologies. Management aims at restoring blood pressure close to what is normal for each patient. Close blood pressure control is indicated following cases such as intracranial aneurysm surgery, creation of vascularized muscular flaps, microvascular surgery, and in patients with severe vascular disease. Resuming chronic antihypertensive therapy is ideal. If needed, the latter can be supplemented or substituted by a fast-onset, short-acting IV or sublingual drug.

   1.   Beta-adrenergic blockers. Labetalol, 5 to 10 mg, propranolol, 0.5- to 1.0-mg increments, and esmolol, 10 to 100 mg IV, are also suitable for continuous infusions.
   2.   Calcium-channel blockers. Verapamil, 2.5- to 5-mg increments IV, and diltiazem, 20-mg increments IV, are suitable for continuous infusions. Nifedipine, 5 to 10 mg sublingually, has a positive chronotropic effect.
   3.   Hydralazine, 5 to 20 mg IV, is a pure vasodilator indicated when a faster heart rate is desirable.
   4.   Nitrates. Nitroglycerin, starting at 25 μg per minute IV, is preferentially a venodilator. Sodium nitroprusside, starting at 0.5 μg/kg per minute IV, is a potent arterial dilator.
   5.   Alpha-adrenergic blockers are used increasingly in the treatment of chronic hypertension. At present, **phentolamine**, 2.5- to 5.0-mg boluses, is the most common IV agent. Intravenous **labetalol** has a 1:7 ratio of α/β-adrenergic blockade activity.
C.   Arrhythmias. Increased sympathetic outflow, hypoxemia, hypercarbia, electrolyte and acid-base imbalance, myocardial ischemia, increased ICP, drug toxicity, and malignant hyperthermia are possible etiologies of perioperative arrhythmias. Premature atrial contractions and unifocal premature ventricular contractions generally do not require treatment. In the presence of more worrisome rhythm disturbances, supplemental O_2 should be delivered and proper treatment begun while the etiology is investigated (see Chapters 18 and 36).
   1.   Common supraventricular arrhythmias
      a.   Sinus tachycardia may be secondary to pain, agitation, hypovolemia, fever, hypoxemia, congestive heart failure, and pulmonary embolism. It should not be treated symptomatically before its etiology is addressed, unless it constitutes a risk for myocardial ischemia.
      b.   Paroxysmal supraventricular tachycardias include paroxysmal atrial tachycardia, multifocal atrial tachycardia, nodal tachycardia, atrial fibrillation, and flutter. These rhythms may cause significant hypotension.
         (1)   Synchronized cardioversion if the rhythm is hemodynamically unstable, starting at 50 joules (100 joules or more for atrial fibrillation).
         (2)   Adenosine, 6 to 12 mg, rapid IV.
         (3)   Verapamil or **diltiazem** (see section V.B.2).
         (4)   Propranolol or **esmolol** (see section V.B.1).
         (5)   Digoxin, 0.25-mg IV increments up to 1.0 to 1.5 mg slows ventricular response but has a delayed onset.
         (6)   Procainamide and other type II-A agents, **quinidine** and **disopyramide**, are effective in restoring sinus rhythm, but have a narrow therapeutic window and require close monitoring.
         (7)   Amiodarone is recommended for the treatment of atrial fibrillation in the setting of a decreased myocardial function (congestive heart failure or ejection fraction less than 40%).
      c.   Sinus bradycardia may result from a high neuroaxial anesthetic block, opioid administration, vagal stimulation, α-adrenergic blockade, and increased ICP. Symptomatic treatment with anticholinergic muscarinic agents, **atropine**, 0.2

to 0.4 mg IV, or **glycopyrrolate**, 0.2 mg IV, is indicated when hypotension is present. Treatment of profound bradycardia is described in Chapter 36.

2. Stable ventricular arrhythmias. If premature ventricular contractions are multifocal, occur in runs, or occur close to the preceding beat's T-wave, they should be treated.

    a. Underlying etiologies such as hypoxemia, myocardial ischemia, acidosis, hypokalemia, and hypomagnesemia should be corrected.

    b. Lidocaine, 1.5 mg/kg IV, followed by an infusion at 1 to 4 mg per minute.

    c. Procainamide, 20 to 30 mg per minute IV, maximum total 17 mg/kg, and 1 to 2 mg per minute infusion, is an effective second-line drug that can be subsequently converted to oral therapy.

3. Unstable ventricular tachycardia and **ventricular fibrillation** are described in Chapter 36.

D. Myocardial ischemia and infarction

1. T-wave changes include inversion, flattening, and pseudo-normalization. They may be associated with myocardial ischemia and infarction, electrolyte changes, hypothermia, surgical manipulation of the mediastinum, or incorrect lead placement. Isolated T-wave changes must be considered within the clinical context because they are common postoperatively and only rarely are caused by myocardial ischemia.

2. ST-segment elevation or depression is highly specific for myocardial infarction and ischemia, respectively. As supplemental O_2 is administered and a 12-lead ECG obtained, possible precipitating factors must be reviewed. Hypoxemia, anemia, tachycardia, hypotension, and hypertension are common causes and must be corrected. If tolerated, **beta blockade** and IV nitroglycerin may be added. In severe cases, a cardiology consultation and transfer to an ICU are indicated, particularly when ongoing ischemia mandates the institution of invasive monitoring and specialized treatment such as thrombolysis, aortic counter-pulsation, percutaneous angioplasty, or revascularization.

VI. Respiratory complications occurred in 1.3% of 24,157 PACU admissions in a study at a Canadian university hospital. The main events were hypoxemia (0.9% of admissions), hypoventilation (0.2%), and upper airway obstruction (0.2%).

A. Hypoxemia. General anesthesia is associated with inhibition of hypoxic and hypercapneic ventilatory drive and a reduction of the pulmonary functional residual capacity. These changes may persist for a variable period of time postoperatively and predispose to hypoventilation and hypoxemia. Physical signs of hypoxemia include dyspnea, cyanosis, altered mental status, agitation, obtundation, tachycardia, hypertension, and arrhythmias. Before instituting symptomatic treatment of any of these common signs, hypoxemia must be excluded. Causes of hypoxemia include the following:

1. Atelectasis is a predictable consequence of a decreased functional residual capacity. Small areas of alveolar collapse can rapidly reexpand with deep breathing and coughing. Occasionally, hypoxemia may persist and a CXR may reveal a segmental or lobar collapse. Chest physiotherapy, fiberoptic bronchoscopy, or both aids in reinflation of the atelectatic segment.

2.   Hypoventilation causes hypoxemia by promoting alveolar collapse and increasing the CO_2 tension of alveolar air.

3.   Diffusion hypoxia may occur during washout of nitrous oxide upon emergence from general anesthesia. High inspired O_2 fraction (FIO_2) by face mask prevents hypoxemia.

4.   Upper airway obstruction is a characteristic complication of awakening from general anesthesia when the patient has not fully recovered control of airway reflexes and tone (see section VI.C).

5.   Bronchospasm may cause hypoventilation, CO_2 retention, and hypoxemia (see section VI.C).

6.   Aspiration of gastric contents (see Chapter 18).

7.   Pulmonary edema may occur as a result of either cardiac failure or increased pulmonary capillary permeability. Cardiogenic edema occurs mostly in individuals with preexisting cardiac disease and is characterized by hypoxemia, dyspnea, orthopnea, jugular venous distention, wheezing, and an S_3 gallop. It may be precipitated by fluid overload, arrhythmias, and myocardial ischemia. A physical exam, CXR, arterial blood gas tensions, and a 12-lead ECG should be obtained. Evaluation by a cardiologist may be indicated, particularly when invasive treatment of conditions such as unstable angina or acute valvular disease is an option. Inotropic agents, diuretics, and vasodilators are the mainstay of treatment. "Permeability" pulmonary edema secondary to sepsis, head injury, aspiration, transfusion reaction, anaphylaxis, or upper airway obstruction is characterized by hypoxemia without the signs of left-ventricular overload. Treatment generally needs to be continued in an ICU (see Chapter 35).

8.   Pneumothorax may cause hypoventilation, hypoxemia, and hemodynamic instability (see section VI.B.2.f).

9.   Pulmonary embolism seldom occurs immediately postoperatively. It should be considered, however, in the differential diagnosis of hypoxemia in patients with deep venous thrombosis, cancer, multiple trauma, and in those who have been at prolonged bed rest.

B.   Hypoventilation is an inappropriately low-minute ventilation and results in hypercapnea and acute respiratory acidosis. When severe, hypoventilation produces hypoxemia, CO_2 narcosis, and ultimately apnea. Etiologies of postoperative hypoventilation may be divided in two groups:

1.   Decreased ventilatory drive

a. All inhaled **halogenated agents** depress ventilatory drive (see Chapter 11) and may produce hypoventilation in the postoperative period. **Opioids** are potent respiratory depressants. All mu-receptor agonists increase the apneic threshold. Overnarcotized patients typically appear pain free, with a slow respiratory rate and a tendency to become apneic if left unstimulated. Large doses of **benzodiazepines** may also inhibit ventilatory drive. The safest treatment of anesthetic-related hypoventilation is to continue mechanical ventilation until breathing is adequate. Alternatively, pharmacologic reversal may be considered.

(1) Opioid-induced hypoventilation can be reversed by **naloxone**, a pure mu-receptor antagonist. Doses of 40 to 80 μg IV are titrated to effect. Reversal occurs within 1 to 2 minutes and lasts for 30 to 60 minutes. Naloxone treatment may cause significant side effects: pain, tachycardia, hypertension, pulmonary edema, and delayed renarcotization. The effects of opioids on respiratory function may outlast a single dose of naloxone. The patient should be monitored for recurrence of opioid-induced hypoventilation.

(2) Hypoventilation secondary to benzodiazepines can be reversed by **flumazenil**, 0.2 mg IV, titrated to 1 mg over 5 minutes to a maximum of 5 mg. The onset of reversal occurs within 1 to 2 minutes with peak effect at 6 to 10 minutes. Side effects of flumazenil are less pronounced than those of the opioid antagonists, but resedation may occur.

b. Less common but life-threatening causes of ventilatory drive depression include complications of **intracranial** and **carotid artery** surgery, **head injuries**, and intraoperative **stroke** (see section VIII).

2. **Pulmonary and respiratory muscle insufficiency**

   a. **Preexistent respiratory disease** may be the most important risk factor for postoperative respiratory complications. **Chronic obstructive pulmonary disease** (COPD; see Chapter 3) alters the match of ventilation and perfusion, resulting in hypoxemia and hypercapnia. Impaired gas exchange and expiratory flow limitation cause a high ventilatory workload under normal circumstances, which is worsened by surgical trauma, anesthesia, airway secretions, and so on. **Restrictive disease** (e.g., pulmonary fibrosis, pleural effusions, obesity, scoliosis, massive ascites, and pregnancy) is associated with fewer complications than COPD, particularly when respiratory muscle strength is preserved and the restrictive defect is extrapulmonary.

   b. **Inadequate reversal of neuromuscular blockade** may be suggested by the observation of shallow breathing, generalized weakness, and spasmodic twitching. Adequacy of muscle strength can be assessed clinically and with a twitch monitor (see Chapter 12). Special situations must be considered: myasthenia gravis and the myasthenic syndromes; pseudocholinesterase deficiency; succinylcholine-induced, phase II block; hypothermia; acid-base and electrolyte imbalance; and anticholinesterase overdose. If muscle weakness persists following adequate pharmacologic reversal (e.g., **neostigmine**, up to 5 mg, and **glycopyrrolate**, up to 1 mg in an adult), it is best to institute or continue mechanical ventilation, administer adequate anxiolysis, and wait for the muscle strength to recover while the appropriate workup is performed.

   c. **Upper airway obstruction** may cause hypercapnea and hypoxemia (see section VI.C).

   d. **Inadequate analgesia** following thoracic or upper abdominal surgery may cause splinting and reduce minute ventilation, resulting in alveolar collapse, hypercapnea, and hypoxemia. This is preventable with early analgesia and encouragement of deep breathing and coughing.

e. Bronchospasm is common in patients with COPD, asthma, or recent respiratory tract infection. It is often precipitated by manipulation of the airway, particularly tracheal intubation. Wheezing may also be heard with pulmonary edema, endobronchial intubation, aspiration pneumonitis, and pneumothorax. Treatment is discussed in Chapter 3.

f. Pneumothorax may complicate a thoracotomy, mediastinoscopy, bronchoscopy, high retroperitoneal dissection for nephrectomy or adrenalectomy, and spinal fusion. Insertion of central venous lines and nerve blocks of the upper extremities are other possible etiologies. A portable CXR in the sitting position will be diagnostic. In the presence of hemodynamic instability (tension pneumothorax), a tube thoracostomy must be performed even without CXR confirmation. Treatment of pneumothorax is illustrated in Chapter 21.

C. Upper airway obstruction may occur during recovery from anesthesia. Principal signs are the lack of adequate air movement, intercostal and suprasternal retractions, and discoordinate abdominal and chest wall motion during inspiration. While **100% O_2** is given by mask, swift airway management is required from the PACU anesthesiologist (see Chapter 13). Common etiologies include:

1. Incomplete recovery from general anesthesia and/or neuromuscular blockade (see section VI.B). A decreased strength and coordination of the intrinsic and extrinsic airway musculature causes the tongue to fall backwards and occlude the airway. Patency is reestablished by inserting a nasal or oral airway, by manually assisting ventilation, or by intubating the trachea.

2. Laryngospasm may be precipitated by light anesthesia and irritation of the glottis by secretions, blood, or a foreign body (see Chapter 18).

3. Airway edema may occur during bronchoscopy, esophagoscopy, and surgery of the head and neck. It may also follow a traumatic intubation, an allergic reaction, the administration of large amounts of IV fluids, and the head-down position. Children are particularly susceptible to airway obstruction from edema because of the small diameter of their upper airway. Treatment of upper airway edema includes:

a. Administration of warmed, humidified **100% O_2** by face mask.

b. Head elevation and **fluid restriction**.

c. Nebulization of racemic **epinephrine** 2.25% solution, 0.5 to 1.0 mL in normal saline, or L-epinephrine, 2.5–5.0 mL of a 1:1000 solution, which may be repeated in 20 minutes if needed.

d. Dexamethasone, 4 to 8 mg IV every 6 hours for 24 hours.

e. Reintubation of the trachea must be considered early, because distortion of airway anatomy occurs rapidly.

4. Wound hematoma. Thyroid and parathyroid surgery, neck dissections, and carotid endarterectomy may be complicated by bleeding at the surgical site. The pressure caused by an expanding hematoma within the neck tissue planes causes obstruction of venous and lymphatic drainage and massive edema. Neck wound hematomas must be treated rapidly. The surgeon must be notified and an OR prepared. The anesthesiologist must support the airway by mask ventilation with **100% O$_2$**, followed by intubation of the trachea under direct vision. If tracheal intubation cannot be rapidly accomplished, the wound must be reopened to relieve tissue congestion and improve airway patency.

5. Vocal cord (VC) paralysis may occur following thyroid, parathyroid, thoracic, and tracheal surgery, or a traumatic endotracheal intubation. VC paralysis may be transient, resulting from manipulation of the recurrent laryngeal nerve, or permanent, from severing the nerve. Unilateral transient VC paralysis is relatively common and the primary concern is potential aspiration of gastric contents. Permanent unilateral VC paralysis is also fairly benign. With time, compensatory action of the contralateral VC minimizes the occurrence of aspiration. Bilateral VC paralysis can occur following radical surgery for thyroid or tracheal cancer, where neoplastic infiltration makes identification of the recurrent laryngeal nerves virtually impossible. Bilateral VC paralysis is a serious complication that leads to complete upper airway obstruction and requires endotracheal intubation. When permanent, it necessitates a tracheotomy.

D. The intubated patient presents special considerations. Spontaneous ventilation through a "T-piece" may be sufficient when prolonged intubation is not foreseen. Some patients require partial or full ventilatory support. The anesthesiologist in the PACU should establish a plan regarding weaning and extubation or, alternatively, possible transfer to an ICU.

1. Delayed emergence from general anesthesia can be due to volatile or intravenous agents. Reversal may be facilitated pharmacologically (see section VI.B.1.a), but generally it is prudent to support ventilation while the respiratory depression resolves spontaneously.

2. Inadequate reversal of neuromuscular blockade. If muscle weakness persists following adequate pharmacologic reversal (see section VI.B.2.b), the patient needs mechanical support until full recovery is achieved.

3. Inadequate gas exchange. Decreased O$_2$ and CO$_2$ exchange often resolves as the effects of anesthesia, surgery, and positioning fade. While supporting ventilation, possible etiologies, discussed in sections V.A and V.B, must be considered.

4. Potential for airway obstruction exists following major head and neck reconstructions, drainage of pharyngeal abscesses, mandibular wiring, and surgery for trauma of the face and neck. These patients should not be extubated until fully awake. If airway edema is suspected, the patient should be treated as outlined in section VI.C.3.

5. The presence of a **full stomach** mandates extra attention to the recovery of consciousness and pharyngeal reflexes before extubation.

6. Hemodynamic instability, when severe, may be associated with a variable degree of impaired gas exchange and/or consciousness that mandates continuation of mechanical ventilation. Such a patient should promptly be transferred to an ICU.

7. Hypothermia may cause muscle weakness, altered mental status, prolonged drug metabolism, hemodynamic instability, coagulopathy, and shivering.

E. Guidelines for extubation. No single value or ventilatory index will predict a successful extubation with certainty. The following principles may help in assessing the readiness of a postoperative patient to resume unassisted ventilation:

1. Adequate **arterial Pao$_2$** or Spo$_2$.

2. Adequate **breathing pattern**. Patients should be able to sustain spontaneous, unlabored ventilation with a slow rate (less than 30 breaths per minute) and sufficient tidal volume (more than 300 mL), as can be easily tested in a 10-minute trial of unsupported breathing.

3. Adequate **level of consciousness** for cooperation and airway protection.

4. Full **recovery of muscle strength**.

5. Before proceeding with **extubation**, the PACU anesthesiologist should be aware of preexistent airway problems in the event that reintubation is necessary. **Supplemental O$_2$** is administered, the endotracheal tube, mouth, and pharynx suctioned, and the tube removed following a positive-pressure breath. Oxygen is then supplied by face mask as indicated, Spo$_2$ monitored, and the patient assessed for signs of airway obstruction or ventilatory insufficiency.

VII. Renal complications. The physiology, diagnosis, and treatment of renal abnormalities are described in Chapter 4. Three main conditions occur postoperatively.

A. Oliguria is defined as a urine output of less than 0.5 mL/kg per hour, but common sense must be used. A patient who received adequate volume replacement and an osmotic load at the time of aortic cross-clamping is expected to produce a brisk diuresis. Following a major lung resection, on the other hand, where IV fluids may be used sparingly, 0.5 mL/kg per hour may be reasonable. **Hypovolemia** is the most frequent cause of postoperative oliguria. Administration of a fluid bolus (250 to 500 mL of crystalloid or a synthetic colloid), even when other etiologies are not yet excluded, is acceptable. If this is fruitless, further diagnostic tests and invasive monitoring should be considered. **Diuretics** (see Chapter 4) should be used only where necessary, such as in congestive heart failure and chronic renal insufficiency. The unwarranted use of diuretics may aggravate existing renal hypoperfusion and worsen kidney damage. Temporary maintenance of urine output via forced diuresis does not improve the prognosis of acute renal failure. The traditional algorithm of pre-, post-, and intra-renal causes is helpful in the approach to the postoperative patient with oliguria.

1. Prerenal oliguria includes conditions that decrease renal perfusion pressure. Besides **hypovolemia**, other causes of a decreased cardiac output must be considered (see section V.A). Compartment syndrome from high intraabdominal pressure (i.e., intraperitoneal hemorrhage or massive ascites) also may reduce renal perfusion. Analysis of urine electrolytes (see Chapter 4) will reveal a low urinary sodium concentration (less than 10 mEq/L).

2. Intrarenal causes of postoperative oliguria include acute tubular necrosis secondary to hypoperfusion (e.g., shock or sepsis), toxins (e.g., nephrotoxic drugs or myoglobinuria) and trauma. Urinalysis may show granular casts.

3. Postrenal causes include urinary catheter obstruction, trauma, and iatrogenic damage.

B. Polyuria, defined as a urine output disproportionately high for a given fluid intake, is less frequent. Symptomatic treatment is based on volume replacement to maintain hemodynamic stability and fluid balance. Electrolyte and acid-base equilibrium may be altered from the etiologic condition or from the large volume losses. The differential diagnosis includes:

1. Excessive volume administration, requiring simple observation in healthy subjects.

2. Pharmacologic diuresis.

3. Postobstructive diuresis following resolution of urinary obstruction.

4. Nonoliguric renal failure. Acute tubular necrosis may cause transient polyuria due to the loss of the concentrating function of the tubules.

5. Osmotic diuresis may be caused by **hyperglycemia,** alcohol intoxication, and administration of hypertonic saline, mannitol, or parenteral nutrition.

6. Diabetes insipidus secondary to the lack of antidiuretic hormone (ADH) may follow head injury or intracranial surgery.

C. Electrolyte disturbances. With renal failure, **hyperkalemia** and acidemia may develop within hours and need to be corrected emergently to avoid ventricular arrhythmias and death (see Chapter 4). Polyuria may cause profound dehydration, with massive potassium losses and alkalemia. **Hypokalemia,** often associated with **hypomagnesemia,** may also trigger atrial and ventricular arrhythmias, but not as severe as those associated with hyperkalemia. Potassium replacement needs to be cautious to avoid overdose. Magnesium replacement may effectively treat atrial and ventricular arrhythmias.

VIII. Neurologic complications

A. Delayed awakening

1. The most frequent cause of a delayed awakening is the **persistent effect of anesthesia** (see sections VI.B and VI.C). Less common but possibly life-threatening causes include the organic cerebral events described below.

2. Decreased cerebral perfusion of sufficient duration, during or after surgery, may cause diffuse or localized cerebral damage responsible for obtundation and delayed awakening. In patients with cerebrovascular disease, short periods of hypotension may cause a critical reduction of cerebral perfusion and brain damage. If such event is suspected, a neurological consultation should be obtained and specific tests (e.g., computed tomography, magnetic resonance imaging, or angiography) considered. If cerebral edema is suspected, treatment should be started immediately (see Chapter 24).

3. Metabolic causes of delayed awakening include hypoglycemia, sepsis, preexisting encephalopathies, and electrolyte or acid-base derangements. Cerebral edema from the inadvertent infusion of hypotonic crystalloid solutions has been reported.

B. Neurologic damage may occur from a **stroke** and may be initially difficult to diagnose because of residual anesthesia.

Strokes can be **thromboembolic** (patients with cerebrovascular disease, hypercoagulable states, or atrial fibrillation) or **hemorrhagic** (patients with coagulopathies, hypertension, arteriovenous malformations, or trauma). Strokes are more frequent following **intracranial surgery, carotid endarterectomy,** or multiple **trauma.** Neurologic consultation is mandatory to guide the possible choice of immediate, lifesaving treatments.

C.   Emergence delirium is characterized by excitement alternating with lethargy, disorientation, and inappropriate behavior. Delirium may occur in any patient, but more frequently in the elderly and in those with a history of drug dependency or psychiatric disorders. Many drugs used perioperatively may precipitate delirium: ketamine, droperidol, opioids, benzodiazepines, large doses of metoclopramide, and atropine. Delirium may be a symptom of ongoing pathology (e.g., hypoxemia, acidemia, hyponatremia, hypoglycemia, intracranial injury, sepsis, severe pain, and alcohol withdrawal). Treatment is symptomatic: supplemental O_2, fluid and electrolyte replacement, and adequate analgesia. An antipsychotic medication such as **haloperidol** (0.5- to 5-mg IV increments every 20 to 30 minutes) may be indicated. Benzodiazepines (**diazepam,** 2.5 to 5 mg IV, or **lorazepam,** 1 to 2 mg IV) may be added if agitation is severe. **Physostigmine** (0.5 to 2.0 mg IV) may reverse anticholinergic delirium.

D.   Peripheral neurologic lesions may follow direct surgical damage and improper intraoperative positioning. The most frequent lesion is the external peroneal palsy (foot drop) associated with the lithotomy position. In a series from the Mayo Clinic, risk factors for a motor neuropathy following surgery in the lithotomy position were a lengthy operation (more than 4 hours), low body mass, and history of smoking. Other sites of possible nerve damage are the elbow (ulnar nerve), wrist (median and ulnar nerve), internal aspect of the arm (radial nerve) and axilla (brachial plexus), and the points of emergence of the main branches of the VII cranial nerve, which are compressible during mask–airway cases. Early neurological consultation for diagnosis and rehabilitation are crucial for a full recovery.

X.   Principles of pain management are described in Chapter 37. Adequate analgesia begins in the OR and continues in the PACU.

A.   Opioids (IV or peridural) are the mainstay of postoperative analgesia. Intramuscular injections, ordered on an "as needed" basis, have essentially no indication in adult PACU patients.

1.   Fentanyl, a potent synthetic opioid, is commonly limited to the operative setting, where airway patency can be strictly controlled. Occasionally, however, small IV doses (25 to 50 μg IV) can be titrated postoperatively to rapidly establish analgesia.

2.   Morphine, 2 to 4 mg IV, may be repeated every 10 to 20 minutes until adequate analgesia is achieved. In children above 1 year of age, 15 to 20 μg/kg IV or IM can be safely administered at 30- to 60-minute intervals.

3.   Meperidine, 25 to 50 mg IV, is similarly effective. It lacks the vagotonic effect of other opiates and may reduce postanesthetic shivering. **Meperidine must be avoided in patients taking monoamine-oxidase inhibitors.**

B.   Nonsteroidal anti-inflammatory drugs (NSAIDs) are an effective complement to opioids. **Ketorolac,** 30 mg IV, followed by

15 mg every 6 to 8 hours, provides potent postoperative analgesia. Other NSAIDs (**ibuprofen**, **acetaminophen**, and **indomethacin**) are also effective. Potential toxicities of all NSAIDs include decreased platelet aggregation and nephrotoxicity. A new class of potent analgesic agents is represented by the **cyclooxygenase inhibitors**. A representative drug is **rofecoxib**. Although available only in an oral preparation at present, they offer effective analgesia without significant respiratory depression. Similar to NSAIDs, cyclooxygenase inhibitors have mild gastrointestinal and platelet toxicity, thus predisposing to bleeding complications. They have a similar degree of nephrotoxicity as the NSAIDs.

C. Adjuvant analgesics include **hydroxyzine**, spasmolytics (**cyclobenzaprine**), and small doses of benzodiazepines and neuroleptics.

D. Regional sensory blocks can be very effective postoperatively (see Chapter 17).

E. Patient-controlled and **continuous epidural analgesia** should be started in the PACU.

XI. Postoperative nausea and vomiting

A. Patients are stratified preoperatively according to their risk of postoperative nausea and vomiting (PONV; Table 34-1). Individuals felt to be at minimal risk, such as young males undergoing minimally invasive procedures (hernia repair), would receive treatment for PONV only if required. Initial treatment utilizes **ondansetron**, 2 mg IV, and **dexamethasone**, 4 mg IV, as a single dose. If PONV continues to be problematic after 30 minutes, patients may receive **promethazine**, 12.5 to 25 mg IV, or **prochlorperazine** suppository, 25 mg per rectum. Individuals at moderate risk for PONV (procedures such as laproscopic cholecystectomy, total abdominal hysterectomy) may receive ondansetron and dexamethasone prophylactically, and promethazine or prochlorperazine may be utilized as salvage therapy. Individuals at highest risk

Table 34-1. **Prophylaxis of postoperative nausea and vomiting**

Risk Class	Definition	Suggested Treatment
Minimal	Hernia repair	None
Moderate	Abdominal hysterectomy	Ondansetron and dexamethasone prophylaxsis with promethazine and ondansetron salvage
Severe	Prior history PONV Major abdominal surgery	Pretreatment with ondansetron, dexamethasone and either promethazine, prochlorperazine, or meclizine

PONV, postoperative nausea and vomiting.

Table 34-2.   **Treatment of postoperative nausea and vomiting**

First episode; no known risk	Ondansetron and dexamethasone
Recurrent episodes	Promethazine or prochlorperazine
Intractable	Consider droperidol (see Appendix 1)

for PONV (major abdominal procedures or a past history of severe PONV) should receive both ondansetron, dexamethasone, and either promethazine, prochlorperazine or **meclizine**, 25 mg orally (ideally in the preoperative setting; see Table 34-1). The incidence is higher in young adults, following eye and ear surgery, laparoscopy, and when opiates and nitrous oxide are used (Table 34-2).

B.   Droperidol (0.625 to 2.5 mg IV) has commonly been used as an antiemetic. Recent concerns over QT-interval prolongation and induction of ventricular arrhythmias now limit its use to patients failing other therapies, and only after it is determined that QT prolongation does not exist. Monitoring for arrhythmias is recommended before treatment and for 2 to 3 hours after treatment (see *Droperidol* in Supplemental Drug Information).

XII.   Body temperature changes.

A.   Postoperative **hypothermia** may cause vasoconstriction, hypoperfusion, and metabolic acidosis; it impairs platelet function, cardiac repolarization, and decreases the metabolism of many drugs. During rewarming, shivering significantly increases O_2 consumption and CO_2 production, which may be undesirable. Hypothermia can be treated with heated blankets, a forced warm air blanket, and warm IV solutions (see Chapter 18, section VII).

B.   Etiologies of **hyperthermia** include infection, transfusion reaction (see Chapter 33, section VIII.A), hyperthyroidism (see Chapter 6, section III), **malignant hyperthermia** (see Chapter 18, section XVII), and neuroleptic malignant syndrome (see Chapter 18, section XVII.F.4). Symptomatic treatment should be limited to situations in which hyperthermia is potentially dangerous, such as in young children or patients with compromised respiratory or cardiac reserve (see Chapter 18, section VIII). **Acetaminophen** (suppositories, 650 to 1,300 mg or 10 mg/kg in children) and cooling blankets are commonly used.

XIII.   Recovery from regional anesthesia

A.   Uncomplicated regional blocks do not require recovery in the PACU. Postoperative monitoring is indicated when heavy sedation was administered, a complication from the block occurred (e.g., intravascular injection of a local anesthetic or pneumothorax), or when required by the nature of the surgery (e.g., carotid endarterectomy).

B.   Recovery from spinal and epidural anesthesia progresses from cephalad to caudad, with sensory blockade weaning first (see Chapter 16). If recovery seems delayed, a neurologic exam should be performed to investigate the possibility of spinal cord damage.

XIV.   Criteria for discharge. At the Massachusetts General Hospital, all patients who receive general anesthesia are observed until ready for discharge, with no preset minimum time. To be discharged from the PACU, patients must be easily arousable and oriented. They should be hemodynamically stable, normothermic, and able to maintain adequate ventilation and protect their airway. Pain and nausea should be under control and appropriate IV access secured. Effective communication with both the surgical team and the ward to which the patient is to be transferred can expedite the discharge of patients from the PACU. This may be most relevant in the setting of a patient having undergone an uncomplicated procedure, with minimal time under anesthesia, and an uneventful emergence.

SUGGESTED READING

American Heart Association in collaboration with the International Liaison Committee on Resuscitation (ILCOR). Guidelines 2000 for cardiopulmonary resuscitation and emergency cardiovascular care. *Circulation* 2000;102[Suppl I]:I-158–I-165.

Cooper JB, Cullen DJ, Nemeskal R, et al. Effects of information feedback and pulse oximetry on the incidence of anesthesia complications. *Anesthesiology* 1987;67:686–694.

Hedenstierna G. Gas exchange during anesthesia. *Acta Anaesthesiol Scand* 1990;34:27–31.

Hill RP, Lubarsky DA, Phillips-Bute B, et al. Cost-effectiveness of prophylactic anti-emetic therapy with ondansetron, droperidol, or placebo. *Anesthesiology* 2000;92:958–967.

Kissin I. Preemptive analgesia. Why its effect is not always obvious [Editorial]. *Anesthesiology* 1996;84:1015–1019.

Lenhardt R, Marker E, Goll V, et al. Mild intraoperative hypothermia prolongs postanesthetic recovery. *Anesthesiology* 1997;87:1318–1323.

O'Keefe ST, Ni Chonghubhair A. Postoperative delirium in the elderly. *Br J Anaesth* 1994;73:673–687.

Pepe PE, Marini JJ. Occult positive end-expiratory pressure in mechanically ventilated patients with airflow obstruction. *Am Rev Respir Dis* 1982;126:166–170.

Rose DK, Cohen MM, De Boer DP. Cardiovascular events in the postanesthesia care unit: contribution of risk factors. *Anesthesiology* 1996;84:772–781.

Rose DK, Cohen MM, Wigglesworth DF, et al. Critical respiratory events in the postanesthesia care unit. Patient, surgical, and anesthetic factors. *Anesthesiology* 1994;81:410–418.

Van den Elsen M, Dahan A, DeGoede J, et al. Influences of subanesthetic isoflurane on ventilatory control in humans. *Anesthesiology* 1995;83:478–490.

Wahba RWM. Perioperative functional residual capacity. *Can J Anaesth* 1991;38:206–210.

Warner MA, Martin JT, Schroeder DR, et al. Lower-extremity motor neuropathy associated with surgery performed in patients in the lithotomy position. *Anesthesiology* 1994;81:6–12.

Warner MA, Warner MB, Weber JG. Clinical significance of pulmonary aspiration during the perioperative period. *Anesthesiology* 1993;78:56–62.

Perioperative Respiratory Failure

Edward E. George and Luca M. Bigatello

I. Anesthesiologists are often consulted to assist with the perioperative management of the airway (Chapter 13), pulmonary problems (Chapter 3), or ventilatory support.

II. Pathophysiology of acute respiratory failure. Gas exchange between the inspired air and the body tissues is governed by three main mechanisms: ventilation, diffusion, and blood flow. Respiratory failure can be viewed as the impairment of one or more of these functions.

  A. Ventilatory failure
   1. Control of ventilation
      a. Central control of ventilation is by chemoreceptors located on the surface of the medulla. Alterations in cerebrospinal fluid (CSF) pH are the major stimuli for these receptors. Acute changes in arterial partial pressure of carbon dioxide ($Paco_2$) rapidly affect cerebrospinal fluid pH, due to the high permeability of the blood–brain barrier to CO_2. The $Paco_2$ is the main determinant of alveolar ventilation. Throughout normal daily activities, $Paco_2$ is kept within a few mm Hg of baseline (40 mm Hg). Alveolar ventilation increases by 1 to 3 L per minute for each 1 mm Hg increase of $Paco_2$. **Peripheral chemoreceptors**, located in the carotid bodies, are sensitive to changes of the arterial partial pressure of oxygen (Pao_2) and, to a lesser extent, $Paco_2$. These receptors are responsible for all the increase of alveolar ventilation that occurs as the Pao_2 decreases below 100 mm Hg. Following bilateral carotid surgery, patients may loose this hypoxic ventilatory response.
      b. Low inspiratory concentrations of all halogenated agents (0.1% to 0.3% of the minimal alveolar concentration) depress hypoxic ventilatory drive (see Chapters 11 and 34). Higher concentrations decrease the minute ventilation and generate a characteristic pattern of rapid, shallow breathing. **Opioids** are potent inhibitors of the hypercapnic ventilatory drive. Overnarcotized patients show a slow respiratory rate and tend to become apneic if unstimulated. **Hypnotics** and **benzodiazepines** also inhibit ventilatory drive and cause hypoventilation, but to a lesser extent than opioids.
      c. Intracranial pathology (e.g., trauma, neoplasm, or major cerebrovascular accidents) that interrupts the vascular supply to the medulla may affect control of ventilation.
   2. Neuromuscular dysfunction
      a. Upper motor neuron lesions can disrupt phrenic nerve (spinal nerves C-3 to C-5) and intercostal and expiratory muscle function (thoracic spinal nerves) resulting in variable de-

grees of ventilatory dysfunction. These lesions include neoplasms, demyelinating disorders, syringomyelia, and trauma.

b. Lower motor neurons supplying the respiratory muscles may be interrupted by trauma or regional anesthesia or affected by diseases including polyneuritis (Guillain-Barré syndrome), amyotrophic lateral sclerosis, and various neuropathies.

c. Disorders of the neuromuscular junction include myasthenia gravis, Eaton-Lambert syndrome, botulinum toxin poisoning, organophosphate overdose, and residual neuromuscular blockade (see Chapter 12).

3. Respiratory muscle dysfunction may result from a number of causes, including pharmacologic neuromuscular blockade, neuromuscular disease, disuse atrophy, chronic mechanical disadvantage of the ventilatory pump (e.g., flattening of the diaphragm with lung hyperinflation in chronic obstructive pulmonary disease [COPD]), hypoperfusion, and malnutrition. A variable degree of respiratory muscle dysfunction is common following thoracic and upper abdominal procedures.

4. Increased ventilatory load. Hypoventilation can occur with an intact neuromuscular axis, when the action of the respiratory muscles is hindered by either an increased airway resistance or a decreased compliance of the respiratory system.

a. Increased airway resistance is commonly caused by bronchospasm, copious bronchial secretions, compression or narrowing of the airway, and inappropriately small endotracheal tubes (see Chapters 3 and 34).

b. Decreased compliance. Pathologic processes of the lung parenchyma (pneumonia and interstitial fibrosis), the pleura (effusions and pneumothorax) and of the musculoskeletal apparatus (kyphoscoliosis and increased intraabdominal pressure) may decrease the compliance of the respiratory system and impair lung inflation.

B. Diffusion impairment. Capillary blood P_{O_2} equilibrates very rapidly with alveolar P_{O_2} (P_{AO_2}), rendering diffusion impairment uncommon. When diffusion is limited, in diseases such as asbestosis, sarcoidosis, collagen vascular diseases, diffuse interstitial fibrosis and alveolar cell carcinoma, supplemental oxygen readily corrects hypoxemia.

C. Ventilation–perfusion ($\dot{V}/\dot{Q}$) mismatch. Optimal gas exchange depends on the precise match of alveolar ventilation and perfusion. The resting minute ventilation in adults is 4 to 5 L per minute and cardiac output approximately 5 L per minute, producing a typical $\dot{V}/\dot{Q}$ ratio of 0.8 to 1.0. At the two pathologic extremes of $\dot{V}/\dot{Q}$ mismatch, alveoli that are ventilated but not perfused represent **dead space**, and alveoli that are perfused but not ventilated represent **true shunt** (see section VII). Dead space mainly causes hypercapnia, and shunt causes hypoxemia. In practice, $\dot{V}/\dot{Q}$ mismatch is far more frequent than true alveolar dead space and shunt as a cause of hypercarbia and hypoxemia. Virtually all lung parenchymal pathology (pneumonia, pulmonary edema, acute respiratory distress syndrome, COPD, interstitial lung diseases, etc.) can result in hypoxemia and hypercapnia secondary to $\dot{V}/\dot{Q}$ mismatch.

D. Decreased oxygen flux in blood

1. Decreased cardiac output may compromise tissue oxygen supply. Etiologies include hypovolemia, congestive heart failure, and shock.

2.   Decreased oxygen-carrying capacity and oxygen delivery (see section VII). The amount of oxygen carried per liter of blood is reduced by anemia, carbon monoxide poisoning, and methemoglobinemia. A shift to the left in the oxygen–hemoglobin dissociation curve facilitates oxygen uptake but attenuates oxygen unloading to tissues. Factors associated with a leftward shift include hypothermia, alkalemia, hypocapnia and 2,3-diphosphoglycerate deficiency.

3.   Increased oxygen demand can cause hypoxemia. Basal oxygen consumption averages in adults 200 to 250 mL per minute. Hypermetabolic conditions such as fever, increased muscle activity from shivering or seizures, hyperthyroidism, and sepsis may increase oxygen consumption two- to ten-fold. In patients with limited reserve, such as those with respiratory failure, coronary artery disease, and cerebrovascular disease, increases in oxygen demand may represent a significant burden and require etiologic treatment.

III.   Diagnosis of respiratory failure

A.   Clinical findings. Signs of impending respiratory failure include dyspnea, tachypnea (a respiratory rate greater than 30 breaths per minute), bradypnea (a respiratory rate less than six breaths per minute), shallow respirations, use of accessory respiratory muscles, discoordinate motions of the chest and abdomen, cyanosis, and obtundation.

B.   Arterial blood gas analysis. A normal **Pao_2** is 90 to 100 mm Hg and decreases slightly with age due to progressive worsening of $\dot{V}/\dot{Q}$ match. A Pao_2 less than 60 mm Hg usually requires treatment and may indicate impending respiratory failure. A normal **$Paco_2$** is 40 mm Hg. An acute increase of a few mm Hg of the $Paco_2$ may indicate impending respiratory failure. A normal **arterial pH** is 7.40 ± 0.02. An acute increase of the $Paco_2$ decreases the arterial pH: As a rule of thumb, for each 10 mm Hg increase of $Paco_2$, the pH decreases by 0.08 units. Chronic CO_2 retention produces less significant pH changes mainly because of increased bicarbonate reabsorption by the kidneys.

C.   A portable, frontal chest radiograph (CXR) obtained at the bedside may reveal acute pathology such as cardiogenic pulmonary edema, pneumonia, lung collapse, pleural effusion, and pneumothorax. More accurate imaging of the thorax can be obtained in the radiology suite by standard radiographs and **computed tomography** (CT). If pulmonary embolism is suspected, a **ventilation/perfusion scan**, **helical CT scan**, and/or **pulmonary angiogram** should be obtained (see Chapter 18). In elderly patients and in those with known risk factors for coronary artery disease, a 12-lead **electrocardiogram** (ECG) may diagnose an acute cardiac event (ischemia, infarction, or arrhythmia) that might have been the cause or a consequence of the acute respiratory failure. **Fiberoptic bronchoscopy** may diagnose lung and airway pathology, provide samples of bronchial secretions for microbiological analysis, and occasionally treat the cause of the acute respiratory decompensation by removing a mucous plug that caused lung collapse. In unstable patients, however, bronchoscopy may precipitate respiratory failure.

IV. Treatment

A. Supplemental oxygen. Hypoxemia is life-threatening and must be treated promptly.

1. Low-flow oxygen (O_2) systems are simple and readily available. They produce a limited and variable inspired oxygen concentration (FIO_2) that is inversely proportional to patient's peak inspiratory flow rate and minute ventilation.

a. Nasal cannulas increase the FIO_2 by approximately 0.04 per liter per minute of oxygen. Flows above 4 L per minute dry the nasal mucosa and may produce nasal irritation and bleeding. The nasal passages must be patent, although nose breathing is not required because of the effective anatomic reservoir of the upper airway.

b. Simple masks increase the FIO_2 to 0.55 or 0.60 by virtue of higher oxygen flow rates and reservoir space.

c. Masks with reservoir bags (nonrebreathing masks) increase FIO_2 further. With a good seal, an FIO_2 of 0.60 to 0.80 can be reached.

d. Venturi masks deliver a more precise FIO_2, from 0.24 to 0.50, by entraining a set ratio of room air along with oxygen. The inspired FIO_2 is independent of the inspiratory flow rate below flow rates of 40 L per minute. As the FIO_2 increases above 0.40, higher oxygen flow rates are required because of the higher oxygen–air entrainment ratio and the actual FIO_2 may be lower than indicated.

2. High-flow systems provide gas flows to meet the patient's peak inspiratory flow rate (30 to 120 L per minute). The maximum FIO_2 depends mainly on the face mask fit and can approach 1.0. High-flow systems can be humidified to provide better comfort.

B. Secretion clearance. Retained secretions increase airway resistance and promote alveolar collapse. Secretion clearance may be facilitated by the following:

1. Humidification and warming of inspired gases. Administration of dry and cold inspired gas mixtures irritates the respiratory mucosa, dries bronchial secretions, and depletes the respiratory system of moisture and heat. Humidifiers evaporate water, facilitating the humidification of the most distal airways. Alternatively, **passive heat and moisture exchangers**, which are hygroscopic membrane filters that trap the humidity of expired air can be placed between the endotracheal tube and breathing circuit.

2. Suctioning. Bronchial ciliary function is compromised following anesthesia, endotracheal intubation, respiratory infections, and smoking. Pain, sedation, and general debilitation can limit patients' ability to cough and expel secretions. Blind nasotracheal suctioning effectively clears tracheal secretions and stimulates coughing, but needs to be used with caution because it may cause hypoxemia, tachycardia, vagal stimulation, bronchospasm, and mucosal trauma.

3. Chest physical therapy. Properly performed percussion, vibration, and postural drainage are effective means of clearing secretions and preventing mucus plugging. Incentive spirometry (maximum deep inspiration with end-inspiratory hold) is also effective.

4.   **Mucolytics.** Local instillation of acetylcysteine (mucomyst, 2 to 5 mL of 5% to 20% solution every 6 to 8 hours) may decrease mucus viscosity by reducing glycoproteins disulfide bonds. When nebulized, however, it may precipitate bronchospasm; mixing with albuterol, 0.5 mL, decreases the incidence of bronchospasm.

5.   **Bronchoscopy** can be employed to remove secretions and thick mucus plugs from the tracheobronchial airways.

C.   **Pharmacologic therapy**

1.   **Reversal of ventilatory depression.** Numerous drugs produce depression of central and peripheral chemoreceptors (see section II.A.1), which can cause hypoventilation and apnea.

2.   **Reversal of residual neuromuscular blockade.** Respiratory muscle weakness from persistent neuromuscular blockade may lead to ventilatory failure and inadequate airway protection (see Chapter 12).

3.   **Analgesia.** Pain from surgical incisions, trauma, and invasive procedures may hinder the effectiveness of ventilation. Numerous analgesic options are available (see Chapter 37).

4.   **Bronchodilation.** Agents used to treat acute bronchospasm can be administered by inhalation, nebulization, or intravenously (see Chapters 3 and 18).

5.   **Treatment of the underlying condition** must be instituted. This includes hemodynamic control, treatment of infections, arrhythmias, myocardial ischemia, anemia, and so forth. Broad-spectrum **antibiotics** are often started immediately as empiric treatment of pneumonia. Within the ensuing 48 hours, however, antimicrobial therapy should be tailored to the known or likely etiologic agent. If no infection is evident, antibiotics should be discontinued.

D.   **Mechanical ventilation** becomes necessary when spontaneous ventilation is insufficient for adequate gas exchange. Mechanical ventilation treats hypoxemia by the delivery of high F_{IO_2} and through alveolar expansion with positive pressure. It regulates CO_2 elimination by providing partial or full support of the minute ventilation.

1.   **Noninvasive ventilation.** Mechanical ventilation can be delivered without intubation of the trachea. Positive pressure ventilation is applied via a tight-fitting mask. Low-flow inspiratory support can be provided by nasal mask in cooperative patients. In critically ill patients, a face mask and a critical-care ventilator can deliver higher levels of support. Noninvasive ventilation effectively avoids endotracheal intubation in many patients with congestive heart failure and exacerbations of COPD. The most common side effect is gastric distention from air insufflation, which can predispose to vomiting and aspiration and can be treated by continuous nasogastric suction. Some of the side effects of mask ventilation may be minimized by using a special hood, which is made of clear plastic and is pressurized by high gas flows, instead of a mask.

2.   **Endotracheal intubation** remains the most common way to deliver positive pressure ventilation during acute respiratory failure (see Chapter 13).

E.   **Modes of mechanical ventilation.** Microprocessor-controlled ventilators provide a variety of gas delivery patterns.

1. **Nomenclature.** Three elements are necessary to define a mode of ventilation.

   a. **What initiates a mechanical breath**, that is, how a ventilator is "triggered." Modes of ventilation triggered by the patient are called **partial** or **assisted** ventilation; modes that are independent of the patient's effort are called **full** or **mandatory** ventilation.

   b. **What determines the size of a mechanical breath**, that is, what is set to "limit" inspiration: a pressure or a volume.

   c. **What ends mechanical inspiration**, that is, how the ventilator "cycles off": by time (most commonly), flow, or volume. Unfortunately, different terms have been used to denote identical modes of ventilation. In the following section, we propose a simple system to denote all currently used modes of ventilation.

2. **Common modes of ventilation.** Current modes of ventilation can be characterized by: the way inspiration is limited, that is, **pressure** versus **volume**; the way breaths are delivered, that is, intermittent mandatory ventilation (**IMV**), assist-control ventilation (**A-C**), and pressure-support ventilation (**PSV**). In the IMV mode, the ventilator delivers a set number of breaths per minute of a set size and the patient may breathe unsupported in between mandatory breaths. In the A-C mode, the ventilator delivers a breath of set size every time the patient initiates a spontaneous breath. In the PSV mode, the ventilator delivers a set pressure every time the patient initiates a spontaneous breath and holds that pressure constant as the inspiratory flow rate declines to a predetermined value (such as 5 L per minute or 25% of the peak inspiratory flow), when inspiration is cycled off. The combination of these variables generates five possible modes of ventilation, illustrated in Table 35-1.

3. **Volume versus pressure ventilation.** The mode of venti-

Table 35-1.   **Nomenclature for common modes of mechanical ventilation**

	What Limits Mechanical Inspiration	
	Volume	Pressure
Intermittent mandatory ventilation (IMV)	Volume-limited IMV	Pressure-limited IMV
Assist-control (A-C) ventilation	Volume-limited A-C	Pressure-limited A-C
Pressure support ventilation (PSV)	—	PSV

Note: In the absence of spontaneous breathing activity, volume versus pressure is the only variable to choose: IMV and AC are indistinguishable and PSV cannot be used. PSV in not currently available in the volume-limited mode.

lation chosen is that which best adapts to the needs of each patient. **Volume ventilation** has the advantage of guaranteeing a set minute ventilation. This, however, may at times produce dangerously high alveolar pressures. **Pressure ventilation** assures a limit of inspiratory pressure. This, however, may occur at the expense of the minute ventilation. A potential advantage of pressure-limited ventilation is that it allows the delivery of **high and variable inspiratory flow rates** (as high as 180 L per minute and more) to reach the set pressure limit. The rate of rise of the inspiratory flow is determined by the capability of the ventilator, the patient's own contribution, and the impedance imposed by the patient. This feature obviates a significant problem of traditional volume ventilation, where the inspiratory flow rate often did not match the patient's demand, resulting in dyssynchrony, excessive respiratory work, and fatigue. Patients can be mechanically ventilated with pressure-limited modes throughout the course of their respiratory illness with a consistent pattern of assisted inspiration, moving from full support to variable degrees of support with the use of IMV, A-C, or PSV.

4. Bi-level positive airway pressure (BIPAP). BIPAP is a pressure-limited mode in which two levels of pressure, high and low, alternate at a set rate. The main difference from traditional pressure-limited ventilation is that the patient can breathe spontaneously (often supported by PSV at one or both levels of pressure). Thus, when the set rate is sufficient to override the patient's own breaths, it is indistinguishable from pressure-limited ventilation. On the other hand, the rate can be set sufficiently low to provide just an occasional large tidal volume ("sigh") to expand collapsed alveoli during low-level, pressure-limited support.

F. Guidelines for perioperative mechanical ventilation. Many postoperative patients require a limited period of mechanical ventilation for reasons such as airway protection, persistent sedation, or neuromuscular blockade. These patients do not have primary respiratory failure and the management of mechanical ventilation can be kept simple. The choice of mode of mechanical ventilation may be dictated by personal experience and convenience. Conversely, in patients with acute respiratory failure, in whom prolonged mechanical ventilation is foreseen, the choice is more complex. The first question to ask is whether the patient requires full or partial ventilatory support.

1. "Full" or "mandatory" mechanical ventilation is reserved for patients whose lung injury is significant enough that their spontaneous respiratory effort is ineffective. In these patients, adequate gas exchange often is achieved through patterns of ventilation that differ substantially from physiologic breathing patterns and can be carried out only with the aid of sedation and, if necessary, neuromuscular blockade. With full ventilation, one has to choose between pressure-limited and volume-limited ventilation, as discussed in section E. Ventilatory settings include:

  a. With **volume ventilation**: FIO_2, tidal volume, respiratory rate, and positive end-expiratory pressure (PEEP).

  b. With **pressure ventilation**: FIO_2, target inspiratory airway pressure, inspiratory time or inspiratory/expiratory time [I:E] ratio, respiratory rate, and PEEP.

2. **"Partial" or "assisted" mechanical ventilation** can be applied to patients who are capable of contributing to their minute ventilation. Partial ventilation preserves ventilatory drive and the patient's breathing pattern, avoids pharmacologic muscle relaxation, limits sedation, and may reduce respiratory muscle atrophy. The choices of the mode of partial ventilation are outlined in section E. Ventilatory settings include:

a. With **IMV**: FiO_2, tidal volume or target airway pressure, respiratory rate, and PEEP.

b. With **A-C**: FiO_2, tidal volume or target inspiratory pressure, duration of inspiration with pressure-limited modes, backup respiratory rate when desired, and PEEP.

c. With **PSV**: FiO_2, target airway pressure, and PEEP. Once the mode of ventilation is selected, the goal in setting the ventilatory parameters is to optimize gas exchange while causing the least possible iatrogenic damage.

3. **Oxygen exchange.** During mechanical ventilation, oxygen exchange can be improved by providing supplemental oxygen and by delivering positive pressure to the airway:

a. FiO_2 is usually set at 1.0 immediately following the institution of mechanical ventilation, then progressively reduced to maintain a PaO_2 above 60 mm Hg and an O_2 saturation above 90%. The effects of decreasing the FiO_2 can be safely monitored by pulse oximetry.

b. **Positive pressure** at the airway promotes expansion and recruitment of collapsed alveoli, thus increasing the PaO_2.

(1) During **inspiration**, airway pressure can be affected by increasing the size of the breath (target pressure or volume) and by prolonging the duration of inspiration (I:E ratio). Both maneuvers increase the **mean airway pressure,** and thus the **mean alveolar pressure**, which correlates with PaO_2.

(2) During **expiration**, airway pressure can be increased by adding **PEEP**, which raises alveolar end-expiratory pressure. The term "continuous positive airway pressure" (**CPAP**) is used when a fixed positive pressure is delivered at the airway and the patients breathes without additional assistance.

4. **CO_2 elimination** is determined by the minute ventilation. Patients with acute respiratory failure generally have an increased dead space and minute ventilation requirements of 8 to 20 L per minute.

G. **Complications of mechanical ventilation**

1. **Oxygen toxicity.** High FiO_2 over long periods is detrimental to lung tissue, causing acute tracheobronchitis, impairment of ciliary motion, alveolar epithelial damage, and interstitial fibrosis. Furthermore, 100% FiO_2 causes alveolar collapse secondary to **absorption of the alveolar gas**, leading to atelectasis. An FiO_2 of 0.6 is generally considered safe. Individual host factors, such as previous bleomycin therapy, may potentiate the adverse effects of oxygen.

2. **Ventilator-induced lung injury (VILI).** Mechanical ventilation can injure the lung. High alveolar pressure caused by large ventilatory volumes can cause pneumothorax, interstitial emphysema, and pneumatoceles. In addition, alveolar pressure values commonly reached during traditional ventilation (25 to 30 cm H_2O) may cause microscopic lung damage, which with time contributes to the persistence and worsening of respiratory failure.

3. Hemodynamic dysfunction

a. Effects of positive intrathoracic pressure. Positive pressure ventilation increases intrathoracic pressure and decreases venous return to the heart.

(1) Right ventricular (RV) filling is limited by reduced venous return. When alveolar pressure exceeds pulmonary vascular pressure, pulmonary blood flow is limited by alveolar pressure rather than left atrial pressure, producing an increase in pulmonary vascular resistance. As a consequence, RV afterload increases and RV ejection fraction decreases.

(2) Left ventricular (LV) filling is limited by reduced RV output. Increased RV size also affects LV performance by shifting the interventricular septum to the left and decreasing LV diastolic compliance.

(3) Intravascular volume replacement counteracts the negative hemodynamic effects of PEEP.

(4) Increased intrathoracic pressure reduces transmural LV pressure and improves LV ejection and stroke volume. This beneficial effect may be especially noticeable in patients with reduced ventricular function.

b. Effects of discontinuing positive intrathoracic pressure. Decreased intrathoracic pressure during weaning redistributes intravascular volume from peripheral to central compartments. As a result, the transmural LV pressure increases. Patients with coronary artery disease and LV dysfunction may not tolerate this sudden increase of venous return and may develop pulmonary edema and/or myocardial ischemia.

H. Infection. Gram-negative bacterial colonization of the upper gastrointestinal tract causes nosocomial pneumonia in patients requiring mechanical ventilation. Noninvasive ventilation may decrease the incidence of nosocomial pneumonia.

I. Less common ventilatory modes and newer ventilatory strategies

1. High-frequency ventilation (HFV) maintains lung inflation and exchanges gas without normal cyclical breathing. Oxygenation occurs by passive insufflation (molecular diffusion) and CO_2 is eliminated by the mixing of gas within the anatomical dead space. Currently, HFV or some variation of it has been shown to be beneficial only in pediatric patients. Accepted indications of HFV include the facilitation of gas exchange during laryngoscopy and bronchoscopy or via a transtracheal catheter following emergency cricothyroidotomy (see Chapters 13 and 21).

2. Pressure-controlled, inverse-ratio ventilation is a pressure-limited mode of full ventilation in which the inspiratory time exceeds expiratory time. The prolonged inspiration increases **mean alveolar pressure** and thus the Pao_2. This may

occur at the expense of decreased venous return and cardiac output because of significantly elevated intrathoracic pressures.
3. Proportional assist ventilation is a mode of partial ventilation where the ventilator, rather than providing a set level of inspiratory pressure or volume, supports ventilation in proportion to the patient's inspiratory effort. This is accomplished through a rapid-response feedback system that senses instantaneous inspiratory flow and volume and amplifies them by a set percentage. The goal is to improve the synchrony between patient and ventilator during partial mechanical support.
J. Hemodynamic support. Therapeutic measures directed toward restoring circulation and improving oxygen delivery include volume replacement and inotropic and vasoactive support. Achieving adequate **intravascular volume resuscitation** can be a difficult issue in patients with acute respiratory failure. While optimal tissue perfusion is desirable, increased pulmonary capillary permeability and pulmonary artery hypertension favor the development of pulmonary edema, which can further compromise of gas exchange. Nevertheless, it is generally advisable to maintain cardiac output and end organ perfusion with volume expansion as long as the additional volume infusion does not produce an excessive increase of pulmonary vascular pressures. Close hemodynamic monitoring, usually with a Swan-Ganz catheter, is necessary.
K. Other therapeutic strategies
  1. "Lung-protective" ventilatory strategies. The accumulating evidence of the significance of VILI (section IV.G.2) in the evolution of acute respiratory failure has led to significant changes in the approach to the way we deliver mechanical ventilation.
    a. The tidal volume should be limited to 6 to 8 mL/kg of body weight (end-expiratory pressure less than or equal to 25 to 30 cm H_2O) to avoid alveolar damage from overstretching.
    b. Collapsed alveoli can be recruited by "**recruitment maneuvers**," that is, occasional large breaths with a prolonged inspiratory time of 15 to 30 seconds or periodic "sighs".
    c. PEEP should be set to greater than 5 cm H_2O to avoid end-expiratory, cyclical alveolar collapse, which also damages the lung.
    d. The most appropriate levels of end-inspiratory and end-expiratory airway pressure should be chosen based on their effect on gas exchange, hemodynamics, and respiratory mechanics. The performance of inspiratory and expiratory volume-pressure curves of the respiratory system is an accepted way to select ventilatory pressures, but these techniques are not simple to perform and interpret. The evaluation and care of these patients are becoming increasingly sophisticated, and are usually performed in specialized care units.
  2. Neuromuscular blockade can facilitate mechanical ventilation by increasing the compliance of the chest wall and eliminating patient effort. Nondepolarizing muscle relaxants can be given by continuous IV infusion and their effects can be monitored clinically and with the help of a twitch monitor (see Chapter 12). The prolonged use of muscle relaxants has been associ-

ated with long-lasting myopathies. In addition, **muscle relaxants do not**:

    a. Cause bronchodilation. On the contrary, they occasionally may cause bronchospasm by direct histamine release from mast cells.

    b. Provide sedation. Pharmacologic neuromuscular blockade **must be accompanied by adequate sedation and analgesia**. An aware and paralyzed patient may suffer severe psychological trauma.

3.   Deliberate hypothermia is occasionally employed in the presence of refractory hypoxemia to decrease oxygen consumption. It must be accompanied by sedation and neuromuscular blockade to avoid shivering. Temperatures less than 32°C may cause arrhythmias.

4.   Extracorporeal membrane oxygenation (ECMO) allows the exchange of oxygen and/or CO_2 through an veno-arterial or veno-veno bypass circuit. The goal of ECMO and similar techniques such as **extracorporeal CO_2 removal** is to avoid lung tissue trauma from mechanical ventilation and fully "rest" the lungs while they heal. Recent technical improvements have decreased the morbidity associated with ECMO. ECMO has been shown to improve the outcome of selected types of acute respiratory failure in children (see Chapter 27). In adults, ECMO techniques occasionally may be useful in selected patients and in centers with a high level of expertise in this complex procedure.

5.   The prone position. Turning the patient prone produces more uniform pulmonary perfusion and increases inflation and recruitment of collapsed alveoli. The prone position often improves Pao_2 in many patients with acute respiratory failure but requires appropriate and specialized nursing care.

6.   Inhaled nitric oxide gas may be useful to improve Pao_2 and selectively reduce pulmonary pressure in some patients with acute respiratory failure, but has not improved outcome in clinical trials in adults.

V.   Weaning from mechanical ventilation. Most patients wean rapidly from ventilatory support once the condition that led to acute respiratory failure is successfully treated. For a small number of patients, withdrawing ventilatory support is difficult. Most of these patients have preexistent pulmonary disease or other ongoing conditions such as heart disease, infection, and malnutrition. There is no "best" weaning method; the goal is to tailor the amount of mechanical support to the needs and pathology of the individual patient. The key to successful weaning is to avoid fatigue, distress, muscle atrophy, and hemodynamic compromise. Two weaning techniques are currently popular:

    A.   Progressive withdrawal of ventilatory support. The patient's contribution to minute ventilation is gradually increased until he or she reaches a level where mechanical support is no longer necessary. This should allow a smooth progression over time while the patient's conditioning improves and other coexisting problems are addressed. **PSV** is a good choice because it allows freedom for the patient to adjust to the mechanical support.

    B.   Alternating unsupported breathing with full mechanical ventilation. This technique provides periods of full rest alternating with increasing periods of unassisted ventilation. The unassisted period provides the clinician with the opportunity to observe the patient's response to withdrawal of mechanical support without removing the endotracheal tube. When the patient seems ready to be weaned by clinical criteria (see section VI.D), a trial of unsupported breathing is usually performed, either with **T-piece** breathing or minimal **CPAP** before removing the endotracheal tube.

C. Measurements of weaning potential. Clinical judgment, knowledge of respiratory physiology, and experience are the best tools to improve the success of weaning from mechanical ventilation. The following clinical parameters are helpful in this decision making:

1. Subjective symptoms of failure include dyspnea, fatigue, anxiety, and restlessness.

2. Objective evaluation includes general well-being as well as assessment of ventilation. Normal ventilatory parameters do not necessarily assure success because they do not test endurance. Desirable clinical parameters in adults include:

a. A tidal volume greater than 5 mL/kg with a respiratory rate less than 30 breaths per minute. A pattern of rapid shallow breathing appears to be the most sensitive and specific early indicator of weaning failure.

b. A vital capacity greater than 10 mL/kg (enough to generate an effective cough).

c. A negative inspiratory force greater than 25 cm H_2O.

d. A minute ventilation less than 10 L per minute and the absence of bronchospasm.

e. A Pao_2 greater than 60 mm Hg on a Fio_2 less than or equal to 0.4 and a PEEP or CPAP of 5 cm H_2O.

f. Hemodynamic and metabolic stability. The adequacy of the volume status, myocardial performance, nutrition, central nervous system function, and the absence of significant infection need to be carefully evaluated.

VI. Chest tubes (Fig. 35-1). Commercial "three-bottle" systems commonly are used to drain the pleural space. The proximal bottle traps the drainage, the middle bottle is the water seal that prevents air and fluid from being drawn into the thorax, and the distal bottle regulates the level of suction applied to the pleural cavity. The negative pressure is independent of strength of the wall suction and depends only on the height of the water column in the suction-control chamber. Chest tubes are connected to the water seal if minimal air or fluid drainage is expected (e.g., immediately following pneumonectomy) or to suction (usually 10 to 20 cm H_2O) when significant drainage is expected or a pneumothorax needs to be drained. When examining a chest tube drainage system, the water seal level should vary with respiration if the chest tube is patent. Bubbling in the water seal chamber with inspiration indicates a bronchopleural leak.

VII. Respiratory function calculations

A. Impedance to airflow and lung expansion is offered by the **compliance** and **resistance** of the respiratory system according to the **law of motion of the respiratory system**. This law states that pressure applied to the respiratory system generates changes in airflow and volume that are proportional to the pressure applied and the respiratory system compliance, and inversely proportional to airway resistance. Keeping this relationship in mind greatly fa-

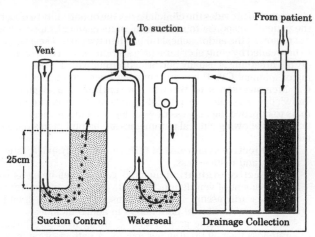

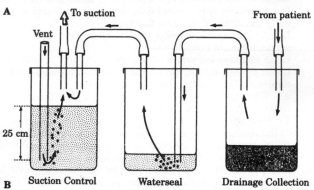

Fig. 35-1.   Chest tube drainage system. A: A commercial apparatus. The proximal chamber is for pleural drainage, the middle chamber (the water seal) prevents air or fluid from being drawn into the thorax, and the distal chamber regulates the level of suction. B: A traditional "three-bottle" system is shown for comparison.

cilitates the understanding of spontaneous and mechanical ventilation.

1.   Measurement of compliance. Compliance of the respiratory system = change in volume / change in pressure. Normal values are approximately 100 mL/cm H_2O, equally shared by lung and chest wall. Assessment of compliance should be made at zero flow, which eliminates the resistive component of breathing. A simple and fairly accurate method is to divide the tidal volume by the airway pressure value determined at end expiration during pressure-limited ventilation when gas flow is at or near zero (**plateau pressure**).

2.   Assessment of resistance. Airway resistance = change in pressure / change in flow. An accurate measure of airway resistance is very difficult because of the need to interrupt flow to correctly measure pressure. A useful estimate of resistance can be made by applying an inspiratory pause at the peak of inspiration during a square-wave, volume-limited breath; the airway pressure will decrease from the peak to the plateau value. The pressure difference between the peak and the plateau pressure is due to airway resistance. Flow rates are determined from the ventilator settings.

B. The alveolar gas equation calculates the alveolar Po_2 (Pao_2):

$$Pao_2 = [(P_{barometric} - P_{water\ vapor}) \times (Fio_2)] - [Paco_2 \times RQ]$$

where RQ = respiratory quotient (usually about 0.8).

C. Oxygen content of arterial blood:

Cao_2

= oxygen bound to hemoglobin + oxygen dissolved in blood

$$Cao_2 = (1.36\ mL\ O_2/g\ Hgb) \times (g\ Hgb/dL) \times (Sao_2)$$

$$+ (Pao_2 \times (0.003\ mL\ O_2/mm\ Hg/dL))$$

D. The Fick equation is used to calculate cardiac output (CO) or oxygen consumption when one of the two variables is known:

CO (dL/min)

$$= O_2\ consumption\ (mL/min)\ /\ (Cao_2 - C\bar{v}o_2\ (mL/dL))$$

where Cao_2 and $C\bar{v}o_2$ are the O_2 contents of arterial and mixed venous blood, respectively. The Fick principle assumes that the amount of oxygen in the inspired gas is constant and equal to the amount added to the blood that flows through the lungs. Oxygen consumption also can be calculated by measuring oxygen differences in inspiratory and expiratory gases.

E. The shunt equation estimates the venous admixture of arterial blood:

$$\dot{Q}_S / \dot{Q}_T = (Cc'o_2 - Cao_2) / (Cc'o_2 - C\bar{v}o_2)$$

$Cc'o_2$ is the O_2 content of pulmonary capillary blood and is calculated from the Pao_2 (as estimated from the alveolar air equation; see VII.B above).

F. $Paco_2$ and minute ventilation relationship:

$$Paco_2 = Paco_2 = CO_2\ production\ /\ alveolar\ ventilation$$

In normal subjects, the $Paco_2$ and $Paco_2$ can be considered identical. The relationship between alveolar ventilation and $Paco_2$ is of practical importance. For example, if the alveolar ventilation is halved, the $Paco_2$ will double (if CO_2 production is constant).

G. Dead space occurs when ventilation is wasted, that is, in the proximal airways (**anatomic dead space**) and in those alveoli that are ventilated and not perfused (**alveolar dead space**). The term **physiologic dead space** includes anatomic and alveolar dead space. Dead space primarily affects CO_2 exchange. Expressed as a fraction of the tidal volume (V_D/V_T), physiologic dead space is a useful measure of lung dysfunction. Values greater than 0.6 are generally incompatible with weaning from mechanical ventilation.

$$V_D / V_T = (\text{Paco}_2 - \text{Peco}_2) / \text{Paco}_2$$

where Peco_2 = mean expired CO_2, obtained by collecting expired gas in a reservoir bag (i.e., Douglas bag) over several breaths. If the Peco_2 is substituted in the equation by the **end-tidal CO_2** (Petco_2), the alveolar dead space can be estimated. Under normal circumstances, Petco_2 is very close to the Paco_2, indicating that there is minimal alveolar dead space. Petco_2 can be measured by capnography when a clear and steady end-expiratory plateau is present.

SUGGESTED READING

ARDSNet Investigators. Ventilation with lower tidal volumes as compared with traditional tidal volumes for acute lung injury and the acute respiratory distress syndrome. *N Engl J Med* 2000;342:301–308.

Artigas A, Bernard G, Carlet J, et al. The American-European Consensus Conference on ARDS. Part II. *Am J Respir Crit Care Med* 1998;157: 1332–1347.

Bernard G, Antigas A, Brigham KL ,et al. The American-European Consensus Conference on ARDS. Part I. *Am J Respir Crit Care Med* 1994; 149:818–824.

Lumb AB, Nunn JF. *Nunn's applied respiratory physiology*, 5th ed. Boston: Butterworth, 1999.

Marini JJ, Kelsen SG. Re-targeting ventilatory objectives in the adult respiratory distress syndrome: new treatment prospects—persistent questions. *Am Rev Respir Dis* 1992;146:2–3.

Tobin MJ. Advances in mechanical ventilation. *N Engl J Med* 2001;344: 1986–1996.

Tobin MJ. *Principles and practice of mechanical ventilation*. New York: McGraw-Hill, 1995.

West J. *Respiratory physiology: the essentials*, 6th ed. Baltimore: Williams & Wilkins, 1999.

Adult, Pediatric, and Newborn Resuscitation

Richard M. Pino

I. Overview. Cardiopulmonary resuscitation (CPR) in the operating room (OR) is the responsibility of the anesthesiologist who knows the location and function of resuscitation equipment, delegates tasks, and instills calmness in assisting personnel. The protocols described below have been modified as appropriate for the anesthesiologist in a hospital setting but closely follow the evidenced-based *Guidelines 2000 for Cardiopulmonary Resuscitation and Emergency Cardiovascular Care.* Table 36-1 lists the classifications for the quality of evidence used to support most of the protocol interventions presented in this chapter.

II. Cardiac arrest

    A. Diagnosis. The absence of a palpable pulse in a major peripheral artery (carotid, radial, or femoral) in an unconscious, unmonitored patient is diagnostic of a cardiac arrest. An electrocardiogram (ECG) may reveal asystole, ventricular fibrillation (VF), ventricular tachycardia (VT) or even an organized rhythm as in pulseless electrical activity.

    B. Etiologies. Common causes of cardiac arrest are:
        1. Hypoxemia.
        2. Acid-base disturbances.
        3. Derangements of potassium, calcium, and magnesium.
        4. Hypovolemia.
        5. Adverse drug effects.
        6. Pericardial tamponade.
        7. Tension pneumothorax.
        8. Pulmonary embolus.
        9. Hypothermia.
       10. Myocardial infarction.

    C. Pathophysiology. With the onset of a cardiac arrest, effective blood flow ceases, and tissue hypoxia, anaerobic metabolism, and accumulation of cellular wastes result. Organ function is compromised and permanent damage ensues unless reversed within minutes. Acidosis from anaerobic metabolism may cause systemic vasodilation, pulmonary vasoconstriction, and decreased responsiveness to the actions of catecholamines.

III. Adult resuscitation

    A. Basic Life Support (BLS) includes basic techniques taught to the general public, but applies equally to OR situations. A cardiac arrest should be suspected in any person unexpectedly found unconscious. If the subject is unarousable, the "ABCDs" (Airway, Breathing, Circulation, Defibrillation) of resuscitation should be followed after first calling for assistance. (The lay public are taught the "phone first/phone fast" [evidence class indeterminate] rule.

Table 36-1. Evidence classification for interventions

Class	Evidence	Clinical Use
I	Excellent	Definitely recommended
IIa	Good/very good	Acceptable, safe, useful
IIb	Fair/good	Acceptable, safe, useful
Indeterminate	Preliminary research stage	May be used
III	Positive evidence absent or strongly suggests or confirms harm	None

For adults, children aged 8 years and older, and all children known to be at high risk for arrhythmias, the emergency medical system (EMS) should be activated before attempts at resuscitation, that is, "phone first." An initial resuscitation attempt followed by the activation of EMS [phone fast] is indicated for children less than 8 years old and for all ages in cases of submersion or near drowning, arrest secondary to trauma, and drug overdose.)

1. Airway and breathing. Spontaneous ventilation is evaluated by observation and auscultation, aided by repositioning or insertion of an oropharyngeal or nasopharyngeal airway. In the absence of effective spontaneous ventilation, rescue breathing is begun (or ventilation by bag-valve mask with 100% O_2). Two slow breaths at low airway pressures to limit gastric distention are delivered initially, followed by 10 to 12 breaths per minute. If ventilation is not possible after these maneuvers, efforts to clear the airway of a suspected foreign body (e.g., Heimlich maneuver, chest compressions, or manual removal) should be attempted.

2. Circulation. The circulation is assessed by palpation of the carotid artery pulse for 5 to 10 seconds. In the absence of a palpable pulse, artificial circulation should be instituted with external chest compressions. (The presence of a pulse does not necessarily mean that an adequate mean arterial pressure is present. Lay rescuers no longer perform pulse checks but are taught to initiate chest compressions in the absence of signs of circulation such as moving, coughing, or breathing.) The patient should be on a firm surface (e.g., backboard) with the head on the same level as the thorax. The rescuer (surgeon in the OR) places the heel of one hand on the patient's sternum two finger-breadths above the xiphoid process and the other hand either on top of the first with interlocked fingers, or grasping the wrist of the first hand. The rescuer's shoulders should be positioned directly over the patient, with the elbows locked for effective compressions. Sternal depression during CPR is to a depth of 1.5 to 2.0 inches in a normal-sized adult, and with a 1:1 compression–relaxation ratio at a rate of 100 compressions per minute. For a prone patient in the OR who cannot be quickly turned supine for CPR, one rescuer can place a clenched fist between the subxiphoid area and the OR table while compressions are administered over the corresponding region of the back. The chest compression to ventilation ratio is 15:2 for resuscitation with one or more than one rescuer.

3. Defibrillation within 3 minutes in the hospital (evidence class I) and 5 minutes after calling the EMS is the major determinant of a successful resuscitation since VF is the most likely etiology of a cardiac arrest in adults. Until recently, defibrillation was taught only to Advanced Cardiac Life Support (ACLS) providers. Public-access defibrillation programs have now enabled "level I" responders (e.g., fire personnel, police, security guards, and airline attendants) to employ readily accessible automated external defibrillators (AEDs). AEDs are small, lightweight defibrillators that use adhesive electrode pads for sensing and delivering shocks. The AED, after analysis of the frequency, amplitude, and slope of the ECG signal, *advises* either "shock indicated" or "no shock indicated." The AED is manually triggered and does not automatically defibrillate the patient.

4. Reassessment. If spontaneous circulation does not return after three shocks or with a "no shock indicated," CPR should be continued for 1 minute followed by ECG analysis. Cardiopulmonary activity should be checked after the first four cycles and every several minutes thereafter if an AED is not used or if defibrillation is not indicated.

B. Advanced Cardiac Life Support is the definitive treatment for cardiac arrest with endotracheal intubation, electrical defibrillation, and pharmacologic intervention.

1. Intubation. Swift control of the airway that does not delay defibrillation will optimize oxygenation and removal of carbon dioxide during resuscitation. Endotracheal intubation (confirmed by capnography) by the most experienced person present should minimally disrupt other resuscitative measures. The endotracheal tube may be used to deliver epinephrine, lidocaine, and atropine if intravenous (IV) access has not been established. Since peak drug concentrations are lower with the endotracheal route compared to IV administration, higher doses (two to three times) diluted in 10 mL of sterile saline should be used.

2. Defibrillation. VT and VF are the most common arrhythmias associated with a cardiac arrest. As the duration of a VF/VT arrest increases, the cardiac activity deteriorates and becomes more difficult to convert to a viable rhythm. A solitary precordial thump is recommended for a witnessed cardiac arrest if a defibrillator is not available. Defibrillation is the priority and can be administered by the anesthetist without compromising the surgical field. Three shocks can be delivered in rapid succession to take advantage of the decrease in transthoracic impedance that occurs with each shock.

a. Monophasic waveform defibrillators deliver a unidirectional current. The energy level for the initial series of unsynchronized, monophasic, damped sinusoidal (MDS) shocks is 200 J followed by 300 J, and 360 J, if needed. Subsequent shocks at 360 J are repeated after every pharmacologic intervention. For recurrent VF following a successful defibrillation, the lowest energy level that was previously useful should be tried first. It is the responsibility of the person operating the defibrillator to ensure that members of the resuscitation team are not in contact with the patient during defibrillation.

b. Biphasic waveform defibrillators deliver current that flows in a positive direction for specified milliseconds followed by reversal of current flow in the negative direction. Although the optimum biphasic energy to terminate VF has not been determined, repeated shocks at 200 J or less appear to be at least as effective as monophasic 200, 300, and 360 J.

c. Cardioversion. Synchronized MDS shocks of 50 to 100 J are used for supraventricular arrhythmias such as paroxysmal supraventricular tachycardia (PSVT) and atrial flutter. Hemodynamically stable VT and atrial fibrillation (AF) can be cardioverted using 100 J as the starting point.

3. Pacing. High-grade heart block with profound bradycardia is an etiology of cardiac arrest. Temporary pacing should be used when the heart rate does not increase with pharmacologic therapy. Transcutaneous pacing is the easiest method to increase the ventricular rate. Esophageal pacing is efficacious for sinus bradycardia with maintained atrioventricular (A-V) conduction and is useful intraoperatively for bradycardia-related hypotension in otherwise stable patients. Transvenous pacing via a temporary wire into the central circulation is a third option to increase heart rate while CPR continues. Special pacing pulmonary artery catheters are capable of A-V pacing.

4. Intravenous access is imperative for a successful resuscitation. The most desirable route is into the central circulation via internal or external jugular, subclavian, or femoral veins, or long peripheral lines inserted based on the anatomy of the patient, experience of the physician, and what is the least disruptive to the resuscitation. The antecubital veins are adequate when an appropriate volume is used to flush the medications toward the central circulation. Fluid replacement is indicated for patients with known or suspected intravascular volume depletion.

5. Drugs. The drugs described below are used in ACLS protocols for the treatment of hemodynamic instability, myocardial ischemia and infarction, and arrhythmias. The doses of drugs used for **Pediatric Advanced Life Support** (PALS) are in parentheses following discussion of adult doses.

    a. Adenosine, an endogenous purine nucleotide with a half-life of 5 seconds, slows A-V nodal conduction and interrupts A-V node reentry pathways to convert a PSVT to a sinus rhythm. It also assists with the diagnosis of supraventricular tachycardias (e.g., atrial flutter with a rapid ventricular response versus PSVT). The initial dose is a 6-mg rapid IV bolus. A brief asystole ensues that is followed by P waves, flutter waves, or AF that are initially without ventricular responses. PSVT is sometimes converted to a sinus rhythm with an initial dose of 6 mg. A second injection of 12 mg may terminate PSVT if the first dose is unsuccessful. Recurrent PSVT, AF, and atrial flutter will require longer half-life drugs for definitive treatment. The dose of adenosine should be increased in the presence of methylxanthines (competitive inhibition) and decreased if dipyridamole (potentiation via blockage of nucleoside transport) has been administered. (PALS: 0.1 mg/kg; repeat dose 0.2 mg/kg; maximum dose 12 mg.)

    b. Amiodarone is the most versatile drug in the ACLS algorithms. It has the properties of all four classes of antiarrhythmics (lengthening of action potential, sodium channel blockade at high frequencies of stimulation, noncompetitive antisynaptic actions, and negative chronotropism) and is preferable for patients with severely impaired cardiac function because of its efficacy and comparative lower incidence of proarrhythmic effects. Amiodarone is indicated for continued unstable VT and for VF after defibrillation and epinephrine treatment (evidence class IIb); rate control of stable monomorphic VT, polymorphic VT (evidence class IIb), and AF (evidence class IIa) to sinus rhythm; ventricular rate control of rapid atrial arrhythmias when digitalis is ineffective (evidence class IIb) and secondary to accessory pathways (evidence class IIb); and as an adjunct to electrical cardioversion of refractory PSVTs (evidence class IIa) and atrial tachycardia (evidence class IIb). The dose for the treatment of unstable VT and VF is 300 mg diluted in 20 to 30 mL of saline or 5% dextrose in water (D5W) administered rapidly. For the treatment of more stable disorders, the dose is 150 mg administered over 10 minutes, followed by an infusion of 1 mg per minute for 6 hours, and then 0.5 mg per minute. The maximum daily dose is 2 grams. Immediate side effects can be bradycardia and hypotension. With chronic use, hypothyroidism, elevation of hepatic enzymes, alveolar pneumonitis, and pulmonary fibrosis may occur. (PALS: loading dose, 5 mg/kg; maximum dose, 15 mg/kg per day.)

c.   Atropine is useful in the treatment of hemodynamically significant bradycardia (evidence class I) or A-V block occurring at the nodal level (evidence class IIa). It increases the rate of sinus node discharge and enhances A-V node conduction by its vagolytic activity. The dose of atropine for bradycardia or A-V block is 0.5 mg repeated every 3 to 5 minutes to a total dose of 0.04 mg/kg. For asystole, atropine is given as a 1-mg bolus repeated in 3 to 5 minutes if needed. Full vagal blockade is obtained at a cumulative dose of 3 mg. (PALS: 0.02 mg/kg; minimum dose, 0.1 mg; maximum single dose, 0.5 mg in child, 1.0 mg in adolescent.)

d.   Beta-adrenergic blocking drugs (atenolol, metoprolol, and propranolol) have established utility (evidence class I) for patients with unstable angina and myocardial infarction. These drugs reduce the rate of recurrent ischemia, nonfatal reinfarction, and post-infarction VF. In contrast to calcium channel blockers, beta-blockers are not direct negative inotropes. Esmolol, in addition the other beta-blockers, is useful for the acute treatment of PSVT, AF, atrial flutter (evidence class I), and ectopic atrial tachycardia (evidence class IIb). Initial and subsequent IV doses, if tolerated, are: atenolol, 5 mg over 5 minutes, repeated once at 10 minutes; metoprolol, three doses at 5 mg every 5 minutes; propranol, 0.1 mg/kg divided into three doses given every 2 to 3 minutes; esmolol, 0.5 mg/kg over 1 minute followed by an infusion starting at 50 μg per minute and titrated as needed to 200 μg per minute. Contraindications include second- or third-degree heart block, hypotension, and severe congestive heart failure. Atenolol and metoprolol, because of their relatively specific β_1-adrenergic blockade, are preferable to propranolol in patients with a history of reactive airway disease. A small number of patients will exhibit bronchospasm with the administration of any beta-blocker. Most patients with chronic obstructive pulmonary disease, however, are able to tolerate beta-blockers.

e.   Calcium is indicated during cardiac arrest only when hyperkalemia, hypermagnesemia, hypocalcemia, or toxicity from calcium channel blockers is suspected. Calcium chloride, 5 to 10 mg/kg IV, can be repeated as necessary. (PALS: 20 mg/kg.)

f. Dopamine has dopaminergic (generally at doses less than 2 μg/kg per minute), beta (2 to 5 μg/kg per minute), and alpha (5 to 10 μg/kg per minute) adrenergic activities. Although the above are "traditional" doses, in practice alpha and beta adrenergic effects can be present at the lowest dosage levels. Therefore, the drug should be started at a low dose (e.g., 150 μg per minute) and titrated until the desired effect (e.g., increased urine output, increased heart rate/inotropy, or increased blood pressure) is seen or undesired side effects (e.g., tachyarrhythmia) occur.

g. In the past, **epinephrine** has been the mainstay of pharmacologic therapy for cardiac arrest. Its α-adrenergic vasoconstriction of noncerebral and noncoronary vascular beds produces compensatory shunting of blood toward the brain and the heart. In high doses, epinephrine may contribute to myocardial dysfunction and is now evidence class indeterminant. Studies have failed to show a significant improvement in the rate of survival to hospital discharge after an arrest. The recommended dose is 1.0 mg IV, repeated every 3 to 5 minutes, or administered by an infusion of 1 to 4 μg per minute. Epinephrine used for symptomatic bradycardia is evidence class IIb. (PALS: bradycardia, 0.01 mg/kg; pulseless arrest, 0.01 mg/kg with subsequent doses up to 0.1 mg/kg.)

h. Ibutilide is used for the acute conversion of AF, either alone or with electrical cardioversion. It prolongs the duration of the action potential and increases the refractory period. The dose of 1 mg given over 10 minutes can be repeated in 10 minutes. The dose for patients weighing less than 60 kg is 0.01 mg/kg. Continuous monitoring of the patient is required during its administration and for at least 6 hours thereafter since the major side effect of ibutilide is polymorphic VT (including torsade de pointes).

i. Isoproterenol is a beta$_1$ and beta$_2$ adrenergic agonist. It is a second-line drug used to treat hemodynamically significant bradycardia that is unresponsive to atropine and dobutamine in the event that a temporarily pacemaker is not available (evidence class IIb). Its beta$_2$ activity can cause hypotension. Isoproterenol is administered by IV infusion at 2 to 10 μg per minute, titrated to achieve the desired heart rate.

j. Lidocaine, the mainstay of ventricular arrhythmia treatment in previous years, has been relegated to an evidence class indeterminate status and is considered a second choice compared with amiodarone, procainamide, and sotalol. It may be useful for the control (not prophylaxis) of ventricular ectopy during an acute myocardial infarction. The initial dose during a cardiac arrest is 1.0 to 1.5 mg/kg IV and may be repeated as a 0.5- to 0.75-mg/kg bolus every 3 to 5 minutes to a total dose of 3 mg/kg. A continuous infusion of lidocaine at a rate of 2 to 4 mg per minute is instituted after successful resuscitation. The lidocaine dose should be decreased for patients with reduced cardiac output, hepatic dysfunction, or advanced age. (PALS: 1 mg/kg; infusion, 20 to 50 μg/kg per minute.)

k. Magnesium is a cofactor in a variety of enzyme reactions including Na + K + -ATPase. Hypomagnesemia can precipitate refractory VF as well as exacerbate hypokalemia. Magnesium replacement is effective for the treatment of drug-induced torsade de pointes. The dose for emergent administration is 1 to 2 grams in 10 mL D5W over 1 to 2 minutes. Hypotension and bradycardia are side effects of rapid administration. (PALS: 25 to 50 mg/kg; maximum dose, 2 g.)

l. Oxygen (100%) should be administered to all cardiac arrest victims by bag-valve mask or endotracheal ventilation and to hemodynamically stable patients by face mask.

m. Procainamide can convert AF and atrial flutter to sinus rhythm (evidence class IIa), control the ventricular response to SVT secondary to accessory pathways (evidence class IIb), and convert wide complex tachycardias of unknown origin (evidence class IIb). The loading dose is a continuous infusion of 20 to 30 mg per minute that is terminated when the arrhythmia is suppressed, hypotension occurs, the QRS complex is widened by 50% of its original size, or a total dose of 17 mg/kg is reached. When the arrhythmia is suppressed, a maintenance infusion of 1 to 4 mg per minute should be initiated, with reduced dose considered in the presence of renal failure. An ECG should be examined for QRS widening at least daily. The therapeutic blood level is the sum of procainamide and its active metabolite, N-acetylprocainamide (NAPA). (PALS: 15 mg/kg.)

n. Sodium bicarbonate administration is detrimental in most cardiac arrests because it creates a paradoxical intracellular acidosis (evidence class III). The few justifications for use are when the standard ACLS protocol has failed in the presence of severe preexisting metabolic acidosis and for the treatment of hyperkalemia or tricyclic antidepressant overdose. The initial dose of bicarbonate is 1 mEq/kg IV, with subsequent doses of 0.5 mEq/kg given every 10 minutes (as guided by arterial blood pH and partial pressure of carbon dioxide [$Paco_2$]). (PALS: 1 mEq/kg.)

o. Vasopressin, a neurohypophyseal-produced antidiuretic, is an evidence class IIb intervention (40 units IV) that is an alternative to epinephrine for the treatment of VF. Endogenous levels of vasopressin are increased in patients undergoing CPR who eventually return to spontaneous circulation. Vasopressin constricts vascular smooth muscle when used in high doses. It is more effective than epinephrine in maintaining the coronary perfusion pressure and has a longer half-life of 10 to 20 minutes.

p. Verapamil and **diltiazem**, calcium-channel blockers that depress A-V nodal conduction, are used to treat hemodynamically stable, narrow-complex PSVTs that are unresponsive to vagal maneuvers or adenosine. The initial verapamil dose is 2.5 to 5.0 mg IV, with subsequent doses of 5 to 10 mg IV administered every 15 to 30 minutes. Diltiazem is given as an initial bolus of 20 mg. An additional dose of 25 mg and an infusion of 5 to 15 mg per hour can be administered if needed. Their vasodilator and negative inotrope properties can cause hypotension, exacerbation of congestive heart failure, bradycardia, and enhancement of accessory conduction in patients with Wolff–Parkinson–White syndrome. The hypotension can often be reversed with calcium chloride, 0.5 to 1.0 g IV.

6. Specific ACLS protocols are shown in Figs. 36-1 through 36-6:

   a. Ventricular fibrillation (Fig. 36-1).
   b. Asystole (Fig. 36-2).
   c. Pulseless electrical activity (Fig. 36-3).
   d. Unstable tachycardia (Fig. 36-4).
   e. Stable tachycardia (Fig. 36-5).
   f. Bradycardia (Fig. 36-6).

7. Open-chest direct cardiac compression is an intervention used at institutions with appropriate resources to manage penetrating chest trauma, abdominal trauma with cardiac arrest, pericardial tamponade, hypothermia, and pulmonary embolism. Direct cardiac compressions also are indicated for individuals with anatomic deformities of the chest that prevent adequate closed-chest compression.

8. Termination of CPR. There are no absolute guidelines to determine when to stop an unsuccessful resuscitation, but there is a very low probability of survival after 30 minutes. It is at the discretion of the physician in charge to determine when the failure of the cardiovascular system to respond to adequately applied BLS and ACLS indicates that the patient has died. There should be a meticulous documentation of the resuscitation, including the reasons for terminating the effort.

9. The advanced directive **"Do not resuscitate" (DNR)** places the anesthesiologist in a key position with respect to intraoperative and postoperative care. It is often incorrectly *assumed* that a DNR order is suspended in the perioperative period. Each institution's written guidelines should be reviewed. In advance of a procedure, physicians and the patient with the DNR status or the patient's health care proxy should clarify any resuscitative measures that would be compatible with the patient's wishes. For example, the use of a pressor to control hypotension following induction of general anesthesia might be permitted in contrast to defibrillation and CPR for spontaneous VF that might be prohibited. When asked to perform an emergent intubation outside of the OR, the anesthesiologist should ask about the patient's code status and is ethically and legally bound to a known decision to limit treatment.

IV. Pediatric resuscitation

   A. Basic life support. The need for CPR in the pediatric age group is rare after the neonatal period. Pediatric cardiac arrests usually result from hypoxemia linked to respiratory failure or airway obstruction. Initial efforts should be directed toward the establishment of a secure airway and adequate ventilation. For children greater than 8 years of age, basic considerations for

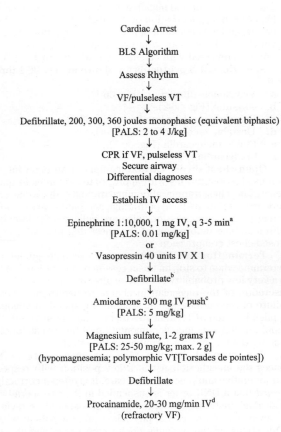

Cardiac Arrest
↓
BLS Algorithm
↓
Assess Rhythm
↓
VF/pulseless VT
↓
Defibrillate, 200, 300, 360 joules monophasic (equivalent biphasic)
[PALS: 2 to 4 J/kg]
↓
CPR if VF, pulseless VT
Secure airway
Differential diagnoses
↓
Establish IV access
↓
Epinephrine 1:10,000, 1 mg IV, q 3-5 min[a]
[PALS: 0.01 mg/kg]
or
Vasopressin 40 units IV X 1
↓
Defibrillate[b]
↓
Amiodarone 300 mg IV push[c]
[PALS: 5 mg/kg]
↓
Magnesium sulfate, 1-2 grams IV
[PALS: 25-50 mg/kg; max. 2 g]
(hypomagnesemia; polymorphic VT[Torsades de pointes])
↓
Defibrillate
↓
Procainamide, 20-30 mg/min IV[d]
(refractory VF)

[a] Defibrillate after each epinephrine administration.
[b] Use the lowest energy that was successful with initial defibrillation.
[c] Amiodarone is diluted in 20-30 ml saline or D5W. If successful, an infusion of 1 mg/min for 6 hours followed by 0.5 mg/hour is given. An additional dose of 150 mg IV push can be administered if VF or pulseless VT recurs. The maximum dose is 2.2 grams over 24 hours.
[d] The maximum dose is 17 mg/kg or termination with arrhythmia suppression, hypotension, or QRS width of 50%. If successful, infuse of 2 mg/kg/hour.

Fig. 36-1.   Protocol for ventricular fibrillation.

Cardiac Arrest
↓
BLS Algorithm
↓
Assess Rhythm
↓
If rhythm is unclear and possible ventricular
fibrillation, defibrillate as for VF
↓
Asystole
↓
Secure airway
↓
Establish IV access
↓
Transcutaneous pacing
↓
Epinephrine 1:10,000, 1 mg IV q 3-5 min
↓
Intubate when possible
↓
Atropine, 1 mg IV q 3-5 min
(total: 0.04 mg/kg)

Fig. 36-2. Protocol for asystole.

Organized ECG activity without pulse
↓
CPR, IV access, intubation
↓
Consider underlying cause:

Hypovolemia (give volume)
Tension pneumothorax (relieve pressure)
Hypoxemia (oxygen)
Cardiac tamponade (pericardiocentesis)
Hypokalemia (give potassium)
Bicarbonate-responsive metabolic acidosis (bicarbonate)
Drug overdose (treatment appropriate to substance)
Myocardial infarction (heparin, thrombolysis, IABP)
↓
Epinephrine 1:10,000, 1 mg IV q 3-5 min
[PALS: 0.01 mg/kg]
↓
Atropine 1 mg IV (if slow PEA rate)
(total: 0.04 mg/kg)

IABP, intra-aortic balloon pump

Fig. 36-3.   Protocol for pulseless electrical activity.

Tachycardia
↓
Ventricular tachycardia
Wide complex of unknown type
Paroxysmal supraventricular tachycardia
Atrial fibrillation
Atrial flutter
↓
Consider unstable if:
Chest pain
Dyspnea
Hypotension
Decreased level of consciousness
Pulmonary edema
Congestive heart failure
Acute myocardial infarction
Hypoxemia
Ventricular rate > 150 bpm
↓
Appropriate sedation and resuscitation equipment present
↓
Synchronous cardioversion
50, 100, 200, 300, 360 joules monophasic (equivalent biphasic)

Fig. 36-4. Protocol for unstable tachycardia in adults.

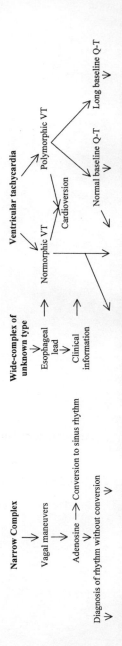

Atrial fibrillation / Atrial flutter	Rhythm	Supraventricular tachycardia EF ≥ 40%	EF < 40%	EF ≥ 40%	EF < 40%	EF ≥ 40%	Consider torsades
Rate Control Diltiazem, β-blocker, Digoxin	*Junctional*	Amiodarone, β-blocker, Diltiazem/verapamil	Amiodarone	*Preferred:* Procainamide, Sotalol	Amiodarone (150 mg) or Lidocaine (0.5–0.75 mg/kg)	Treat ischemia	
Rate control / Conversion Amiodarone, Procainamide	*Paroxysmal*	Diltiazem/verapamil, β-blocker, Digoxin, DC cardioversion, Consider: procainamide, amiodarone, sotalol	Amiodarone, Digoxin, Diltiazem	*Acceptable:* Amiodarone, Lidocaine	Synchronized cardioversion	Correct electrolytes	Correct electrolytes
Conversion DC cardioversion, Ibutilide	*Ectopic or multifocal atrial*	Diltiazem/verapamil, β-blocker, Amiodarone	Amiodarone, Diltiazem			*One of the following:* β-blocker, Lidocaine, Amiodarone, Procainamide, Sotalol	*One of the following:* Magnesium, Overdrive pacing, Isoproterenol, Phenytoin, Lidocaine

Fig. 36-5.   Protocol for stable tachycardia in adults.

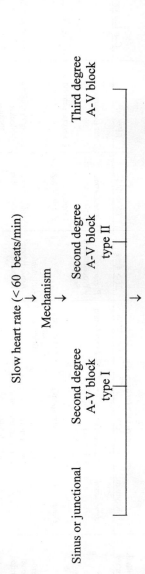

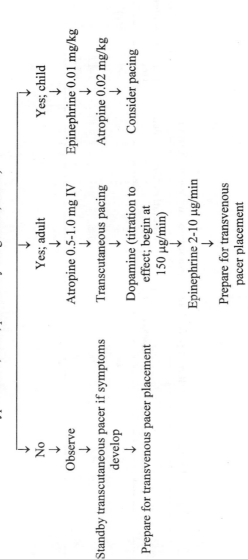

Fig. 36-6. Protocol for bradycardia.

Table 36-2. Adult and pediatric cardiopulmonary resuscitation

Age	Ventilations/min	Compressions/min	Ventilation: Compression Ratio	Depth of Compressions (Inches)
Neonate	30–60	120	3:1	$\frac{1}{3}$–$\frac{1}{2}$ chest depth
Infant (<1 yr)	20	>100	5:1	0.5–1
Child (1–8 yr)	20	100	5:1	1–1.5
Adult and child >8 yr	12	100	5:1	1.5–2

resuscitation are the same as for the adult. As discussed above, the "phone first" rule applies. "Phone fast" applies to children less than 8 years of age, and any child with suspected drowning, traumatic arrest, drug overdose, or at high risk for arrhythmias. Modifications of the rate and magnitude of compressions and ventilations, as well as of the hand position for compressions, are necessary because of anatomic and physiologic differences (Table 36-2). Differences between pediatric and adult resuscitation techniques are detailed below.

1. **Airway and breathing.** Maneuvers to establish an airway are the same as in the adult, with a few caveats. For children less than 1 year old, abdominal thrusts are not used since the gastrointestinal tract can be damaged easily. Hyperextension of an infant's neck for the head tilt/chin lift may lead to airway obstruction because of the small diameter and ease of compression of the immature airway. Submental compression while performing the chin lift can also lead to airway obstruction by pushing the tongue into the pharynx. Ventilations should be given slowly with low airway pressures to avoid gastric distention and should be of sufficient volume to cause the chest to rise and fall.

2. **Circulation.** The brachial or femoral artery is used for pulse assessment in infants (less than 1 year old) because the carotid artery is difficult to palpate. Upon determination that a pulse is absent, chest compressions should be initiated. The compression/relaxation ratio is 1:1. Chest compressions in infants are delivered using two fingertips applied to the sternum or by encircling the chest with both hands and using the thumbs to depress the sternum one fingerbreadth below the intermammary line. In older children, the correct hand position is determined as for adults, only with one hand depressing the sternum. Both one- and two-rescuer scenarios use a 5:1 compression/ventilation ratio with a pause at the end of the fifth compression to allow for adequate ventilation. Return of spontaneous cardiopulmonary activity should be assessed after ten cycles. Thereafter, resuscitation attempts should be interrupted every several minutes for reassessment.

B. **Pediatric advanced life support.** Most pediatric cardiac arrests present as asystole and bradycardia, rather than ventricular arrhythmias, and in infants less than 1 year old. Respiratory and idiopathic (sudden infant death syndrome) etiologies predominate. Anatomic and physiologic differences from the adult require defibrillator settings and drug doses to be weight based.

1. **Intubation.** The endotracheal tube size is based on the patient's age (tube size [mm ID] = 4 + (age / 4) for children over 2 years old). Atropine, epinephrine, and lidocaine can be administered via the endotracheal tube prior to the establishment of IV access.

2. **Defibrillation.** Defibrillator paddles used for infants are 4.5 cm in diameter and those used for older children are 8 cm in diameter. The energy level for the initial shock is 2 J/kg. If this energy level is unsuccessful, it should be increased to 4 J/kg and repeated twice, if necessary. Hypoxemia, acidosis, or

hypothermia should be considered as treatable causes of an arrest if the defibrillation attempts are unsuccessful. After each pharmacologic manipulation, repeat defibrillation should be attempted with an energy level of 4 J/kg or the lowest level that was previously successful. For cardioversion, the starting energy is 0.2 J/kg, with escalation to 1.0 J/kg if needed. The configuration for pediatric paddles varies among defibrillators. AEDs are not indicated for children less than 8 years of age. Recommendations for biphasic defibrillator use in children are still pending.

3.   Intravenous access. Central venous access is preferred, but existing peripheral IVs should be used without delay. The femoral vein can be used with a catheter of suitable length. The intraosseous route may also be used in children. A bone marrow biopsy needle or spinal needle is inserted into the tibial shaft away from the epiphyseal plates to gain access to the large venous sinuses of the bone marrow. If none of the above are available, the endotracheal tube may be used to deliver essential medications if they are diluted in 2 to 5 mL of normal saline to ensure their delivery to the pulmonary vasculature.

4.   Medications. Many of the drugs described in the adult ACLS section (III.B.5) apply to PALS with doses adjusted to the child's weight.

5. Specific ACLS protocols for the adult also apply to the pediatric patient with weight-related adjustments of defibrillation energies and drugs. Protocols pertaining to the pediatric patient are illustrated in Figs. 36-1, 36-2, 36-3, and 36-7.

   a.   Ventricular fibrillation (see Fig. 36-1).
   b.   Asystole (see Fig. 36-2).
   c.   Pulseless electrical activity (see Fig. 36-3).
   d.   Tachycardia (Fig. 36-7).

V.   Neonatal resuscitation. The neonatal period extends through the first 28 days of life. Someone who is skilled in resuscitation of newborns should be present at every delivery. Resuscitation is divided into four phases: stimulation and suctioning, airway management, chest compressions, and delivery of resuscitation drugs and fluids. Resuscitation is often needed during an emergent cesarean section for fetal distress. In the event that the anesthesiologist is the only one available to treat the newborn, the neonatal warmer should be brought to the head of the OR table to facilitate the treatment and monitoring the mother and child until the pediatrician arrives.

A.   Assessment. Immediate neonatal resuscitation is crucial, since profound hypoxemia occurs rapidly and will be exacerbated by respiratory acidosis, which contributes to the persistence of fetal circulation and right-to-left shunting. A neonate who requires resuscitation will likely have a significant right-to-left shunt.

1. The **Apgar score** is an objective assessment of the physiologic well-being of the child that is done at 1 and 5 minutes after birth (Table 27-2).

2. An Apgar score of 0 to 2 mandates immediate CPR. Neonates with scores of 3 to 4 will need bag and mask ventilation and may require more extensive resuscitation. Supplemental oxygen and stimulation are normally sufficient for newborns with

Apgar scores of 5 to 7. Respiratory activity should be evaluated by watching chest excursions and by auscultation. The heart rate is assessed by auscultation or by palpation of the umbilical pulse.

B. **Four phases of newborn resuscitation**

1. Stimulation and suctioning. The cold-intolerant neonate should be dried thoroughly after birth and placed in a pre-warmed environment to minimize heat loss and the exacerbation of acidosis. Placement in the lateral Trendelenberg position will assist with the drainage of secretions. The mouth and nose should be suctioned with a bulb syringe to remove blood, mucus, and meconium. Suctioning should be limited to 10 seconds with oxygen supplied between attempts. During suctioning, the heart rate should be monitored, because bradycardia can occur from hypoxemia or from vagal reflexes to pharyngeal stimulation. Drying and suctioning usually provide adequate respiratory stimulation. Additional measures include gently rubbing the newborn's back and slapping the soles of the feet. **To remove thick meconium,** the hypopharynx is first suctioned by the obstetrician using a DeLee trap after delivery of the head, but before delivery of the thorax. Immediately after delivery, the neonate is brought to the warmer, the trachea is intubated, and, since thick meconium is too viscous to be aspirated through a suction catheter, low suction is applied directly to the endotracheal tube as it is removed. Suctioning is repeated, quickly to avoid bradycardia, until the trachea is cleared of meconium. Thin meconium does not warrant endotracheal intubation.

2. Airway management. Positive pressure ventilation with 100% oxygen is used for apnea, cyanosis, and heart rates below 100 beats per minute. Bag and mask ventilation should be attempted initially. The initial breath may require airway pressures as high as 30- to 40-cm H_2O held for 2 seconds to permit adequate lung expansion. All breaths should be at the lowest pressure possible (while ensuring adequate chest expansion) to prevent gastric distention that may lead to further respiratory compromise. Assisted ventilation is continued until there are adequate spontaneous breaths and a heart rate greater than 100 beats per minute. Endotracheal intubation is used when mask ventilation is ineffective, tracheal suctioning is needed (e.g., meconium aspiration), or prolonged ventilatory assistance is anticipated.

3. Chest compressions. For initial heart rates less than 100 beats per minute, the heart rate is reassessed after adequate ventilation with 100% oxygen has been performed for 30 seconds. If the heart rate is less than 80 beats per minute and not increasing, or less than 60 beats per minute, chest compressions are required in addition to continued assisted ventilation. The sternum should be depressed 0.5 to 0.75 inch at a rate of 120 times per minute. The compression/ventilation ratio in neonates is 3:1 and compression is 50% of the entire compression–relaxation cycle. The compressions are stopped periodically to check the spontaneous heart rate and should be terminated when the intrinsic rate is greater than 80 beats per minute.

4. Delivery of resuscitation drugs and fluids. Resuscita-

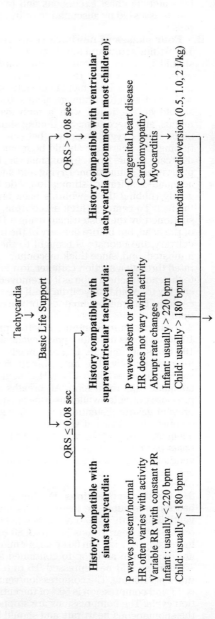

Tachycardia

Basic Life Support

QRS ≤ 0.08 sec

History compatible with sinus tachycardia:

P waves present/normal
HR often varies with activity
Variable RR with constant PR
Infant : usually < 220 bpm
Child: usually < 180 bpm

History compatible with supraventricular tachycardia:

P waves absent or abnormal
HR does not vary with activity
Abrupt rate changes
Infant: usually > 220 bpm
Child: usually > 180 bpm

QRS > 0.08 sec

History compatible with ventricular tachycardia (uncommon in most children):

Congenital heart disease
Cardiomyopathy
Myocarditis

Immediate cardioversion (0.5, 1.0, 2 J/kg)

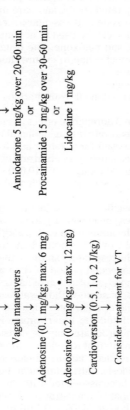

Consider and treat possible causes:
hypoxemia, hypovolemia, hyperthermia
metabolic disorders, toxins/drugs/poisons
tamponade, tension pneumothorax, thromboembolism

Vagal maneuvers →

Adenosine (0.1 mg/kg; max. 6 mg) →

Adenosine (0.2 mg/kg; max. 12 mg) →

Cardioversion (0.5, 1.0, 2 J/kg) →

Consider treatment for VT →

Amiodarone 5 mg/kg over 20-60 min
or
Procainamide 15 mg/kg over 30-60 min
or
Lidocaine 1 mg/kg

Fig. 36-7. Protocol for tachycardia in children.

tion drugs should be administered when the heart rate remains below 80 beats per minute despite adequate ventilation with 100% oxygen and chest compressions. The umbilical vein, the largest and thinnest of the three umbilical vessels, provides the best vascular access for resuscitation of the newborn. It is cannulated with a 3.5- to 5.0-French umbilical catheter after the umbilical cord stump has been prepped with an antiseptic and trimmed. Sterile umbilical tape placed at the base of the cord will prevent bleeding. The catheter should be placed below the skin level with blood aspirated freely, and care must be taken not to permit air into the system. If vascular access is unavailable, the endotracheal tube can be used to administer epinephrine, atropine, lidocaine, and naloxone. The drugs may be diluted in 1 to 2 mL of normal saline to ensure their delivery to the pulmonary vasculature.

5. **Drug and fluid dosages**

   a. **Oxygen** (100%) is used in all resuscitations without concern for toxicity.

   b. **Epinephrine.** The β-adrenergic effect of epinephrine increases the intrinsic heart rate during neonatal resuscitation. Epinephrine should be used for asystole and for heart rates less than 80 despite adequate oxygenation and chest compressions. The dose is 10 to 30 μg/kg of a 1:10,000 solution IV or via endotracheal tube; doses can be repeated every 3 to 5 minutes, as needed.

   c. **Naloxone** is a specific opiate antagonist used for neonatal respiratory depression secondary to narcotics administered to the mother. The initial dose is 10 μg/kg IV, intramuscularly, subcutaneously, or via endotracheal tube, repeated every 2 to 3 minutes. The respiratory status of the child should be monitored for an extended period of time after narcotic reversal, because the duration of action of naloxone is shorter than that of narcotics. An acute withdrawal reaction may be precipitated in the child of a narcotic-addicted mother.

   d. The routine use of **sodium bicarbonate** is not recommended. The use of bicarbonate may be considered during prolonged arrests in an attempt to relieve depression of myocardial function and reduced action of catecholamines induced by marked acidosis. Intraventricular hemorrhage in premature infants has been associated with the osmolar load occurring with bicarbonate administration. A neonatal preparation of sodium bicarbonate (4.2% or 0.5 mEq/mL) should be used to prevent this from occurring. The initial dose is 1 mEq/kg IV given over 2 minutes. Subsequent doses of 0.5 mEq/kg may be given every 10 minutes and should be guided by arterial blood pH and $Paco_2$.

   e. **Atropine, calcium, and glucose** are not recommended for use in neonatal resuscitation unless specifically indicated.

   f. **Fluids.** Hypovolemia should be considered in the setting of peripartum hemorrhage, hypotension, weak pulses, and persistent pallor, despite adequate oxygenation and chest compressions. Albumin 5%, lactated Ringer's solution, or O-negative whole blood cross-matched with maternal blood may be used for resuscitation. The volume infused should be 10 mL/kg and repeated as necessary.

SUGGESTED READING

International Consensus on Science. Guidelines 2000 for cardiopulmonary resuscitation and emergency cardiovascular care. *Circulation* 2000;102[Suppl I].

Pain

Joshua Bloomstone and David Borsook

I. Pain is a sensory and emotional experience. The pain system provides information on noxious stimuli that allows the body to respond to the injury (immediate: e.g., withdrawal from the noxious source; longer term: e.g., protection of the injured part by guarding and so forth). Pain may be somatic, visceral, neuropathic, or sympathetically maintained.

A. Somatic pain that results from tissue injury is aching, gnawing, and/or sharp in quality; generally well localized; and initiated by nociceptor activation in cutaneous and deep tissues. Examples include acute postoperative pain and bone fractures.

B. Visceral pain is also associated with tissue injury, specifically infiltration, compression, or distention of viscera. It is usually dull and aching in quality, poorly localized, and may be referred to other sites. Examples include shoulder pain after laparoscopic surgery.

C. Neuropathic pain results from injury to the peripheral or central nervous system (CNS) (the very pain system that is responsible for transmission of acute pain). Shooting, electrical, or burning pain often is superimposed on a chronic background of burning and aching sensations. Examples include postherpetic neuralgia (PHN) and diabetic neuropathy. **Chronic regional pain syndrome** (sympathetic maintained pain or causalgia) is associated with a host of signs and symptoms that develop over time. Like neuropathic pain, there is an initial nerve insult, which is followed by the development of painful sensations that are augmented by continuous efferent sympathetic discharge.

II. The neural basis for pain

A. The anatomy and physiology of pain are complex. Although simplified, it is easiest to examine the anatomy of the system in terms of the four major physiologic processes that are involved:

1. Transduction (nociceptors).

2. Transmission (primary afferent fibers, dorsal horn, ascending tracts).

3. Interpretation (cortical processing, limbic processing).

4. Modulation (descending control and neurohumoral mediators).

B. Nociceptors

1. Potentially tissue damaging sensory information is conveyed to the CNS by way of free nerve endings located within cutaneous and noncutaneous tissue (viscera and somatic tissue). These free nerve endings are referred to as nociceptors. The sensory information gathered by these receptors is relayed to the dorsal horn of the spinal cord by way of rapidly conduct-

ing, small-diameter, unmyelinated C-fibers and by thinly myelinated A-delta-fibers.

2. C-fibers exhibit polymodal responses that allow the individual to discriminate among mechanical, thermal, and chemical
injuries. When tissue damage occurs, a host of chemical mediators are released in the area of damage, leading to the classic
findings of inflammation. Certain of these mediators lead to nociceptor hypersensitivity; this is referred to as **primary hyperalgesia**.

3. Often, the tissue surrounding the area of damage is also
sensitive, and this is referred to as **secondary hyperalgesia**.
Studies have demonstrated that nociceptors found within damaged tissue demonstrate decreased threshold responses, increased responses to suprathreshold stimuli, and both basal and
spontaneous fiber discharge, causing pain.

C. Primary afferent fibers:

1. The **primary afferent axons** activated by nociceptors are
the free nerve endings of myelinated A-delta-fibers and unmyelinated C-fibers (see Chapter 15, Table 15-1). The majority of
nociceptive input to the CNS is carried by C-fibers. The cell
bodies of these primary afferents are located within the **dorsal
root ganglion**. A-delta-fibers conduct relatively rapidly (5 to 25
m per second), while C-fibers are have a slower conduction
velocity (less than 2 m per second). This difference is the basis
for "first" and "second" pain. The next key step in nerve transmission occurs at the synapse between these primary afferent
fibers and neurons found within the dorsal horn. **Cutaneous
pain fibers** travel in the sensory nerves. **Visceral afferent pain
fibers** travel in the parasympathetic and sympathetic nerves
(the cell bodies of these are also located in the DRG). Numerous
neuromodulators, including peptides, are located in neurons
within the DRG. Significantly, primary afferent fibers play an
important role in hyperalgesia; for example, substance P and
CGRP are both released from the nerve terminals to potentiate
the inflammatory response.

2. Neurotransmitters. Numerous neurotransmitters are involved in pain pathways. Essentially, these can be divided into
rapidly acting excitatory (aspartate and kainate) or inhibitory
(gamma-aminobutyric acid and glycine) amines or more slow-
acting excitatory (substance P) or inhibitory (enkephalin and
galanin) modulators. Some of these are neurotoxic at high levels
(e.g., following nerve transection or damage), while others are
neuroprotective (e.g., galanin and enkephalin). Numerous receptors are present in these pathways. Some unusual ones include capsaicin-specific receptors and cannabinoid receptors.
Finally, some receptors are present in the peripheral nerve
under normal conditions (e.g., N-methyl-D-aspartate receptors)
or following nerve damage (e.g., opioid receptors).

D. Dorsal horn. Nociceptive afferents enter the spinal cord
by way of the dorsal root ganglion to terminate on neurons within
the dorsal horn. The dorsal horn is divided into several layers
based on neuron morphology and arrangement. Specifically, the
gray matter of the dorsal horn is divided into ten layers referred to

as **Rexed's laminae** (see Fig. 37-1). C-fibers terminate principally within lamina II (substantia gelatinosa); those of A-delta-fibers terminate within lamina I and V. These fibers synapse onto interneurons and second-order neurons; the latter form ascending tracts. These neurons have been divided into categories based on their responses to pain:

   1.   Wide–dynamic-range neurons respond to mechanical as well as noxious stimuli and are located mainly in Rexed's laminae I, II, and V.

   2.   Nociceptive-specific neurons are activated only by painful stimuli and are found in a number of lamina.

   3.   The axons from these second order neurons, cross the spinal cord to the anterolateral segment and ascend to higher brain structures. The classic tract is the **spinothalamic tract** (STT); however, other tracts including spinohypothalamic, spinoreticular, and spinopontoamygdala tracts also exist.

E.   Ascending tracts. Of the four ascending tracts listed above, the STT, located in the ventro-lateral aspect of the spinal cord, is the most important. Most of the peripheral afferents cross the spinal cord within one or two segments of entry, and after synapsing within the dorsal horn, ascend to higher centers within the CNS. The first cortical synapse is within the thalamus; from here third-order neurons send axons to the somatosensory cortex (from the lateral thalamus) or regions of the brain involved in affective responses to pain (from the medial thalamus or limbic system including the cingulate cortex). Other tracts involved in the autonomic response to pain project to the hypothalamus (e.g., stress response and sleep-wake response). In this way, the CNS is "wired" to allow for a sensory and emotional response to an acute, painful stimulus.

F.   Pain modulation and descending analgesia. The periaqueductal gray (located in the midbrain) and raphe magnus (located in the medulla) are not the only areas involved in pain modulation. Stimulation of specific thalamic and hypothalamic nuclei also produce analgesia. Key elements within this system include opioid, central noradrenergic, and serotonergic systems. Receptors for these mediators have been found within pain modulating areas and, when stimulated, cause analgesia that is effectively reversed by pharmacologic antagonists. Axons descend in the dorsolateral funiculus to terminate in the dorsal horn where they directly (onto STT neurons) or indirectly (via interneurons) modulate afferent input from the periphery.

G.   Changes in the nervous system producing chronic (neuropathic) pain

   1.   Neuropathic pain results from either central or peripheral neuronal injury. It is often severe, debilitating, delayed in onset, and may be burning or electrical in quality. Pain often occurs in the absence of the original injury.

   2.   Chronic pain often follows minor trauma, medical diseases, such as rheumatoid arthritis, or nerve damage. Research has demonstrated a number of abnormal neuronal functions in chronic pain conditions:

      a.   Ephaptic cross-talk is the development of abnormal contacts (ephapsis) between axons after injury. Activity in one nerve leads to the activation of another.

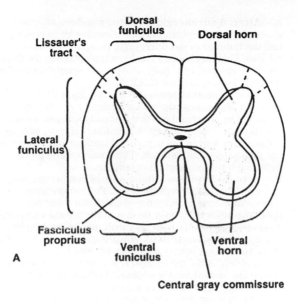

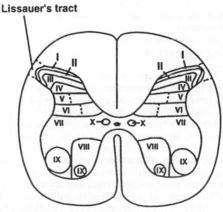

Fig. 37-1. (A) Diagrammatic cross-section of the spinal cord. (B) Rexed's laminae I to X of the spinal cord.

b. Altered adrenergic receptor number. After injury, regenerating nociceptors become sensitive to norepinephrine and the number of α-1 adrenergic receptors on the axons increases. This mechanism has been implicated in the development of sympathetic pain states (see sympathetic-afferent coupling below, section II.G.2.e).

c. Altered neural connectivity. A-delta and C-fibers make contacts predominantly within laminae I and II. Light touch is carried by A-beta-fibers that normally synapse within laminae III and IV. After injury, A-beta-fibers sprout, making new connections within the superficial laminae and synapsing on the pain projecting neurons. Thus, pain can be produced by light touch in neuropathic conditions.

d. Ectopic impulses. Under normal conditions, neuromodulators keep pain fibers quiescent. Following damage, abnormal spontaneous activity develops within these nerves. This spontaneous activity may be due to the release of excitatory neuromodulators such as glutamate and substance P.

e. Sympathetic-afferent coupling. Under normal conditions, the sympathetic system has no effect on primary afferent neurons. After nerve injury, noradrenergic axons sprout within the dorsal root ganglion and form basket-like structures around injured neurons. As described above, the injured neurons develop adrenergic receptors, which completes the coupling of the two systems. Now, with sympathetic activation the pain system becomes activated. Conversely, with sympathetic blockade, pain is inhibited (hence, sympathetically maintained pain).

H. Central nervous system plasticity and preemptive analgesia

1. Preemptive analgesia is a concept based on experiments which suggest that analgesic intervention before a noxious stimulus reduces or eliminates subsequent pain. Noxious impulses from deep tissues can trigger prolonged changes in spinal cord excitability, which often require significant doses of opioid to be blunted. Hyperexcitability may be prevented if small doses of local anesthetic or opioid are administered before the stimulus.

2. Centralization of pain occurs when damage in the periphery alters function in more central pathways (e.g., the thalamus) where spontaneous abnormal activity may be present.

3. The concept of plasticity within the CNS underlies the concept of preemptive analgesia. Plasticity specifically refers to a process of structural and functional changes that take place after nerve damage in conditions of neuropathic pain. The exact biological significance of these changes in humans is not clear. If these changes in pain pathways can be prevented by the administration of an analgesic before surgery, it is likely that preemptive analgesia may prevent CNS hyperexcitability, leading to reduced postoperative analgesic requirements or inhibition of the development of neural plasticity.

I. Opioid agonism of mu receptors inhibits activation through enzyme-linked systems. Presynaptic mu agonism inhibits calcium influx, which is necessary for signal transduction to occur. Postsynaptic mu agonism produces hyperpolarization by increasing potassium permeability. The combined effect of reduced neurotransmitter release and postsynaptic hyperpolarization leads to less excitation, resulting in less pain transmission. In addition, morphine increases α-2 adrenergic receptor activation in the spinal cord, which further inhibits sensory processing.

III. **Clinical issues of pain management**

A. **Basic issues regarding pain management**

1. **Acute (somatic) pain usually is responsive to opioids**.

2. Neuropathic pain is difficult to treat and requires trials of different medications.

3. The **Visual Analogue Scale** (0 to 10 scale) is critical in assessing a patient's pain; in general, a pain level of less than 5 out of 10 is considered acceptable and correlates with increased activity, sleep, and so forth. Of course, we strive to produce pain levels of 0 out of 10 with minimal side effects.

4. There are occasions where a patient's **anxiety** is more of an issue than the pain. Adjuvant medications such as haloperidol or lorazepam can be extremely useful.

5. Patients addicted to opioids should be treated similarly to any other acute pain patient, except that tolerance will increase the amount of opioid that needs to be given to manage baseline requirements.

B. **Acute postoperative pain management**. **Acute pain** follows injury to the body and generally disappears with wound healing. It often is associated with physical signs of autonomic hyperactivity. Unfortunately, the most common reason for unrelieved pain is the failure of medical staff to routinely and systematically evaluate the patient's pain and pain relief. One study of analgesic practice in a busy emergency department reported that 50% of patients who presented with an acutely painful condition had no analgesics administered. Of those treated, 50% waited more than 1 hour for an analgesic, and 32% received suboptimal doses.

C. A simplified **approach to the pharmacologic agents** often used to treat acute pain includes the following:

1. **Nonopioid analgesics** (aspirin [ASA] or acetaminophen).

2. **Nonsteroidal anti-inflammatory drugs** (NSAIDs): Cyclooxygenase (Cox) I and II nonselective inhibitors (ibuprofen, naproxyn, and ketorolac) and Cox II selective inhibitors (rofecoxib and celecoxib).

3. **Opioid analgesics** (codeine, oxycodone, hydromorphone, meperidine, morphine, and fentanyl).

4. **Opioid agonist–antagonist analgesics** (pentazocine, nalbuphine, and butorphanol [these are rarely used]).

5. **Local anesthetics** (lidocaine and bupivacaine).

6. **Analgesic adjuvants** (benzodiazepines, caffeine, dextroamphetamine, mexilitene, phenytoin [dilantin], carbamazepine [tegretol], phenothiazines, gabapentin, lamotrigine, and clonidine).

D. **Aspirin and nonsteroidal anti-inflammatory drugs.** Aspirin, acetaminophen, and the NSAIDs are all useful in the management of acute and chronic pain (Table 37-1). These agents differ significantly from opioid analgesics: There is a **ceiling effect** to analgesia; there is **no tolerance** or physical dependence, and they are **antipyretic**. Both ASA and the NSAIDs work by inhibiting the cyclooxygenase pathway, which in turn stops the production of various prostaglandins that can sensitize free nerve endings to

Table 37-1.   Selected nonopioid analgesics: analgesic dosage and comparative efficacy to standards

Drug	Proprietary Names (not all-inclusive)	Average Analgesic Dose (mg)	Dose Interval (hrs)	Maximal Daily Dose (mg)	Pediatric Dose (mg/kg)	Analgesic Efficacy Compared with Standards	Plasma Half-life (hrs)	Comments
Acetaminophen	Numerous	500–1,000 PO	4–6	4,000	10–15 PO q4–6h	Comparable to aspirin 650 mg	2–3	Rectal suppository available for children and adults
Salicylates Aspirin	Numerous	500–1,000 PO	4–6	4,000	10–15 PO q4–6h	—	0.25	Because of risk of Reye's syndrome, do not use in children under 12 yr with possible viral illness; rectal suppository available for children and adults

Diflunisal	Dolobid	1,000 PO initial, 500 PO subsequent	8–12	1,500	—	500 mg superior to aspirin 650 mg, with slower onset and longer duration; initial dose of 1,000 mg significantly shortens time to onset	8–12	—
Choline magnesium trisalicylate	Trilisate	100–1,500 PO	12	2,000–3,000	25 PO bid	Longer duration of action than aspirin 650 mg	9–17	—
NSAIDs *Propionic acids* Ibuprofen	Motrin, Rufen, Nuprin, Advil, Medipren	200–400 PO	4–6	2,400	10 PO q6–8h	Superior at 200 mg to aspirin at 650 mg	2–2.5	—

(continues)

Table 37-1. *(Continued)*

Drug	Proprietary Names (not all-inclusive)	Average Analgesic Dose (mg)	Dose Interval (hrs)	Maximal Daily Dose (mg)	Pediatric Dose (mg/kg)	Analgesic Efficacy Compared with Standards	Plasma Half-life (hrs)	Comments
Naproxen	Naprosyn	500 PO initial; 250 PO subsequent	6–8	1,250	5 PO bid	—	12–15	—
Naproxen sodium	Anaprox	550 PO initial; 275 PO subsequent	6–8	1,375	5 PO bid	275 mg comparable to aspirin 650 mg, with longer slower onset and duration; 550 mg superior to aspirin 650 mg	—	—
Fenopren	Nalfon	200 PO	4–6	800	—	Comparable to aspirin 650 mg	2–3	—
Ketoprofen	Orudis	25–50 PO	6–8	300	—	Superior at 25 mg to aspirin 650 mg	1.5	—

Indolacetic acids								
Indomethacin	Indocin	25 PO	8–12	100	—	Comparable to aspirin 650 mg	2	Not routinely used because of high incidence of side effects; rectal, IV forms available for adults
Pyrrolacetic acids								
Ketorolac	Toradol	30 mg IM initial; 15 or 30 mg IM subsequent	6	150 first day, 120 thereafter	—	In the range of 6–12 mg of morphine	6	Not >5 days PO
COX II Inhibitors								
Rofecoxib	Vioxx	12.5 mg–50 mg PO	q24	50 mg	—	—	17	—
Celecoxib	Celebrex	100 mg–200 mg PO	q12	400 mg	—	—	11	Not to be taken if sulfa allergic
Anthranilic acids								
Mefenamic acid	Ponstel	500 PO initial; 250 PO subsequent	6	1,500	—	Comparable to aspirin 550 mg	2	In U.S. use is restricted to interval of 1 week

COX, cyclooxygenase; h, hour(s); bid, twice a day; IM, intramuscularly; IV, intravenous; NSAIDs, nonsteroidal anti-inflammatory drugs; PO, orally; q, every.

painful stimuli. The mechanism of analgesia produced by acetaminophen is not known. As a general rule, even when a patient's pain is bad enough to require opioid analgesics, they will do better if a nonopioid agent is also administered.

1. Aspirin. Gastritis and functional thrombocytopenia are common with therapeutic doses of ASA. With children less than 12 years of age, the administration of ASA in the setting of a viral syndrome (particularly varicella) is contraindicated. Hypersensitivity to ASA is well described. Patients may develop respiratory symptoms with rhinitis, asthma, and nasal polyps. They may also develop urticaria, angioneurotic edema, and shock. Patients who are sensitive to ASA may also be sensitive to NSAIDs.

2. Acetaminophen has no antiplatelet effects, minimal anti-inflammatory effects, and minimal effects on gastric mucosa. Patients with liver disease may develop severe hepatic failure when usual therapeutic doses of acetaminophen are taken.

3. NSAIDs. These agents are useful analgesics in most acute pain states, but often are overlooked in the postoperative period. Unless there is a specific contraindication, these drugs should be routinely considered.

   a. Analgesia. Some NSAIDs are equivalent to ASA. Others, such as ketorolac (15 to 30 mg every 8 hours intramuscularly or intravenously [IV]), are equivalent to a few milligrams of morphine. Since patients vary in their response to these agents, it is prudent to try a different agent if the first is unsuccessful.

   b. Hematological effects. Unlike ASA, NSAIDs reversibly inhibit platelet aggregation. This inhibition lasts only as long as there is an effective serum drug concentration. NSAIDs cause an excessive prolongation of the prothrombin time in those individuals taking oral anticoagulants.

   c. Gastrointestinal effects. Dyspepsia, gastritis, and duodenitis have been reported. The concomitant use of prophylactic regimen again gastrointestinal erosion, such as an antacid drug, is recommended. The use of alcohol should also be avoided, since hepatitis has been reported with this combination.

   d. Renal effects. Renal insufficiency has been described in patients taking NSAIDs. Risk factors include hypovolemia, congestive heart failure, chronic renal insufficiency, cirrhosis with ascites, systemic lupus erythematosus, diuretic use, peripheral vascular disease, and multiple myeloma. Allergic nephritis, renal tubular acidosis with hyperkalemia, and enhanced secretion of antidiuretic hormone activity with significant hyponatremia have been reported. The putative mechanism of the renal insufficiency is decreased synthesis of renal vasodilator prostaglandins, impaired renin secretion, and enhanced tubular water and sodium reabsorption. The newer COX II inhibitors, celecoxib and rofecoxib, are associated with fewer side effects (notably a lower incidence of gastrointestinal symptoms), but are only available in oral formulations.

E. Opioid analgesics. Systemic opioids have long been the treatment of choice for acute postoperative pain (Table 37-2). The

Table 37-2. Opioid analgesics

Name	Equianalgesic Dose (mg)		Starting Oral Dose		Time (h)
	Oral	Parenteral[a]	Adults (mg)	Children (mg/kg)	
Morphine	30	10	15–30	0.3	2–3.5
Hydromorphone (Dilaudid)	7.5	1.5	4–8	0.06	3–12
Oxycodone	30	—	15–30	0.3	2–3
Methadone (Dolophine)	20	10	5–10	0.2	12–16
Levorphanol (Levo-Dromoman)	4	2	2–4	0.04	3–4
Fentanyl	—	0.1	—	—	
Oxymorphone (Numorphan)	—	1	—	—	
Meperidine (Demerol)	300	75	Not recommended		

[a] These are standard intramuscular (IM) doses for acute pain in adults and also may be used to convert doses for intravenous (IV) infusions and repeated small IV boluses. For single IV boluses, use half the IM dose. IV doses for children <6 months of age = parenteral equianalgesic dose × weight (kg)/100.

route, dosage, and schedule of opioids should be individualized to rapidly and safely achieve pain control. Routes of administration include:

   1.   **Oral administration.** The oral route is optimal for patients with chronic pain because of its convenience and steady blood levels. For patients who cannot swallow, many opioids are available as elixirs. Others can be easily crushed and put into concentrated emulsions. With the exception of sustained release formulations, most of the oral opioids reach peak effect within 30 to 60 minutes. This may not be acceptable for those patients with rapidly fluctuating pain.

   2.   **Intramuscular injection.** Although commonly used, painful intramuscular injections rarely are necessary in a postoperative patient. In addition, intramuscular injections may cause subcutaneous or muscle fibrosis, and sterile abscesses.

   3.   **Intravenous bolus, continuous IV infusion, and patient-controlled analgesia (PCA).** Bolus administration is the fastest route to analgesia. Time to peak effect is determined by the lipid solubility of the drug. Onset time ranges from 1 to 5 minutes with fentanyl and 10 to 15 minutes with morphine. PCA is a technique that combines continuous availability of medication with the rapid analgesic effect of bolus administration. Commonly used opioids and their doses for PCA are summarized in Table 37-3.

   a.   Morphine is most commonly used. It is a naturally occurring, inexpensive opioid. As a mu-receptor agonist, its effects

Table 37-3.   Adult patient-controlled analgesia

Requirements	Drug		
	Morphine	Hydromorphone	Meperidine
Concentration (mg/mL)	1	0.5	10
Demand dose (mL)	1	0.5	1
Range (mL)	0.5–2.0	0.5–2.0	0.5–2.0
Lockout interval	6 min	10 min	6 min
Basal rate (mL/hr)			
Day	0	0	0
Night	0.5	0.5	0.5
Hourly limit (mL)	<12	<6	<10
Loading dose (mg) (every 5 min until comfortable)	2 mg	0.5 mg	2.0 mg
Maximum loading dose (mg)	10–15 mg	2–4 mg	75–150 mg

Note: These suggested dosages are based on those required by a healthy, 55–70-kg, opioid-naive adult. Adjustments must be made according to the condition of the patient, his or her prior opioid use, and the recent (preoperative) use of opioids.

and side effects are well understood. There are rare circumstances, such as the occurrence of unacceptable side effects, when drugs other than morphine should be considered. For PCA with morphine, we generally use a 1 mg/mL dose, a demand dose of 1 mL, a lockout interval of 6 minutes, and a basal rate of 0 to 1 mL per hour during sleep.

b. **Hydromorphone** (dilaudid) is the second drug of choice for PCA. It is more potent that morphine and is often tolerated in patients who have side effects from morphine. A typical PCA dosage is 0.5 mg/mL, a demand dose of 0.5 to 1 mL, a lockout interval of 10 minutes, and a basal rate of 0 to 1 mL per hour during sleep.

c. **Meperidine** continues to be widely utilized for acute pain and is useful in some patients. Its use is complicated by its toxicities, including the accumulation of the epileptogenic metabolite normeperidine, which may be particularly problematic in patients with renal dysfunction and in patients taking monoamine oxidase inhibitors (MAOIs). A typical PCA dosage is 10 mg/mL, a demand dose of 1 mL, a lockout interval of 6 minutes, and a basal rate of 0 to 1 mL per hour during sleep.

d. The **side effects of opioids** are well described. Respiratory depression is a true risk of opioid treatment and the respiratory rate of all patients, especially in the postoperative period, should be monitored. Severe depression of respiration should be treated with naloxone.

e. **Fear of patient addiction** is widespread among health care providers and among patients and their families. Although most patients who take opioids daily for more than a month develop some degree of tolerance and physical dependence, the available data suggests that the risk of addiction should not be a primary concern in the treatment of acute pain.

f. **PCA may be used in children** (see Table 37-4). It is important that the child understand the relationship between a stimulus (pain), a response (pushing the button), and a delayed result (pain relief) for PCA to be effective. Opioid dosing for children is not as well established as for adults. For babies and infants with acute postoperative pain, continuous morphine infusions (10 to 25 μg/kg per hour) without a bolus is used.

4. **Transdermal fentanyl.** Fentanyl is lipid soluble and is readily absorbed through skin. A fentanyl patch is extremely convenient since steady blood levels are attained with a system that is only changed every three days. A 25-μg-per-hour patch is equivalent to 10 mg of IV morphine administered every 8 hours. Peak effect after the initial administration ranges from 24 to 72 hours. After removal, serum drug levels drop by 50% after an average of 17 hours. Given the lag time to peak effect, this method of drug delivery is not commonly used in the acute pain setting.

5. **Rectal administration of opioids.** Although not commonly used, rectal administration is a good alternative when there is no other access. The vascular anatomy of the rectum allows for opioids to be rapidly absorbed.

Table 37-4. Patient-controlled analgesia (PCA) or continuous infusion of morphine for pediatric cases

Children Under 7 Years of Age
(Use Dilute Solution: 0.2 mg/mL)

Requirements	Dose (mg/kg)	Example: For a 10-kg Child, Using 0.2 mg/mL
Basal rate (per hour)	0.01–0.05	0.1 mg = 0.5 mL
Hourly limit	0.03	0.3 mg = 1.5 mL
Initial bolus (every 5 min until comfortable)	0.02	0.2 mg = 1 mL
Maximum bolus	0.1	1 mg = 5 mL
For increasing pain	2 to 3 times basal rate	
For nonfunctioning IV, if morphine morphine needed	0.05–0.10	

Children 7 to 11 Years of Age
(These Children Can Usually Cope With Patient-Controlled
Dosing; Use Dilute Solution: 0.2 mg/mL)

Age Range (yrs)	Approximate Weight (kg)	PCA Setting[a] Using 0.2 mg/mL
7–8	20	1/6/0
9–11	30	2/6/0

Children 12 to 15 Years of Age
(These Children Cope Well With PCA; Use Standard
Solution (1 mg/mL); Over 15 Years of Age, Treat as Adults)

Age Range (yrs)	Approximate Weight (kg)	PCA Setting[a] Using 1 mg/mL
12–14	40–50	0.5/6/0
15	>50	1/6/0

[a] PCA setting: demand dose mL/lockout interval (min)/basal rate (mL/h).

6. **Epidural analgesia** can provide excellent intraoperative as well as postoperative analgesia.

a. **Epidural catheters** commonly are placed in the following groups of patients:

(1) Patients undergoing thoracic or upper abdominal surgery.

(2) Patients undergoing thoracic, upper or lower abdominal surgery, and who have significant pulmonary disease.

(3) Patients having lower limb surgery in whom early mobilization is important.

(4) Patients undergoing lower-extremity vascular procedures in whom a sympathectomy is advantageous.

b. A common infusion for postoperative epidural therapy is a mixture of 0.1% bupivacaine with 0.02 mg/mL hydromorphone. Fentanyl (2 to 10 μg/mL) is chosen for patients such as the very young or the very old who may be particularly sensitive to opioid effects. Its short duration of action and its greater lipophilicity (compared with hydromorphone and morphine) contribute to its tendency to bind locally to spinal cord receptors, rather than floating cephalad toward vital respiratory centers within the brain. In elderly patients, patients with marginal respiratory status, and in patients aged 1 through 7 years, a mixture of 0.1% bupivacaine with 2 μg/mL fentanyl is recommended. Infants under 1 year of age should not have fentanyl added to the epidural mixture, since this age group is particularly sensitive to the depressant effects of opioids. Table 37-5 describes suitable epidural orders for adults and children. Other drugs may be used for epidural analgesia, including morphine and the α-2–adrenergic agonist, clonidine.

c. **Management problems.** The keys to epidural management are proper placement of the catheter (which should be at least 3 cm in the epidural space), testing that the catheter is functioning before the patient is anesthetized, and proper postoperative care.

(1) **Inadequate analgesia.** When pain is not well controlled with an epidural infusion, the infusion rate or concentration can be increased, and supplemental parenteral opioids may be administered within a monitored setting (e.g., operating room, postanesthesia care unit [PACU], or intensive care unit [ICU]). Concentrated local anesthetics can be administered to test the catheter; otherwise, a bolus of 5 to 10 mL of the epidural solution that the patient is receiving can be administered. If there is no response within 10 to 20 minutes, the catheter should be replaced or the patient started on alternative systemic analgesia.

(2) **Catheter disconnections.** After a witnessed "disconnect," the distal inch of catheter can be cleaned with an alcohol swab, cut off, and a new sterile adapter hub attached to the freshly cut end. After an unwitnessed disconnection, the catheter should be removed and then replaced, or the patient can be placed on systemic analgesics. Epidural catheter insertion sites should be inspected daily for signs of infection. Catheters usually are removed after 4 to 7 days of use.

Table 37-5.   **Suitable regimens for epidural infusions in adults and children**

Solutions

<1 yr old: 0.1% bupivacaine *without* fentanyl

1 to 7 yr of age: 0.1% bupivacaine with 2 µg/mL fentanyl

>7 yr of age or adult: 0.1% bupivacaine with 20 µg/mL hydromorphone

Special indications: fentanyl or hydromorphone without bupivacaine

Rate of infusion

Adults

  Starting rate, 2 to 10 mL/h

  For increasing pain, increase in increments of up to 10 mL/h

  For decreasing pain or for side effects, decrease in increments down to 1 mL/h

Children

  Starting rate, 0.1 mL/kg per hour of appropriate solution (see above)

  For increasing pain, increase in increments up to 0.3 mL/kg per hour

  For bolusing catheter:

    ≥6 kg, 1 mL of 1% lidocaine with 1:200,000 epinephrine

    6 to 15 kg, 2 mL of 1% lidocaine with 1:200,000 epinephrine

    >15 kg, 5 mL of 1% lidocaine with 1:200,000 epinephrine

Note: Pediatric mixtures of bupivacaine and fentanyl may be indicated in special circumstances for adult patients.

(3)   **Treatment of side effects.** Pruritus, urinary retention, and nausea are easily treated with the opioid antagonist **naloxone** (0.04 to 0.1 mg IV as needed). Profound sedation and respiratory depression may require higher doses (0.1 to 0.4 mg IV as needed). These doses may also partially reverse analgesia. A continuous, titrated naloxone infusion (5 to 10 µg/kg per hour) is often useful to reverse respiratory depression while permitting continued analgesia. The risk of delayed respiratory depression after epidural opioids is inversely proportional to the lipid solubility of the drug. This risk is greatest for epidural morphine, but it is still a rare event with an incidence of less than 1%. The risk of delayed respiratory depression after epidural opioids is potentiated by coadministered CNS depressants such as parenteral opioids, barbiturates, and benzodiazepines. Additional risk factors include advanced age, respiratory disease, and factors that encourage the cephalad spread of drug such as increased intrathoracic and abdominal pressure, a more cephalad level of injection, and a larger doses of opioid.

(4)   **Discontinuing epidural analgesia.** Epidural analgesia is converted to oral analgesics (e.g., acetaminophen 325 mg with oxycodone, 5 mg) when the patient can tolerate oral intake.

7. Intrathecal catheters may be used for both short- and long-term analgesia (also see Chapter 16, section IV.C.3.g). Commonly used catheters are 20-gauge, 28-gauge, or 32-gauge. They are used most frequently for obstetric procedures; orthopedic, general, and vascular surgery; and cancer pain. Spinal opioids are chosen based on length of analgesia desired, potency, and potential side effects. This mode of analgesia is usually restricted to patients in a monitored setting (e.g., PACU, ICU) or for those with cancer pain.

    a. Preservative-free morphine (Duramorph or Astramorph, 0.25 to 1.0 mg). Characteristics include low lipid solubility, slow onset (30 to 60 minutes), long duration (12 to 24 hours), and a high potential for side effects.

    b. Meperidine (preservative-free, 25 to 50 mg) has both opioid and local anesthetic properties and is most commonly used as an anesthetic for obstetric, perineal, and lower-abdominal procedures. Characteristics include high lipid solubility, fast onset (4 minutes), short duration (90 minutes), and a moderate incidence of side effects.

    c. Fentanyl (5 to 25 μg) is commonly administered along with spinal local anesthetic to prolong the duration of a primary anesthetic. It is also used for postoperative analgesia and cancer pain. Characteristics include high lipid solubility, fast onset (minutes), moderate duration (1.5 to 3.0 hours), and a low incidence of side effects.

    d. Sufentanil (3 to 10 μg) is used in a fashion similar to that of fentanyl. Characteristics include high lipid solubility, fast onset (minutes), short duration (1 to 2 hours), and a low incidence of side effects.

8. Opioid tolerance and dependence. Patients who have previously been receiving opioids sometimes can be inappropriately undertreated. In general, the patient's usual maintenance dose should be given as a baseline; additional dosing should be administered for the acute event (i.e., perioperative pain). The following definitions may be useful:

    a. Tolerance is a reduced effect on repeated exposure to a drug at a constant dose.

    b. Dependence is the need for continued exposure to a drug to avoid a withdrawal syndrome.

    c. Addiction is a biological and psychological behavior of serious compulsive use of a substance despite adverse consequences.

    d. Withdrawal is a syndrome that follows cessation of a drug or administration of an opioid antagonist, which is characterized by sympathetic overdrive and symptoms such as hyperpyrexia, diarrhea, and hyperalgesia.

9. Basic opioid conversions

    a. Converting from IV to oral dosing. An equivalent oral opioid dose usually is three times the IV dose (see Table 37-2).

    b. Converting from one opioid to another. As a rough guide, 10 mg of morphine sulfate is equivalent to 10 mg methadone, 1.5 mg hydromorphone, 75 mg meperidine, or 2 mg levorphanol. An IV infusion of 1 mg morphine per hour is equivalent to 50 μg fentanyl per hour.

    c. Discontinuing opioids. Decreasing the dose by 1/3 each day is a safe way of weaning opioids; it is also relatively safe to decrease the total dose to 10% to 20% of the dose if rapid removal of opioids is necessary. Administration of clonidine can help ameliorate withdrawal symptoms.

IV. Chronic pain. Chronic pain syndromes are varied and complex in their manifestations. Before starting any therapy, a careful review of the history, physical findings, other diagnostic studies, and opinions of other consultants is necessary. Significant behavioral changes often are present when pain of any etiology has persisted for more than a few months. Irritability, insomnia, dependency on family members, dependency on drugs, and lack of motivation are common. **Depression** is frequent enough to warrant empiric therapy. Tricyclic antidepressants and MAOIs not only act on analgesic pathways directly, but also affect neuromodulators such as endorphins. Side effects include drowsiness, which is helpful when these drugs are administered at bedtime. **Neurosurgical procedures** (e.g., percutaneous neurectomy, dorsal rhizotomy, or cordotomy) have been employed to treat refractory benign and malignant pain.

    A. Low back pain occurs at some time in at least 50% of all adults due to multiple, often coexistent mechanisms. Occult disease (e.g., retroperitoneal tumor) must be excluded, anatomic derangements (e.g., bony fragments) characterized, and surgical options (e.g., foraminotomy) considered with orthopedists or neurosurgeons before selecting nonsurgical management. Sensorimotor function, including tenderness and pain on flexion or extension of the spine and extremities, should be documented at each stage of treatment. Bowel or bladder dysfunction argues for aggressive surgical intervention, as does a persistent decrease in motor power or sensation.

    1. Epidural steroid injections

        a. Indications for epidural steroid therapy for low back pain include patients with disk herniation and the postlaminectomy syndrome. Each of these conditions may cause nerve root irritation with subsequent edema and swelling. Epidural steroid administration will decrease pain and inflammation in many patients and is especially attractive when coexistent disease places the patient at increased operative and anesthetic risk.

        b. Protrusion of the intervertebral disk may lead to nerve compression or cauda equina syndrome. Pain and paresthesias in the lower extremities may ensue and progress to muscle weakness and paralysis, as well as loss of sexual function, bowel, and bladder control. Acute nerve entrapment leading to sudden progression of neurologic symptoms should be considered a neurosurgical emergency, and immediate consultation must be obtained.

        c. Spinal stenosis is produced by either congenital, traumatic, or degenerative narrowing of the spinal canal. This narrowing usually is accompanied by painless bilateral leg weakness and/or neurogenic claudication relieved with rest.

        d. When a patient with low back pain fails more conservative treatment and there has been no progression of neurologic symptoms (e.g., foot drop or bowel and bladder dysfunction), epidural steroid injection is indicated.

e. Technique. With the patient in the prone position, a 22-gauge 2- or 3-inch spinal needle (Quincke point) is advanced under fluoroscopic guidance into the epidural space. A permanent radiograph is taken to verify needle placement. After an appropriate test dose, 75 mg of triamcinolone (3 mL of Aristocort 2.5%) in 10 mL of 0.125% or 0.25% bupivacaine is injected, and the patient is observed for signs of adverse reaction. Local trauma due to needle insertion may produce an exacerbation of back pain for a few days following the injection. Patients are reevaluated in 2 weeks. If the patient is substantially improved and satisfied with this level of improvement, no further therapy is needed. If there is only some improvement or the symptoms have returned, a repeat block is indicated. If pain is worse after the first injection, a different modality (e.g., substitution of one brand of glucocorticoid for another or injection at a different site) should be tried. No more than three injections in a 12-week period should be performed, since significant blunting of the hypothalamic-pituitary axis may take place.

2. Paravertebral spinal nerve root block

    a. Indications are to determine the contribution of a particular nerve root to a patient's overall pain syndrome and to reduce pain due to irritation of a previously identified root.

    b. Technique. With the patient prone, a skin mark is made above the root foramen (the lateral margin of the vertebral body as it joins the transverse process). Using fluoroscopy, a 10-cm, 22-gauge needle is inserted 5 to 8 cm lateral to the midline and advanced toward the skin mark at an angle of 45 degrees posterior to the plane of the back. When the transverse process is reached, the needle is withdrawn and redirected caudally until a paresthesia is elicited. Once the needle tip is confirmed to be near the foramen by fluoroscopy, 1 to 2 mL of either lidocaine (1% with epinephrine 1:200,000) or bupivacaine (0.5% with epinephrine 1:200,000) is injected in divided doses, and the patient is observed for a change in pain intensity. Ideal dermatomal anesthesia may not result from injection of a single root. Any extreme pain during injection may indicate an intraneural injection and mandates immediate repositioning of the needle. A permanent radiograph is taken for verification of needle position. A corticosteroid may be added to the local anesthetic to reduce edema and scarring.

3. Facet joint injections

    a. Indications. Facet joint pathology is suspected when low back pain is referred to the buttock or thighs and the patient is able to perform forward flexion but is limited in extension and rotation of the spine.

    b. Technique. With the patient prone or turned slightly lateral with one knee drawn toward the chest to open the facet maximally, a 10-cm, 22-gauge spinal needle is advanced into the facet joint under fluoroscopic guidance. A characteristic loss of resistance is felt when penetration is achieved. Verification is accomplished by obtaining lateral fluoroscopic views. A dose of 1 to 2 mL of bupivacaine (0.5% with 1:200,000 epinephrine) or tetracaine (1% with 1:200,000 epinephrine) is administered, and a permanent radiograph is obtained. A corticosteroid may be added for therapeutic effect.

B. Myofascial pain

1. Myofascial pain can be quite debilitating and confused with disk or facet joint disease. It is important to distinguish discrete trigger points from a diffuse myofascial pain syndrome, since the latter may be a symptom of systemic disease. Hyperirritable sites in muscle and connective tissue, termed trigger points, result from trauma, fatigue, or tension, and can produce reflex muscle spasm, ischemia, and pain. Trigger point injections may be beneficial.

2. Anesthetic technique. A 1- to 3-ml dose of local anesthetic (either 1% lidocaine or 0.5% bupivacaine) with corticosteroid (triamcinolone 0.1% or 0.25%) in a mixture of 10 to 25 mg (i.e., 1 mL) of steroid plus 9 mL of anesthetic is injected into each trigger point. Injections may be repeated 5 to 7 days apart to deliver up to 75 mg per month for no more than 3 months. Patients should respond quickly to therapy. The need for frequent treatments may indicate misdiagnosis or concomitant psychological dysfunction. Use of NSAIDs, muscle relaxants (benzodiazepines), or cooling and stretching of trigger points also may be used.

C. Occipital neuralgia

1. Pain involving the occipital nerve frequently follows neck injury and can be treated with selective nerve blocks. Patients usually complain of aching pain in the suboccipital region that may radiate across the scalp or into the neck and have a lancinating retroorbital component.

2. Anesthetic technique. The greater occipital nerve is blocked as it crosses a line drawn from the greater occipital protuberance to the mastoid process (superior nuchal line). After palpation of the occipital artery, 3 to 5 mL of either 1% lidocaine, 0.25% bupivacaine, or a 50:50 mixture of 0.5% bupivacaine and 1% lidocaine with 10 to 20 mg of triamcinolone (Aristocort 1%, 1 to 2 mL) is injected on either side of the arterial pulse. A paresthesia or pressure dysesthesia may or may not be elicited. Generally, a series of three injections is sufficient to provide pain relief for an extended period of time.

D. Chronic regional pain syndromes (reflex sympathetic dystrophy [RSD]) typically occurs following a trivial injury or obvious nerve trauma and is associated with an alteration of the nervous system, resulting in heightened sympathetic outflow. When this alteration follows direct nerve trauma, the term **causalgia** is used.

1. The hallmark of this syndrome is **an exquisitely painful body part** (usually a limb). The pain is characterized as a burning sensation with exquisite sensitivity to stimuli (**hyperesthesia**) and progression of pain with repetitive innocuous stimuli (**hyperpathia**). Single innocuous stimuli (e.g., light touch) may also produce pain (**allodynia**). Typically starting in a small, discrete area, the pain intensifies over time and spreads proximally from its origin.

2. Characteristic changes are noted when RSD becomes progressive. The skin, which is typically cold, adopts a smooth, glassy appearance and has decreased hair growth and sweating.

The end stage is significant for disuse atrophy and marked osteoporosis.

3. Anesthetic technique. Diagnosis and treatment of RSD and causalgia depend on relief of pain following sympathetic blockade.

  a. Stellate ganglion (cervicothoracic) block

   (1) With the patient in the supine position, a 22-gauge 1- or 2-inch needle is advanced under fluoroscopic guidance posteriorly between the trachea and carotid artery. The target is the prevertebral fascia on the anterolateral surface of the C-7 vertebra. A 15-ml dose of 1% lidocaine, 0.25% bupivacaine, or a 50:50 solution of 1% lidocaine and 0.5% bupivacaine is slowly injected. Cervical plexus, phrenic, superficial, or recurrent laryngeal nerve anesthesia is common. **Horner's syndrome** (ptosis, enophthalmos, miosis, and anhidrosis) is typically seen, although this sign alone is not pathognomonic for successful sympathetic blockade of the upper extremity.

   (2) Postblock alterations. The **galvanic skin response** is a change in voltage potential of the hand or foot in response to an abrupt noise or painful stimulus. Abolition of the galvanic skin response and an increase in skin temperature of 10°F or higher are evidence of sympathetic blockade.

   (3) This block can be performed intermittently or continuously through a catheter. A total of 5 to 10 mL of 0.25% bupivacaine can be injected three to four times a day at a rate of 1 mL per minute.

  b. Sympathetic blockade of the upper extremity also may be achieved with placement of local anesthetic into the interpleural space. Bupivacaine, 75 to 100 mg in either 0.25% or 0.5% concentration, can be given four times a day.

  c. Lumbar sympathetic block. The L-2 vertebra is identified with fluoroscopy and the skin marked in the manner described in section IV.A.2.b for paravertebral spinal nerve root block. A 10- to 15-cm, 22- or 20-gauge needle is inserted just below the twelfth rib and directed toward the body of the L-2 vertebra with the needle bevel facing laterally. When the transverse process is encountered, the needle is redirected cephalad to contact the vertebral body. The needle tip is advanced slightly beyond the anterior projection of the vertebral body and confirmed with fluoroscopy. A total of 15 to 30 mL of 1% lidocaine, 0.25% bupivacaine, or a 50:50 solution of 1% lidocaine and 0.5% bupivacaine is given in divided doses and the limb monitored for effect. This technique may be performed using a catheter technique to provide intermittent injections (10 to 20 mL of 0.5% bupivacaine four times a day) or a continuous infusion (4 to 8 mL per hour of 0.125% to 0.25% bupivacaine). A minimum treatment duration of 7 days with aggressive physical therapy is recommended.

  d. Intravenous regional sympathetic block. Adrenergic-antagonist drugs may alter the sensitivity of nociceptors. Potential agents include guanethidine, reserpine, labetalol (10 to 30 mg in 30 to 50 mL of normal saline), or 0.5% lidocaine in a tourniquet-isolated limb for a minimum of 20 minutes.

Most commonly, 35 to 70 mg of lidocaine is used as an IV challenge dose, depending on the size of the patient and the medical history.

E.   Postherpetic neuralgia

1.   PHN is an extremely painful complication of **acute vari- cella zoster infection**, occurring most commonly in the elderly and immunocompromised patients. The patient experiences persistent severe burning pain in the same distribution as the original infection. Currently, medical therapies appear to be more beneficial than blockade, although blocks can produce long-lasting effects in some patients.

2.   Anesthetic techniques. PHN has been reported to re- spond to sympathetic blocks as described above, provided these blocks are performed during or shortly after (less than 6 weeks) the acute attack. PHN in the thoracic distribution may be treated with intermittent intercostal or interpleural nerve blocks or con- tinuously with epidural local anesthetic infusions. Long-estab- lished PHN is difficult to treat and is usually managed in the same way as neuropathic pain.

F.   Neuropathic pain results from an aberration of nerve physi- ology or anatomy, and can be seen with alcoholic or diabetic neu- ropathies as well as following amputation or partial spinal cord damage.

1.   Lancinating pain, secondary to the spontaneous firing of nociceptors or nerve fibers, is treated with anticonvulsants such as carbamazepine, phenytoin, or clonazepam. **Burning dyses- thesias** are commonly treated with tricyclic antidepressant drugs such as amitriptyline or doxepin. **For refractory pain**, a combination of amitriptyline and fluphenazine has been tried with success. An added benefit of sedating antidepressants is to give an evening dose to prevent the insomnia commonly seen with neuropathic and other forms of chronic pain.

2.   Intravenous infusion of local anesthetic may be used as a diagnostic test or to treat neuropathic pain, particularly if associated with mononeuropathies (e.g., in diabetes mellitus). If an IV infusion of 100 to 300 mg of 1% lidocaine over 20 to 30 minutes provides long-lasting relief, the patient may benefit from a trial of oral mexiletine hydrochloride, 150 to 200 mg three or four times a day. Careful follow-up with periodic blood levels is prudent.

V.   Cancer pain. Treatment of cancer pain is multifaceted and may require pharmacologic intervention combined with counseling, nursing care, pastoral and social services, nerve blockade, surgery, radiation therapy, chemotherapy, and hospice care. Cancer pain often is a dynamic process with remissions and exacerbations paral- leling the disease course.

A.   Pharmacologic therapy

1.   NSAIDs are a useful first line of therapy in cancer pain, particularly since metastatic lesions to bone often cause prosta- glandin-mediated inflammation and pain.

2.   Oral opioids. Propoxyphene and codeine are initiated first. Addition of more potent opioids such as methadone or time- released morphine (MS Contin) may follow. Every effort is made to keep the outpatient comfortable for as long as possible on oral medications administered "by the clock." As-needed "rescue" doses of short-acting medications such as immediate-release morphine tablets or elixir, oxycodone, or hydromorphone may be required (see Table 37-2). Opioid dosage may be increased until either pain is successfully treated or side effects interfere. Sedation is a common problem and can be treated with the addition of dextroamphetamine (5 mg every 6 hours). An added benefit of this combination is increased analgesia.

3. Parenteral opioids are used when oral medications fail. The appropriate parenteral dosage is calculated using oral to parenteral conversion data (see Table 37-2), and the patient is started on an intermittent IV or subcutaneous regimen. Since patients develop significant tolerance to opioids after prolonged therapy, withdrawal must be anticipated and avoided when changing the route of a patient's medication (see section IV.B). PCA with the help of skilled outpatient nursing services lends itself well to treating severe cancer pain.

4. Alternate routes. Transdermal delivery of opioids, such as the fentanyl patch, is an alternative to the oral route for the treatment of cancer patients. **Transdermal fentanyl** is available in doses that deliver 25, 50, 75, and 100 μg per hour. Patches are worn for 48 to 72 hours and achieve a steady-state blood level within 12 to 24 hours. The consistency of blood levels and the circumvention of an unreliable oral route without resort to injections may be ideal. Unfortunately, transdermal opioids appear to induce tolerance as quickly as continuous infusions, and nausea remains a frequent side effect. Rectal and sublingual opioid administration are other alternatives.

5. Long-term neuraxial opioids

   a. High systemic doses of opioids can be avoided with the introduction of neuraxial opioids through a temporary epidural catheter. **Preservative-free morphine** (2 to 4 mg) is started on a twice-daily dosing schedule. The dosage is increased by 1 mg per dose and/or the schedule is changed (e.g., to three times a day) as needed. Parenteral or oral rescue doses (e.g., 10 to 20 mg of morphine elixir every 2 hours as needed) are administered during the epidural trial protocol. Patients should be kept on a minimum of 25% of their regular daily dose of systemic opioid to prevent the abstinence syndrome. Combinations of opioids and local anesthetics provide excellent analgesia and allow opiate receptors to "reset" and become more sensitive to opioids.

   b. If a trial of epidural opioids is successful, **the catheter may be tunneled or surgically implanted** for long-term use over several months. Patients are sent home or to a hospice with a dosing schedule in place, and require close follow-up by a skilled nursing service.

6. Side effects. All opioids, especially when given in high dosage, generate side effects. Constipation is controlled by initiating bowel stimulants and stool softeners whenever opioid therapy is begun. Urecholine may be required to treat urinary retention.

B. Neurolytic blocks. The decision to perform a neurolytic block is based on the nature of the patient's malignancy, anticipated life expectancy, medical status, and response to other therapeutic options. Any neurolytic block first must be simulated using local anesthetic alone to assess a particular nerve's contribution to cancer pain. Neurolytic blocks then can be performed with 50% to 100% ethanol or 6% to 10% phenol. Ethanol is more likely to have a permanent effect, but has a higher tendency to produce painful neuropathies.

C.   Celiac plexus blockade is performed to relieve visceral pain caused by pancreatic and upper abdominal tumors.

    1.   Technique. Under fluoroscopic guidance and with the patient prone, 15-cm, 20-gauge needles are inserted bilaterally just below the twelfth rib and directed medially to contact the body of the L-1 vertebra. The left-sided needle is advanced cephalad to the transverse process 1 to 2 cm anterior to the L-1 vertebral body or until aortic pulsations are felt. Renograffin dye (50%), 2 to 5 mL, mixed 1:1 with sterile saline is instilled to demonstrate a periaortic outline. The right-sided needle is advanced 1 to 2 cm. Undiluted renograffin, 2 to 5 mL, is injected to demonstrate a pericaval outline. An irregular outline on either side mandates repositioning of the needle to avoid a psoas muscle injection. Tracking of dye under the diaphragm or toward spinal roots also mandates repositioning. Either 25 mL of 0.25% bupivacaine with 1:200,000 epinephrine or a 50:50 mixture of 1% lidocaine with 1:200,000 epinephrine and 0.5% bupivacaine with 1:200,000 epinephrine is injected in divided doses through each needle. If pain is relieved, this may be followed after 24 hours by 25 mL per needle of 50% alcohol in 1% lidocaine or 7% phenol in water.

    2.   Complications include temporary (although sometimes persistent) hypotension and diarrhea. Intrathecal, epidural, or intramuscular injection of a neurolytic agent may result in sexual dysfunction, lower-extremity dysesthesias, or paraplegia secondary to spinal artery syndrome. Pneumothorax, bowel perforation, kidney or liver puncture, and retroperitoneal hemorrhage may occur.

SUGGESTED READING

Anand KJ, Arnold JH. Opioid tolerance and dependence in infants and children. *Crit Care Med* 1994;22:334–342.

Ballantyne J, Fishman SM, Abdi S. *The Massachusetts General Hospital handbook of pain management*, 2nd ed. Philadelphia: Lippincott Williams & Wilkins, 2002.

Brown DL. *Atlas of regional anesthesia*, 2nd ed. Philadelphia: WB Saunders, 1999.

Carr DB, Goudas LC. Acute pain. *Lancet* 1999;353:2051–2058.

Collins JJ, Grier HE, Kinney HC, et al. Control of severe pain in children with terminal malignancy. *J Pediatr* 1995;126:653–657.

Ferrante FM. Principles of opioid pharmacotherapy: practical implications of basic mechanisms. *J Pain Symptom Manage* 1996;11:265–273.

Galer BS. Neuropathic pain of peripheral origin: advances in pharmacologic treatment. *Neurology* 1995;45:S17–25, S35–S36.

Latarjet J, Choinere M. Pain in burn patients. *Burns* 1995;21:344–348.

Mather CM, Ready LB. Management of acute pain. *Br J Hosp Med* 1994; 51:85–88.

McQuay H. Opioids in pain management. *Lancet* 1999;353:2229–2232.

McQuay H, Carroll D, Jadad AR, et al. Anticonvulsant drugs for management of pain: a systematic review. *BMJ* 1995;311:1047–1052.

Portenoy RK. Tolerance to opioid analgesics: clinical aspects. *Cancer Surv* 1994;21:49–65.

Portenoy RK, Kanner RM. Pain management: theory and practice. Philadelphia: FA Davis Co, 1996.

Stanton-Hicks M, Janig W, Hassenbusch S, et al. Reflex sympathetic dystrophy: changing concepts and taxonomy. *Pain* 1995;63:127–133.

Waldman SD. *Interventional pain management,* 2nd ed. Philadelphia: WB Saunders, 2001.

Wall PD, Melzak R. *Textbook of pain,* 4th ed. Philadelphia: WB Saunders, 1999.

Woolf CJ, Mannion RJ. Neuropathic pain: aetiology, symptoms, mechanisms, and management. *Lancet* 1999;353:1959–1964.

Woolf CJ, Salter MW. Neuronal plasticity: increasing the gain in pain. *Science* 2000;288:1765–1769.

Complementary and Alternative Medicine

Margaret Gargarian and P. Grace Harrell

I.   Complementary and alternative medicine (CAM). Complementary and alternative therapies encompass a broad range of therapeutic modalities, and can be integrated into Western medicine. CAM offers patients treatment options, especially when dealing with chronic illness and symptom alleviation. As physicians, the more comfortable and informed we are about CAM, the more effectively we can help our patients make safe and intelligent decisions. As anesthesiologists, we should ask about CAM use during our standard history taking, especially the use of herbs. Knowledge of CAM use can help prevent potential hazards during surgery, and can assist with the management of pain, anxiety, and nausea and vomiting.

A.   Definitions of CAM

1.   Practices that are not accepted as correct or in conformity with the beliefs of the dominant group of medical practitioners in a society.

2.   Interventions neither taught widely in medical schools nor generally available in hospitals.

B.   CAM includes a spectrum of practices and beliefs. Many may become "mainstream" when proved safe and effective.

C.   Categories of CAM practices. The National Center for Complementary and Alternative Medicine, which is a subdivision of the National Institutes of Health, has grouped CAM practices into five major subdivisions:

1.   Alternative medical systems are complete systems of theory and practice that have evolved in various cultures, mostly before the inception of conventional medicine. An example is traditional oriental medicine, which uses acupuncture, herbal medicine, massage, and qi gong.

a.   Acupuncture emphasizes the proper flow of qi (a vital energy) and involves the insertion of fine, solid needles into specific points on the body, to produce a therapeutic result. Acupuncture influences the nervous system at multiple levels, and causes release of endorphins, serotonin, norepinephrine, and cortisol. Many of these substances reduce inflammation and pain sensation.

b.   Ayurveda is India's traditional system of medicine, which emphasizes the equal importance of body, mind, and spirit. It utilizes diet, exercise, meditation, herbs, massage, and controlled breathing.

2.   Mind–body interventions use techniques to facilitate the mind's ability to affect bodily functions. Examples include hypnosis, meditation, prayer, and mental healing.

3.   Biologically based treatments overlap with conventional medicine's use of dietary supplements. They include herbal therapy (see section III), special diets, shark cartilage to treat cancer, and bee pollen to treat autoimmune diseases.

4. Manipulative and body-based methods use movement or manipulation of the body to restore health. An example is chiropractic medicine, which believes that realigning the spine allows the "innate intelligence" of the body to restore itself to health. Other examples are massage therapy and osteopathic manipulation.

5. Energy therapies focus on energy fields originating within the body (biofields) or those from other sources (electromagnetic fields). Examples are qi gong, reiki, and therapeutic touch. **Qi gong** combines movement, meditation, and regulation of breathing to enhance the flow of qi and improve circulation. **Reiki** is based on channeling spiritual energy through the practitioner to heal the spirit and in turn heal the body. **Therapeutic touch** involves a practitioner focusing on the intent to heal, while lightly touching or passing hands over the patient, to identify energy imbalances.

II. Prevalence of CAM

A. In 1997, there were 629 million CAM visits in the United States, compared with 386 million primary care physician visits. Visits to chiropractors and massage therapists accounted for nearly half of all CAM visits. Total out-of-pocket expense for CAM in 1997 was $27 billion, which was comparable to money spent on visits to U.S. physicians. The out-of-pocket total for CAM included $3 billion on vitamins, and $5 billion on herbs.

B. Most CAM therapies are used for chronic conditions, especially back and neck problems, depression, anxiety, and chronic fatigue. Symptom relief is the main benefit reported. The vast majority of people use CAM in conjunction with conventional therapies.

C. Seventy-five U.S. medical schools offer coursework in alternative medicine, and many U.S. hospitals now have complementary medicine departments.

D. Disclosure rates. Only 40% of patients tell their doctors about the CAM therapies that they are using. This places the burden on the physician to elicit this information from their patients. A physician informed about alternative medicine can help their patients avoid dangerous side effects, and also help them make safe and intelligent choices.

III. Herbal therapy and anesthesia

A. Herbal medicines are plants or parts of plants that contain biologically active components. There is tremendous variability in the purity and potency of herbal preparations. The amount of active component can vary widely within the same species depending on growing conditions. Herbal products have been adulterated with foreign substances, including drugs, bacteria, and toxic metals.

B. Herbal medicines are currently regulated in the category of "dietary supplements" along with compounds such as vitamins and amino acids. The manufacturer does not have to prove efficacy or safety of a compound before it is marketed, and products are not scrutinized via the same stringent testing placed on drugs.

Some companies are now using techniques such as chromatography to identify and standardize herbal preparations.

C.   Many herbs can be dangerous when used in combination with prescription or over-the-counter drugs. They can alter the metabolism of important medications, and many herbs have anticoagulant effects. The American Society of Anesthesiologists recommends discontinuing herbal remedies 2 weeks before elective surgery.

D.   It has been estimated that one in five Americans taking prescription drugs are also taking vitamins or herbal supplements. The most frequently used herbs are echinacea, gingko biloba, St. John's wort, garlic, and ginseng.

E.   Commonly used herbs and possible anesthetic interactions

   1.   Echinacea (*Echinacea purpura* purple cone flower)

   a.   Uses: for common colds, wounds and burns, urinary tract infections, coughs, and bronchitis (immunostimulation via enhanced phagocytosis and nonspecific T-cell stimulation).

   b.   Problems and interactions: may cause hepatotoxicity or potentiate hepatotoxic effects of anabolic steroids, amiodarone, ketoconazole, or methotrexate. By inhibiting microsomal enzymes, can precipitate toxicity of drugs dependent on hepatic metabolism (e.g., phenytoin, rifampin, or phenobarbital). May decrease effectiveness of corticosteroids and cyclosporine.

   2.   Ephedra (*Ephedra sinica*, Ma Huang)

   a.   Uses: in over-the-counter diet aids; for bacteriostatic, antitussive actions (sympathomimetic with positive inotropic/chronotropic effects; α- and β-adrenergic agonist).

   b.   Problems and interactions: potential interactions with cardiac glycosides and halothane (arrhythmias); guanethidine (enhanced sympathomimetic effects); monoamine oxidase inhibitors (MAOIs; enhanced sympathomimetic effects); oxytocin (hypertension); intraoperative hypotension better treated with phenylephrine than ephedrine.

   3.   Feverfew (*Tanacetum parthenium*)

   a.   Uses: as migraine prophylactic, and antipyretic (inhibits serotonin release from aggregating platelets via inhibition of arachidonic acid release).

   b.   Problems and interactions: can inhibit platelet activity (potentiate anticoagulants); rebound headache with sudden cessation; 5% to 15% develop aphthous ulcers or gastrointestinal irritation. Like other tannin-containing herbs, feverfew can interact with iron preparations and decrease bioavailability.

   4.   Garlic (*Allium sativum*)

   a.   Uses: for lipid lowering, vasodilatory, antihypertensive, antiplatelet, antioxidant, and antithrombotic/fibrinolytic qualities.

   b.   Problems and interactions: may potentiate effects of warfarin. A case of spontaneous epidural hematoma has been reported.

   5.   Ginger (*Zingiber officinalis*)

   a.   Uses: for antiemetic, antivertigo, and antispasmodic effects.

   b.   Problems and interactions: potent inhibitor of thromboxane synthetase; can potentiate anticoagulant effects of other medications.

6. **Ginkgo** (*Ginkgo biloba*, maidenhair tree)
   a. Uses: as a circulatory stimulant; antioxidant; for intermittent claudication, tinnitus, vertigo, memory loss, dementia, and sexual dysfunction (inhibits platelet-activating factor, modulates nitric oxide, has anti-inflammatory effects).
   b. Problems and interactions: may enhance bleeding in patients already on anticoagulant or antithrombotic therapy (e.g., aspirin, nonsteroidal anti-inflammatory drugs, warfarin, heparin). Cases of spontaneous subarachnoid hemorrhage and subdural hematomas have been reported. May decrease effectiveness of anticonvulsant drugs (e.g., carbamazepine, phenytoin, and phenobarbital).

7. **Ginseng** (*Panax ginseng*)
   a. Uses: to enhance energy level, and for antioxidant and reported aphrodisiac effects (thought to augment adrenal steroidogenesis via a centrally mediated mechanism).
   b. Problems and interactions: "ginseng abuse syndrome" (more than 15 g per day) characterized by sleepiness, hypertonia, and edema. May see tachycardia or hypertension with other stimulants; hypotension intraoperatively; mastalgia; postmenopausal bleeding; mania in patients on MAOIs (phenelzine); and decreased effectiveness of warfarin. Hypoglycemic effect may necessitate monitoring in diabetics or neurosurgical patients receiving steroids.

8. **Goldenseal** (*Hydrastis canadensis*, turmeric root)
   a. Uses: as diuretic, anti-inflammatory, laxative.
   b. Problems and interactions: functions as an oxytocic; overdose may cause paralysis (amount not known); free water diuresis (no sodium excreted, just free water); electrolyte abnormalities; hypertension.

9. **Kava-kava** (*Piper methysticum*)
   a. Uses: as anxiolytic, treatment for gonorrhea, skin diseases.
   b. Problems and interactions: thought to inhibit norepinephrine; potentiates sedating effects of barbiturates, benzodiazepines; can potentiate ethanol effects. Increased suicide risk in patients with endogenous depression.

10. **Licorice** (*Glycyrrhiza glabra*)
    a. Uses: for gastritis, gastric, and duodenal ulcers; and cough and bronchitis.
    b. Problems and interactions: glycyrrhizic acid in licorice may cause hypertension, hypokalemia, and edema. Contraindicated in many chronic liver conditions, renal insufficiency, hypertonia, hypokalemia.

11. **Saw palmetto** (*Serenoa repens*, cabbage palm)
    a. Uses: for treatment of benign prostatitic hypertrophy; has an antiandrogenic effect.
    b. Problems and interactions: may see additive effects with other hormone therapies (including oral contraceptives and estrogen replacement therapy).

12. **St. John's wort** (*Hypericum perforatum*, goat weed)
    a. Uses: for depression, anxiety, sleep disorders, vitiligo

(may inhibit monoamine oxidase, gamma-aminobutyric acid, and serotonin receptors).

b. Problems and interactions: possible interaction with MAOIs, may prolong effects of anesthesia, and may photosensitize. Potential serotoninergic syndrome (tremors, hypertonicity, autonomic dysfunction, and hyperthermia) with concomitant beta-sympathomimetic amines or selective serotonin reuptake inhibitors, including fluoxetine, paroxetine.

   13. Valerian (*Valeriana officinalis*, all-heal, vandal root)

   a. Uses: has mild sedative and anxiolytic properties.

   b. Problems and interactions: potentiates effects of barbiturates, may decrease symptoms of benzodiazepine withdrawal, and prolong anesthetic actions.

SUGGESTED READING

American Society of Anesthesiologists. What you should know about your patient's use of herbal medicines. Available at *http://www.asahq.-org*. Accessed on April 29, 2002.

Astin JA. Why patients use alternative medicine: results of a national study. *JAMA* 1998;279:1548–1553.

Eisenberg DM. Advising patients who seek alternative medical therapies. *Ann Intern Med* 1997;27:61–69.

Eisenberg DM, Davis RB, Ettner SL, et al. Trends in alternative medicine use in the United States, 1990–1997: results of a follow-up national survey. *JAMA* 1998;280:1569–1575.

Jonas W, Levin J, eds. *Essentials of complementary and alternative medicine.* Philadelphia: Williams & Wilkins, 1999.

Kuhn M. *Complementary therapies for health care providers.* Baltimore, MD: Lippincott Williams & Wilkins, 1999.

Meurisse M, Hamoir E, Defechereaux T, et al. Bilateral neck exploration under hypnosedation: a new standard of care in primary hyperparathyroidism. *Ann Surg* 1999;229:401–408.

Miller LG. Herbal medicinals: selected clinical considerations focussing on known or potential drug-herb interactions. *Arch Intern Med* 1998;158:2200–2211.

National Center for Complementary and Alternative Medicine. Major domains of complementary and alternative medicine. Available at: *http://www.nccam.nih.gov*. Accessed on April 29, 2002.

Tsen LC, Segal S, Pothier M, et al. Alternative medicine use in presurgical patients. *Anesthesiology* 2000;93:148–151.

Ethical and End-of-Life Issues

William E. Hurford and Rae M. Allain

This chapter explores ethical issues that frequently arise in anesthetic practice. Customs, laws, ethical beliefs, and religious practices vary among cultures and societies. This chapter describes the prevailing practice at the Massachusetts General Hospital in Boston, Massachusetts.

I. Decisions concerning treatment

A. Patient autonomy (i.e., respect for an individual's preferences) is a highly valued guiding ethical principle in U.S. medicine. Competent adult patients can and may choose to accept or refuse medical therapies. If a patient's competence is questionable, a psychiatrist should evaluate the patient to determine if he or she has decision-making capacity. This requires an ability to receive and understand medical information, to discern the various options presented, and to choose a course based on the information offered and one's values.

B. Autonomy is best preserved by obtaining the patient's **informed consent** for procedures and therapies whenever possible (see Chapter 1). Frequently, critically ill patients are incompetent to make medical decisions because of the gravity of their illness or because of sedative/analgesic medications employed to diminish suffering.

1. An **advance directive** (**or "living will"**), a document specifying the types of treatment that the patient wishes to receive or reject should future need arise, is very useful in this circumstance.

2. In addition to or in the absence of an advance directive, a patient may designate a **surrogate** (health care proxy or health care power of attorney) who is charged with executing the patient's wishes should he or she become incompetent. The surrogate offers **substituted judgment** for the patient, providing decisions that the patient would make if competent. If the patient has not designated a surrogate prior to becoming incompetent, the next of kin may become the de facto surrogate. In some circumstances where no family is living or available, a trusted friend may act as the patient's surrogate.

3. A court-appointed legal **guardian** may be necessary in rare instances where no family member or friend is able to make decisions in the best interest of the patient.

C. Conflict is best resolved via ongoing discussion with the individuals involved. The anesthetist must recognize and respect cultural differences that influence a patient's decisions. Unresolvable conflict among family members, health care team members, or between the family and the medical care team often is best addressed by the institutional ethics committee (see below).

D. The institutional ethics committee is generally comprised of a group of health care professionals trained in medical ethics.

1. The purpose of the ethics committee is to educate and advise clinicians regarding ethical dilemmas and to enable resolution of ethical conflicts. The ethics committee offers an objective analysis of the patient's case and may draw upon basic ethical principles to guide the patient, physician, and family to a consensus about the therapeutic course. Ideally, the ethics committee should be accessible to all members of the health care team and to the patient and family. This diminishes inequalities of power present in the hospital environment and promotes a climate of respect for all viewpoints.

2. When the ethics committee is requested to consult on a case, the question to be answered or the nature of the conflict should be clearly stated. The patient's condition and prognosis should be documented. Members of the ethics committee may help organize and/or attend a family meeting in order to facilitate decision making.

3. The ethics committee uses guiding ethical principles to make recommendations to the health care team, the patient, and/or the family. The role is one of expert consultant, not arbiter in a dispute. In rare situations where irreconcilable differences exist between the physician and the patient and/or family, care of the patient may be transferred to another accepting attending physician. It is even more extraordinary for ethical conflicts to reach resolution by judicial intervention.

E. The pediatric patient deserves special consideration when ethical issues are confronted. Legally, such decisions are deferred to the parents. Ethically, the child may participate in these decisions depending upon his or her developmental level and decision-making capacity. If the child is too immature to participate in decisions, parents are relied upon to make decisions in the child's best interest by weighing the benefit versus burden of the planned therapy. Pediatric anesthetists must be sensitive to individual family dynamics and parenting styles when approaching such discussions.

F. Jehovah's Witness patients generally may refuse to receive blood or blood products (e.g., fresh-frozen plasma, platelets, cryoprecipitate, or albumin) based on their religious beliefs, even if such refusal results in death. Some patients may accept autotransfused or chest-tube–salvaged autologous blood, especially if it remains in contiguous circulation with their vasculature. Special considerations regarding homologous transfusion may apply if the patient is a minor, is incompetent, or has responsibilities for dependents, and in certain emergency circumstances. An ethical dilemma may present when unexpected hemorrhage is encountered following a preoperative agreement not to transfuse. Careful documentation of preoperative discussions and informed consent is mandatory. Legal precedent generally supports patient autonomy regarding the acceptance of transfusion.

G. "Do not resuscitate (DNR)" orders in the operating room are not automatically suspended, as is often thought. Each institution should have written guidelines on this situation. In advance of a procedure, physicians and the patient with the DNR status or the patient's health care proxy should clarify any resuscitative measures that would be compatible with the patient's wishes and the demands of the planned procedure (see also Chapter 36, section III.B.8).

II. Determination of death using brain criteria

    A. "**Brain death**" is a term used to connote that death had been determined via evaluation of brain function. Brain death must be understood to be no different from a diagnosis of death made by cardiac criteria. Practically, the diagnosis of brain death means that a patient can potentially become an organ donor on the conditions of consent and medical acceptability. **Locally accepted guidelines** are used to establish the diagnosis of brain death. Diagnostic criteria for the clinical diagnosis of brain death in adults, adapted from those used at the Massachusetts General Hospital, are summarized below. Other institutions may have different criteria.

    B. **Brain death is a clinical syndrome** of coma or unresponsiveness, absence of brain stem reflexes, and apnea in which the proximate cause is known and demonstrably irreversible. Prerequisites include:

        1. Evidence of an acute central nervous system catastrophe that is compatible with brain death.

        2. Exclusion of complicating medical conditions that may confound clinical assessment (e.g., severe electrolyte, acid-base, or endocrine disturbance).

        3. No evidence of drug intoxication or poisoning.

        4. Demonstrated absence of neuromuscular blockade if the patient has had recent or prolonged use of muscle relaxants.

        5. Core temperature greater than 32°C (90°F).

        6. In the presence of confounding variables, brain death may still be determined with the aid of ancillary testing (see below). A period of observation of at least 24 hours without clinical neurologic change is necessary if the cause of the coma is unknown.

    C. **Many clinical conditions may interfere** with the clinical diagnosis of brain death, so that the diagnosis cannot be made with certainty on clinical grounds alone. In such cases, confirmatory tests are recommended.

    D. **Confirmatory laboratory tests** that may support the diagnosis of brain death include angiography, electroencephalography, transcranial Doppler ultrasonography, and technetium 99m hexamethylpropyleneamine oxime (HMPAO) brain scanning.

III. Organ donation. Some patients declared brain dead, usually those suffering from traumatic head injury or devastating intracranial event, may be eligible for tissue or organ donation.

    A. **Conversations with the family** regarding organ donation must be done tactfully and in consultation with trained professionals from the regional organ procurement agency. Ideally, the discussion should be coordinated by a physician with whom the family has developed a rapport. The topic may be introduced by asking the family if the deceased had ever expressed an opinion regarding use of his organs after death. Many families are consoled by the thought that their loved one's body parts may be lifesaving to another individual and may in some sense carry on the life that has been lost.

    B. **Early contact** with the organ procurement agency is important in cases of potential organ donors. Organ procurement agencies generally have specific preferences regarding medications (such as vasopressors and diuretics), mechanical ventilator settings, and laboratory blood work to be performed. These should be known to the anesthetist.

C. **Care of the patient** for organ donation is challenging. Problems frequently encountered include hypotension, arrhythmias, hypoxemia, and diabetes insipidus. If a successful donation is to occur, a vigilant anesthetist, in concert with direction from the organ procurement agency, is necessary.

D. If the institutional transplant team will participate in harvesting or transplanting organs, it is prudent to establish contact with the team and immediately apprise them of any change in the donor's condition that might warrant expedited harvest.

IV. **Supporting survivors**

A. **Support** of the patient's survivors following a death begins with honest, frequent, and compassionate communication from the medical team.

B. **Cultural background and individual values** will affect each conversation. The medical team should strive for flexibility when presented with each situation.

1. The medical social worker may an important source for understanding the family's religious and cultural background.

2. Many patients and families find solace in the presence of clergy. If so, arrangements should be made for the patient's own religious representative or a hospital-based chaplain to be available.

V. **Legal considerations.** Physicians who engage in honest, open communication with patients and their families about ethical and end-of-life issues should rarely find themselves resolving such issues in a court of law. Nevertheless, several recent judicial rulings have implications that may prove useful to the clinician when confronted with ethical issues.

A. **Patient autonomy is primary in decision making.** That patients may refuse life-sustaining or other therapies has been repeatedly affirmed. Wishes of the patient may be expressed via advance directives or, lacking this, via prior voiced opinion. The role of a surrogate in providing substituted judgment has been supported.

B. **Human life has qualification beyond mere biologic existence.** Thus, a surrogate's decision to withdraw care may be based on the potential for meaningful existence ("**quality of life**").

C. **Care once rendered may be withdrawn.** The idea that a life-sustaining therapy that has been implemented can never be stopped is not valid.

D. **End-of-life decisions are best addressed by the physician and the patient and/or family** with help from institutional facilitators (e.g., ethics committee) as needed. Permission to withdraw or withhold a therapy does not require a "court order."

E. **Withdrawal of hydration or nutritional support is not legally different from withdrawal of other life support.** In addition to legal decisions, this stance has been supported by numerous medical societies, including the American Medical Association and the American Academy of Neurology.

F. **Physicians are not bound to provide care that they deem**

futile. While still somewhat controversial, the latter was supported by a jury decision involving a patient at the Massachusetts General Hospital from whom ventilatory support was withdrawn despite the objection of one family member. It is advisable for a physician, however, to pursue every avenue of conflict resolution, including removing herself or himself from the care of a patient, before exercising this dictum against a family's wishes.

G.   For unusual or questionable cases, it is appropriate to seek the advice of the institutional legal counsel before acting on decisions.

SUGGESTED READING

Brody H, Campbell ML, Faber-Langendoen KF, et al. Withdrawing intensive life-sustaining treatment: recommendations for compassionate clinical management. *N Engl J Med* 1997;336:652–656.

Luce JM. Physicians do not have a responsibility to provide futile or unreasonable care if a patient or family insists. *Crit Care Med* 1995; 23:760–766.

Luce JM. Withholding and withdrawal of life support: ethical, legal, and clinical aspects. *New Horiz* 1997;5:30–37.

Meisel A. Legal myths about terminating life support. *Arch Intern Med* 1991;151:1497–1502.

Murphy DJ, Burrows D, Santilli S, et al. The influence of the probability of survival on patients' preferences regarding cardiopulmonary resuscitation. *N Engl J Med* 1994;330:545–549.

Prendergast TJ. Resolving conflicts surrounding end-of-life care. *New Horiz* 1997;5:62–71.

Schneiderman LJ, Jecker NS, Jonsen AR. Medical futility: its meaning and ethical implications. *Ann Intern Med* 1990;112:949–954.

Todres ID, Armstrong A, Lally P, et al. Negotiating end-of-life issues. *New Horiz* 1998;6:374–382.

Supplemental Drug Information

Abiciximab (Reopro)

Indications	Prevents thrombus formation after percutaneous transluminal coronary angioplasty (PTCA) and after stent placement.
Dosage	Bolus (0.25 mg/kg) administered 10–60 min prior to PTCA.
Effect	Inhibits glycoprotein IIB/IIIA; prevents platelet adhesion and aggregation.
Clearance	Remains in circulation for ≥15 days in a platelet-bound state.
Comments	Anaphylaxis may occur; hypotension with bolus dose. Bleeding complications and thrombocytopenia are common side effects.

Acetazolamide (Diamox)

Indications	Respiratory acidosis with metabolic alkalosis. Increased intraocular and intracranial pressures.
Dosage	125–500 mg IV over 1 to 2 min or PO not to exceed 2 g in 24 h.
Effect	Inhibits carbonic anhydrase, which results in increased excretion of bicarbonate.
Clearance	70% to 100% excreted unchanged in the urine within 24 h.
Comments	May increase insulin requirements in diabetic patients; cause renal calculi in patients with past history of calcium stones; cause hypokalemia, thrombocytopenia, aplastic anemia, increased urinary excretion of uric acid, and hyperglycemia. Initial dose may produce marked diuresis. Tolerance to desired effects of acetazolamide occurs in 2 to 3 days. Rare hypersensitivity reaction in patients with sulfa allergies.

Adenosine (Adenocard)

Indications	Paroxysmal supraventricular tachycardia, Wolff–Parkinson–White syndrome.
Dosage	Adult: 6–12 mg IV bolus. Pediatric: 50 μg/kg IV.
Effect	Slows or temporarily blocks AV node conduction and conduction though reentrant pathways.
Clearance	RBC and endothelial cell metabolism.
Comments	The effects of adenosine are antagonized by methyl-

xanthines such as theophylline. Adenosine is contraindicated in patients with second- or third-degree heart block or sick sinus syndrome. When large doses are given by infusion, hypotension can occur. Not effective in atrial flutter or fibrillation. Asystole for 3–6 s after administration is common.

Albuterol (Proventil, Ventolin)

Indications	Bronchospasm.
Dose	Aerosolized: 2.5 mg in 3 mL saline via nebulizer; 180 or 200 μg (2 puffs) via inhaler. PO: 2.5 mg. Pediatric: 0.1 mg/kg (syrup 2 mg/5 mL).
Effect	Beta$_2$-receptor agonist.
Comments	Possible β-adrenergic overload, tachyarrhythmias.

Aminocaproic Acid (Amicar)

Indications	Hemorrhage due to fibrinolysis.
Dosage	5 g/100–250 mL of NSS IV to load, followed by 1 g/h infusion.
Effect	Stabilizes clot formation by inhibiting plasminogen activators and plasmin.
Clearance	Primarily renal elimination.
Comments	Contraindicated in disseminated intravascular coagulation.

Aminophylline (Theophylline Ethylenediamine)

Indications	Bronchospasm, infantile apneic spells.
Dosage	Adult: LOAD—5.0 mg/kg IV at <25 mg/min; MAINT—0.5–0.7 mg/kg/h IV. Lower dose in elderly, CHF, hepatic disease. Pediatric: 1 mo–1 yr, 0.16–0.7 mg/kg/h; 1–9 yr, 0.8 mg/kg/h.
Effect	Inhibits phosphodiesterase, antagonizes adenosine, resulting in bronchodilation and positive inotropic and chronotropic effects.
Clearance	Hepatic metabolism; renal elimination (10% unchanged).
Comments	May cause tachyarrhythmias. Therapeutic concentration, 10–20 μg/mL. Aminophylline 100 mg = Theophylline 80 mg.

Amiodarone (Cordarone)

Indications	Refractory or recurrent ventricular tachycardia or ventricular fibrillation.

Dosage	LOAD: 800–1,600 mg/day PO × 1–3 weeks, then 600–800 mg/day PO × 4 weeks; MAINT: 100–400 mg/day PO; IV: 150 to 300 mg over 10 min (15 mg/min), 360 mg over the next 6 h (1 mg/min), then 540 mg over the next 18 h (0.5 mg/min).
Effect	Depresses the sinoatrial node and prolongs the PR, QRS, and QT intervals; produces α- and β-adrenergic blockade.
Clearance	Biliary elimination.
Comments	May cause severe sinus bradycardia, ventricular arrhythmias, AV block, liver and thyroid function test abnormalities, hepatitis, and cirrhosis. Pulmonary fibrosis can result from long-term use. Increases serum levels of digoxin, oral anticoagulants, diltiazem, quinidine, procainamide, and phenytoin.

Amrinone (Inocor)

Indication	Acute ventricular failure.
Dosage	0.75 mg/kg IV bolus over several minutes, then infuse at 5–10 μg/kg/min. Infusion mixtures (usually 100 mg in 250 mL) must not contain dextrose.
Effect	Inhibits phosphodiesterase, which results in increased cardiac output, increased contractility, and direct vasodilation.
Clearance	Variable hepatic metabolism; renal/fecal excretion.
Comments	May cause hypotension, thrombocytopenia, and anaphylaxis (contains sulfites).

Aprotinin (Trasylol)

Indications	Prophylactic reduction in perioperative blood loss in patients undergoing cardiopulmonary bypass.
Dosage	Supplied as 10,000 KIU (Kallikrein inhibitor units)/mL or 1.4 mg/mL. One-milliliter test dose followed by LOAD: 1–2 million KIU (100–200 mL) IV over 20–30 min; "pump prime": 1–2 million KIU; MAINT: 250,000–500,000 KIU/h (25–50 mL/h).
Effect	Protease inhibitor of trypsin, plasmin, and kallikrein. Antifibrinolytic. Protects glycoprotein Ib receptor on platelets during cardiopulmonary bypass.
Clearance	Renal elimination.
Comments	Rapid administration may cause transient hypotension. Anaphylactic reaction in <0.5% of patients.

Atenolol (Tenormin)

Indications	Hypertension, angina, postmyocardial infarction (MI).

Dosage	PO: 50–100 mg/day. IV: 5 mg prn.
Effect	Beta$_1$-selective adrenergic receptor blockade.
Clearance	Renal, intestinal elimination.
Comments	High doses block β$_2$-adrenergic receptors. Relatively contraindicated in congestive heart failure, asthma, and heart block. Caution in patients on calcium-channel blockers. Rebound angina can occur with abrupt cessation.

Atropine

Indications	**1.** Antisialagogue. **2.** Bradycardia.
Dosage	Adult: **1.** 0.2–0.4 mg IV. **2.** 0.4–1.0 mg IV. Pediatric: **1.** 0.01 mg/kg/dose IV/IM (<0.4 mg). **2.** 0.02 mg/kg/dose IV (<0.4 mg).
Effect	Competitive blockade of acetylcholine at muscarinic receptors.
Clearance	50%–70% hepatic metabolism; renal elimination.
Comments	May cause tachyarrhythmias, AV dissociation, premature ventricular contractions, dry mouth, or urinary retention. CNS effects occur at high doses.

Bicarbonate, Sodium (NaHCO$_3$)

Indications	Metabolic acidosis.
Dosage	IV dose in mEq NaHCO$_3$ = (base deficit × weight [kg] × 0.3) (subsequent doses titrated against patient's pH).
Effect	H+ neutralization.
Clearance	Plasma metabolism; pulmonary, renal elimination.
Comments	May cause metabolic alkalosis, hypercarbia, and hyperosmolality. In neonates, can cause intraventricular hemorrhage. Crosses placenta. An 8.4% solution is approximately 1.0 mEq/mL; a 4.2% solution is approximately 0.5 mEq/mL.

Bumetanide (Bumex)

Indications	Edema, hypertension, intracranial hypertension.
Dosage	0.5–1.0 mg IV, repeated to a maximum of 10 mg/day.
Effect	Loop diuretic with principal effect on the ascending limb of the loop of Henle. Causes increased excretion of Na$^+$, K$^+$, Cl$^-$, and H$_2$O.
Clearance	Hepatic metabolism; 81% renal excretion (45% unchanged).
Comments	May cause electrolyte imbalance, dehydration, and deafness. Patients who are allergic to sulfonamides

may show hypersensitivity to bumetanide. Effective in renal insufficiency.

Calcium Chloride (CaCl$_2$); Calcium Gluconate (Kalcinate)

Indications	Hypocalcemia, hyperkalemia, hypermagnesemia.
Dosage	Calcium chloride: 5–10 mg/kg IV prn (10% CaCl$_2$ = 1.36 mEq Ca^{2+}/mL). Calcium gluconate: 15–30 mg/kg IV prn (10% calcium gluconate = 0.45 mEq Ca^{2+}/mL).
Effect	Maintains cell membrane integrity, muscular excitation–contraction coupling, glandular stimulation–secretion coupling, and enzyme function. Increases blood pressure.
Clearance	Incorporated into muscle, bone, and other tissues. Renal excretion.
Comments	May cause bradycardia or arrhythmia (especially with digitalis). Irritating to veins. Ca^{2+} less available with calcium gluconate than with calcium chloride due to binding of gluconate.

Captopril (Capoten)

Indications	Hypertension, congestive heart failure.
Dosage	LOAD: 12.5–25.0 mg PO bid; MAINT: 25–150 mg PO bid.
Effect	Angiotensin I-converting enzyme inhibition decreases angiotensin II and aldosterone levels. Reduces both preload and afterload in patients with congestive heart failure.
Clearance	Hepatic metabolism; 95% renal elimination (40%–50% unchanged).
Comments	May be used in hypertensive emergency. May cause neutropenia, agranulocytosis, hypotension, or bronchospasm. Avoid in pregnant patients. Exaggerated response in renal artery stenosis and with diuretics.

Cimetidine (Tagamet)

Indications	Pulmonary aspiration prophylaxis (reduction of gastric volume and acidity), gastroesophageal reflux, gastric acid hypersecretion, anaphylaxis prophylaxis.
Dosage	300 mg q 6h IV/IM/PO (q 12h in renal failure).
Effect	Antagonizes action of histamine on H$_2$ receptors, with inhibition of gastric acid secretion.

Clearance	Hepatic metabolism; 75% renal elimination (unchanged) (IV dose).
Comments	May cause small increases in creatinine levels, increases concentration of many drugs due to inhibition of oxidative drug metabolism. Can produce confusion or somnolence with repeated dosing. Venous irritation.

Chlorothiazide (Diuril)

Indications	Edema in heart failure, acute or chronic renal failure; hypertension.
Dosage	Adult: 250–500 mg IV bolus at 50–100 mg/min, 2 g maximum over 24 h. Pediatric: oral, 20 mg/kg/day in two divided doses every 12 h.
Effect	Thiazide diuretic.
Clearance	Renal elimination.
Comments	Enhances activity of antihypertensives, digoxin. May enhance activity of loop diuretics in renal failure. May increase insulin requirements in diabetic patients.

Citrate, Sodium Dihydrate/Citric Acid Monohydrate (Bicitra)

Indications	Gastric acid neutralization.
Dosage	15 mL in 15 mL water PO (500 mg sodium citrate, 334 mg citric acid per 5 mL).
Effect	Absorbed and metabolized to sodium bicarbonate.
Clearance	Oxidation; 5% excreted in urine (unchanged).
Comments	Contraindicated in patients with sodium restriction or severe renal impairment. Do not use with aluminum-based antacids.

Clonidine (Catapres)

Indications	Hypertension; autonomic hyperactivity secondary to drug withdrawal.
Dosage	0.1–1.2 mg/day PO in divided doses (2.4 mg/day maximum dose). Also available as a transdermal patch delivering 0.1, 0.2, or 0.3 mg/day for 7 days.
Effect	Central α_2-adrenergic agonist; decreases systemic vascular resistance and heart rate.
Clearance	50% hepatic metabolism; elimination 20% biliary, 80% renal.
Comments	Abrupt withdrawal may cause rebound hypertension or arrhythmias. Can cause drowsiness, nightmares, restlessness, anxiety, or depression. Intravenous in-

jection may cause transient peripheral α-adrenergic stimulation.

Dalteparin (Fragmin)

Indications	**1.** Prophylaxis of deep venous thrombosis. **2.** Acute coronary syndromes. **3.** Deep venous thrombosis.
Dosage	**1.** 2,500–5,000 units SC qd. **2.** 120 units/kg (maximum dose 10,000 units) SC q 12h × 5–8 days with concurrent aspirin therapy. **3.** 100 units/kg SC bid or 200 units/kg SC qd.
Effect	Anticoagulant; inhibits both factor Xa and factor IIa. See heparin.
Clearance	Hepatic; renal excretion.
Comments	Equally effective as unfractionated heparin; more predictable dose–response characteristics. Spinal and epidural hematomas have been associated with spinal and epidural anesthesia and lumbar punctures in patients receiving fractionated heparins or heparinoids. The risk of epidural hematoma formation is increased in patients who have indwelling epidural catheters or are also receiving other drugs that may adversely affect hemostasis. Safety and efficacy in pediatric patients not established. Rarely causes thrombocytopenia.

Danaparoid (Orgaran)

Indications	**1.** Prophylaxis of deep venous thrombosis following elective hip replacement surgery. **2.** Systemic anticoagulation for patients with heparin-induced thrombocytopenia.
Dosage	**1.** 750 anti-Xa units SC bid. **2.** IV or SC; dose is dependent on indication and patient weight, and generally guided by monitoring anti-Xa activity.
Effect	Anticoagulant; prevents fibrin formation via thrombin generation inhibition by anti-Xa and anti-IIa effects,.
Clearance	Renal elimination.
Comments	Bleeding can occur, as with other anticoagulants. Monitoring accomplished by measuring anti-Xa activity. Monitoring PT and aPTT is not necessary. Spinal and epidural hematomas have been associated with spinal and epidural anesthesia and lumbar punctures in patients receiving fractionated heparins or heparinoids. The risk of epidural hematoma formation is increased in patients who have indwelling epidural catheters or are also receiving other drugs that may adversely affect hemostasis. Safety and efficacy in pediatric patients not established. Rarely causes thrombocytopenia.

Dantrolene (Dantrium)

Indications	Malignant hyperthermia (MH); skeletal muscle spasticity.
Dosage	Mix 20 mg in 60 mL of sterile water. At first signs of MH, 2.5 mg/kg IV bolus; if signs persist after 30 min, repeat dose, up to 10 mg/kg. Prophylactic IV treatment is not recommended.
Effect	Reduces Ca^{2+} release from sarcoplasmic reticulum.
Clearance	Hepatic metabolism; renal elimination.
Comments	Dissolves slowly into solution. May cause muscle weakness, gastrointestinal upset, drowsiness, sedation, or abnormal liver function (chronically). Additive to effects of neuromuscular blocking agents. Tissue irritant.

Desmopressin Acetate (DDAVP)

Indications	1. Treatment of coagulopathy in von Willebrand's disease, hemophilia A, renal failure. 2. Antidiuretic.
Dosage	Adult: 1. 0.3 µg/kg IV (diluted 50 mL NSS), infused over 15–30 min. 2. 2–4 µg/day usually in two divided doses. Pediatric: <10 kg, dilute adult dose in 10 mL NSS; >10 kg, see adult dose.
Effect	Increases plasma levels of factor-VIII activity by causing release of von Willebrand's factor from endothelial cells; increases renal water reabsorption.
Clearance	Renal elimination.
Comments	Chlorpropamide, carbamazepine, and clofibrate potentiate the antidiuretic effect. Repeat doses q 12–24h will have diminished effect compared with initial dose.

Dexamethasone (Decadron)

Indications	Cerebral edema from CNS tumors; airway edema.
Dosage	LOAD: 10 mg IV. MAINT: 4 mg IV q 6h (tapered over 6 days).
Effect	See hydrocortisone. Has 25 times the glucocorticoid potency of hydrocortisone. Minimal mineralocorticoid effect.
Clearance	Primarily hepatic metabolism; renal elimination.
Comments	See hydrocortisone.

Dextran 40 (Rheomacrodex)

Indications	Inhibition of platelet aggregation; improvement of blood flow in low-flow states (e.g., vascular surgery); intravascular volume expansion.

Dosage	Adult: LOAD: 30–50 mL IV over 30 min; MAINT: 15–30 mL/h IV (10% solution). Pediatric: <20 mL/kg/ 24 h of 10% dextran.
Effect	Immediate, short-lived plasma volume expansion; adsorption to RBC surface prevents RBC aggregation, decreases blood viscosity and platelet adhesiveness.
Clearance	Renal elimination.
Comments	Administer Promit (dextran monomer), 20 mL IV, prior to giving dextran 40 to minimize the risk of anaphylaxis. May cause volume overload, anaphylaxis, bleeding tendency, interference with blood cross-matching, or false elevation of blood sugar. Renal failure has been reported.

Digoxin (Lanoxin)

Indications	Heart failure, tachyarrhythmias, atrial fibrillation, atrial flutter.
Dosage	Adult—LOAD: 0.5–1.0 mg/d IV or PO in divided doses; MAINT: 0.125–0.5 mg IV or PO qd. Pediatric (IV/IM in divided doses)—LOAD: Total daily doses usually divided into two or more doses. Neonates, 15–30 µg/kg/day; 1 month–2 yr, 30–50 µg/kg/day; 2–5 yr, 25–35 µg/kg/day; 5–10 yr, 15–30 µg/kg/day; >10 yr, 8–12 µg/kg/day. MAINT: 20%–35% of LOAD qd (reduce in renal failure).
Effect	Increases myocardial contractility; decreases conduction in AV node and Purkinje fibers.
Clearance	Renal elimination (50%–70% unchanged).
Comments	May cause gastrointestinal intolerance, blurred vision, ECG changes, or arrhythmias. Toxicity potentiated by hypokalemia, hypomagnesemia, hypercalcemia. Use cautiously in Wolff–Parkinson–White syndrome and with defibrillation. Heart block potentiated by beta blockade and calcium-channel blockade.

Diltiazem (Cardizem)

Indications	Angina pectoris, variant angina from coronary artery spasm, atrial fibrillation/flutter, paroxysmal supraventricular tachycardia, hypertension.
Dosage	PO: 30–60 mg q 6h. IV: 20 mg bolus then 10 mg/h infusion.
Effect	Calcium channel antagonist that slows conduction though sinoatrial and AV nodes, dilates coronary and peripheral arterioles, and reduces myocardial contractility.
Clearance	Primarily hepatic metabolism; renal elimination.
Comments	May cause bradycardia and heart block. May interact

with beta-blockers and digoxin to impair contractility. Causes transiently elevated liver function tests. Avoid use in patients with accessory conduction tracts, AV block, IV beta-blockers, or ventricular tachycardia. Active metabolite has $\frac{1}{4}$–$\frac{1}{2}$ of the coronary dilation effect.

Diphenhydramine (Benadryl)

Indications	Allergic reactions, drug-induced extrapyramidal reactions; induction of sedation.
Dosage	Adult: 10–50 mg IV q 6–8h. Pediatric: 5.0 mg/kg/day IV in 4 divided doses (maximum 300 mg).
Effect	Antagonizes action of histamine on H_1 receptors; anticholinergic; CNS depressant.
Clearance	Hepatic metabolism; renal excretion.
Comments	May cause hypotension, tachycardia, dizziness, urinary retention, seizures.

Dobutamine (Dobutrex)

Indications	Heart failure, hypotension.
Dosage	Infusion mix: 250 mg in 250 mL of 5% D/W or NSS. Adult: Begin infusion at 2 µg/kg/min and titrate to effect. Pediatric: 5–20 µg/kg/min.
Effect	Beta$_1$-adrenergic agonist.
Clearance	Hepatic metabolism; renal elimination.
Comments	May cause hypertension, arrhythmias, or myocardial ischemia. Can increase ventricular rate in atrial fibrillation.

Dopamine (Intropin)

Indications	1. Hypotension, heart failure. 2. Oliguria.
Dosage	Infusion mix: 200–800 mg in 250 mL of 5% D/W or NSS. 1. Infusion at 5–20 µg/kg/min IV titrate to effect. 2. Infusion at 1–3 µg/kg/min IV.
Effect	Dopaminergic; α- and β-adrenergic agonist.
Clearance	MAO/COMT metabolism.
Comments	May cause hypertension, arrhythmias, or myocardial ischemia. Primarily dopaminergic effects (increased renal blood flow) at 1–5 µg/kg/min. Primarily α- and β-adrenergic effects at ≥10 µg/kg/min.

Doxazosin (Cardura)

Indications	Hypertension.
Dosage	Starting 1 mg PO qd, may be slowly increased (over

weeks) to 4 to 16 mg PO qd depending on individual patient's response.

Effect   Alpha$_1$ (postjunctional) adrenergic antagonist.

Clearance   Hepatic metabolism predominates.

Comments   Significant "first-dose" effect with marked postural hypotension and dizziness. Maximum reductions of blood pressure with 2 to 6 h of dosing.

Droperidol (Inapsine)

Indications   1. Nausea, vomiting. 2. Agitation; adjunct to anesthesia.

Dosage   Adult: 1. 0.625–2.5 mg IV prn. 2. 2.5–10 mg IV prn. Pediatric: 1. 0.05–0.06 mg/kg q 4–6 h.

Effect   Dopamine (D$_2$) receptor antagonist. Apparent psychic indifference to environment, catatonia, antipsychotic, antiemetic.

Clearance   Hepatic metabolism; renal excretion.

Comments   Cases of QT prolongation and/or torsades de pointes have been related to droperidol use, even at doses at or below the recommended range; some cases have been fatal. Droperidol is contraindicated in patients with known or suspected QT prolongation. Droperidol should be reserved for patients failing other therapies, and only after determining that QT prolongation does not exist. Electrocardiographic monitoring is recommended prior to treatment and for 2 to 3 hours after treatment.

Enalapril/Enalaprilat (Vasotec)

Indications   Hypertension, congestive heart failure.

Dosage   PO: LOAD, 2.5–5.0 mg qd; MAINT, 10–40 mg qd; IV, 0.125–5.0 mg q 6h (as enalaprilat).

Effect   Angiotensin-converting enzyme inhibitor; synergistic with diuretics.

Clearance   Hepatic metabolism of enalapril to active metabolite (enalaprilat); renal and fecal elimination.

Comments   Causes increased serum potassium, increased renal blood flow, volume-responsive hypotension. Subsequent doses are additive in effect. Can cause angioedema, blood dyscrasia, cough, lithium toxicity, or worsening of renal impairment.

Enoxaparin (Lovenox)

Indications   1. Prophylaxis of deep venous thrombosis. 2. Acute coronary syndromes. 3. Deep venous thrombosis.

Dosage	**1.** 30 mg SC bid or 40 mg SC qd. **2.** 1 mg/kg SC bid for a minimum of 2 days, in conjunction with aspirin therapy. **3.** 1 mg/kg SC q 12h or 1.5 mg/kg SC qd.
Effect	Anticoagulant; inhibits both factor Xa and factor IIa. See heparin.
Clearance	Hepatic; renal excretion.
Comments	More predictable dose–response characteristics than unfractionated heparin. Appears superior to unfractionated heparin in aspirin-treated patients with unstable angina or non–Q-wave myocardial infarction. Spinal and epidural hematomas have been associated with spinal and epidural anesthesia and lumbar punctures in patients receiving fractionated heparins or heparinoids. The risk of epidural hematoma formation is increased in patients who have indwelling epidural catheters or are also receiving other drugs that may adversely affect hemostasis. Safety and efficacy in pediatric patients not established. Rarely causes thrombocytopenia.

Ephedrine

Indication	Hypotension.
Dosage	5–50 mg IV prn.
Effect	Alpha- and β-adrenergic stimulation; norepinephrine release at sympathetic nerve endings.
Clearance	Mostly renal elimination (unchanged).
Comments	May cause hypertension, arrhythmias, myocardial ischemia, CNS stimulation, decrease in uterine activity, and mild bronchodilation. Minimal effect on uterine blood flow. Avoid in patients taking MAO inhibitors. Tachyphylaxis with repeated dosing.

Epinephrine (Adrenalin)

Indications	**1.** Heart failure, hypotension, cardiac arrest. **2.** Bronchospasm, anaphylaxis.
Dosage	Infusion mix: 1 mg in 250 mL of 5% D/W or NSS. Adult: **1.** 0.1–1 mg IV or 1 mg intratracheal q 5 min prn. **2.** 0.1–0.5 mg SC, 0.1–0.25 mg IV, or 0.25–1.5 μ/min IV infusion. Pediatric: **1.** Neonates, 0.01–0.03 mg/kg IV or intratracheal q 3–5 min; children, 0.01 mg/kg IV or intratracheal q 3–5 h (up to 5 mL 1:10,000). **2.** 0.01 mg/kg IV up to 0.5 mg. 0.01 mg/kg SC q 15 min × 2 doses up to 1 mg/dose.
Effect	Alpha- and β-adrenergic agonist.
Clearance	MAO/COMT metabolism.
Comments	May cause hypertension, arrhythmias, or myocardial ischemia. Arrhythmias potentiated by halothane. Topical or local injection (1:80,000–1:500,000) causes vasoconstriction. Crosses the placenta.

Epinephrine, Racemic (Vaponefrin)

Indications	Airway edema, bronchospasm.
Dosage	Adult: Inhaled via nebulizer—0.5 mL of 2.25% solution in 2.5–3.5 mL of NSS q 1–4h prn. Pediatric: Inhaled via nebulizer—0.5 mL of 2.25% solution in 2.5–3.5 mL of NSS q 4h prn.
Effect	Mucosal vasoconstriction (see also epinephrine [adrenalin]).
Clearance	See epinephrine.
Comments	See epinephrine.

Ergonovine (Ergotrate)

Indication	Postpartum hemorrhage due to uterine atony.
Dosage	For postpartum hemorrhage: IV (emergency only), 0.2 mg in 5 mL of NSS ≥1 min; IM, 0.2 mg q 2–4h prn for ≤5 doses, then PO: 0.2–0.4 mg q 6–12h for 2 days or prn.
Effect	Constriction of uterine and vascular smooth muscle.
Clearance	Hepatic metabolism; renal elimination.
Comments	May cause hypertension from systemic vasoconstriction (especially in eclampsia and hypertension), arrhythmias, coronary spasm, uterine tetany, or gastrointestinal upset. Intravenous route is only used in emergencies. Overdosage may cause convulsions or stroke.

Esmolol (Brevibloc)

Indications	Supraventricular tachyarrhythmias, myocardial ischemia.
Dosage	Start with 5–10 mg IV bolus and increase q 3 min prn to total 100–300 mg; infusion 1–15 mg/min.
Effect	Selective β_1-adrenergic blockade.
Clearance	Degraded by RBC esterases; renal elimination.
Comments	May cause bradycardia, AV conduction delay, hypotension, congestive heart failure; beta$_2$ activity at high doses.

Ethacrynic Acid (Edecrin)

Indications	Edema, congestive heart failure, acute/chronic renal failure.
Dosage	Adult: oral, 50–200 mg/day in 1–2 divided doses; IV, 25–100 mg IV over 5–10 min; 24-h cumulative dose,

400 mg. Pediatric: oral, 25 mg/day to start, increase by 25 mg/day until response is obtained (maximum, 3 mg/kg/day); IV, 1 mg/kg/dose (repeat doses with caution due to potential for ototoxicity).

Effect   Diuretic.

Clearance Hepatically metabolized to active cysteine conjugate (35% to 40%); 30% to 60% excreted unchanged in bile and urine.

Comments May potentiate the activity of antihypertensives, neuromuscular blocking agents, digoxin, and increase insulin requirements in diabetic patients.

Famotidine (Pepcid)

Indications Pulmonary aspiration prophylaxis, peptic ulcer disease.

Dosage 20 mg IV/PO q 12h (dilute in 1–10 mL of 5% D/W or NSS).

Effect Antagonizes action of histamine on H_2 receptors.

Clearance 30%–35% hepatic metabolism; 65%–70% renal elimination.

Comments May cause confusion. Rapid IV administration may increase risk of cardiac arrhythmias and hypotension.

Flumazenil (Mazicon)

Indication **1.** Reversal of benzodiazepine sedation. **2.** Reversal of benzodiazepine overdose.

Dosage **1.** 0.2–1.0 mg IV q 20min at 0.2 mg/min. **2.** 3–5 mg IV at 0.5 mg/min.

Effect Competitive antagonism of CNS benzodiazepine receptor.

Clearance 100% hepatic metabolism; 90%–95% renal elimination of metabolite.

Comments Duration of action dependent on dose and duration of action of administered benzodiazepine and on dose of flumazenil. May induce CNS excitation including seizures, acute withdrawal, nausea, dizziness, and agitation. Does not reverse nonbenzodiazepine induced CNS depression.

Furosemide (Lasix)

Indications Edema, hypertension, intracranial hypertension, renal failure, hypercalcemia.

Dosage Adult: 2–40 mg IV (initial dose, dosage individualized). Pediatric: 1–2 mg/kg/day.

Effect	Increases excretion of Na^+, Cl^-, K^+, PO_4^{3-}, Ca^{2+}, and H_2O by inhibiting reabsorption in loop of Henle.
Clearance	Hepatic metabolism; 88% renal elimination.
Comments	May cause electrolyte imbalance, dehydration, transient hypotension, deafness, hyperglycemia, or hyperuricemia. Sulfa-allergic patients may exhibit hypersensitivity to furosemide.

Glucagon

Indications	1. Duodenal or choledochal relaxation. 2. Refractory β-adrenergic blocker toxicity.
Dosage	1. 0.25–0.5 mg IV q 20min prn. 2. 5 mg IV bolus, with 1–5 mg/h titrated to patient response.
Effect	Catecholamine release. Positive inotrope and chronotrope.
Clearance	Hepatic and renal proteolysis.
Comments	May cause anaphylaxis, nausea, vomiting, hyperglycemia, or positive inotropic and chronotropic effects. High doses potentiate oral anticoagulants. Use with caution in presence of insulinoma or pheochromocytoma.

Glycopyrrolate (Robinul)

Indications	1. Decrease gastrointestinal motility, antisialagogue. 2. Bradycardia.
Dosage	Adult: 1. 0.1–0.2 mg IV/IM/SC; 1–2 mg PO. 2. 0.1–0.2 mg/dose IV. Pediatric: 0.004–0.008 mg/kg IV/IM up to 0.1 mg.
Effect	See atropine.
Clearance	Renal elimination.
Comments	See atropine. Better antisialagogue with less chronotropy than atropine. Does do not cross blood–brain barrier or placenta. Erratic oral absorption.

Haloperidol (Haldol)

Indications	Psychosis, agitation.
Dosage	0.5–2 mg PO/IM/IV prn (dosage individualized).
Effect	Antipsychotic effects due to dopamine (D_2) receptor antagonism. CNS depression.
Clearance	Hepatic metabolism; renal/biliary elimination.
Comments	May cause extrapyramidal reactions or mild α-adrenergic antagonism. Can prolong QT interval and pro-

duce ventricular arrhythmias, notably torsade de pointes, and lower seizure threshold. May precipitate neuroleptic malignant syndrome. Contraindicated in Parkinson's disease.

Heparin

Indications	Anticoagulation for: **1.** Thrombosis, thromboembolism. **2.** Cardiopulmonary bypass. **3.** Disseminated intravascular coagulation. **4.** Thromboembolism prophylaxis.
Dosage	Adult: **1.**LOAD, 50–150 units/kg IV; MAINT, 15–25 units/kg/h IV. Titrate dosage with partial thromboplastin time or activated clotting time. **2.** LOAD, 300 units/kg IV; MAINT, 100 units/kg/h IV, titrate with coagulation tests. **3.** LOAD, 50–100 units/kg IV. Pediatric: LOAD, 50 units/kg IV; MAINT, 15–25 units/kg/h IV; titrate with coagulation tests. **4.** 5,000 units q 8–12 h SC.
Effect	Potentiates action of antithrombin III; blocks conversion of prothrombin and activation of other coagulation factors.
Clearance	Primarily by reticuloendothelial uptake, hepatic biotransformation.
Comments	May cause bleeding, thrombocytopenia, allergic reactions, and diuresis (36–48 h after a large dose). Half-life increased in renal failure and decreased in thromboembolism and liver disease. Does not cross placenta. Reversed by protamine. Spinal and epidural hematomas have been associated with spinal and epidural anesthesia and lumbar punctures in patients receiving fractionated heparins or heparinoids. The risk of epidural hematoma formation is increased in patients who have indwelling epidural catheters or are also receiving other drugs that may adversely affect hemostasis.

Hydralazine (Apresoline)

Indication	Hypertension.
Dosage	2.5–20.0 mg IV q 4h or prn (dosage individualized).
Effect	Reduces vascular smooth muscle tone (arteriole more than venule).
Clearance	Extensive hepatic metabolism; renal elimination.
Comments	May cause hypotension (diastolic more than systolic), reflex tachycardia, systemic lupus erythematosus syndrome. Increases coronary, splanchnic, cerebral, and renal blood flows.

Hydrocortisone (Solu-Cortef)

Indications	Adrenal insufficiency, inflammation and allergy, cerebral edema from CNS tumors, asthma.
Dosage	10–100 mg IV q 8h. Physiologic replacement: IV, 0.25–0.35 mg/kg/day; PO, 0.5–0.75 mg/kg/day.
Effect	Anti-inflammatory and antiallergic effect; mineralocorticoid effect; stimulates gluconeogenesis; inhibits peripheral protein synthesis; has membrane stabilizing effect.
Clearance	Hepatic metabolism; renal elimination.
Comments	May cause adrenocortical insufficiency (Addisonian crisis) with abrupt withdrawal, delayed wound healing, CNS disturbances, osteoporosis, or electrolyte disturbances.

Hydroxyzine (Vistaril, Atarax)

Indications	Anxiety, nausea and vomiting, allergies, sedation.
Dosage	PO, 25–200 mg q 6–8h; IM, 25–100 mg q 4–6h. Not an IV drug.
Effect	Antagonizes action of histamine on H_1 receptors. CNS depression, antiemetic.
Clearance	Hepatic (P-450) metabolism; renal elimination.
Comments	May cause dry mouth. Minimal cardiorespiratory depression. Intravenous injection may cause thrombosis. Crosses the placenta.

Indigo Carmine

Indications	Evaluation of urine output. Localization of ureteral orifices during cystoscopy.
Dosage	40 mg IV slowly (5 mL of 0.8% solution).
Effect	Rapid glomerular filtration produces blue urine.
Clearance	Renal elimination.
Comments	Hypertension from α-adrenergic stimulation, lasts 15–30 min after IV dose.

Indocyanine Green (Cardio-Green)

Indications	Cardiac output measurement by indicator dye dilution.
Dosage	5 mg IV (diluted in 1 mL of normal saline) rapidly injected into central circulation.

Effect   Almost complete binding to plasma proteins, with
                    distribution within plasma volume.
Clearance   Hepatic elimination.
Comments   May cause allergic reactions or transient increases
                    in bilirubin levels. Absorption spectra changed by
                    heparin. Cautious use in patients with iodine allergy
                    (contains 5% sodium iodide).

Insulin

Indications   1. Hyperglycemia. 2. Diabetic ketoacidosis.
Dosage   1. (Individualized): usually 5–10 units IV/SC prn (reg-
                    ular insulin). 2. LOAD, 10–20 units IV (regular insu-
                    lin); MAINT: 0.05–0.1 units/kg/h IV (regular insulin),
                    titrated against plasma glucose level.
Effect   Facilitates glucose transport intracellularly. Shifts
                    K^+ and Mg^{2+} intracellularly.
Clearance   Hepatic and renal metabolism; 30%–80% renal elimi-
                    nation. Unchanged insulin is reabsorbed.
Comments   May cause hypoglycemia, allergic reactions, or syn-
                    thesis of insulin antibodies. May be absorbed by plas-
                    tic in IV tubing.

Isoproterenol (Isuprel)

Indications   Heart failure, bradycardia.
Dosage   Adult: 2 μg/min titrated up to 10 μg/min. Pediatric:
                    Start at 0.1 μg/kg/min; titrate to effect.
Effect   Beta-adrenergic agonist; positive chronotrope and in-
                    otrope.
Clearance   Hepatic and pulmonary metabolism; 40%–50% renal
                    excretion (unchanged).
Comments   May cause arrhythmias, myocardial ischemia, hyper-
                    tension, or CNS excitation.

Isordil (Isosorbide Dinitrate)

Indications   Angina, hypertension, myocardial infarction, conges-
                    tive heart failure.
Dosage   5–20 mg PO q 6h.
Effect   See nitroglycerin.
Clearance   Nearly 100% hepatic metabolism; renal elimina-
                    tion.
Comments   See nitroglycerin. Tolerance may develop.

Ketorolac (Toradol)

Indications	Nonsteroidal, anti-inflammatory analgesic (NSAID) for moderate pain. Useful adjunct for severe pain when used with parenteral or epidural opioids.
Dosage	PO: 10 mg q 4–6h. IM/IV: 30–60 mg, then 15–30 mg q 6h.
Effect	Limits prostaglandin synthesis by cyclooxygenase inhibition.
Clearance	Less than 50% hepatic metabolism, renal metabolism; 91% renal elimination.
Comments	Adverse effects are similar to those with other NSAIDs: peptic ulceration, bleeding, decreased renal blood flow. Duration of treatment not to exceed 5 days.

Labetalol (Normodyne, Trandate)

Indications	Hypertension, angina, controlled hypotension.
Dosage	IV: 5–10-mg increments at 5-min intervals, to 40–80 mg/dose. Infusion: 5 mg/mL mix; start at 0.05 µg/kg/min.
Effect	Selective α_1-adrenergic blockade with nonselective β-adrenergic blockade. Ratio of α/β blockade = 1:7.
Clearance	Hepatic metabolism; renal elimination.
Comments	May cause bradycardia, AV conduction delays, bronchospasm in some asthmatics, and postural hypotension. Crosses the placenta.

Levothyroxine (Synthroid)

Indications	Hypothyroidism.
Dosage	Adjust according to individual requirements and response. Adults: PO, 0.1–0.2 mg/day; IV, 75% of adult oral dose. Pediatric: PO—0–6 months, 25–50 µg/day or 8–10 µg/kg/day; 6–12 months, 50–75 µg/day or 6–8 µg/kg/day; 1–5 years, 75–100 µg/day or 5–6 µg/kg/day; 6–12 years, 100–150 µg/day or 4–5 µg/kg/day; >12 years, over 150 µg/day or 2–3 µg/kg/day. IV—75% of oral dose.
Effect	Exogenous thyroxine.
Clearance	Metabolized in the liver to triiodothyronine (active); eliminated in feces and urine.
Comments	Contraindicated with recent myocardial infarction, thyrotoxicosis, or uncorrected adrenal insufficiency. Phenytoin may decrease levothyroxine levels. Increases effects of oral anticoagulants. Tricyclic antidepressants may increase toxic potential of both drugs.

Lidocaine (Xylocaine)

Indications	1. Ventricular arrhythmias. 2. Cough suppression. 3. Local anesthesia.
Dosage	Adult: 1. LOAD, 1 mg/kg IV × 2 (2nd dose 20–30 min after 1st dose); MAINT, 15–50 μg/kg/min IV (1–4 mg/min). 2. 1 mg/kg IV. 3. 5 mg/kg maximum dose for infiltration or conduction block. Pediatric: 1. LOAD, 0.5–1 mg/kg IV (2nd dose 20–30 min after 1st dose); MAINT, 15–50 μg/kg/min IV. 2. 1 mg/kg IV. 3. 5 mg/kg maximum dose for infiltration or conduction block.
Effect	Decreases conductance of sodium channels. Antiarrhythmic effect; sedation; neural blockade.
Clearance	Hepatic metabolism to active/toxic metabolites; renal elimination (10% unchanged).
Comments	May cause dizziness, seizures, disorientation, heart block (with myocardial conduction defect), or hypotension. Crosses the placenta. Therapeutic concentration = 1–5 mg/L. Avoid in patients with Wolff–Parkinson–White syndrome.

Magnesium Sulfate

Indications	1. Preeclampsia/eclampsia. 2. Hypomagnesemia. 3. Polymorphic ventricular tachycardia (torsade de pointes).
Dosage	1. LOAD, 1–4 g (8–32 mEq) IV (10% or 20% solution); MAINT, 1–3 mL/min (4 g/250 mL of 5% D/W or NSS). 2. 1–2 g (8–16 mEq) every 6–8 h, prn. 3. 1–2 g in 10 mL D/W over 1–2 min; 5–10 g may be administered for refractory arrhythmias.
Effect	Repletes serum magnesium; prevents and treats seizures or hyperreflexia associated with preeclampsia/eclampsia.
Clearance	100% renal elimination for IV route.
Comments	Potentiates neuromuscular blockade (both depolarizing and nondepolarizing agents). Potentiates CNS effects of anesthetics, hypnotics, and opioids. Toxicity occurs with serum concentration ≥10 mEq/L. May alter cardiac conduction in digitalized patients. Avoid in patients with heart block. Caution in patients with renal failure.

Mannitol (Osmitrol)

Indications	1. Increased intracranial pressure. 2. Oliguria or anuria associated with acute renal injury.
Dosage	Adult: 1. 0.25–1.0 g/kg IV as 20% solution over 30–60

min (in acute situation, can give bolus of 1.25–25.0 g over 5–10 min). **2.** 0.2 g/kg test dose over 3–5 min, then 50–100 g IV over 30 min if adequate response. Pediatric: **1.** 0.2 g/kg test dose, then 2 g/kg over 30–60 min.

Effect Increases serum osmolality, which reduces cerebral edema and lowers intracranial and intraocular pressure; also causes osmotic diuresis and transient expansion of intravascular volume.

Clearance Renal elimination.

Comments Rapid administration may cause vasodilation and hypotension. May worsen or cause pulmonary edema, intracranial hemorrhage, systemic hypertension, or rebound intracranial hypertension.

Methylene Blue (Methylthionine Chloride, Urolene Blue)

Indications **1.** Surgical marker for genitourinary surgery. **2.** Methemoglobinemia.

Dosage **1.** 100 mg (10 mL of 1% solution) IV. **2.** 1–2 mg/kg IV of 1% solution over 10 min; repeat q 1h, prn.

Effect Low dose promotes conversion of methemoglobin to hemoglobin. High dose promotes conversion of hemoglobin to methemoglobin. Less useful than sodium nitrate and amyl nitrite.

Clearance Tissue reduction; urinary and biliary elimination.

Comments May cause RBC destruction (prolonged use), hypertension, bladder irritation, nausea, diaphoresis. May inhibit nitrate-induced coronary artery relaxation. Interferes with pulse oximetry for 1–2 min. Can cause hemolysis in patients with glucose-6 phosphate-dehydrogenase deficiency.

Methylergonovine (Methergine)

Indication Postpartum hemorrhage.

Dosage IV (*emergency only*, after delivery of placenta): 0.2 mg in 5 mL of NSS/dose over ≥1 min. IM: 0.2 mg q 2–4h, prn (<5 doses). PO (after IM or IV doses): 0.2–0.4 mg q 6–12h × 2–7 days.

Clearance Hepatic metabolism; renal elimination.

Comments See ergonovine. Hypertensive response less marked than with ergonovine.

Methylprednisolone (Solu-Medrol)

Indications See hydrocortisone. Spinal cord injury.

Dosage Adult: 40–60 mg IV q 6h. Higher doses in transplant patients. Pediatric: 0.16–0.8 mg/kg/day. Status asthmaticus: LOAD, 2 mg/kg; MAINT, 0.5–1 mg/kg q 6h. Spinal cord injury: LOAD, 30 mg/kg IV over 15 min; after 45 min begin MAINT, 5.4 mg/kg/h × 23 or 47 h.

Effect   See hydrocortisone; has five times the glucocorticoid potency of hydrocortisone. Almost no mineralocorticoid activity.

Clearance   Hepatic metabolism; renal elimination (dose and route dependent).

Comments   See hydrocortisone.

Metoclopramide (Reglan)

Indications Gastroesophageal reflux, diabetic gastroparesis, pulmonary aspiration prophylaxis, antiemetic.

Dosage   Adult: 10 mg IV or PO. Pediatric: 0.1 mg/kg IV or PO.

Effect   Facilitates gastric emptying by increasing gastric motility; relaxes pyloric sphincter and increases peristalsis in the duodenum and jejunum. Increases resting tone of the lower esophageal sphincter. Antiemetic effects appear secondary to antagonism of central and peripheral dopamine receptors.

Clearance   Hepatic metabolism; renal elimination.

Comments   Avoid in patients with GI obstruction, pheochromocytoma, or Parkinson's disease. Extrapyramidal reactions occur in 0.2%–1% of patients. May exacerbate depression.

Metoprolol (Lopressor)

Indications Hypertension, angina pectoris, arrhythmia, hypertrophic cardiomyopathy, myocardial infarction, pheochromocytoma.

Dosage   50–100 mg PO q 6–24h. 2.5–5 mg IV boluses q 2 min, prn, up to 15 mg.

Effect   Beta$_1$-adrenergic blockade (β_2-adrenergic antagonism at high doses).

Clearance   See labetalol.

Comments   May cause bradycardia, clinically significant bronchoconstriction (with doses >100 mg/day), dizziness, fatigue, insomnia. Can increase risk of heart block. Crosses the placenta and blood–brain barrier.

Milrinone (Primacor)

Indications Congestive heart failure.

Dosage   LOAD: 50 µg/kg IV over 10 min. MAINT: titrate 0.375–0.750 µg/kg/min to effect.

Effect	Phosphodiesterase inhibition causing positive inotropy and vasodilation.
Clearance	Renal elimination.
Comments	Short-term therapy. May increase ventricular ectopy, may aggravate outflow tract obstruction in IHSS. Not recommended for acute MI.

Nadolol (Corgard)

Indications	Angina pectoris, hypertension.
Dosage	40–240 mg/day PO.
Effect	Prolonged (approximately 24 h) nonselective β-adrenergic blockade.
Clearance	No hepatic metabolism; renal elimination.
Comments	May cause bronchospasm in susceptible patients (see propranolol).

Naloxone (Narcan)

Indications	Reversal of systemic opioid effects.
Dosage	Adult: 0.04–0.4 mg doses IV, titrated q 2–3 min. Pediatric: 1–10 μg/kg IV (in increments) q 2–3 min (up to 0.4 mg).
Effect	Antagonizes effects of opioids by competitive inhibition.
Clearance	Hepatic metabolism (95%); primarily renal elimination.
Comments	May cause hypertension, arrhythmias, rare pulmonary edema, delirium, reversal of analgesia, or withdrawal syndrome (in opioid-dependent patients). Renarcotization may occur because antagonist has short duration. Caution in hepatic failure.

Nifedipine (Procardia)

Indications	Coronary artery spasm, hypertension, myocardial ischemia.
Dosage	10–40 mg PO tid. 10–20 mg SL, prn (extracted from capsule).
Effect	Blocks slow calcium channels, which produces systemic and coronary vasodilation and can increase myocardial perfusion.
Clearance	Hepatic metabolism.
Comments	May cause reflex tachycardia, gastrointestinal upset, and mild negative inotropic effects. Little effect on

automaticity and atrial conduction. May be useful in asymmetric septal hypertrophy. Drug solution is light sensitive. May rapidly produce severe hypotension in some patients, especially with sublingual administration.

Nitroglycerin (Glycerol Trinitrate, Nitrostat, Nitrol, Nitro-Bid, Nitrolingual)

Indications	Angina, myocardial ischemia or infarction, hypertension, congestive heart failure, controlled hypotension, esophageal spasm.
Dosage	IV infusion initially at 10 µg/min. Titrate to effect. Customary mix: 30–50 mg in 250 mL of 5% D/W or NSS. SL: 0.15–0.6 mg/dose. Topical: 2% ointment, 0.5–2.5 inches q 6–8 h.
Effect	Produces smooth muscle relaxation by enzymatic release of NO, causing systemic, coronary, and pulmonary vasodilatation (veins more than arteries); bronchodilation; biliary, gastrointestinal, and genitourinary tract relaxation.
Clearance	Nearly complete hepatic metabolism; renal elimination.
Comments	May cause reflex tachycardia, hypotension, or headache. Tolerance with chronic use may be avoided with a 10- to 12-h nitrate-free period. May be absorbed by plastic in IV tubing. May cause methemoglobinemia at very high doses.

Nitroprusside (Nipride, Nitropress)

Indications	Hypertension, controlled hypotension, congestive heart failure.
Dosage	IV infusion initially at 0.1 µg/kg/min, then titrated to patient response to maximum 10 µg/kg/min. Customary mix: 50 mg in 250 mL of 5% D/W or NSS.
Effect	Direct NO donor causing smooth muscle relaxation (arterial more than venous).
Clearance	RBC and tissue metabolism; renal elimination.
Comments	May cause excessive hypotension, reflex tachycardia. Accumulation of cyanide with liver dysfunction; thiocyanate with kidney dysfunction. Cyanide/thiocyanate buildup with prolonged infusion. Avoid with Leber's hereditary optic atrophy, tobacco amblyopia,

hypothyroidism, or vitamin-B12 deficiency. Solution and powder are light sensitive and must be wrapped in opaque material.

Norepinephrine (Levarterenol, Levophed)

Indication	Hypotension.
Dosage	1–8 μg/min IV, then titrate to desired effect. Customary mix: 4 mg in 250 mL of 5% D/W or NSS.
Effect	Both α- and β-adrenergic activity, with α-adrenergic activity predominating.
Clearance	MAO/COMT metabolism.
Comments	May cause hypertension, arrhythmias, myocardial ischemia, increased uterine contractility, constricted microcirculation, or CNS stimulation.

Octreotide (Sandostatin)

Indication	**1.** Upper gastrointestinal tract bleeding, acute variceal hemorrhage. **2.** Control of symptoms in patients with metastatic carcinoid and vasoactive intestinal peptide-secreting tumors (VIPomas); pancreatic tumors, gastrinoma, secretory diarrhea. **3.** Unlabeled uses include AIDS-associated secretory diarrhea, cryptosporidiosis, Cushing's syndrome, insulinomas, small bowel fistulas, postgastrectomy dumping syndrome, chemotherapy-induced diarrhea, graft-versus-host-disease (GVHD)–induced diarrhea, Zollinger–Ellison syndrome.
Dosage	**1.** 25–50 μg IV bolus followed by continuous IV infusion of 25–50 μg/h. **2. and 3.** Carcinoid: 100–600 μg/day in 2–4 divided doses. VIPomas: 200–300 μg/day in 2–4 divided doses. Diarrhea: 50–100 μg IV q 8h; increased by 100 μg/dose at 48–h intervals; maximum dose: 500 μg q 8h. Pediatric: 1–10 μg/kg q 12h beginning at the low end of the range and increasing by 0.3 μg/kg/dose at 3-day intervals.
Effect	Somatostatin analogue that suppresses release of serotonin, gastrin, vasoactive intestinal peptide, insulin, glucagon, and secretin.
Clearance	Hepatic and renal (32% eliminated unchanged); decreased in renal failure.
Comments	May cause nausea, decreased GI motility, transient hyperglycemia. Duration of therapy should be no

longer than 72 h because of lack of documented efficacy beyond this time.

Omeprazole (Losec, Prilosec)

Indications	Gastric acid hypersecretion or gastritis, gastroesophageal reflux.
Dosage	20–40 mg PO qd.
Effect	Inhibits H^+ secretion by irreversibly binding H^+/K^+ ATPase.
Clearance	Extensive hepatic metabolism; 72%–80% renal elimination; 18%–23% fecal elimination.
Comments	Increases secretion of gastrin. More rapid healing of gastric ulcers than with H_2 blockers. Effective in ulcers resistant to H_2 blocker therapy. Inhibits some cytochrome P450 enzymes.

Ondansetron Hydrochloride (Zofran)

Indications	Prophylaxis and treatment of perioperative nausea and vomiting.
Dosage	Adult: 4 mg IV over >30 s or 8 mg PO. Pediatric: 4 mg PO.
Effect	Selective $5\text{-}HT_3$-receptor antagonist.
Clearance	Hepatic, 95%; 5% renal excretion.
Comments	Used in much higher doses for chemotherapy-induced nausea. Mild side effects include headache and reversible transaminase elevation.

Oxytocin (Pitocin, Syntocinon)

Indications	1. Postpartum hemorrhage, uterine atony. 2. Augmentation of labor.
Dosage	1. 10 units IM or 10–40 units in 1,000 mL of crystalloid-infused IV at rate necessary to control atony (e.g., 0.02–0.04 units/min). 2. Labor induction: 0.0005–0.002 units/min, increasing until contraction pattern established or maximum dose of 20 milliunits/min reached.
Effect	Reduces postpartum blood loss by contraction of uterine smooth muscle. Renal, coronary, and cerebral vasodilation.
Clearance	Tissue metabolism; renal elimination.

Comments   May cause uterine tetany and rupture, fetal distress, or anaphylaxis. Intravenous bolus can cause hypotension, tachycardia, arrhythmia.

Phenobarbital

Indications   1. Sedation, hypnosis. 2. Seizures.
Dosage   1. Adult and pediatric: 1–3 mg/kg PO, IM, or IV. 2. Adult and pediatric: LOAD, 10–20 mg/kg IV, additional 5 mg/kg doses q 15–30 min for control of status epilepticus, maximum 30 mg/kg; MAINT, 3–5 mg/kg/day PO or IV in divided doses.
Clearance   Hepatic metabolism; 25%–50% renal elimination (unchanged).
Comments   May cause hypotension. Multiple drug interactions through induction of hepatic enzyme systems. Therapeutic anticonvulsant concentration 15–40 µg/mL at trough (just before next dose).

Phenoxybenzamine (Dibenzyline)

Indication   Preoperative preparation for pheochromocytoma resection.
Dosage   10–40 mg/day PO titrated (start at 10 mg/day and increase dosage by 10 mg/day every 4 days prn).
Effect   Nonselective noncompetitive α-adrenergic antagonist.
Clearance   Hepatic metabolism; renal/biliary excretion.
Comments   May cause orthostatic hypotension (which may be refractory to norepinephrine), reflex tachycardia. Nasal congestion expected.

Phentolamine (Regitine)

Indications   1. Hypertension from catecholamine excess as in pheochromocytoma, 2. Extravasation of alpha-agonist.
Dosage   1. 1–5 mg IV prn for hypertension. 2. 5–10 mg in 10 mL of NSS SC into affected area within 12 h of extravasation.
Effect   Nonselective, competitive α-adrenergic antagonist.
Clearance   Unknown metabolism; 10% renally eliminated (unchanged).
Comments   May cause hypotension, reflex tachycardia, cerebro-

vascular spasm, arrhythmias, stimulation of gastrointestinal tract, or hypoglycemia.

Phenylephrine (Neo-synephrine)

Indication	Hypotension.
Dosage	10 µg/min IV initially, then titrated to response; IV bolus 40–100 µg/dose. Customary mix: 10–30 mg in 250 mL of 5% D/W or NSS.
Effect	Alpha-adrenergic agonist.
Onset	Rapid.
Duration	5–20 min.
Clearance	Hepatic metabolism; renal elimination.
Comments	May cause hypertension, reflex bradycardia, microcirculatory constriction, uterine contraction, or uterine vasoconstriction.

Phenytoin (Diphenylhydantoin, Dilantin)

Indications	1. Seizures. 2. Digoxin-induced arrhythmias. 3. Refractory ventricular tachycardia.
Dosage	Adult: **1.** LOAD, 10–15 mg/kg IV at <50 mg/min (up to 1,000 mg cautiously, with ECG monitoring); for neurosurgical prophylaxis, 100–200 mg IV q 4h (at <50 mg/min). **2. and 3.** For arrhythmias: 50–100 mg IV at <50 mg/min q 10–15 min until arrhythmia is abolished, side effects occur, or a maximal dose of 10–15 mg/kg is given.
	Fosphenytoin can be substituted for phenytoin for IV or IM injection. Fosphenytoin injections appear to be better tolerated and have fewer side effects compared with phenytoin, which uses propylene glycol as a vehicle. Fosphenytoin is a product of phenytoin, with 1.5 g of fosphenytoin yielding 1 g of phenytoin. Fosphenytoin is prescribed as phenytoin-equivalent units (PEs).
Effect	Anticonvulsant effect via membrane stabilization. Antiarrhythmic effect similar to those of quinidine or procainamide.
Clearance	Hepatic metabolism; renal elimination (enhanced by alkaline urine).
Comments	May cause nystagmus, diplopia, ataxia, drowsiness, gingival hyperplasia, gastrointestinal upset, hyperglycemia, or hepatic microsomal enzyme induction. Intravenous bolus may cause bradycardia, hypotension, respiratory arrest, cardiac arrest, or CNS depression. Tissue irritant. Crosses the placenta. Significant interpatient variation in dose needed to

achieve therapeutic concentration = 7.5–20.0 μg/mL. Determination of unbound phenytoin levels may be helpful in patients with renal failure or hypoalbuminemia.

Phosphorus (Phospho-Soda, Neutra-Phos, Potassium Phosphate, Sodium Phosphate)

Indications	**1.** Treatment and prevention of hypophosphatemia. **2.** Short-term treatment of constipation. **3.** Evacuation of the colon for rectal and bowel exams.
Dosage	**1.** Mild to moderate hypophosphatemia: children <4 years, 250 mg (phosphorus) PO 3–4 times/day; >4 years and adults, 250–500 mg (phosphorus) PO 3 times/day or 0.08–0.15 mmol/kg IV over 6 h. Moderate to severe hypophosphatemia: children <4 years, 0.15–0.3 mmol/kg IV over 6 h; >4 years and adults, 0.15–0.25 mmol/kg IV over 6–12 h. **2.** Laxative (Phospho-Soda): children 5–9 years, 5 mL PO as a single dose; 10–12 years, 10 mL PO as a single dose; children >12 years and adults, 20–30 mL PO as a single dose. **3.** Colonoscopy preparation (Phospho–Soda): oral, adults, 45 mL diluted to 90 mL with water PO the evening prior to the examination and repeated the following morning.
Effect	Electrolyte replacement.
Clearance	Kidneys reabsorb 80% of dose.
Comments	Infuse doses of IV phosphate over a 4–6 h period; risks of rapid IV infusion include hypocalcemia, hypotension, muscular irritability, calcium deposition, renal function deterioration, and hyperkalemia. Orders for IV phosphate preparations should be written in mmol (1 mmol = 31 mg). Use with caution in patients with cardiac disease and renal insufficiency. Do not give with magnesium- and aluminum-containing antacids or sucralfate, which can bind with phosphate.

Physostigmine (Antilirium)

Indications	Postoperative delirium, tricyclic antidepressant overdose, reversal of CNS effects of anticholinergic drugs.
Dosage	0.5–2.0 mg IV q 15min prn.
Effect	Central and peripheral cholinergic effects; inhibits cholinesterase.
Clearance	Cholinesterase metabolism.
Comments	May cause bradycardia, tremor, convulsions, hallucinations, CNS depression, mild ganglionic blockade,

or cholinergic crisis. Crosses blood–brain barrier. Antagonized by atropine. Contains sulfite.

Potassium (KCl)

Indication	Hypokalemia, digoxin toxicity.
Dosage	Adult: 20 mEq of KCl administered IV over 30–60 min; Usual infusion 10 mEq/h. Pediatric: 0.02 mEq/kg/min.
Effect	Electrolyte replacement.
Clearance	Renal.
Comments	Intravenous bolus administration may cause cardiac arrest; infusion rate should not exceed 1 mEq/min in adults. A central venous line is preferable for administration of concentrated solutions.

Procainamide (Pronestyl)

Indications	Atrial and ventricular arrhythmias.
Dosage	Adult: LOAD, 20 mg/min IV, up to 17 mg/kg, until toxicity or desired effect occurs. Stop if ≥50% QRS widening, or PR lengthening occurs. MAINT, 1–4 mg/min. Pediatric: LOAD, 3–6 mg/kg over 5 min, not to exceed 100 mg/dose; repeat q 5–10 min to maximum dose of 15 mg/kg; MAINT, 20–80 μg/kg/min; maximum of 2 g/24 h.
Effect	Blocks sodium channels; class I-A antiarrhythmic.
Clearance	Hepatic conversion of 25% to active metabolite N-acetyl procainamide (NAPA), a class-III antiarrhythmic; renal elimination (50%–60% unchanged).
Comments	May cause increased ventricular response with atrial tachyarrhythmias unless receiving digitalis; asystole (with AV block); myocardial depression; CNS excitement; blood dyscrasia; lupus syndrome with + ANA; liver damage. Intravenous administration can cause hypotension from vasodilation, accentuated by general anesthesia. Decrease LOAD by one-third in congestive heart failure or shock. Reduce doses in hepatic or renal impairment. Therapeutic concentration = 4–10 μg/mL (procainamide); 15–25 μg/mL (NAPA); 10–30 μg/mL (combined). Contains sulfite.

Prochlorperazine (Compazine)

Indications	Nausea and vomiting.
Dosage	5–10 mg/dose IV (≤40 mg/day); 5–10 mg IM q 2–4h prn; 25 mg PR q 12h prn.
Effect	Central dopamine (D_2) antagonist with neuroleptic

and antiemetic effects. Also antimuscarinic and anti-
histaminic (H_1) effects.

Clearance   Hepatic metabolism; renal and biliary elimination.

Comments   May cause hypotension (especially when given IV),
extrapyramidal reactions, neuroleptic malignant syndrome, leukopenia, and cholestatic jaundice. Contains sulfites. Caution in liver disease. Less sedating
than chlorpromazine.

Promethazine (Phenergan)

Indications   Allergies, anaphylaxis, nausea and vomiting, sedation.

Dosage   Adult: 12.5–50.0 mg IV q 4–6h prn. Pediatric: 0.1–1
mg/kg IV, IM, PO, PR q 4–6 h prn.

Effect   Antagonist of H_1, D_2, and muscarinic receptors. Antiemetic and sedative.

Clearance   Hepatic metabolism; renal elimination.

Comments   May cause mild hypotension or mild anticholinergic
effects. Crosses the placenta. May interfere with
blood grouping. Extrapyramidal effects rare. Contains sulfite. Intraarterial injection can cause gan-
grene.

Propranolol (Inderal)

Indications   Hypertension, atrial and ventricular arrhythmias,
myocardial ischemia or infarction, hypertension, thyrotoxicosis, hypertrophic cardiomyopathy, migraine
headache.

Dosage   Adult: Test dose of 0.25–0.5 mg IV, then titrate ≤1
mg/min to effect; PO, 10–40 mg q 6–8 h, increased
prn. Pediatric: 0.05–0.1 mg/kg IV over 10 min.

Effect   Nonspecific β-adrenergic blockade.

Clearance   Hepatic metabolism; renal elimination.

Comments   May cause bradycardia, AV dissociation, and hypoglycemia. Bronchospasm, congestive heart failure,
and drowsiness can occur. Crosses the placenta and
blood–brain barrier. Abrupt withdrawal can precipitate rebound angina.

Prostaglandin E_1 (Alprostadil, Prostin VR)

Indications   Pulmonary vasodilator, maintenance of patent ductus arteriosus.

Dosage   Starting dose 0.05–0.1 µg/kg/min. Titrate to effect or

	maximum or 0.6 μg/kg/min. Customary mix: 500 μg/ 250 mL of NSS or 5% D/W.
Effect	Vasodilation, inhibition of platelet aggregation, vascular smooth muscle relaxation, and uterine and intestinal smooth muscle stimulation.
Clearance	Pulmonary metabolism; renal elimination.
Comments	May cause hypotension, apnea, flushing, and bradycardia.

Protamine

Indication	Reversal of the effects of heparin.
Dosage	1 mg/100 units of heparin activity IV at ≤5 mg/min.
Effect	Polybasic compound forms complex with polyacidic heparin.
Clearance	Fate of the heparin–protamine complex is unknown.
Comments	May cause myocardial depression and peripheral vasodilation with sudden hypotension or bradycardia. May cause severe pulmonary hypertension, particularly in the setting of cardiopulmonary bypass. Protamine–heparin complex antigenically active. Transient reversal of heparin may be followed by rebound heparinization. Can cause anticoagulation if given in excess relative to amount of circulating heparin (controversial). Monitor response with activated partial thromboplastin time or activated clotting time.

Quinidine Gluconate (Quinaglute)

Indications	Atrial and ventricular arrhythmias.
Dosage	For acute arrhythmias: 800 mg IV in 50 mL of 5% D/W; LOAD, 200–400 mg/dose at ≤10 mg/min; may require as much as 500–750 mg; stop IV infusion if arrhythmia is gone or toxicity occurs (25%–50% QRS widening, HR >120, or loss of P waves); MAINT, quinidine–gluconate sustained-release tablets 324 mg PO tid; therapeutic concentration = 3–6 mg/L; toxic concentration >8 mg/L.
Effect	Class I-A antiarrhythmic; blocks Na channels.
Clearance	Hepatic metabolism; renal elimination (10%–50% unchanged).
Comments	May cause hypotension (from vasodilation and negative inotropic effects), increased ventricular response in atrial tachyarrhythmias, AV block, QT prolongation, congestive heart failure, mild anticholinergic effects, increase in serum digoxin level, cinchonism, or gastrointestinal upset. Hemolysis in G-6-P-D deficient patients. May potentiate action of oral anticoagulants.

Ranitidine (Zantac)

Indications	Duodenal and gastric ulcers, esophageal reflux; reduction of gastric volume, increasing gastric pH.
Dosage	IV: 50–100 mg q 6–8h. PO: 150–300 mg q 12h.
Effect	Histamine H_2-receptor antagonist. Inhibits basal, nocturnal, and stimulated gastric acid secretion.
Clearance	Renal elimination of 70% (unchanged).
Comments	Doses should be reduced by 50% with renal failure.

Scopolamine (Hyoscine)

Indications	Antisialagogue, sedative, antiemetic, motion sickness.
Dosage	0.3–0.6 mg IV/IM.
Effect	Peripheral and central cholinergic (muscarinic) antagonism.
Clearance	Hepatic metabolism; renal elimination.
Comments	Excessive CNS depression can be reversed by physostigmine. May cause excitement, delirium, transient tachycardia, hyperthermia, or urinary retention. Crosses the blood–brain barrier and placenta.

Streptokinase (Streptase)

Indications	**1.** Thrombolytic agent used in treatment of recent severe or massive deep-vein thrombosis; pulmonary emboli. **2.** Myocardial infarction. **3.** Occluded arteriovenous cannulas.
Dosage	Adult: **1.** Thromboses: 250,000 units IV over 30 min, then 100,000 units/h for 24–72 h. **2.** Myocardial infarction: 1.5 million units IV over 1 h; if hypotension develops, decrease infusion rate by 50%; standard concentration is 1.5 million units/250 mL. **3.** Cannula occlusion: 250,000 units into cannula, clamp for 2 h, then aspirate contents and flush with normal saline. Use with caution, considering risk of potentially life-threatening adverse reactions (e.g., hypersensitivity or bleeding). Pediatric: Safety and efficacy not established; limited studies have used 3,500–4,000 units/kg over 30 min followed by 1,000–1,500 units/kg/h.
Effect	Thrombolytic agent.
Clearance	Eliminated by circulating antibodies and via the reticuloendothelial system.
Comments	Best results are realized if used within 5–6 h of myocardial infarction; has been demonstrated to be effective up to 12 h after coronary artery occlusion and onset of symptoms; give aspirin (325 mg) at the start

of streptokinase infusion; begin heparin therapy (800–1,000 units/h) at the end of streptokinase infusion. Avoid intramuscular injections and vascular punctures at noncompressible sites before, during, and after therapy. Contraindicated with recent administration of streptokinase (antibodies to streptokinase remain for 3–6 months after initial dose), recent *Streptococcus* infection; active internal bleeding, recent CVA (within 2 months), or intracranial or intraspinal surgery. Relatively contraindicated following major surgery within the last 10 days, GI bleeding, recent trauma, or severe hypertension. Fibrinolytic effects last only a few hours, while anticoagulant effects can persist for 12–24 h.

Terbutaline (Brethine, Bricanyl)

Indications	1. Bronchospasm. 2. Tocolysis (inhibition of premature labor).
Dosage	1. Adult: 0.25 mg SC; repeat in 15 min prn (use <0.5 mg/4 h); 2.5–5.0 mg PO q 6h prn (<15.0 mg/day). Pediatric: 3.5–5.0 µg/kg SC. 2. 2.5–10 µg/min IV infusion. Titrate upwards as necessary; usually maximal dose of 17.5–30 µg/min.
Effect	Beta$_2$-selective adrenergic agonist.
Clearance	Hepatic metabolism; renal elimination.
Comments	May cause arrhythmias, pulmonary edema, hypertension, hypokalemia, or CNS excitement.

Tissue Plasminogen Activator (Alteplase, Activase, t-PA)

Indications	1. Lysis of coronary arterial thrombi in hemodynamically unstable patients with acute myocardial infarction. 2. Management of acute massive pulmonary embolism (PE) in adults. 3. Acute embolic stroke.
Dosage	1. LOAD: 15 mg (30 mL of the infusion) IV over 1 min followed by 0.75 mg/kg (not to exceed 50 mg) given over 30 min. MAINT: 0.5 mg/kg IV up to 35 mg per hour for 1 h immediately following the loading dose. Total dose not to exceed 100 mg. 2. 100 mg IV continuous infusion over 2 h. 3. Total dose of 0.9 mg/ kg IV (maximum 90 mg); administer 10% as a bolus and the remainder over 60 min.
Effect	Tissue plasminogen activator (tPA).
Clearance	Rapid hepatic clearance.
Comments	Tissue plasminogen activator (alteplase) has not been demonstrated to be superior to streptokinase for thrombolysis in acute myocardial infarction. Aspi-

rin (325 mg) should be given at the initiation of therapy; heparin should be started (1,000 units/h) by continuous infusion 1 h from the initiation of alteplase. Use within 6 h of coronary occlusion for best results. Doses above 150 mg have been associated with an increased incidence of intracranial hemorrhage. Contraindicated with active internal bleeding, history of hemorrhagic stroke, intracranial neoplasm, aneurysm, or recent (within 2 months) intracranial or intraspinal surgery or trauma. Should be used with caution in patients who have received chest compressions, and patients who are currently receiving heparin, coumadin, or antiplatelet drugs.

Trimethaphan (Arfonad)

Indications   Hypertension, controlled hypotension.
Dosage   Adult: 0.5–2 mg/min IV, titrated to effect (usually about 0.3–6 mg/min). Pediatric: 50–150 μg/kg/min. Customary mix: 500 mg in 500 mL of 5% D/W.
Effect   Blocks nicotinic receptors at autonomic ganglia; direct-acting vasodilator.
Clearance   Primarily pseudocholinesterase metabolism; renal elimination (mostly unchanged).
Comments   Mild decrease in cardiac contractility thought to be useful in patients with dissecting aortic aneurysms. May cause prolonged hypotension (especially with high doses), bradycardia in elderly, tachycardia in the young. Histamine release, urinary retention, mydriasis, tachyphylaxis. Potentiates the effects of succinylcholine.

Tromethamine (Tris [Tris(hydroxymethyl-aminomethane)] Buffer, THAM)

Indications   Metabolic acidosis.
Dosage   Adult and pediatric: Dose depends on buffer base deficit; tromethamine (mL of 0.3 M solution) = body weight (kg) × base deficit (mEq/L). If base deficit is not known, 3–6 mL/kg/dose. Pediatric: maximal recommended pediatric dose, 33–40 mL/kg/day or 500 mg/kg/dose.
Effect   Organic proton acceptor (buffer).
Clearance   Rapidly eliminated by kidneys (>75% in 3 h).
Comments   Use with caution in patients with renal impairment or chronic respiratory acidosis. 1 mEq THAM (0.3 M tromethamine) = 3.3 mL = 120 mg tromethamine.

Urokinase (Abbokinase)

Indications	Treatment of: **1.** recent myocardial infarction, **2.** deep vein thrombosis, **3.** severe or massive pulmonary emboli, **4.** occluded intravenous cannulas, **5.** loculated pleural effusions and empyemas.
Dosage	Adults: **1.** Myocardial infarction: 6,000 units/min intracoronary for up to 2 h. **2.** Deep-vein thrombosis: 4,400 units/kg/h IV for 12 h. **3.** Clot lysis (large-vessel thrombi): LOAD, 4,000 units/kg/dose IV over 10 min; MAINT, 4,400–6,000 units/kg/h adjusted to achieve clot lysis or patency of affected vessel; doses up to 50,000 units/kg/h have been used. Therapy should be initiated as soon as possible after diagnosis of thrombi and continued until clot is dissolved (usually 24–72 h). **4.** Occluded IV catheters: 5,000 units into the catheter, then aspirate; may repeat every 5 min for 30 min; if still occluded, cap and leave in catheter for 30 min to 1 h, then aspirate contents and flush with normal saline. **5.** 80,000 units/50 mL instilled into a chest tube.
Effect	Thrombolytic agent.
Clearance	Hepatic; a small amount is excreted in urine and bile.
Comments	Contraindicated with recent *Streptococcus* infection, any internal bleeding, CVA (within 2 months), and brain carcinoma. Use with caution in patients with severe hypertension, recent lumbar puncture, and patient receiving intramuscular injections. Increased bleeding with anticoagulants, antiplatelet drugs, aspirin, indomethacin, and dextran. Avoid intramuscular injections and vascular punctures at noncompressible sites before, during, and after therapy.

Vasopressin (Antidiuretic Hormone, Pitressin)

Indications	**1.** Diabetes insipidus. **2.** Upper GI hemorrhage. **3.** Pulseless ventricular tachycardia or ventricular fibrillation. **4.** Shock refractory to fluid and vasopressor therapy (controversial).
Dosage	**1.** 5–10 units IM/SC q 8–12 h. **2.** 0.1–0.4 units/min IV infusion. **3.** 40 units IV bolus (single dose). **4.** 0.04 units/min IV infusion.
Effect	Increases urine osmolality and decreases urine volume; smooth muscle constriction; vasoconstriction of splanchnic, coronary, muscular, and cutaneous vasculature.
Clearance	Hepatic and renal metabolism; renal elimination.
Comments	May cause oliguria, water intoxication, pulmonary edema; hypertension, arrhythmias, myocardial is-

chemia; abdominal cramps (from increased peristalsis); anaphylaxis; contraction of gallbladder, urinary bladder, or uterus; vertigo or nausea. Patients with coronary artery disease are often treated with concurrent nitroglycerin.

Verapamil (Isoptin, Calan)

Indications	Supraventricular tachycardia, atrial fibrillation or flutter, Wolff–Parkinson–White syndrome, Lown–Ganong–Levine syndrome.
Dosage	Adult: 2.5–10.0 mg (75–150 µg/kg) IV over ≥2 min. If no response in 30 min, repeat 10 mg (150 µg/kg). Pediatric: 0–1 yr, 0.1–0.2 mg/kg IV; 1–15 yr, 0.1–0.3 mg/kg IV. Repeat once if no response in 30 min.
Effect	Blocks slow calcium channels in heart. Prolongs PR and AH intervals. Negative inotrope and chronotrope; systemic and coronary vasodilator.
Clearance	Hepatic metabolism; renal elimination.
Comments	May cause severe bradycardia, AV block (especially with concomitant β-adrenergic blockade), excessive hypotension, or congestive heart failure. May increase ventricular response to atrial fibrillation or flutter in patients with accessory tracts. Active metabolite has 20% of the antihypertensive effect of the parent compound.

Vitamin K (Phytonadione, AquaMEPHYTON)

Indication	Deficiency of vitamin K-dependent clotting factors, reversal of warfarin anticoagulation.
Dosage	2.5–10 mg IM/SC/PO, or 1–10 mg IV at ≤1 mg/min (with caution). If prothrombin time is not improved 8 h after initial dose, repeat prn.
Effect	Promotion of synthesis of clotting factors II, VII, IX, X.
Clearance	Hepatic metabolism.
Comments	Excessive doses can make patient refractory to further oral anticoagulation. May fail with hepatocellular disease. Rapid IV bolus can cause profound hypotension, fever, diaphoresis, bronchospasm, anaphylaxis, and pain at injection site. Crosses the placenta.

Warfarin (Coumadin)

Indication	Anticoagulation.
Dosage	LOAD: 5 mg PO × 2–5 days; MAINT: 2–10 mg PO,

	titrated to prothrombin time (international normalized ratio [INR] should be 2 to 3, based on indication).
Effect	Interferes with utilization of vitamin K by the liver, and inhibits synthesis of factors II, VII, IX, X.
Clearance	Hepatic metabolism; renal elimination.
Comments	May be potentiated by ethanol, antibiotics, chloral hydrate, cimetidine, dextran, thyroxine, diazoxide, ethacrynic acid, glucagon, methyldopa, monoamine oxidase inhibitors, phenytoin, prolonged use of narcotics, quinidine, sulfonamides, congestive heart failure, hyperthermia, liver disease, malabsorption, and so on. May be antagonized by barbiturates, chlordiazepoxide, haloperidol, oral contraceptives, hypothyroidism, hyperlipidemia. Crosses the placenta.

Key to Abbreviations

AV, atrioventricular; CNS, central nervous system; COMT, catechol-O-methyltransferase; D/W, dextrose in water; ECG, electrocardiogram; GI, gastrointestinal; IM, intramuscularly; IV, intravenously; LOAD, loading dose; MAINT, maintenance dose; MAO, monoamine oxidase; NPH, neutral protamine Hagedorn; NSS, normal saline solution; PO, orally; prn, as needed or indicated; RBCs, red blood cells; SC, subcutaneously; SL, sublingually.

Table I-1.   Common intravenous antibiotics

Drug	Usual Adult IV Dose	Usual Dose Interval	Comments
Amikacin	300 mg	q8h	Preferred for infections resistant to other aminoglycosides.
Amphotericin B (Fungizone)	Initial dose: 0.25 mg/kg administered over 6 h; dose should be gradually increased, ranging up to 1 mg/kg/d or 1.5 mg/kg on alternate days	q1–2d	Broad-spectrum antifungal. Initial test dose: 1 mg infused over 30 min to 1 h. Do not exceed 1.5 mg/kg/d. Because of the nephrotoxic potential of amphotericin, other nephrotoxic drugs should be avoided.
Ampicillin	1 g	q4h	May induce interstitial nephritis. Combined with sulbactam is Unasyn.
Ampicillin-sulbactam (Unasyn)	3 g	q6h	Not effective against *Pseudomonas* spp.
Aztreonam	1 g	q8h	Can be used for patients allergic to penicillins or cephalosporins.
Cefazolin (Ancef, Kefzol)	1 g	q4–8h	First generation cephalosporin. Adjust dosage in renal disease.
Cefotetan (Cefotan)	1–2 g	q12h	Second generation cephalosporin. Possible disulfiram-like reaction.

Ceftazidime	1 g	q8h	Preferred for *Pseudomonas aeruginosa* infections and neutropenic patients with fever.
Ceftriaxone	1 g	q24h	Preferred for empiric coverage for bacterial meningitis.
Cefuroxime	750 mg	q8h	Preferred for community-acquired pneumonia.
Chloramphenicol	0.25–1 g	q6h	Adjust dose according to serum concentration.
Ciprofloxacin	400 mg	q12h	Good absorption via oral route (500 mg q12h).
Clindamycin (Cleocin)	600 mg	q8h	Associated with *C. difficile* colitis. May prolong neuromuscular blockade.
Doxycycline	100 mg	q12h	Possible hepatoxocity. Can cause benign intracranial hypertension with vitamin A. See tetracycline.
Erythromycin	0.5–1 g	q6h	Bacteriostatic. Gastritis with oral route. Venous irritation.
Fluconazole	200–400 mg	q24h	Well absorbed orally.
Gentamicin	60–120 mg (3–5 mg/kg/d)	q8–12h	Decrease dosage in renal failure. Renal toxicity and ototoxicity. Precipitates with heparin. May cause/prolong neuromuscular blockade.

(continues)

Appendix I. (Continued)

Drug	Usual Adult IV Dose	Usual Dose Interval	Comments
Imipenem-cilastatin	500 mg	q6h	Preferred for multiple-drug resistant gram-negative bacterial infections. May cause seizures, expecially in renal failure.
Levofloxacin	500 mg	qd	Pure L-isomer of ofloxacin. Well absorbed orally.
Meropenem	0.5–1 g	q8h	Less likely to cause seizures than imipenem.
Metronidazole (Flagyl)	500 mg	q8h	Possible disulfiram-like reaction, leukopenia, leukopenia, convulsions, acute toxic psychosis with disulfiram.
Nafcillin	1–2 g	q4h	Preferred for antistaphlyococcal coverage.
Penicillin G[a]	500,000–2,000,000 U	q4h	Hypersensitivity is common. May induce seizures at high doses and induce interstitial nephritis.
Piperacillin	4 g	q6h	Usually combined with aminoglycoside for treatment of *Pseudomonas*.
Piperacillin-tazobactam (Zosyn)	3.375 g	q6h	Tazobactam expands activity of piperacillin to include beta-lactamase producing strains of *S. aureus, H. influenzae, Enterobacteriaceae, Pseudomonas, Klebsiella, Citrobacter, Serratia, Bacteroides,* and other gram-negative anaerobes.

Tetracycline	250–500 mg	q12h	Contraindicated in pediatrics (tooth discoloration). Antagonism with penicillins. Crosses placenta.
Ticarcillin	3 g	q4h	Anti-Pseudomonal penicillin of choice. May cause bleeding abnormalities.
Ticarcillin-clavulanate (Timentin)	3.1 g	q4h	—
Trimethoprim/ sulfamethoxazole (Bactrim, Septra)	8–10 mg/kg/d (based on trimethoprim component)	q6–12h	Allergic reactions common. Interferes with elimination of creatinine and potassium; values may increase.
Tobramycin	60–120 mg (3–5 mg/kg/d over 15–20 min)	q8h	See gentamicin.
Vancomycin (Vancocin)	500 mg–1 g over 30–60 min	q6–12h	Preferred for oxacillin-resistant staphylococcal infections and patients with penicillin allergy. Decrease dose in renal disease. Histamine release ("red man syndrome"), renal damage, deafness. May precipitate with other medications.

[a] Five to ten percent of penicillin-allergic patients will react to cephalosporins.

Note: Adult doses are those usually given to healthy 70-kg patients and may vary with the patient's condition or concomitant drug intake. Older or debilitated patients may require smaller doses.

Normal Laboratory Values for Blood

Chemistry

Albumin:	3.1–4.3 g/dL
Alkaline phosphatase:	
Female	30–100 U/L
Male	45–115 U/L
Ammonia, plasma:	12–48 μmol/L
Amylase, serum:	53–123 U/L
Anion gap (calculated):	5–15 mmol/L
Arterial blood gas tensions and pH	
Pao_2:	80–100 mmHg
$Paco_2$:	35–45 mmHg
pH:	7.35–7.45
Bicarbonate (CO_2):	22–26 mEq/L
Bilirubin, direct:	<0.4 mg/dL
Bilirubin, total:	<1.0 mg/dL
Blood urea nitrogen (BUN):	8–25 mg/dL
Calcium:	8.5–10.5 mg/dL
Calcium, ionized:	1.14–1.30 mmol/L
Chloride:	100–108 mmol/L
Cholesterol	
Desirable:	<200 mg/dL
Borderline:	200–239 mg/dL
High:	>240 mg/dL
Creatine kinase (CK)	
Female:	40–150 U/L
Male:	60–400 U/L
Creatine kinase isoenzyme index:	0%–2.5% relative index
Creatine kinase isoenzymes, MB fraction:	0–5 ng/mL
Creatinine:	0.6–1.5 mg/dL
Globulin:	2.6–4.1 g/dL
Glucose (fasting):	70–110 mg/dL
Iron, serum:	30–160 μg/dL
Lactate dehydrogenase (LDH):	110–210 U/L
Lactic acid, plasma:	0.5–2.2 mmol/L
Lipase:	3–19 U/dL
Magnesium:	1.4–2.0 mEq/L
Osmolality:	280–296 mOsm/kg
Phosphorus:	2.6–4.5 mg/dL
Potassium:	3.5–5.0 mmol/L
Protein, total:	6.0–8.0 g/dL
SGOT (aspartate aminotransferase [AST])	
Female:	9–25 U/L
Male:	10–40 U/L
SGPT (alanine aminotransferase [ALT])	
Female:	7–30 U/L
Male:	10–55 U/L

Sodium:	135–145 mmol/L
Thyroid function tests	
Thyroid hormone binding index:	0.77–1.23
Thyroid-stimulating hormone (TSH):	0.5–5.0 μU/mL
Thyroxine, total (T_4):	4.5–10.9 μg/dL
Triiodothyronine, total (T_3):	60–181 ng/dL
Triglycerides (fasting):	40–150 mg/dL
Troponin T:	<0.1 ng/mL
Uric acid	
Female:	2.3–6.6 mg/dL
Male:	3.6–8.5 mg/dL
Venous blood gas tensions, mixed	
Pmv_{O_2}:	50 mm Hg
Pmv_{CO_2}:	40–50 mm Hg
pH:	7.32–7.42

Hematology and Coagulation Values

D-dimer:	0.0–0.5 μg/mL
Erythrocyte count (RBC)	
Female:	$4.1–5.1 \times 10^6/mm^3$
Male:	$4.5–5.3 \times 10^6/mm^3$
Erythrocyte sedimentation rate (ESR)	
Female:	1–25 mm/h
Male:	1–17 mm/h
Fibrin degradation products (FDP):	0–2.5 μg/mL
Fibrinogen:	175–400 mg/dL
Hematocrit	
Female:	36%–46%
Male:	37%–49%
Hemoglobin	
Female:	12–16 g/dL
Male:	13–18 g/dL
Iron:	30–150 μg/dL
Iron binding capacity (TIBC):	226–428 μg/dL
Leukocyte count (WBC):	$4.5–11 \times 10^3/mm^3$
Neutrophils:	45%–75%
Bands:	0%–5%
Lymphocytes:	16%–46%
Monocytes:	4%–11%
Eosinophils:	0%–8%
Basophils:	0%–3%
Mean corpuscular hemoglobin (MCH):	25–35 pg/cell
Mean corpuscular hemoglobin concentration (MCHC):	31–37 g/dL
Mean corpuscular volume (MCV):	78–100 μm^3

Partial thromboplastin time, activated (aPTT):	22.1–34.1 s
Platelet count:	150–350 × 10³/mm³
Prothrombin time (PT):	11.2–13.2 s
Reticulocyte count:	0.5%–2.5%

Reference: Kratz A, Lewandrowski KB. Case records of the Massachusetts General Hospital. Weekly clinicopathological exercises. Normal references laboratory values. *N Engl J Med* 1998;339: 1063–1072.

Subject Index

Page numbers followed by f and t indicate figures and tables, respectively.

699